WC
178
4/04

HIV & AIDS:

A foundation for nursing and healthcare practice

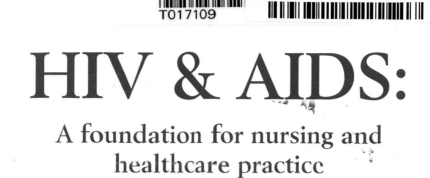

5TH EDITION

Robert J. Pratt

CBE FRCN RN BA MSc RNT DN (Lond) PGDARM
Professor of Nursing, Director, Richard Wells Research Centre,
Faculty of Health & Human Sciences, Thames Valley University, London, UK

A member of the Hodder Headline Group
LONDON

First published in Great Britain in 1986
Second edition 1988
Third edition 1991
Fourth edition 1995
This fifth edition published in 2003 by Arnold,
a member of the Hodder Headline Group,
338 Euston Road, London NW1 3BH

http://www.arnoldpublishers.com

Distributed in the United States of America by
Oxford University Press Inc.,
198 Madison Avenue, New York, NY10016
Oxford is a registered trademark of Oxford University Press

Whilst the advice and information in this book are believed to be true and
accurate at the date of going to press, neither the authors nor the publisher
can accept any legal responsibility or liability for any errors or omissions
that may be made. In particular (but without limiting the generality of the
preceding disclaimer) every effort has been made to check drug dosages;
however, it is still possible that errors have been missed. Furthermore,
dosage schedules are constantly being revised and new side-effects
recognized. For these reasons the reader is strongly urged to consult the
drug companies' printed instructions before administering any of the drugs
recommended in this book.

British Library Cataloguing in Publication Data
A catalogue record for this book is available from the British Library

Library of Congress Cataloging-in-Publication Data
A catalog record for this book is available from the Library of Congress

ISBN 0340 70639 2

1 2 3 4 5 6 7 8 9 10

Commissioning Editor: Georgina Bentliff
Development Editor: Heather Smith
Project Editor: Wendy Rooke
Production Controller: Lindsay Smith
Cover Design: Amina Dudhia

Typeset in Berling Roman by Phoenix Photosetting, Chatham, Kent
Printed and bound in Malta

What do you think about this book? Or any other Arnold title?
Please send your comments to feedback.arnold@hodder.co.uk

Contents

Contributors

Karen Gibson RN, BSc, MSc, PGDipEd
Senior Lecturer (Sexual Health), Thames Valley University, London, UK

Heather Loveday MA, RN, RNT, PGCARM
Principal Lecturer (Research), Richard Wells Research Centre, Thames Valley University, London, UK

Carol Pellowe MA (Ed), BA (Hons), RN, RNT, PGDARM
Deputy Director, Richard Wells Research Centre, Thames Valley University, London, UK

Nicola Robinson PhD, BSc (Hons) Lic Ac, Hon MFPHM
Head of Centre for Complementary Health Care & Integrated Medicine, Faculty of Health & Human Sciences, Thames Valley University, London, UK

Tim Stephens BA (Hons) Nursing, RN
Staff Nurse, Intensive Care Unit, Royal London Hospital, London, UK

Foreword to the fifth edition

In the UK, London has always been the epicentre of our national epidemic of human immunodeficiency virus (HIV) infection and disease. Here, we now have almost a quarter of a century of collective experience in caring for and supporting large numbers of people who are living with HIV/AIDS. Our knowledge of the underlying science and pathology that underpin this disease continues to increase dramatically in leaps and bounds. Today's great success story of this epidemic, at least here in Europe and in North America, Australasia and other resource-rich nations, has been the development of sophisticated and effective antiretroviral treatment strategies that delay end-stage disease and significantly improve the quality of life for those living with HIV. However, no biomedical 'cure' for this disease has yet emerged and, although several candidate vaccines are now in clinical trials, it may be years before an effective vaccine to prevent HIV disease is available. **The need for nurses to 'care' is as urgent now as it was when this disease first surfaced**.

Since its first edition in 1986, this book has established itself as the premier reference text in Europe on the nursing care of people with HIV disease. Now completely rewritten and updated, the fifth edition includes important new chapters reflecting the changing face of HIV/AIDS.

Using the latest available research evidence, Robert Pratt outlines a new understanding of the science behind the disease and the factors driving the epidemic. Complex subjects are made understandable as he describes more comprehensively the biology of HIV, the natural history of HIV infection and disease and our evolving perception of the immunological responses to infection. Key clinical issues are extensively described, such as HIV-related tuberculosis, viral hepatitis and nervous system pathology.

Important new chapters on the management of occupational exposure to blood-borne pathogens, preventing mother-to-child HIV transmission and the complexities of antiretroviral therapy are included in this new edition. Of particular value has been the opportunity for nurse clinicians, educationalists and researchers to input into this extensively used text.

Tim Stephens and Karen Gibson have co-authored with Robert Pratt the core chapter on the individualized nursing care of patients with HIV disease. As in previous editions, the focus of this chapter is firmly on the unique role of the nurse in caring for individuals with HIV disease. The authors develop a behavioural and needs-based model of nursing to set the scene for an in-depth exploration of the actual and potential care requirements of people requiring in-patient care.

In response to the changing needs and expectations of patients, Dr Nicola Robinson has co-authored with Robert Pratt a new chapter on complementary and alternative approaches to care, describing the best available evidence of efficacy for each therapy.

Heather Loveday provides a thoughtful and immensely helpful chapter on the central importance of supporting adherence to therapy. Recognizing the international distribution of this text and the global reach of AIDS, a new chapter by Carol Pellowe focuses on important nursing care issues in the resource-poor regions of the industrially developing world.

Each chapter begins with a description of the intended learning outcomes and is complemented by extensive references, recommended further reading and, importantly, comprehensive and relevant internet resources and associated website addresses.

Robert Pratt has been associated with the issues surrounding the nursing care of patients with HIV disease since the very beginning of the pandemic and he has made a major contribution in facilitating the nursing profession's effective response to the challenges of HIV disease, both in the UK and internationally. As a Consultant to the World Health Organization and the British Council, he has for many years directed HIV-related nursing and medical education and action research projects in Africa, Asia, the Arabian Gulf and Eastern Europe. He is an adviser to a variety of government and non-governmental organizations, including the Chief Medical Officer's Expert Advisory Group on AIDS at the Department of Health (England). He is also the President of the Infection Control Nurses Association of the British Isles and Patron of the UK National HIV Nurses Association. In 1998, he was conferred with the Fellowship of the Royal College of Nursing for his international contribution to promoting sexual health. In recognition of his unique contribution to nursing education, in 2003 he was appointed a Commander of the Order of the British Empire by Her Majesty, Queen Elizabeth II.

Drawing on his experience of working in London at the very heart of the UK epidemic, he offers a clear, easy to understand, yet comprehensive reference text for nurses and other healthcare professionals who need ready access to current nursing and scientific information. Having been published in five different languages, including a special Arabic edition published by the World Health Organization, the continuing popularity of this book reflects how effectively it meets the needs of nurses and other healthcare professionals around the world.

Effective nursing care is based on research, knowledge, skill, compassion and integrity, and all of these elements are consistently reflected throughout this text. I commend this new edition to you as the definitive reference guide for professional nurses and other healthcare practitioners striving to deliver confident, competent and compassionate support within the arena of HIV patient care.

Professor Christine Beasley CBE
Partnership Development Director
NHS Modernisation Agency

July 2003, London

Acknowledgements

I am grateful to many colleagues for their help in developing this new edition, including my new chapter co-authors, **Carol Pellowe, Heather Loveday, Dr Nicky Robinson, Tim Stephens** and **Karen Gibson**, all at Thames Valley University, London. **Professor Clive Loveday** and **Professor John M. Grange** in London and **Dr Roger Woodruff** in Melbourne, Australia, were invaluable in providing scientific and medical advice. **Ian O'Reilly** and **Simon Jones** at Thames Valley University and **Anne Wadmore** in London vastly improved the material in this edition by their skilful artwork. I am also grateful to the staff at Hodder Arnold and the freelances who have worked on this book, especially **Georgina Bentliff** (commissioning editor), **Laurence Errington** (indexer), **Wendy Rooke** (project editor), **Heather Smith** (development editor), **Jane Smith** (copy-editor) and **Harriet Stewart-Jones** (proofreader). Finally, I am especially thankful to my colleague and good friend **Carol Pellowe** for reviewing chapter drafts and advising on style.

This text is dedicated to all my friends, colleagues, students and patients whose lives have been affected by AIDS, principally remembering **Werner, David, John** and **Michael**. They were my friends, my first patients and, ultimately, my teachers. Finally, remembering always the outstanding contribution made to our profession by the late **Richard Wells FRCN**, at the Royal College of Nursing, I especially dedicate this text to his memory, and to the memory of **Maurice Jeffery**.

Introduction

HIV infection and AIDS – 25 years on . . .
As the fifth edition of this text is published, the global pandemic of HIV infection and AIDS continues to escalate and hardly anywhere seems untouched by the scourge of this, the most important public health disaster of our lifetimes. For almost a quarter of a century, we have experienced the collective and personal tragedy that is AIDS – 25 years of fear, 25 years of illness, 25 years of death and 25 years of courage. It is important to recall what has happened in those long 25 years – the first decades of AIDS.

Although undeniably present in the world long before 1981, it was in that year, almost 25 years ago, that AIDS came slipping and sliding into our world with reports from the Centers for Disease Control (CDC) in America of five cases of *Pneumocystis carinii* pneumonia (PCP) among previously healthy young men.[1] They had developed this pneumonia because their immune systems had been attacked and fatally damaged by some unknown assailant. This report was followed within weeks by further reports of more cases of PCP and Kaposi's sarcoma in more young men who had the same curious immune system lesion,[2] but . . . no one then, no one the following year, or even a few years later, could imagine the magnitude of what was about to happen to our world.

That was only 25 years ago and look what's happened to our world since then. Within just two and a half short decades, HIV infection would come to establish itself as a dominant force for ill-health, making sick and then killing over 20 million people around the world. Within just these few years, HIV would infect 60 million people, changing their destinies and assigning almost everyone who becomes infected to the nightmare of AIDS. Today, as we applaud the amazing scientific and technological progress made in the industrially developed nations of the world in preventing infection and in the clinical management of people with HIV disease, it is important to remember that for most of the more than 40 million people currently living in that 'other world' with HIV/AIDS, nothing has changed – nothing. Although this text can only touch on the clinical issues of HIV disease in the developing world, we need to remember that this is where the tragedy of AIDS is being played out; this is where the vast majority of affected people live, where they suffer, where they yearn for care and where they die.

But here in our world, the industrially developed world, progress during the last 25 years has been absolutely startling. Within just a few months after our realization of the epidemic, nurses, doctors and scientists all over the world began a complex journey of coming to understand what was happening.

By the beginning of 1982, a case definition for AIDS was developed by CDC in America[3] and global surveillance began. To everyone's amazement, AIDS was being found practically everywhere one looked, especially in sub-Saharan Africa, Western Europe, North America and Australasia.

By 1983, the potential for a wild-fire global pandemic was first recognized, and just as quickly denied by many. While policy makers and scientists debated, AIDS quickly spread around the world until today, just 25 years since this began, AIDS is found in every community in every country in every region throughout the world.

The ways in which HIV is transmitted from person to person were rapidly established –

it was clear that this was a blood-borne and sexually transmitted infection and, as early as 1983, the means to avoid becoming infected were known. But that knowledge would not stop 60 million people becoming infected during the first 9000 days of the global pandemic and it would not stop more then 20 million men, women and children dying from this new infection during these first years.

Also in 1983, French scientists at the Pasteur Institute in Paris identified the virus that causes AIDS,[4] and a basic understanding of how this virus infects host cells and replicates was quickly forthcoming. Having many early names, this virus would eventually become known as the human immunodeficiency virus (HIV) – a truly new 'horseman of the apocalypse'.

Two years later, in 1985, a test for HIV infection was developed and deployed, allowing blood transfusions and other tissue and organ donations to be screened for the presence of HIV infection. Following its introduction, this test would be used and abused in a variety of situations, and millions upon millions of people would receive the lonely news that they were infected with HIV.

Meanwhile, in the developed world, most care and treatment was directed at managing the opportunistic events associated with a decline in immunity, and many of these illnesses, such as Kaposi's sarcoma and HIV-associated dementia, were particularly feared.

Then, in 1987, the first truly effective drug that suppressed viral replication was introduced into clinical practice – zidovudine, or AZT as it was first known. The early results showed that it was effective in reducing HIV-associated illnesses and deaths from AIDS. To patients, it was startling – improvements were often dramatic, as was the hope that this infection could, after all, be managed. However, the drug was initially scarce, side effects were significant and any clinical improvements were short lived. It did buy some time for our friends and neighbours, for our patients and colleagues, but not much – perhaps only 6 months or so.

The development of new, more robust and effective antiretroviral agents was dependent upon a better, more sophisticated understanding of how HIV infects and kills host cells in the immune system. This understanding of the pathogenesis of HIV disease evolved from the late 1980s to the mid-1990s, when scientists were able to plot the clinical consequences of the results of a changing inverse relationship between a rising viral load and a falling CD4+ T-lymphocyte count. The stages and events of HIV disease then became utterly and depressingly predictable. However, so too did the opportunities for interventions.

By the mid-1990s, a range of antiretroviral drugs attacking the virus at different stages of its replication cycle became available to treat HIV disease and, by 1995–6, the world looked entirely different for those infected – well, at least in our world, the industrially developed world, things looked entirely different. That other world, the developing world, peopled with the poor and the disempowered, those with no hope, that world looked the same. But here, more drugs similar to zidovudine were introduced (the nucleoside reverse transcriptase inhibitors), followed by the powerful protease inhibitors and then the non-nucleoside reverse transcriptase inhibitors. Regimens were developed that consisted of various combinations of these drugs and the result was absolutely dramatic – patients got better, they returned to work, they got their lives back, dedicated in-patient facilities were scaled down or closed altogether, and an air of real optimism, based on solid science, permeated the world of HIV/AIDS.

It almost seemed feasible then, in the early to mid-1990s, that intensive combination therapy that effectively suppressed viral replication below the level of detection for as long as the longest lived infected cell could survive would ultimately lead to viral eradication. But the dream of eradication was short lived, and we all know now that this will probably never be achieved.

However, other successes were soon forthcoming; one of the most important was the development of strategies to prevent infected women transmitting HIV infection to their newborn children. These strategies focused on three aspects:

1. various obstetric interventions to reduce the risk of transmission, such as caesarean section rather than routine vaginal delivery;
2. avoiding breastfeeding and substituting safe alternative infant feeding;
3. most importantly, treating the mother for HIV infection, or at least giving appropriate antiretroviral chemoprophylaxis to prevent mother-to-child transmission.

These strategies would reduce the risk of mother-to-child transmission in the industrially developed world from more than 30 per cent to less than 5 per cent. However, all these interventions depended upon identifying HIV infection in women during the antenatal period. In the UK and the USA all women are now offered and encouraged to undergo testing for HIV – for their benefit, and for the benefit of their babies, and mother to-child transmission is becoming uncommon.

Other equally dramatic interventions are on the horizon with the introduction of new drugs able to brake the ability of HIV to replicate and to prevent further immune system damage. A new generation of antiretroviral agents is currently in development and these drugs should be available within the next few years. They include better nucleoside and non-nucleoside reverse transcriptase inhibitors and protease inhibitors, which will have better absorption potentials, simpler dosing requirements and fewer side effects. Also in development are new drugs, including entry blockers such as fusion inhibitors, able to stop HIV from infecting cells and, the most elusive of all, integrase inhibitors, capable of preventing the integration of the proviral DNA into the nucleus of the host cell, and more refined biological agents, such as cytokines, able to stimulate a damaged immune system to fight off the ongoing assault by HIV.

Although these drugs will be available to us in the industrially developed world, they will not save everyone. The only scientific intervention that can do that is the global deployment of an effective vaccine able to modify the biological and clinical consequences of HIV infection. Several candidate vaccines are currently in clinical trials and hopes are high that effective vaccines will soon be available.

As we continue through the first years of the new millennium, the excitement of these new developments needs to be tempered with an understanding of the challenges we continue to face on a daily basis

The incidence of new infections is rising all over the world and this means an increasing number of people seeking treatment and care within the context of a decreasing number of nurse specialists and dwindling healthcare resources.

Globally, the projected incidence of new infections and end-stage disease is shocking – the numbers becoming so large as to be almost devoid of meaning. Today, AIDS is the number 1 killer in Africa, soon it will be the number 1 killer in South Asia and it is already the number 4 killer of young adults throughout the world.[5] HIV infection causes the death of more people each year throughout the world then any other pathogenic microorganism. Having now caused the deaths of more then 20 million people, the total death rate will soon exceed the total number of deaths caused by the greatest of past plagues. Challenges indeed – these projections are breathtaking.

Another great worry is the anticipated increases in drug resistance. HIV infection requires lifelong treatment with powerful drugs with equally powerful side effects. It requires total adherence – the consequences of even mild deviations from the prescribed regimen are invariably drug resistance. Not only will drug resistance foreclose on that individual's treatment options, it will also limit treatment options for those who become infected with drug-resistant variants of HIV. Nurse researchers throughout the world are engaged in trying to develop tools that will identify those patients who need the greatest support to adhere to prescribed therapy. In this arena, adherence is everything, and this issue will continue to dominant research agendas well into the future.

Finally, only recently have we become aware of the serious long-term side effects of current antiretroviral treatment regimens; no one yet knows if it is possible to keep individuals on these regimens for their entire lives – the betting is that it is probably not. In the meantime, nurse researchers are exploring strategies to prevent and manage the long-term side effects of these powerful drugs.

So far in this introduction, I have discussed yesterday and today. But what of tomorrow – what has AIDS taught us and what does it demand from us?

Michael Gottlieb – the physician who uncovered the first cluster of those five young men with PCP in 1980 that alerted us to this new pandemic – has been reflecting on his more than two decades of experience in caring for AIDS patients, and these reflections have touched familiar places in the hearts of many nurses. Michael feels that *'For many doctors and nurses, the AIDS epidemic has been a proving ground where character, beliefs and values are tested. It has taught us about the nature and diversity of love, about courage, compassion, and caring. As a result of treating patients with HIV, many of us have matured into more skilful healthcare professionals than we might otherwise have been.'*[6] My colleagues and I work in a university nursing research centre that is named in honour of the outstanding contribution to HIV nursing care in the UK made by our dear friend and close colleague the late Richard Wells, a Fellow of The Royal College of Nursing and the College's Professional Nurse Adviser. Richard was an early master of sound bites and some of these seemingly throwaway lines were so pertinent, so exactly right, that they touched the hearts of many and influenced a generation of nurses. Richard said that *'AIDS has a habit of bringing out the best and the worst in everyone – let it bring out the best in you'*. I know I work very hard to have it bring out the best in me, and I'm equally confident that you, the reader, do too.

The first edition of this text was published in 1986 to share information, to encourage nurses to engage in the issues associated with HIV disease and to continue to help ensure that all patients, including those with HIV disease, receive quality nursing care when they need it, from confident, competent and compassionate nurses. Almost 20 years on, the goals are the same, the dangers are still real, the challenges are still there and nurses, the largest healthcare force in the world, have a unique historical opportunity to make the defining difference in this pandemic. I hope that this text, by providing a reference guide for nurses, will help in your professional quest to make that difference.

Robert J. Pratt CBE FRCN
July 2003,
London

REFERENCES

1.   Centers for Disease Control (CDC). Pneumocystis pneumonia. Los Angeles. *Morbidity and Mortality Weekly Report (MMWR)* 5 June 1981; **30**:250–2.

2. CDC. Kaposi's sarcoma and pneumocystis pneumonia among homosexual men. New York City and California. *Morbidity and Mortality Weekly (MMWR)* 3 July 1981; **30**:305–8.

3. CDC. Update on acquired immune deficiency (AIDS) United States. *Morbidity and Mortality Weekly (MMWR)* 1982; **31**:507–14.

4. Barre-Sinoussi F, Chermann JC, Rey F et al. Isolation of a T-lymphotropic retrovirus from a patient at risk for acquired immune deficiency syndrome (AIDS). *Science* 1983; **220**:868–71.

5. UNAIDS/WHO. *AIDS Epidemic Update* (UNAIDS/02.58E). Geneva: Joint United Nations Programme on HIV/AIDS and the World Health Organization, December 2002. Available online from: http://www.unaids.org

6. Gottlieb MS. AIDS – past and future. *New England Journal of Medicine* 2001; **344**:1788–91.

CHAPTER 1

The evolution of a pandemic

With time, the HIV/AIDS pandemic is unfolding and revealing its secrets. Paradoxically, the pandemic is becoming simultaneously more difficult and simpler to comprehend. A modern understanding of the pandemic requires two levels of awareness. First, it is essential to appreciate the enormously complex histories of individual HIV/AIDS epidemics at the community or national level. Yet this level of information is insufficient. It is also necessary to recognize the common features among the HIV/AIDS epidemics which, at a deeper level, provide insight into the natural history and the shape of the slowly maturing pandemic.

Jonathan Mann and Daniel Tarantola[1]

Introduction

Now in the third decade of our experience with this pandemic, to many of us, acquired immunodeficiency syndrome (AIDS) seems to have always been here, always stalking us, always part of our lives, always the principal focus of our personal and professional activities. Nurses and other healthcare professionals working in this field today are involved in a rapidly accelerating spiral of dynamic developments: evolving science, new drugs, new prevention strategies, ever-moving political agendas, changing vulnerabilities and the restructuring of models for the provision of care. In our lifetimes, AIDS is perhaps the ultimate epidemic, reshaping our world beyond recognition, bringing out both the best and the worst in humankind. To be actively involved in this great event and to be positioned to influence outcomes, nurses need to continue to develop their insights into the entire spectrum of this epidemic . . . and that insight begins with an understanding of the changing shape of the global pandemic and the diverse human circumstances, behaviours and vulnerabilities that drive national epidemics around the world.

Learning outcomes

At the end of reviewing and reflecting on the material in this chapter you will be able to:

- describe the history and evolution of human immunodeficiency virus (HIV) infection and AIDS as a global pandemic;
- define common terms associated with describing epidemics;
- discuss the dynamics of the continuing growth of the epidemic in different regions throughout the world.

THE BEGINNING ...

It is sometimes difficult to recall how all this started, how we arrived at this stage of our journey through a global disaster, engaging one of the most serious threats to public health in our lifetimes. The story began a long time ago . . .

Early summer 1981 – the United States of America

AIDS was to enter the world's consciousness and become part of the vocabulary of the human soul as a result of a dawning awareness of the advent of a strange new disease first reported in California in 1981.

In the early months of that year, five young men were admitted to various hospitals in Los Angeles, suffering from an unusual type of pneumonia caused by a commonly occurring microorganism, specifically a fungus known as *Pneumocystis carinii*. Previously, pneumonia caused by *P. carinii* had only been seen in patients who were immunocompromised, for example infants born with a **primary immune deficiency**, such as severe combined immune deficiency (SCID), or adults whose immune system had become deficient due to other causes, i.e. **secondary immune deficiency** states. Most cases of pneumonia caused by *P. carinii* had been observed in renal transplant units, where patients had received immunosuppressant chemotherapy following kidney transplants, or in oncology units, where patients had been immunosuppressed as a result of receiving anti-cancer chemotherapy. People in countries in the Western world have frequently been exposed to this microbe and it is often part of the normal flora in the respiratory system in many people. It is harmless in individuals with a competent immune system. Only in those with an impaired immune system can it cause disease, in which case the treatment of choice was a little-used antibiotic, manufactured in the UK and known as pentamidine isetionate.

The physician in charge of the first cases in Los Angeles was puzzled. These five patients were all young men who had evidence of a widespread immunodeficiency without any apparent reason. They had evidence of other infections and, coincidentally, they were all homosexuals, i.e. 'gay men'. The Centers for Disease Control and Prevention (CDC) in Atlanta, Georgia, was notified and supplies of pentamidine were requested, although by this time two of the five patients had died. The CDC, which has as part of its function the task of monitoring the trends of infectious diseases throughout the USA and its territories, published an account of these five cases in its weekly bulletin, the *Morbidity and Mortality Weekly Report (MMWR)*, on 5 June 1981. In this report it was noted that the occurrence of pneumonia caused by *P. carinii* (pneumocystosis) in five previously healthy individuals, who had no known reason for their defective immune status, was unusual. The report questioned whether their homosexual lifestyle, or a disease acquired through sexual contact among men having sex with men, could be associated with the development of the defects in the immune system which led to pneumocystosis.[2]

Probably then no one actually suspected the magnitude of the epidemic that was in the making. However, evidence of the gathering storm was soon arriving.

At about the same time as physicians in Los Angeles had reported the cluster of cases of pneumocystosis, other physicians in New York City and California notified the CDC of the occurrence of a severe form of Kaposi's sarcoma in 26 young men. Kaposi's sarcoma is a vascular neoplasm, uncommon in the USA and in Western Europe, being seen mainly in elderly men, in whom it is manifested by skin and visceral lesions and a chronic clinical course. However, in 1978, Kaposi's sarcoma had been described in patients who had undergone renal transplants and had received immunosuppressant therapy and in others who were iatrogenically immunosuppressed.

Of the 26 patients reported to the CDC in July 1981, all had evidence of an immunodeficiency not related to any known cause and several had other serious infections (four having pneumocystosis). All were homosexual men.[3]

Simultaneously, an additional ten cases of pneumocystosis in previously healthy young gay men in Los Angeles and San Francisco were reported, two of whom also had Kaposi's sarcoma. All these patients had evidence of an immunodeficiency with no known underlying cause. The following month saw an additional 70 cases of these two conditions.[4] It was then clear that a new potential epidemic was brewing.

Extremely alarmed, the CDC instituted a nationwide surveillance programme in July 1981. The new disease was termed the **acquired immune deficiency syndrome (AIDS)** and it was characterized as the occurrence of unusual (opportunistic) infections or cancers in previously healthy individuals, due to an acquired immunodeficiency of unknown cause. The CDC developed and published the first surveillance definition for this new disease, which was used throughout the Western world and in Australasia.[5]

ARC, PGL and LAS

In addition to cases of fully expressed AIDS, many homosexual men were presenting for investigation and/or treatment with what seemed a lesser form of AIDS, which came to be referred to as the **AIDS-related complex (ARC)**. Individuals with ARC often had a combination of various indicators of ill-health without having frank opportunistic infections or other conditions described in the surveillance definition for AIDS. Frequently they presented with unexplained persistent and generalized swollen lymph glands. This by itself became known as in the USA and UK as **persistent generalized lymphadenopathy (PGL)** or, in France, the **lymphadenopathy syndrome (LAS)**, almost always including cervical and axillary lymph nodes.[6] Individuals with ARC frequently complained of fever, profuse night sweats, fatigue and weight loss. All these patients showed abnormalities in tests for cell-mediated immunity and the vast majority of them would, in time, progress to AIDS. In the first few years of the USA epidemic, for every case of AIDS, there would be ten cases of ARC. The numbers started to look astronomical.

Data coming into the CDC from investigators all over the USA showed that the incidence of AIDS was roughly doubling every 6 months. By 1992, the prevalence of human immunodeficiency virus (HIV) infection in the USA was estimated to be between 650 000 and 900 000.[7] By the beginning of 2003, almost a million people were living with HIV/AIDS in North America.[8]

That same summer in Western Europe ...

Within just a few weeks of the first report of American AIDS cases, patients with AIDS were being identified in Denmark and France and, within a year, AIDS cases would be identified in all countries in Western, Southern and Northern Europe.[9,10]

And in the UK that summer ...

In the late summer of 1981, a patient was diagnosed as suffering from AIDS in a London hospital.[11] AIDS had arrived in the UK. Throughout 1982, new cases were identified and, by the end of September 2002, the total reported number of people diagnosed with HIV infection would rise to 52 729.[12]

A pandemic gathers

Within the first 4 years of our knowing that AIDS was here, cases were being reported from every geographical region in the world.[13] In each country where it appeared, it would become entrenched, silently moving and growing, spawning a conundrum of social, political and scientific reactions. This, the last great pandemic of the twentieth century, and our responses to it are redefining the very fabric of society throughout the world during this new millennium.

TERMINOLOGY

In describing the changing patterns of HIV infection as it swarms over the world, two terms are frequently used: prevalence and incidence.

Prevalence is the term used to describe the number of persons who have a specific disease or condition in a defined population at one specific point in time. An example of prevalence would be the total number of men and women between the ages of 14 and 65, residing in London, known to be infected with HIV and alive by the end of July 2003.

Incidence is the rate at which a certain event occurs in a defined population during a specific period of time, e.g. the number of new cases of HIV infection that occurred in the UK during 2003.

Other important terms used in describing the epidemiology of infectious diseases include endemic, epidemic and pandemic.

Endemic is the term used to describe the diseases present (or usually prevalent) in a population or geographical area all of the time. For example, a certain level of hepatitis C infection is always present (endemic) in injecting drug users in London.

An **epidemic** is a sudden increase in the incidence of an endemic disease (or condition), or the occurrence of a new disease with a high incidence introduced into a population. An example of an epidemic might be a sudden and significant increase in the incidence of tuberculosis (a low-prevalence disease which is always present in the UK population) during a specified period of time, e.g. the last quarter of 2003. Another example of an epidemic disease might be a new strain of influenza virus introduced during the winter of 2002–03 in London, which caused an **outbreak** (rapid and significant incidence) of influenza.

Finally, a **pandemic** refers to an epidemic disease distributed or occurring widely throughout a region, country, continent or globally. HIV/AIDS is a global pandemic composed of a plethora of local epidemics, all with their own unique characteristics, driven nationally by varied but similar human behaviours and societal conditions.

THE DEVELOPING GLOBAL PANDEMIC OF HIV INFECTIUN AND AIDS

Each year the Joint United Nations Programme on HIV/AIDS (UNAIDS), in collaboration with the World Health Organization (WHO), publishes a report on the status of the global HIV/AIDS pandemic. Their report at the end of December 2002 made sombre reading.[8] The global estimates of the HIV/AIDS epidemic as of the end of 2002 are described in Table 1.1.

TABLE 1.1 Global summary of the HIV/AIDS epidemic as of December 2002[8]

Number of people living with HIV/AIDS at the end of 2002	Total	**42 million**
	Adults	38.6 million
	Women	19.2 million
	Children <15 years	3.2 million
People newly infected with HIV during 2002	Total	**5.0 million**
	Adults	4.2 million
	Women	2.0 million
	Children <15 years	800 000
AIDS deaths during 2002	Total	**3.1 million**
	Adults	2.5 million
	Women	1.2 million
	Children <15 years	610 000

The UNAIDS report at the end of 2002 described a world in which **42 million people were now living with HIV/AIDS**, where **20 million people had already died** from this infection and where HIV, the virus that causes AIDS, continued to spread in all countries.[8] The regional prevalence of adults and children living with HIV/AIDS is reflected in Figure 1.1. **During 2002, over 14 000 people became infected with HIV every day**, accounting for **5 million new infections** in that year alone (Figure 1.2). While all these people were becoming exposed to and infected with HIV during that year, **3.1 million children and adults who had been previously infected, died** from HIV-related illnesses (Figure 1.3).

Adult men and women

By the end of 2002, 38.6 million adults, the majority of them in the most sexually active age bracket (15–49 years), were living with HIV/AIDS but only a tiny fraction of them even know they are infected. Worldwide, AIDS is among the top five causes of death in adults and is the number one cause of death from an infectious microorganism.

Children

Over 3.2 million children under the age of 15 years were living with HIV/AIDS by the end of 2002 and, during that year, 610 000 died from AIDS.

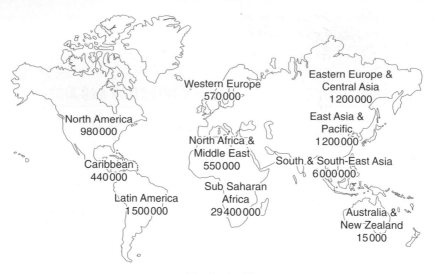

Total: 42 million

FIGURE 1.1 *Adults and children estimated to be living with HIV/AIDS, end 2002. (Courtesy of UNAIDS.)*

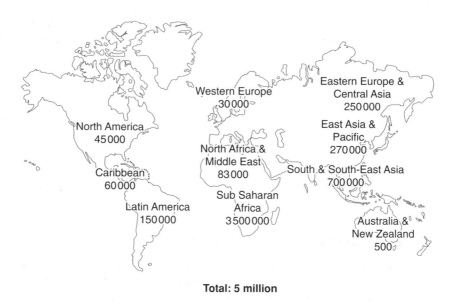

Total: 5 million

FIGURE 1.2 *Estimated number of adults and children newly infected with HIV during 2002. (Courtesy of UNAIDS.)*

Orphans

As of June 2002, more then 13 million children around the world had lost one or both parents to AIDS, over 90 per cent of them living in sub-Saharan Africa. By the year 2010, UNAIDS anticipates the total number of 'AIDS orphans' will exceed 25 million children.[14]

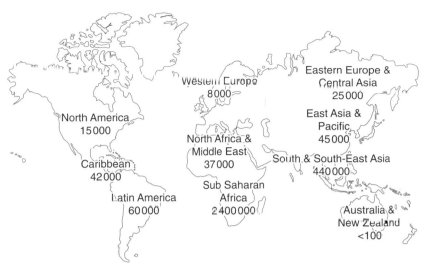

Total: 3.1 million

FIGURE 1.3 *Estimated adult and child deaths due to HIV/AIDS during 2002. (Courtesy of UNAIDS.)*

Extended family structures, once capable of caring for these children, are being weakened by the huge increase in death rates among younger adults, urbanization and the migration of labour. As the number of orphans continues to grow, the number of people available to care for them is rapidly diminishing.

Regional pandemics

The global pandemic of HIV infection and AIDS is composed of a variety of regional pandemics which, in turn, consist of national and local epidemics, all swirling around, each with its own unique characteristics: differing epidemiological time frames, incidence rates, societal factors, population risk behaviours, vulnerabilities and transmission models. The spread of HIV throughout the world has occurred in at least two distinct waves, each wave consisting of quite unique epidemiological patterns.[1]

The first wave of the pandemic (mid-1970s to late 1980s)

HIV began to spread extensively in the mid to late 1970s in North America, Western Europe, Australasia, Latin America and the Caribbean, and throughout sub-Saharan Africa. Very few AIDS cases were identified outside of these regions during this first wave. By 1997, only 1 per cent of AIDS cases were identified in other countries or regions and most of them had had sexual contact with people in those first-wave countries.

In this first wave of the epidemic, two distinct patterns were identified. Although these patterns applied generally, different patterns could co-exist within any one country.

Pattern I

During the first wave of the pandemic, in North America, Western Europe, Australasia and in many urban areas in Latin America, HIV was being transmitted sexually, principally by homosexual and bisexual men having sex with other men (men having sex with men, or MSM). Heterosexual transmission was also occurring but, in these regions in the early years of the pandemic, the numbers of people infected from heterosexual exposure was small. As few women were infected, perinatal transmission was initially uncommon. Some individuals were becoming infected as a result of being recipients of HIV-contaminated human blood or blood products, although their numbers were small compared to the growth of the epidemic among MSM. Injecting drug users (IDUs) were vulnerable to infection as a result of sharing HIV-contaminated injecting equipment, and the numbers of IDUs becoming infected during this first wave quickly escalated.

Pattern II

During this same period, i.e. the first wave of the pandemic, HIV was spreading rapidly throughout sub-Saharan Africa, but here, heterosexual transmission was the dominant force driving national epidemics. Latin America and the Caribbean also shared the same pattern.

Drug-injection behaviour was uncommon in most of these countries and was not a significant factor in the growth of the epidemic.

Transmission from HIV-contaminated blood transfusions or blood products, or from unsterile needles or other HIV-contaminated healthcare equipment, was also a significant factor in fuelling the epidemic.

Female commercial sex workers became infected early in the first wave of the pandemic in these countries, exposing their clients to HIV, who then became infected and, in turn, infected their wives and girlfriends.

As many more women were infected in these countries, perinatal transmission was common, and increasing numbers of children were being born already infected with HIV, or became infected by their HIV-infected mothers in the early post-natal period from breast milk.

The second wave of the pandemic (the 1990s)

During the last decade of the twentieth century, the pandemic broadened out from those countries affected during the first wave. During this period, AIDS established dramatic footholds in those regions that were spared during the 1980s: South and South East Asia, Eastern Europe and Central Asia, north and south Africa, the Middle East, and East Asia and the Pacific region. In these previously HIV-naïve populations, there was an accelerated, almost unchecked transmission of HIV, with a momentum established in which incidence rates of new infections spiralled out of control.

In addition, regional pandemics continued throughout Western Europe, North America, the Caribbean, Latin America, Australasia and, in the worst affected region, sub-Saharan Africa.

THE SHAPE OF THE GLOBAL PANDEMIC IN 2003

By the beginning of 2003, the shape of the global pandemic was well documented (Table 1.2).[8] The number of people living with HIV disease is concentrated in the industrially developing world, mostly in those resource-deprived countries least able to afford to care for HIV-infected people. Sub-Saharan Africa and the developing countries of Asia, which

TABLE 1.2 Regional HIV/AIDS statistics and features at the end of 2002[a]

Region	Epidemic started	Adults and children living with HIV/AIDS	Adults and children newly infected with HIV in 2002	Adult prevalence rate (%)[a]	Percentage of HIV-positive adults who are women	Main mode(s) of transmission[b] for adults living with HIV/AIDS[b]
Sub-Saharan Africa	Late 1970s–early 1980s	29.4 million	3.5 million	8.8	58	Hetero
North Africa and Middle East	Late 1980s	550 000	83 000	0.3	55	Hetero, IDU
South and South East Asia	Late 1980s	6.0 million	700 000	0.6	36	Hetero, IDU
East Asia and Pacific	Late 1980s	1.2 million	270 000	0.1	24	IDU, hetero, MSM
Latin America	Late 1970s–early 1980s	1.5 million	150 000	0.6	30	MSM, IDU, hetero
Caribbean	Late 1970s–early 1980s	440 000	60 000	2.4	50	Hetero, MSM
Eastern Europe and Central Asia	Early 1990s	1.2 million	250 000	0.6	27	IDU
Western Europe	Late 1970s–early 1980s	570 000	30 000	0.3	25	MSM, IDU
North America	Late 1970s–early 1980s	980 000	45 000	0.6	20	MSM, IDU, hetero
Australia and New Zealand	Late 1970s–early 1980s	15 000	500	0.1	7	MSM
Total		**42 million**	**5 million**	**1.2**	**50**	

[a]The proportion of adults (15–49 years of age) living with HIV/AIDS in 2002, using 2002 population numbers.

[b]Hetero, heterosexual transmission; IDU, transmission through injecting drug use; MSM, sexual transmission among men who have sex with men.

between them only account for less than 10 per cent of the global Gross National Product, are home to over 90 per cent of all people who are living with HIV disease today.

Estimates of new HIV infections in industrially developing regions in most parts of the world describe aggressive national epidemics with large numbers of people becoming infected (and then infecting others) each day, each week, each month: 14 000 people become infected every day – most of them in countries in the developing world.

As the natural history of HIV disease changes, principally due to the advent of highly active antiretroviral therapy (HAART), countries in the resource-rich industrialized world now tend to concentrate on identifying new HIV infections rather than following AIDS cases. These new surveillance strategies will track both the prevalence and incidence of infection, more accurately reflecting trends in epidemics. Data on AIDS cases will continue to be important as an indicator of severe HIV-related morbidity in populations and to represent populations in which treatments have failed or those which were not tested or treated prior to a diagnosis of AIDS.

The number of new AIDS cases in many industrialized regions (North America, Western Europe, Australasia) is falling, due to the increasing use of HAART regimens and to the continuing decline in vertical (perinatal) transmission by the identification and treatment of mothers in the antenatal period. These treatment advances have changed the shape of the epidemic in industrialized countries, altered the natural history of HIV disease, and led to an increase in the numbers of people in these regions living with HIV/AIDS but not yet progressing to end-stage disease, i.e. AIDS.

Additionally, primary prevention initiatives (health education, condom use) are reducing the incidence of HIV infection in industrialized countries to a significant extent.

Consequently, a two-world situation has developed: a continuing and dramatic increase in the incidence of HIV in the poorer regions of the world, ultimately leading to staggering increases in AIDS cases and deaths, and a stabilizing and falling rate in new infections, AIDS cases and deaths in wealthier regions of the world.

THREE PANDEMICS IN TWO WORLDS

Acting in synergy and firing the global pandemic of HIV/AIDS are two other conditions: the global pandemics of sexually transmitted infections (STIs) and tuberculosis (TB).

Sexually transmitted infections

Each year, an estimated 250 million new cases of STI occur throughout the world and the global prevalence and incidence of these infections are rising.[1] The USA has the highest rates of STIs in the industrialized world.[15] and many countries in the developing world experience continuing high incidence and prevalence of potentially curable STIs.[1] Adding to the burden of the new cases of STIs each year are the tremendous underlying prevalence of people with subclinical infections who are not diagnosed and treated and the large number of people with a curable STI who are inadequately treated and not cured.

Throughout the HIV/AIDS pandemic, researchers have consistently presented evidence for a strong epidemiological association between HIV/AIDS and other STIs. Both ulcerative and inflammatory STIs are co-factors for HIV transmission, dramatically increasing the infectiousness of HIV transmission and the susceptibility to HIV infection on exposure.[1,15]

Consequently, the increasing global incidence and prevalence of STIs are accelerating the continuing high incidence of HIV infection, the two pandemics acting in synergy, mutually reinforcing each other.

Tuberculosis

The danger of the growing global HIV/AIDS pandemic is further compounded by the re-emergence, out of the shadows, of one of the great killers of the past – TB.

One-third of the world's population (i.e. 2 billion people), including more than 10 million HIV-infected individuals, are infected with *Mycobacterium tuberculosis*, the causative agent of TB. From this large pool of infected people, over 8 million succumb to active TB every year, 95 per cent of them in the developing world, and 2–3 million of them die from this disease.[16,17]

When a person who is latently infected with TB becomes infected with HIV, the resultant depression of their immune system causes TB to reactivate, causing disease and making that person infectious to others. TB is the most common opportunistic infection in HIV-infected people and one of the few infections that can be transmitted to others.

Additionally, if an HIV-infected person becomes infected with *M. tuberculosis*, he or she is 30 times more likely to have active TB than a person who is not infected with HIV.

One-third of the growing incidence in TB all over the world during the last 5 years of the twentieth century can be attributed to the global HIV pandemic and, in turn, TB accounts for almost one-third of AIDS deaths worldwide.[18]

The two diseases, forming a dangerous liaison, and having been termed 'the cursed duet',[19] make the future for humankind somewhat more precarious than most had expected.

TWO WORLDS

The global pandemic of HIV/AIDS is widening the division between the industrially developed and the industrially developing worlds, i.e. between rich and poor countries.

Comprehensive and sustainable health education, early identification of infection, effective prophylaxis and treatment of HIV-related opportunistic infections, highly active antiretroviral therapy with appropriate laboratory monitoring, high-quality outpatient and inpatient care and the protection of children from vertical transmission are only possible in the industrially developed world. However, 90 per cent of all those people living with HIV reside in sub-Saharan Africa and the developing countries of Asia, which between them account for less than 10 per cent of the global Gross National Product.[13] They do not have the resources to manage their own national epidemics and this disparity between these two worlds widens by the day.

Summary

Seemingly coming out of nowhere two decades ago, HIV/AIDS now poses one of the most significant threats to public health for this generation, and perhaps for generations to come.

We already have the means to prevent infection, e.g. health education, behavioural change, antenatal screening and screening donated blood and organs. However, the entire continuum of humanity remains at risk. In no country on this planet can it be said that this epidemic is under control. It continues as a volatile, unstable and escalating situation.

This global pandemic will only be brought under control when all the issues that are factored into its continuing escalation are confronted: sexual and drug-taking behaviour and individual responsibility; political and institutional structures at all levels; healthcare resources and the provision of meaningful high-quality care; discrimination, poverty, ignorance and malnutrition. Only then will humankind be safe from the further destructive forces of these three great pandemics – truly plagues of our time.

Prologue to Chapter 2

As this global pandemic is caused by people becoming infected with a lethal virus, it is essential that nurses and other healthcare professionals understand the biology of viruses in general, and retroviruses in particular, in order to make sense of the anticipated clinical outcomes of infection and strategies for primary prevention, infection control and antiretroviral treatment. The next chapter provides a basic review of the biology of viruses, preparing the reader for a more detailed introduction to retroviruses, particularly the human immunodeficiency viruses.

REFERENCES

1. Mann JM, Tarantola DJ (eds). *AIDS in the World II: A Global Dimensions, Social Roots, and Responses*. New York: Oxford University Press, 1996.
2. Centers for Disease Control (CDC). Pneumocystis pneumonia. Los Angeles. *Morbidity and Mortality Weekly Report (MMWR)* 5 June 1981; **30**:250–2.
3. CDC. Kaposi's sarcoma and pneumocystis pneumonia among homosexual men. New York City and California. *Morbidity and Mortality Weekly Report (MMWR)* 3 July 1981; **30**:305–8.
4. CDC. Follow-up on Kaposi's sarcoma and pneumocystis pneumonia. *Morbidity and Mortality Weekly Report (MMWR)* 28 August 1981; **30**:409–10.
5. CDC. Update on acquired immune deficiency (AIDS). United States. *Morbidity and Mortality Weekly Report (MMWR)* September 24 1982; **31**:507–14.
6. CDC. Persistent, generalized lymphadenopathy among homosexual males. *Morbidity and Mortality Weekly Report (MMWR)* 21 May 1982; **31**:249–51.
7. Karon JM, Rosenberg PS, McQuillan G, Khare M, Gwinn M, Petersen LR. Prevalence of HIV Infection in the United States, 1984 to 1992. *Journal of the American Medical Association* 1996; **276**:126–31.
8. UNAIDS/WHO. *AIDS Epidemic Update* (UNAIDS/02.58E). Geneva: Joint United Nations Programme on HIV/AIDS and the World Health Organization, December 2002. Available online from: http://www.unaids.org
9. Leibowitch J. *Un virus étrange venu d'ailleurs*. Paris: Grasset; 1984. American edition: *A Strange Virus of Unknown Origin*. New York: Ballantine, 1985.
10. Grmek MD. *History of AIDS: Emergence and Origin of a Modern Pandemic*. Oxford: Princeton University Press, 1990.
11. Dubois RM, Branthwaite MA, Mikhail JR, Batten JC. Primary *Pneumocystis carinii* and cytomegalovirus infection. *Lancet* 1981; **ii**:1339.
12. Communicable Disease Surveillance Centre (CDSC). AIDS and HIV infection in the United Kingdom: monthly report. *Communicable Disease Report – CDR Weekly* [serial online] 2003; **13**. Cited 14 January 2003. Available from: http://www.phls.co.uk/publications/cdr/pages/hiv.html
13. Joint United Nations Programme on AIDS (UNAIDS), World Health Organization (WHO). *Report on the Global HIV/AIDS Epidemic*. Geneva: UNAIDS and WHO, June 2000. UNAIDS/00.13E, 135 pp. Available from UNAIDS: http://www.unaids.org/
14. UNAIDS. *Children on the Brink 2002*. A joint USAID/UNICEF/UNAIDS Report on Orphan Estimates and Program Strategies. Geneva: UNAIDS, 2002. Available online at: http://www.unaids.org/barcelona/presskit/childrenonthebrink.html
15. CDC. HIV prevention through early detection and treatment of other sexually transmitted diseases – United States: Recommendations of the Advisory Committee for HIV and STD Prevention. *Morbidity and Mortality Weekly Report (MMWR)* 31 July 1998; **47**(RR-12):1–25.
16. Kochi A. The global tuberculosis situation and the new control strategy of the World Health Organization. *Tubercle* 1991; **72**:1–6.
17. Snider DE. Tuberculosis: the world situation. History of the disease and efforts to combat it. In: Porter JDH, McAdam KPWJ (eds), *Tuberculosis: Back to the Future*. Chichester: John Wiley & Sons, 1994, 22–4.

18. WHO Global Tuberculosis Programme. *TB Advocacy – A Practical Guide 1999.* Geneva: WHO GPA, WHO/TB/98.239, 1998. Available from: fightTB@who.ch

19. Chretien J. Tuberculosis and HIV. The cursed duet. *Bulletin of the International Union against Tuberculosis and Lung Disease* 1990; **65**:25–8.

FURTHER READING

Grmek MD. *History of AIDS: Emergence and Origin of a Modern Pandemic.* Oxford: Princeton University Press, 1990, 279 pp, ISBN 0-691-08552-8.

Mann JM, Tarantola DJ (eds). *AIDS in the World II: Global Dimensions, Social Roots, and Responses.* Oxford: Oxford University Press, 1996, 616 pp, ISBN 0-674-01266-6.

Mulhall A. *Epidemiology, Nursing and Health Care: A New Perspective.* London: Macmillan Press Ltd, 1996, 240 pp, ISBN 0-333-62252-9.

Shilts R. *And The Band Played On: Politics, People and the AIDS Epidemic.* London: Viking (The Penguin Group), 1987, 630 pp, ISBN 0-670-82270-1.

INTERNET RESOURCES

United Kingdom

■ Public Health Laboratory Service AIDS Centre (HIV/STI Division, Communicable Disease Surveillance Centre) and the Scottish Centre for Infection & Environmental Health.
AIDS/HIV Quarterly Surveillance Tables (Official UK Government HIV/AIDS Data and Statistics).
Communicable Disease Report Weekly (CDR Weekly) publishes online the weekly notifications of infectious diseases, including a monthly report on *HIV-1 Infection and AIDS in the United Kingdom.*
Both of the above publications are easily accessed from the CDSC worldwide web site (home page): http://www.phls.co.uk/

Europe

World Health Organization – European Region.

■ WHO publishes communicable disease surveillance news gathered from public health centres in the European Union (EU) in its bulletin *Eurosurveillance Weekly.* The site is updated a minimum of once a week, giving reports on outbreaks as they unfold.

■ Surveillance of HIV/AIDS in Europe is conducted by 48 countries of the WHO European Region. Anonymous individual data on AIDS cases are compiled by the European Centre for the Epidemiological Monitoring of AIDS and presented in the quarterly report *HIV/AIDS Surveillance in Europe.* This report is accessed through the above CDSC home page.

United States of America

- *The HIV/AIDS Surveillance Report*: http://www.cdc.gov/hiv/stats/hasrlink.htm
  This report contains tabular and graphic information about US AIDS and HIV case reports, including data by state, metropolitan statistical area, mode of exposure to HIV, sex, race/ethnicity, age group, vital status, and case definition category. It is published semi-annually by the Division of HIV/AIDS Prevention, Nation Center for HIV, STD, and TB Prevention at the Centers for Disease Control and Prevention (CDC) in the USA.
- *Morbidity & Mortality Weekly Report (MMWR)*:
  http://www.cdc.gov/epo/mmwr/
  Similar to the *CDR Weekly* in the UK and publishes current AIDS updates and statistics in many issues throughout the year.

Africa

- General epidemiological data can be found in the Africa-focused website maintained by the Center for Molecular Medicine and Genetics at Wayne State University in Detroit, Michigan, USA:
  http://cmmg.biosci.wayne.edu/asg/hivafrica.html

Joint United Nations Program on AIDS (UNAIDS)

- Publishes regular reports and press releases in relation to the global epidemiology of the pandemic. Also publishes an annual *Report on the Global HIV/AIDS Epidemic* (usually in June each year):
  http://www.unaids.org/

The tables and figures in this chapter are also available as PowerPoint slides from:
http://www.unaids.org/worldaidsday/2002/press/graphics.html

Understanding the cause of AIDS – the biology of viruses

Individual viruses have evolved interesting and unique lifestyles. One consequence is that battles have been won or lost when a particular virus infected one army but not its adversaries. Viruses have depleted the native populations of several continents. Entire countries have been changed geographically, economically, and religiously as a result of sweeping virus infections that were impervious to known cures.

Michael Oldstone, 1998[1]

Introduction

From the beginning of the epidemic, AIDS exhibited all the classic signs of an infectious disease, and the only convincing explanation for its cause was the emergence of a new infectious agent. An infective aetiology was consistent with the geographical clustering of early cases and epidemiological evidence of case-to-case contact, the newness of the disease, the pattern of groups at risk, its occurrence within the same time scale in the diverse groups affected and, finally, its exponential spread.

In 1983, just 2 years after our awareness of AIDS as a new disease in our communities, French scientists at the Pasteur Institute in Paris discovered a previously unknown virus that was associated with AIDS.[2] During the following year, research in the USA further confirmed that this new virus was indeed the cause of AIDS.[3,4] Although originally referred to by a variety of terms, by early 1986, the AIDS-causing viruses were officially designated as **human immunodeficiency viruses (HIV)**. This has become the standard term for the viruses that can cause immunosuppression and ultimately AIDS in HIV-infected humans and refers to two closely related viruses: **HIV-1**, the predominant

AIDS-related virus in the world, and **HIV-2**, a genetically similar but biologically distinct second type of AIDS-related virus. These viruses are described in more detail in the next chapter, but first it is important that nurses have a basic understanding of the general characteristics of viruses before we examine the more specialist group of retroviruses which cause AIDS and other diseases in humans.

Learning outcomes

After studying and reflecting on the material in this chapter, you will be able to:

- discuss the general characteristics of viruses and describe their varying composition and structure, which allows them to be classified;
- explain how different viruses infect and replicate within host cells.

VIRUSES – A GENERAL OVERVIEW

In the late nineteenth century, scientists were able to extract bacteria by filtration, i.e. passing fluid containing microorganisms through a filter, such as porcelain. Bacteria (and protozoa), being fairly large microorganisms, remained on or in the filter following filtration. However, scientists observed that in some instances, the filtered fluid, i.e. the filtrate, still contained unidentified substances, clearly smaller than bacteria and able to pass through the filter, which could cause disease. By the early 1900s, these minute infectious particles were termed filterable viruses (Latin *virus* – poison) and, by 1935, scientists were able to isolate and, using an electron microscope, visualize these tiny microorganisms.

All viruses have certain characteristics that distinguish them from other microorganisms, such as bacteria, fungi and protozoa, and that also provide a means by which to describe and classify them (Table 2.1). These characteristics are related to their structure, the composition and polarity of their genome (see below), the shape of their nucleocapsid, method of replication, size, viral attachment sites and the surface receptors on host cells that they are attracted to.

TABLE 2.1 How viruses are described and/or classified

- The nucleic acid composition of their genome, i.e. DNA or RNA
- The number of strands of nucleic acid and their arrangement, i.e. linear, circular, single stranded, double stranded
- For ssRNA viruses, the polarity of their genome, i.e. the RNA is either positive or negative stranded
- The specific base sequence of the genome that will characterize specific viruses (and even subpopulations of those specific viruses)
- The shape (symmetry) of their nucleocapsid
- The presence or absence of an outer envelope composed of a lipid–protein–carbohydrate complex
- Method of replication
- Viral attachment sites and associated host cell surface receptors

Viruses are not classified as true cells as they do not contain a limiting plasma membrane, cytoplasm, ribosomes, mitochondria, enzymes to generate high-energy bonds, or muramic acid in their outer coverings. Unlike living cells, viruses do not possess the critical enzymes needed to perform independent cellular metabolic processes and cannot reproduce independently. However, because they contain nucleic acid, i.e. deoxyribonucleic acid (**DNA**) or ribonucleic acid (**RNA**), the fundamental property of life, they are able to replicate, but *only inside a living host cell that they have infected*, thus being obligatory intracellular parasites.

THE CHARACTERISTICS OF VIRUSES

The viral genome

The central core of a virus is referred to as the **genome** and it contains the genetic material, i.e. the complete gene complement, that the virus uses to survive and to replicate. Unlike living cells that contain *both* DNA *and* RNA, the genome of a virus is composed of a single type of nucleic acid, i.e. *either* DNA *or* RNA but *never* both. The composition of the viral nucleic acid genome is the most important way in which viruses are classified, i.e. they are *either* DNA *or* RNA viruses.

The molecules that make up the viral nucleic acid in the genome are arranged in a precise sequence within either a single or a double strand. Consequently, the viral genome is described as being either **single stranded (ss)** or **double stranded (ds)**. These strands may be circular, linear, in one piece (continuous) or in several pieces (segmented).

All DNA viruses (except parvoviruses) are double stranded and, with just one exception (reoviruses), the genome of all RNA viruses is single stranded. RNA viruses may have one single strand of nucleic acid, or they may have two copies of this single strand; in both instances they are classified as being single-stranded RNA viruses.

The capsid

The viral genome is enclosed within and intimately attached to a protein shell, known as the **capsid**. The capsid is made up of numerous smaller protein subunits called **capsomeres** (Figure 2.1). The function of the capsid is to protect the delicate nucleic acid which makes up the viral genome.

The nucleocapsid

The capsid and genome of the virus are closely integrated to form a **nucleocapsid** of an *exactly defined symmetry*, i.e. **shape**. The nucleocapsids of different viruses have different shapes. Some are **icosahedral** (cubical) in shape, some are **helical** (like a spiral staircase) and still others have a nucleocapsid that is composed of extremely **complex** structures. Most viruses have a nucleocapsid that has either a spiral or cubical shape. This provides an additional way of describing viruses: they have either an icosahedral or helical nucleocapsid (or, more unusually, a nucleocapsid with a complex shape).

The envelope

Some viruses are enclosed in a **lipoprotein envelope** (or **coat**), made up of some combination of lipids (fat), proteins and carbohydrates. The envelope is derived from material (nuclear and cytoplasmic membranes) from the cells that viruses infect and that clings to them when

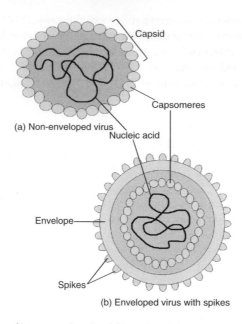

FIGURE 2.1 *General structure of (a) non-enveloped and (b) enveloped viruses.*

they exit these cells by the process of **budding**. The envelopes of some viruses are covered with **spikes** that project outwards from the surface of the virus. These spikes are composed of a complex of protein and carbohydrates, i.e. **glycoproteins**, manufactured by the host cell and incorporated into a newly assembled virus towards the end of its intracellular replication cycle (Figure 2.1).

The virion

The genome in the core surrounded by the capsid (and the envelope, if present) comprises the complete infective viral particle and is known as a **virion**. The virion is the *extracellular form of the virus* and can be found prior to the virus entering and infecting a cell. The virion serves as a transportation mechanism, carrying the viral genome to other cells targeted for invasion.

Size of virions

Virions are extremely small, varying in diameter from **18** to **300 nanometres**. A nanometre (nm) is one millionth of a millimetre (mm) or one-thousandth of a micrometre (µm). Virions are amongst the smallest microorganisms that infect humans.

Polarity of ssRNA viral genomes

During replication, the genome of some ssRNA viruses is able to act directly as **messenger RNA (mRNA)**, i.e. it can be translated (changed) into viral proteins by cell ribosomes. This type of viral genome is referred to as being **positive stranded**.

Other ssRNA viruses cannot do this. They use a viral enzyme (**RNA polymerase**) to make an identical positive-stranded copy of their original negative strand of RNA. This new mirror-image copy then acts as mRNA and is used to synthesize new viral proteins. These viruses are known as **negative-stranded** viruses.

The **polarity** of the ssRNA viral genome is classified as being either positive or negative.

Viral replication

DNA viruses replicate their nucleic acid within the nucleus of the host cell they have infected, but the manufacture of their capsid and other viral proteins occurs in the cytoplasm of that cell.

RNA viruses behave differently. They multiply within the cytoplasm of the host cell, where they hijack cellular components, e.g. ribosomes, to make new viral proteins.

An important family of RNA viruses (and the family of viruses which HIV belongs to) known as *Retroviridae* (**retroviruses**) replicate quite differently. The genome of retroviruses consists of two identical molecules of positive-stranded, single-strand RNA (+ssRNA). Once they gain entry into a cell, they use a special viral enzyme (**reverse transcriptase**) to transcribe (change) one of their single strands of positively charged RNA (+ssRNA) to produce an identical, single strand of negatively charged DNA (−ssDNA). The remaining +ssRNA and the newly transcribed −ssDNA then form a **DNA–RNA hybrid**. The +ssRNA in this hybrid is eventually digested away by the activity of ribonuclease H (**RNase H**), a subunit of the viral enzyme reverse transcriptase. Another subunit of reverse transcriptase is known as **DNA polymerase**, which, using the remaining −ssDNA as a template, facilitates the generation of a second DNA copy, to form a double-stranded DNA molecule (dsDNA) that is then incorporated into the cell's nucleus (which, of course, is composed of DNA). The subsequent steps in viral replication for this family of viruses are discussed in more detail in the following chapter.

Viral attachment sites and cell receptors sites

As described earlier, all viruses have proteins distributed over their surface that contain their **attachment sites**. The structures of the sites have evolved to match specific receptors on the surface of different host cells and vary on different types of viruses. They usually take the form of pockets or various types of bulges or protuberances, e.g. spikes, on the surface of the virus. The attachment sites (also known as a **receptor-binding sites**) contain the docking elements that viruses use to attach and bind themselves to complementary **cell surface receptors** on host cells the virus has targeted for infection. Cell surface receptors consist of complexes of protein and glycoprotein adhesion molecules on the host cell's surface plasma membrane and are inherited characteristics of the host.

The viral attachment sites can be thought of as **keys** and the host cell surface receptors as **locks**. The keys and locks are complex. Each key is composed of several protein characters (like fingers on a hand) and each lock consists of multiple complexes of molecules that match the proteins that make up the key.

Each virus that successfully infects humans has keys for certain locks, but not all locks. When a virion enters the human body, it searches for those host cells that have locks its keys will fit. By using these keys, the virus can open the locks and enter and infect the host cell.

Summary

Viruses are extremely small life forms, the genome of which is composed of molecules of nucleic acid (either DNA or RNA, but never both). A protein outer shell (the capsid) surrounds the genome, and together they are referred to as a nucleocapsid, which, in different viruses, is structured in varying but exactly defined shapes (symmetry). Additionally, the nucleocapsid of some viruses is itself surrounded by an envelope made up of a complex of fat, protein and carbohydrates. In order for viruses to replicate, they must first infect a living cell. When viruses infect humans, they search for host cells that contain specific cell surface receptors to which their attachment sites can bind and then penetrate and infect that cell. Different viruses have different attachment sites and therefore are attracted to different host cells. This attraction for specific host cells that have complementary receptor sites is known as **tropism**.

Prologue to Chapter 3

Although not all viruses are harmful, many hundreds are capable of causing severe disease in humans, animals and plants. One of the most significant discoveries in virology during the last 25 years has been the identification of a previously unknown group of retroviruses that are able to infect humankind efficiently and cause a fatal immunosuppression. The resultant concoction of consequent illnesses makes up a well-defined syndrome that we now call AIDS. Within just a quarter of a century, these AIDS-causing viruses have now seeded the whirlwind of a global pandemic that continues to rage unabated in nations throughout the world.

The next chapter provides a comprehensive review of these retroviruses, enabling the reader better to comprehend the following discussions related to HIV prevention, infection, testing, clinical outcomes, treatment and antiretroviral prophylaxis.

REFERENCES

1. Oldstone MBA. *Viruses, Plagues, & History*. Oxford: Oxford University Press, 1998, 211 pp.
2. Barre-Sinoussi F, Chermann JC, Rey F et al. Isolation of a T-lymphotropic retrovirus from a patient at risk for acquired immune deficiency syndrome (AIDS). *Science* 1983; **220**:868–71.
3. Gallo RC, Salahuddin SZ, Popovic M et al. Frequent detection and isolation of cytopathic retroviruses (HTLV-III) from patients with AIDS and at risk from AIDS. *Science* 1984; **224**:500–3.
4. Levy JA, Hoffman AD, Kramer SM et al. Isolation of lymphocytopathic retroviruses from San Francisco patients with AIDS. *Science* 1984; **225**:840–2.

FURTHER READING

Collier L, Oxford J. *Human Virology*, 2nd edn. Oxford: Oxford University Press, 2000, 284 pp, ISBN 0-19-262820-8.
Wilson J. *Clinical Microbiology: An Introduction for Healthcare Professionals*, 8th edn. London: Baillière Tindall, 2000, 410 pp, ISBN 0-7020-2316-7.

CHAPTER 3

Retroviruses – the cause of AIDS

The evidence that AIDS is caused by HIV-1 or HIV-2 is clear-cut,
exhaustive and unambiguous, meeting the highest standards of science.

The Durban Declaration 2000 South Africa[1]

Introduction

When the viruses that cause AIDS were discovered in 1983/84,[2–4] healthcare
professionals all over the world soon needed to become well acquainted with a relatively
unfamiliar family of viruses that most had thought were harmless to humans. Today, we
have a clearer understanding of how these viruses infect and cause illness in humans and
the unique threat to global health they now pose.

Learning outcomes

After reviewing Chapter 2 and studying and reflecting on the material in this chapter, you will
be able to:

- outline the general features of retroviruses, particularly those that infect and cause
  disease in humans;
- describe the structure and biology of human immunodeficiency viruses (HIV), including
  the mechanisms they use to infect and replicate within host cells;
- discuss the origins of HIV;
- compare and contrast HIV-1 and HIV-2 and describe HIV-1 subtypes (clades).

RETROVIRUSES

Human immunodeficiency viruses belong to that large family of RNA viruses previously mentioned, the *Retroviridae* (retroviruses). Most retroviruses are associated with disease in fish, reptiles, birds and mammals. Only a few retroviruses are associated with infection and disease in human and non-human primates.

Retroviruses are divided into seven distinct groups (genera) according to the relationships and sequencing of nucleotides in and the structure of their genome.[5] Two groups of retroviruses are particularly important as they cause human disease: **lentiviruses** and the **HTLV-BLV** group of retroviruses.

Lentiviruses

Viruses in the genus *Lentivirus* (Latin *lentus* – 'slow' virus) are characterized by the absence of a cancer-causing gene (oncogene) in their genome and their association with slowly progressive disease in some animals and humans. The viruses **HIV-1** and **HIV-2** are important members of this genus, as are other viruses that infect, and in some instances cause disease in, non-human primates and other animals. These include: **SIV** (simian immunodeficiency viruses), infecting many species of free-ranging monkeys in sub-Saharan Africa; **EIAV** (equine infectious anaemia virus), causing disease in horses; **FIV** (feline immunodeficiency virus), causing disease in cats (not to be confused with another retrovirus, the feline leukaemia virus, or FeLV); **BIV** (bovine immunodeficiency virus), causing disease in cattle; **CAEV** (caprine arthritis-encephalitis virus), causing diseases in goats; and **visna maedi virus**, which causes disease in sheep.

HTLV-BLV group

The genome of the HTLV-BLV group of retroviruses possesses an oncogene, and viruses within this genus are associated with T-cell lymphoma and neurological diseases in humans (**HTLV-I** and **HTLV-II** – human T-cell leukaemia or lymphotropic viruses) and B-cell lymphoma in cattle (**BLV** – bovine leukaemia virus).

HISTORY OF HUMAN RETROVIRUSES

Retroviruses were initially known as RNA tumour viruses and are among the earliest known viruses, being first described in 1911 when they were associated with causing sarcomas, a type of cancer, in chickens.[6] For many years they were known to cause disease in some animals but they were not thought to be involved in causing human illness. In 1979, a new retrovirus associated with the aetiology of an aggressive adult T-cell leukaemia, and named the human T-cell leukaemia/lymphoma virus (now referred to as HTLV-I), was isolated by Robert Gallo.[7] In 1982, Gallo's group identified another similar, but distinct, retrovirus from a patient with hairy cell leukaemia. This was named the human T-cell leukaemia/lymphoma virus, type II (HTLV-II).[8] HTLV are especially (but not exclusively) attracted to T-lymphocytes of the helper subgroup (**CD4+ T-lymphocytes**), which become their targets. This attraction (tropism) for these particular cells made them likely candidates for investigation as a potential cause of AIDS, as it was known that people with this disease have a decreased number of CD4$^+$ T-lymphocytes. The term HTLV was eventually redefined as **human T-cell leukaemia/lymphotropic viruses**.

Robert Gallo first reported the possibility that a retrovirus was involved in the aetiology of AIDS in February 1902.[9] In 1983, Francoise Barre-Sinoussi and Luc Montagnier at the Institut Pasteur in Paris discovered a novel retrovirus associated with AIDS which they named the **lymphadenopathy-associated virus (LAV)**.[2] A year later, Robert Gallo's group also identified what they thought was a different retrovirus in patients with AIDS and they concluded (incorrectly as it turned out) that this was a new type of human T-cell leukaemia/lymphotropic virus (which they named **HTLV-III**).[3] In that same year, Jay Levy in San Francisco also identified a new type of retrovirus in people with AIDS that he termed the **AIDS-associated retrovirus (ARV)**.[4] Within 2 years, all three of these viruses were conclusively shown to be associated with AIDS and it became clear that they were all different isolates of the virus originally discovered by Montagnier's group in Paris. However, unlike HTLV (the cancer-causing viruses within the HTLV-BLV group of retroviruses), this new retrovirus was a **lentivirus**. It was subsequently renamed the human immunodeficiency virus, type 1 (**HIV-1**).

During 1985/86, a second biologically distinct AIDS-related retrovirus was identified in patients in different countries in West Africa and this virus became known as human immunodeficiency virus, type 2 (**HIV-2**).[10] Although HIV-2 is closely related to HIV-1, it is even more closely related to (and often indistinguishable from) several strains of SIV.[11]

SPECIAL CHARACTERISTICS OF HIV

Structure

HIV-1 and HIV-2 are morphologically similar. Both are approximately 110 nanometres in diameter and are spherical structures consisting of an outer **envelope** composed of a double lipid membrane with glycoprotein molecules protruding from it. Enclosed within the sphere is a cubical (icosahedral) **shell** made up of matrix protein. Within this shell is a vase-shaped conical (helical) structure, constructed of a protein and known as a **capsid**. Within the vase (capsid) is the diploid RNA **genome**. The vase and genome together form the viral **nucleocapsid** (Figure 3.1).

The proteins that make up various parts of the virus are referred to by their molecular weight (mass), in thousands of daltons (kilodaltons), which are arbitrary units of molecular weight or mass. For example, **p17** refers to a protein with a molecular weight of between 17 and 18 kilodaltons; **gp120** refers to a **glycoprotein** (protein–carbohydrate complex) with a molecular weight of 120 kilodaltons.

HIV genome

Like all retroviruses, the genome of HIV is **diploid**. This means that it is composed of two identical copies of single-stranded RNA, both with positive polarity. Because many graphical representations of HIV clearly illustrate these two single-stranded molecules of RNA in the viral genome, a common misconception is to think of HIV as a double-stranded RNA virus. HIV is, as described above, a single-stranded RNA virus; it just has two copies of single-stranded RNA in its genome.

The viral RNA is composed of at least nine different **genes**, of which the major three (*gag,*

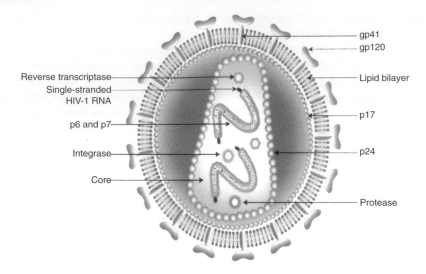

FIGURE 3.1 *Structural features of the human immunodeficiency virus. The glycoprotein (gp) molecules protrude through a lipid membrane (bilayer). An icosahedral protein shell (p17) underlies the membrane and itself encloses a vase-shaped protein structure (p24).The diploid RNA genome is enclosed in the 'vase' (viral core), along with viral enzymes and other core proteins (p6, p7).*

pol and *env*) are common to all retroviruses. These genes provide genetic information and instructions that allow the virus to make either **structural** or **regulatory proteins**, which it uses to replicate. This process is known as **encoding**.

The gene composition of the human immunodeficiency viruses has been mapped and is well understood (Figure 3.2).[12–14]

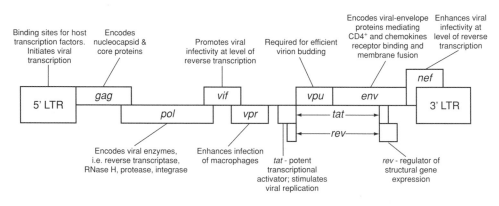

FIGURE 3.2 *Genetic structure of the HIV-1 genome.*[12–14]

- Genes encoding **structural proteins** include:
  1. the *env* gene that encodes the surface-coat glycoproteins gp41 and gp120 in the viral envelope;
  2. the *gag* gene that encodes the internal capsid (nucleocapsid) and core proteins in the virus (p6, p7, p17, p24);

3. the *pol* gene that encodes **viral enzymes**, i.e. reverse transcriptase (p66/p51), RNase H, protease (p10) and integrase (p32);

- Genes encoding for **early regulatory proteins**, important for viral replication, are: *tat* (p14) and *rev* (p19), which, when switched on, increase viral replication, and *nef* (p27), which, when activated, enhances HIV infectivity (see below).
- Other genes that encode for **late regulatory proteins** include *vif* (p23) and, in HIV-1 (but not in HIV-2), *vpu* (p15), which are necessary for the efficient release of budding virions from the cell (see below).
- Another gene, *vpr* (p15), encodes for **accessory proteins** and is important for efficient infection and viral replication in the natural target cells, such as macrophages. *vpx* (p16) is another gene that encodes for accessory proteins, but only in HIV-2; it is not found in HIV-1 (see below).

The genomes of all retroviruses contain **long terminal repeat (LTR)** elements, generated during reverse transcription and only completely present in the DNA copy of the viral genome. LTRs do not encode for protein, but are binding sites that are essential for the initiation of viral transcription and the regulation of viral gene expression.

Core proteins, glycoproteins and the viral envelope

Surrounding the viral genome is a double protein coat consisting of specific **core proteins**. The outermost layer of this double coat is the icosahedral shell. Icosahedral means that the shell has a geometric shape consisting of 20 sides or faces. This shell contains the inner helical (spiral shape, like a winding staircase) cone-shaped vase that encloses the viral genome (see Figure 3.1). The vase is constructed of a **capsid protein** known as **p24**, and the cubical (icosahedral) shell that contains the vase consists of a **matrix protein** known as **p17**. The matrix protein lines and interacts with the inner surface of the lipid bilayer (viral envelope).

Two nucleocapsid proteins are also present in the genome: **p7**, which is a binding protein for the two single strands of RNA; and **p6**, another binding protein which also plays a critical role in virion assembly and release.

Viral enzymes

The two molecules of single-stranded RNA are attached to molecules of the enzyme **reverse transcriptase (RT)**, which transcribes the viral RNA into proviral DNA once the virus has entered a cell. Other enzymes are also found within the viral genome, including **integrase** and **protease**, and these are discussed in more detail in Chapter 6, where viral replication and cellular pathogenesis are described.

Lipid bilayer and envelope glycoproteins

These core proteins are surrounded by a fatty membrane (**lipid bilayer**) with **glycoprotein structures** (proteins linked to carbohydrates) attached to and embedded in it. The **surface (SU) glycoprotein**, known as **gp120 SU**, is the external portion of the viral envelope, and the **transmembrane (TM) glycoprotein**, known as **gp41 TM**, spans the lipid bilayer and anchors the glycoprotein complex to the surface of the virion.

The lipid bilayer, derived from human cells and carrying host antigens, is the viral envelope. It is externally studded with cellular proteins, including β2-microglobulin and proteins of human origin, known as **class I** and **class II major histocompatibility complex** molecules. These proteins are discussed in more detail in Chapter 6.

These proteins and glycoproteins form the **viral attachment sites**, i.e. the 'keys' that will enable HIV to dock onto the **host cell receptor sites**, i.e. the 'locks' on the surface of those cells that HIV has targeted for infection. Exactly how HIV does this is discussed in detail in Chapters 5 and 6.

THE ORIGINS OF HIV

It may be that the exact origins of HIV will never be completely elicited. There are, however, certain facts that have led to a more or less general agreement among scientists as to the source of this epidemic. It is plausible to conclude that HIV is a pathogen new to the human race, the first documented cases of what is now known to have been HIV-1 infection in humans occurring in central Africa in 1959.[15,16]

HIV infection of humans probably resulted from a non-pathogenic, subhuman primate retrovirus, which made a species jump from African monkeys and chimpanzees to humans. There is widespread evidence that many Old World primates in sub-Saharan Africa, e.g. chimpanzees, mandrills, sooty mangabeys and African green monkeys, have been infected with retroviruses similar to HIV for thousands of years, although they are non-pathogenic and do not cause disease in these animals.[11] These viruses are referred to as simian immunodeficiency viruses. They have the same complex genomic structure as HIV, share 40–50 per cent homology (genomic similarity) with HIV and infect T-lymphocytes through the CD4$^+$ cell-surface receptor, just as HIV does. It is probable that these retroviruses are the progenitor viruses from which HIV either mutated or recombined into the human population.

Humans may have been exposed to these viruses as a result of killing and butchering monkeys. In doing so, blood from an SIV-infected non-human primate could have infected a human through non-intact skin on the hands. Once SIV had gained entry to the human body, it found it could thrive in what was, after all, simply a closely related primate species. This concept of cross-species transmission, i.e. a **zoonosis**, refers to any disease or infection that may be transmitted between animals and humans under natural conditions. Several other infectious diseases of humans have a zoonotic origin, e.g. tuberculosis, rabies, brucellosis, Lassa fever and various tropical haemorrhagic fevers.

The species leap may have occurred, from time to time, for many hundreds of years. However, HIV infection (and subsequent disease) remained episodic. Because of the rural (village) lifestyle, short life span and restriction of the number of different sexual partners in the past, the infection was not widely transmitted to other humans and remained localized to the village. Several factors conspired to change this episodic infection, first to an epidemic and then to a pandemic infection, including the migration of rural populations into cities, changes in sexual behaviour and increasing sexual freedom leading to more frequent changes in sexual partners, improved road, rail and air travel routes and international travel. In addition, increasing reliance on non-barrier forms of contraception, i.e. 'the pill', and injecting drug use also hastened the spread of HIV infection. There is no evidence to support the theory that oral polio vaccines used in Africa during the 1960s and 1970s had been accidentally contaminated during manufacture with the chimpanzee strain of SIV and may have contributed to the rapid spread of human HIV infection in Africa.[17]

Cases of AIDS in sub-Saharan Africa came to light at about the same time (1981) as American and European cases, although it is likely that human HIV infection existed in Africa long before the disease was recognized.[15,16] HIV infection and AIDS are now epidemic in all Central and East African countries (Zambia, Zaire, Rwanda, Uganda and Tanzania) and have now moved aggressively into West, North and Southern Africa. The current pandemic probably began in Africa and spread simultaneously to the USA and Europe. It is likely that the initial spread of HIV infection into the UK occurred via British tourists returning from American holidays. Although this equally accounted for much of the spread of HIV infection into the rest of Europe, many European countries also experienced increased numbers of new infections as a result of their traditional African links. It then took less than 10 years for HIV infection to spread to the most densely populated areas of the world, i.e. Latin America, the Caribbean, India and South East Asia, where the pandemic is currently rapidly accelerating out of control.

HIV-1 AND HIV-2

There are two major **types** of HIV, HIV-1 and HIV-2, and each type has recognized **subtypes**. Serologic surveys in Dakar, Senegal (West Africa), in 1985 identified antibody patterns in female sex workers that indicated infection with a virus closely related to HIV.[18] In 1986, a retrovirus similar to but distinct from HIV was isolated from patients ill with an AIDS-like illness in Guinea-Bissau and the Cape Verde Islands in West Africa.[10] This was originally referred to as LAV-2, but is now known as HIV-2. Although similar to HIV-1, HIV-2 has a different sequence of nucleotides in its genome. In addition, HIV-1 has one gene (*vpu*) that is not found in HIV-2, and the latter has a gene (*vpx*) that is not found in HIV-1 but is found in SIV.[19] Studies focused on the structural similarity (homology) of the viral genome of each virus, i.e. HIV-1 and HIV-2, suggest that they both evolved from SIV, but from different simian species. HIV-1 diverged from chimpanzee SIV and HIV-2 diverged from sooty mangabey SIV.[11,20-22]

Seroprevalence surveys have shown HIV-2 infection in most West African countries, the highest prevalence being in Guinea-Bissau, Gambia, Côte d'Ivoire, Mali, Angola, Mozambique and Burkina Faso.[23,24] Some individuals are infected with both viruses and although HIV-1 was introduced much later than HIV-2, in some countries, e.g. Côte d'Ivoire, it is now present at higher levels than HIV-2. HIV-2 infection in Europe, Central or East Africa and North America is uncommon and individuals who are infected with HIV-2 are almost always West African immigrants or those who have had sexual contact (directly or indirectly) with West Africans.

Both HIV-1 and HIV-2 have the same method of transmission, i.e. close, intimate contact where blood or semen is exchanged, and both target the same host cells for infection.

HIV-2 is significantly less transmissible than HIV-1, both from mother to child (vertical transmission) and between sexual partners. HIV-2 infection, unlike HIV-1 infection, is frequently seen in older people, confirming that it is spread less efficiently than HIV-1, i.e. it takes more exposures over a longer period of time to become infected with HIV-2. Following infection with HIV-2, the level of virus in the blood is much lower than in those infected with HIV-1. HIV-2 also seems less virulent than HIV-1, but still causes disease. Once infected with HIV-2, progression to end-stage disease, i.e. AIDS, is much slower than with HIV-1 infection.[19,24]

VIRAL VARIATION

HIV is a rapidly replicating virus and, similar to other retroviruses, the enzyme that copies the RNA in HIV (reverse transcriptase) is prone to making errors. This **fast rate of viral replication** (billions of new virions being produced each day), along with its inherent tendency to produce **mutations** and **recombinant forms**, results in the generation of a plethora of slightly different, i.e. genetically distinct, variants (strains) of HIV-1. Genetic diversity is a characteristic of all lentiviruses and HIV-1 is no exception.[25] The ability of lentiviruses to continuously generate seemingly endless variations of themselves may confer on them a survival advantage as they adapt to different local environments or respond to selection pressures in individuals. Viral variations occur within each infected individual (intra-host diversity), where they are referred to as a **quasispecies**. Geographical diversity also occurs, and viral variations exist as HIV subtypes. Different HIV-1 subtypes are prevalent in different populations within diverse geographical areas.

Viral diversity in individuals (intra-host diversity)

Within every infected person, there will be a unique population of viral variants known as a quasispecies.[26] Because there are so many isolates of HIV being produced every day in an infected person, it is not possible to categorize each and every one of them. However, medical scientists distinguish viral variants by a wide variety of characteristics, including syncytium-inducing (SI) capacity, cell tropism, and resistance to antiretroviral therapy. These characteristics are discussed in more detail in Chapter 6.

Viral diversity in geographical regions (geographical diversity)

HIV-1 is divided into three groups: **Group M** (for major), **Group O** (for outlier) and **Group N** (for non-M, non-O strains).

- **Group M viruses** are separated into ten different subtypes (**clades**) distinguished by capital alphabetical letters **A** to **J**.
- **Group O viruses** consist of a pool of highly divergent, genetically related strains with no defined subtypes.
- Those rare (but increasingly being identified) variants of HIV that cannot be assigned to either group are now designated as **Group N viruses**.[27]

Individual subtypes may be associated with different transmission potentials and differences in virulence between HIV-1 variants.[27]

In some regions of the world, a specific subtype can be identified as the dominant clade infecting most people. For example, in North America, Western Europe and East Asia, HIV-1 Group M clade B is the dominant subtype, while in Thailand it is HIV-1 Group M clade E, and clade C predominates in Southern Africa, the Horn of Africa and West Asia. In some regions, mixtures of clades are found, e.g. Eastern Europe and sub-Saharan Africa.[28] Most subtypes are found in Africa, as you would expect, as this was the origin of HIV.

Because HIV-1 Group O differs significantly from HIV-1 Group M clades, infection with this variant was not always detected by some HIV antibody tests. In the past, this represented a potential risk to public health, particularly in relation to maintaining the safety of blood products. However, all current assays have now been modified to take account of Group O strains. Antibody tests may not, however, detect the more rarely occurring Group N strains of HIV-1. It is probable that other variants of HIV may emerge, and medical scientists all over the world are engaged in co-operative, active surveillance for the early detection of new variants and the appropriate modification of test kits so that all HIV variants can be serologically identified.

Subtypes have also been recognized and described for HIV-2 (designated A to E), but these have been based on studies of limited number of isolates.[19]

Summary

Until relatively recently, retroviruses were thought to cause disease only in animals, not humans. Following the recognition of AIDS in 1981, scientists in France and the USA quickly identified new retroviruses that caused fatal lesions in the immune system that led to the development of AIDS, and in time these viruses became known as HIV-1 and HIV-2. In this chapter, we have reviewed the biological characteristics of HIV, including the genetic structure of the RNA viral genome. We have also noted the functions of viral enzymes such as reverse transcriptase, integrase and protease and their role in viral replication. Additionally, we discussed the origins of HIV, compared and contrasted HIV-1 and HIV-2, and finally focused on the diversity of these viruses, both in individuals with the development of quasispecies, and geographical diversity, with the development of different groups and subtypes of HIV.

Prologue to Chapter 4

Having acquired a general understanding of the biology of HIV, in the following chapter we will review how these viruses are transmitted from person to person and examine the diverse vulnerabilities to infection among individuals and communities. We will further extend our understanding of basic retrovirology in Chapter 6, when we explore the pathogenesis of HIV disease, that is, the calamitous impact HIV has on the immune system and individual health.

REFERENCES

1. Anonymous. The Durban Declaration. *International AIDS Society Newsletter* 2000; **17**:14.
2. Barre-Sinoussi F, Chermann JC, Rey F et al. Isolation of a T-lymphotropic retrovirus from a patient at risk for acquired immune deficiency syndrome (AIDS). *Science* 1983; **220**:868–71.
3. Gallo RC, Salahuddin SZ, Popovic M et al. Frequent detection and isolation of cytopathic retroviruses (HTLV-III) from patients with AIDS and at risk from AIDS. *Science* 1984; **224**:500–3.
4. Levy JA, Hoffman AD, Kramer SM et al. Isolation of lymphocytopathic retroviruses from San Francisco patients with AIDS. *Science* 1984; **225**:840–2.
5. Coffin JM. Retrovirology: an overview. In: Wormser GP (ed.), *AIDS and Other Manifestations of HIV Infection*, 3rd edn. Philadelphia: Lippincott-Raven, 1998, 41–121.
6. Rous P. A sarcoma of the fowl transmissible by an agent separable from the tumor cells. *Journal of Experimental Medicine* 1911; **13**:397.

7. Poiesz BJ, Ruscetti FW, Gazdar AF, Bunn PA, Minna JD, Gallo RC. Detection and isolation of type-C retrovirus particles from fresh and cultured lymphocytes of a patient with cutaneous T-cell lymphoma. *Proceedings of the National Academy of Sciences, USA* 1980; **77**:7415–19.
8. Kalyanaraman VS, Sarngaddharan MG, Robert-Gurogg M et al. A new subtype of human T-cell leukemia virus (HTLV-II) associated with a T-cell variant of hairy cell leukemia. *Science* 1982; **218**:571–3.
9. Gallo RC, Essex M, Gross L. *Human T-cell Leukemia/Lymphoma Virus*. Cold Spring Harbor, NY: Cold Spring Harbor Press, 1982.
10. Clavel F, Guétard D, Brun-Vézinet F et al. Isolation of a new human retrovirus from West African patients with AIDS. *Science* 1986; **233**:343–6.
11. Essex M. Origin of acquired immunodeficiency syndrome. In: DeVita VT Jr, Hellman S, Rosenberg SA (eds), *AIDS: Etiology, Diagnosis, Treatment and Prevention*, 4th edn. Philadelphia: JB Lippincott-Raven, 1997, 3–14.
12. Stevenson M. Viral genes and their products. In: Merigan TC Jr, Bartlett JG, Bolognesi D (eds), *Textbook of AIDS Medicine*, 2nd edn. Baltimore: Williams & Wilkins, 1999, 23–48.
13. Pavlakis GN. The molecular biology of human immunodeficiency virus type 1. In: DeVita VT Jr, Hellman S, Rosenberg SA (eds), *AIDS: Etiology, Diagnosis, Treatment and Prevention*, 4th edn. Philadelphia: JB Lippincott-Raven, 1997, 45–74.
14. Geleziunas R, Greene WC. Molecular insights into HIV-1 infection and pathogenesis. In: Sande MA, Volberding PA (eds), *The Medical Management of AIDS*, 5th edn. Philadelphia: WB Saunders Co., 1999, 22–39.
15. Nahmias AJ, Weiss J, Yao X et al. Evidence for human infection with an HTLV-III/LAV-like virus in Central Africa, 1959. *Lancet* 1986; **I**:279.
16. Zhu T, Ho D, Nahmias A. An African HIV-1 sequence from 1959 and implications for the origin of the epidemic. *Nature* 1998; **391**:531–2.
17. Weiss RA. Polio vaccines exonerated. *Nature* 2001; **410**:1035–6.
18. Barin F, M'Boup S, Denis F et al. Serological evidence for virus related to simian T-lymphotropic retrovirus III in residents of West Africa. *Lancet* 1985; **ii**:1387–9.
19. Essex M, Kanki PJ. Human immunodeficiency virus type 2 (HIV-2). In: Merigan TC Jr, Bartlett JG, Bolognesi D (eds), *Textbook of AIDS Medicine*, 2nd edn. Baltimore: Williams & Wilkins, 1999, 985–1001.
20. Hahn B. The origin of HIV-1: a puzzle solved? 6th Conference on Retroviruses and Opportunistic Infections, Chicago, IL, January 31–February 4, 1999, Abst S2.
21. Gao F, Bailes E, Robertson DL et al. Origin of HIV-1 in the chimpanzee *Pan troglodytes troglodytes*. *Nature* 1999; **397**:436–41.
22. Hirsch VM, Olmsted RA, Murphey-Corb M, Purcell RH, Johnson PR. An African primate lentivirus (SIVsm) closely related to HIV-2. *Nature* 1989; **339**:389–92.
23. Hu DJ, Dondero TJ, Mastro TD, Gayle HD. Global and molecular epidemiology of HIV. In: Wormser GP (ed.), *AIDS and Other Manifestations of HIV Infection*, 3rd edn. Philadelphia: Lippincott-Raven, 1998, 27–40.
24. Kanki PJ. Virologic and biologic features of HIV-2. In: Wormser GP (ed.), *AIDS and Other Manifestations of HIV Infection*, 3rd edn. Philadelphia: Lippincott-Raven,1998, 161–73.
25. Coffin JM. Genetic diversity and evolution of retroviruses. *Current Topics in Medical Immunology* 1992; **176**:143–64.
26. Eigen M. Viral quasispecies. *Scientific American* 1993; **269**:42–9.

27. Simon F, Maculère P, Roques P et al. Identification of a new human immunodeficiency virus type 1 distinct from Group M and Group O. *Nature Medicine* 1998; **4**:1032–7.
28. Burke DS, McCutchan FE. Global distribution of human immunodeficiency virus-1 clades. In: DeVita VT Jr, Hellman S, Rosenberg SA (eds), *AIDS: Etiology, Diagnosis, Treatment and Prevention,* 4th edn. Philadelphia: JB Lippincott-Raven, 1997, 119–26.

FURTHER READING

Coffin JM. Retrovirology: an overview. In: Wormser GP (ed.), *AIDS and Other Manifestations of HIV Infection,* 3rd edn. Philadelphia: Lippincott-Raven, 1998, 11–121, ISBN 0-397-58760-0.

Collier L, Oxford J. *Human Virology,* 2nd edn. Oxford: Oxford University Press, 2000, 284 pp, ISBN 0-19-262820-8.

Weiss RA, Wain-Hobson S (eds). Origins of HIV and the AIDS epidemic. Papers of a Discussion Meeting. *Philosophical Transactions of The Royal Society* 29 June 2001; **356**:777–977. Available from The Royal Society, 6 Carlton House Terrace, London SW1Y 5AG, UK; e-mail: sales@royalsoc.ac.uk or from the website: www.pubs.royalsoc.ac.uk

INTERNET RESOURCES

- To review an animated version of HIV replication, visit Roche Pharmaceuticals' *HIV Focus* website on:
  http://www.roche-hiv.com

HIV transmission

In this global emergency, prevention of HIV infection must be our greatest worldwide public health priority. Science will one day triumph over AIDS, just as it did over smallpox. Curbing the spread of HIV will be the first step. Until then, reason, solidarity, political will and courage must be our partners.

The Durban Declaration 2000 South Africa[1]

Introduction

The continuing perpetuation of the global pandemic of HIV disease and the ever-increasing incidence of new HIV infections every year throughout the world, as reviewed in Chapter 1, are inextricably linked to the different ways in which this virus is transmitted among people. Understanding the means by which people can become exposed to and infected with HIV is central to developing strategies for patient education focused on primary prevention. In this chapter we explore these different domains of exposure and the risk factors in each domain associated with an increased vulnerability for HIV infection in both individuals and communities.

Learning outcomes

After studying and reflecting on the material in this chapter, you will be able to:

- describe the principal means by which people become exposed to and infected with HIV;
- identify risk factors associated with each of these transmission categories;
- discuss the varying patterns of HIV transmission in different regions of the world.

DOMAINS OF EXPOSURE

Now, at the beginning of the third decade of our experience with this disease, the known means of viral transmission are well understood. HIV is a blood-borne virus and has been isolated from blood,[2] semen,[3] pre-ejaculatory fluid,[4] saliva,[5] tears,[6] breast milk[7] and cerebrospinal fluid.[8]

HIV is transmitted through sexual activity and exposure to infected blood or blood components and, perinatally, from mother to infant. Transmission potentials can be conveniently categorized into five domains of possible exposure as outlined in Figure 4.1.

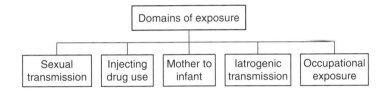

FIGURE 4.1 *Domains of exposure.*

The global pandemic is a composite of many individual, though overlapping, smaller epidemics, each with its own dynamics and differing population vulnerabilities. Although most people become infected with HIV as a result of sexual exposure, there are varied and changing patterns of risk events and behaviours in different regions, different localities within a country, even in different populations within a community. For example, where HIV infection is commonly acquired in one community as a result of exposure to HIV-contaminated blood from injecting drug use, it can be rare in a neighbouring community or country due to a lower prevalence of injecting drug use or HIV infection or the implementation of more effective primary prevention strategies, e.g. needle exchange programmes. Another example is mother-to-infant HIV transmission – relatively uncommon in most industrially developed countries, such as the UK, but more frequent in resource-poor countries in the industrially developing world with a higher prevalence of HIV infection and limited resources to prevent perinatal infection. Varying exposure patterns in different parts of the world resulting in infection and end-stage disease – AIDS – are reflected in Table 4.1.[9]

SEXUAL TRANSMISSION

Most people throughout the world who have become infected with HIV have done so as a result of being sexually exposed to this virus. Because HIV can be present in seminal, pre-ejaculatory, vaginal and cervical secretions, and in saliva (and other body fluids, especially blood) in infected individuals, a variety of sexual behaviours can efficiently facilitate viral transmission and these behaviours can occur in both heterosexual and homosexual encounters. Globally, **unprotected penetrative heterosexual vaginal intercourse** with an HIV-infected partner **is the most common means by which the vast majority of people become infected with HIV.**[10] 'Unprotected' means the male insertive partner not using, or not correctly using, an intact latex or polyurethane condom, or the female partner is not using,

TABLE 4.1 Reported AIDS cases by assumed mode of transmission (%)[a]

Region	Heterosexual	Homo/bi-sexual (MSM)	Injecting drug use	Blood/blood products	Mother to infant	Other
Sub-Saharan Africa	91	0	0	1	8	0
Americas[b]	64	22	6	1	5	2
Asia	69	11	16	1	2	1
Industrialized countries[c]	33	37	27	2	2	0
Eastern Europe	29	27	35	1	2	6
North Africa & Middle East	65	10	12	10	2	0
Oceania	48	41	4	1	7	0

[a]Data reported by 15 November 2000; excludes cases with unknown mode of transmission; percentages do not always add up to 100% due to rounding.[9]
[b]Excluding Canada and the USA.
[c]Western Europe, Canada and the USA.

or not correctly using, an intact polyurethane female condom, for example the Femidom® or Reality® female condom.

In addition to unprotected penetrative heterosexual vaginal intercourse, HIV can also be easily transmitted during unprotected insertive and receptive heterosexual or homosexual **anal intercourse**[11,12] and, less efficiently, during **oral sex** (fellatio, cunnilingus).[13]

In Western Europe, North America and Australasia, homosexual or bisexual men, that is, **men who have sex with men (MSM)**, constitute the largest group of individuals who have, so far, become infected with HIV. This is due to the high risk of viral transmission associated with anal sex, the propensity for this sexual practice among MSM, the multiplicity of sexual partners often associated with this group, and biological factors associated with rectal trauma during penile insertion that allow rectal mucosal cells to be directly infected.[12] The breakdown of cumulative HIV infection in the UK by exposure categories is described in Figure 4.2.[14]

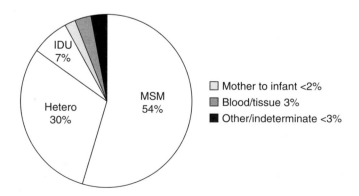

FIGURE 4.2 *HIV infections in the UK by exposure categories, to end September 2002.*[14] *(MSM, men who have sex with men; IDU, injecting drug users; Hetero, heterosexual.)*

In sub-Saharan Africa, the Caribbean and South East Asia, HIV is principally a heterosexually spread infection and this is also how most people in North East Asia, Latin America, the south east Mediterranean and Western Europe become exposed and infected.[10] The incidence of heterosexual transmission is increasing in Western Europe and North America,[10]

Risk factors for sexual transmission

The principal sexual activities that are associated with sexually transmitting HIV are unprotected insertive and receptive vaginal and anal intercourse. Several factors (risk factors) may increase the likelihood or risk that an uninfected person may become exposed and subsequently infected with HIV during vaginal, anal and sometimes oral sexual intercourse (Table 4.2).

TABLE 4.2 Factors that can increase the risk of infection associated with sexual exposure to HIV

- Likelihood that sexual partner is infected with HIV
- Type of sexual activity
- Disease stage of the infected partner
- Presence of other sexually transmitted infections
- Frequency of partner change
- Biological factors
- Lack of male circumcision
- Viral variants
- Host infectiousness

Likelihood that sexual partner is infected with HIV

For HIV to be sexually transmitted, clearly one of the sexual partners needs to be infected. Consequently, a principal risk is the likelihood (risk) that one's sexual partner is infected with HIV. In different communities, different individuals may engage in various sexual practices or other behaviours that increase their likelihood of being infected. For example, commercial sex workers (CSW) and their clients, MSM and injecting drug users all have a high probability of having been infected with HIV. Having sexual intercourse with a person who has a history of these risk behaviours, or who resides in or has had sexual contact with people in regions with a high prevalence of HIV infection, for example Africa or South Asia, increases the likelihood of being exposed to HIV.

Type of sexual activity

Male-to-female vaginal and anal intercourse and insertive male-to-receptive male homosexual anal intercourse are the most efficient ways in which HIV can be transmitted. This is chiefly because the volume and concentration of virus in semen ejaculated into the vagina or rectum are generally greater than those found in cervical or vaginal secretions, and because of the increased contact time with infectious semen.[12] Consequently, an **HIV-infected male insertive partner is more likely to transmit infection to an uninfected receptive partner**. However, an infected woman can just as efficiently transmit HIV to an uninfected man if there is an increased number of HIV-infected white blood cells and macrophages in cervical or vaginal secretions as a result of chronic pelvic inflammatory disease, e.g. sexually transmitted infections (STIs). If either partner is exposed to HIV-infected blood during sexual intercourse, e.g. vaginal intercourse during menstruation or rectal trauma during anal intercourse, the risk of the insertive partner becoming infected will be enhanced.

In addition, there is a risk of HIV transmission during unprotected **oral sex**, especially receptive fellatio if the male insertive partner is infected with HIV, but this risk is less than that from unprotected penetrative vaginal or anal sexual intercourse.[13] However, ejaculation of semen into the mouth or oral contact with pre-ejaculatory fluid, and oral contact with blood if oral sex with a woman (cunnilingus) takes place during menstruation, significantly heightens the risk of HIV transmission. Additionally, the presence of oral infections, lesions or inflammatory conditions, bleeding gums (for example after brushing teeth) will increase the risk of HIV transmission. As more people change from higher to lower risk sexual behaviours, oral sex may become more frequent and, consequently, play a larger role in propagating the epidemic.

Disease stage of HIV-infected sexual partner and viral load

As discussed further in Chapters 6 and 7, the amount of virus present in the blood varies over time with the disease stage of an infected person. For example, there is a high level (or titre) of virus in the blood during primary infection (the first 3–4 months following initial infection) and later, during end-stage disease (AIDS) when the immune system becomes so compromised it can no longer check continuing rapid tempo viral replication. The titre of virus in peripheral blood is measured by doing a viral load test, which is described in Chapter 20. A person with a high viral load can more efficiently transmit HIV during vaginal, anal and oral sex than a person with a low or undetectable viral load.[15–17]

Presence of other sexually transmitted infections

Other untreated sexually transmitted infectious diseases, especially ulcerative conditions such as syphilis, genital herpes or chancroid, and also inflammatory sexually transmitted diseases (STDs) such as gonorrhoea are important risk factors for HIV infection. Their presence in a person who is not infected with HIV increases the probability that they will become infected with HIV when sexually exposed to this virus. A person who is already infected with HIV and acquires a new STI, or has a chronic, untreated STD, will be more efficient at transmitting HIV to his or her sexual partners.[18,19] However, the beneficial effects of comprehensive STI treatment programmes on the incidence of HIV infection remain unproven.[20]

Frequency of partner change

A direct relationship exists between the number of different sexual partners and the probability of contracting HIV infection during unprotected, penetrative sexual activity.

Biological factors

There are several biological factors that may increase the risk of infection when exposed to HIV. Some individuals lack a critical host cell receptor (called CCR5) that HIV uses to dock onto and infect cells. This makes these individuals more resistant to becoming infected with HIV-1 when sexually exposed. It is thought that up to 20 per cent of the white population carries the defective CCR5 gene that results in this deletion, which affords them substantial but certainly not complete protection from becoming sexually infected with HIV-1.[21]

Cervical ectopy is a condition in which there is exocervical exposure of the columnar epithelium along the exposed junction known as the transformation zone, normally found within the relatively protected endocervical region. Because these displaced (or ecotopic) endocervical cells are unprotected, they have an increased susceptibility to HIV infection. This condition is a normal developmental variation in many female adolescents, in whom cervical ectopy may involve up to half of the cervix. Cervical ectopy is also associated with the use of oral contraceptives.[12] Consequently, sexually active adolescent girls, and girls and women using oral contraceptives, are more likely to become infected on exposure to HIV.

Male circumcision

Circumcised men are less likely to become infected when exposed to HIV than are men who are not circumcised.[22-24] This is due to the ease with which HIV can infected Langerhans' cells (epithelial CD4+ dendritic cells), found in abundance on the inner mucosal surface of the non-keratinized foreskin. These cells are not present on the tougher keratinized, stratified squamous epithelium that covers the penile shaft and outer surface of the foreskin and the epithelium of the glans penis. During penetrative sexual intercourse, the foreskin is retracted back down the shaft of the penis, and the entire inner surface of the foreskin is exposed to vaginal secretions, providing a large area where HIV transmission could take place.[24]

Viral variants

There is a significant variation in the diverse range of viral isolates which evolve in an infected person. Some of these variants may have greater **infectivity** (i.e. a greater ability to infect host cells) and/or be more **virulent** (i.e. have a greater ability to replicate in and destroy host cells) than other variants, although this is difficult to quantify. It is also difficult to know with certainty if specific subtypes of HIV have greater infectivity than others.[25]

Host infectiousness

Some HIV-infected individuals may be significantly more infectious than others, becoming highly effective disseminators of infection, and conversely, some infected individuals may be significantly less infectious than others, becoming relatively or completely non-infectious.[25]

DRUG USE

HIV transmission among individuals who use injectable drugs, that is, **injecting drug users (IDUs)**, account for a third or more of all individuals with AIDS in the industrialized countries of Western Europe and North America and in Eastern Europe.[9] In the UK, the known prevalence of HIV infection among IDUs remains lower than in some other European countries and this mode of transmission accounted for just under 7 per cent of the cumulative HIV infections reported by the end of December 2000.[14]

Risk factors associated with drug use

HIV infection is efficiently transmitted by sharing blood-contaminated needles, syringes and injecting paraphernalia, a common phenomenon among IDUs. However, drug users are, by and large, sexually active individuals, and may also acquire HIV infection as a result of sexual exposure. Other, non-injectable, drugs, for example alcohol, amphetamine-based drugs ('speed', 'whizz', 'ecstasy') and LSD, often remove protective behavioural inhibitions, which may increase the exposure of drug users to infection, as will trading or selling sex for drugs or money. Smoking 'crack' cocaine is associated with an increased risk of becoming infected with HIV.[26] Finally, the chaos in which many drug users live, e.g. homelessness, unemployment, poverty, may make it difficult for them to access prevention and healthcare services and may prevent them from incorporating effective harm reduction strategies into both their sexual and drug-taking behaviours.

MOTHER-TO-INFANT HIV TRANSMISSION

AIDS in children was first reported in 1982.[27,28] Since then, millions children throughout the world have become infected with HIV, most from mother-to-child transmission. By Christmas 2002, 3.2 million children were living with HIV/AIDS and, during that year, 610 000 children died from AIDS.[29] Infants born to HIV-infected women can become infected with HIV during pregnancy or childbirth or as a result of breastfeeding (Figure 4.3). This mode of transmission is referred to as mother-to-infant transmission (also called perinatal or vertical transmission).

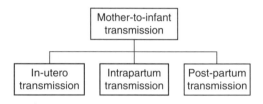

FIGURE 4.3 *Mother-to-infant transmission.*

Risk factors for mother-to-infant transmission

Most pregnant women become infected with HIV following sexual exposure. Any factor that predisposes women to becoming sexually infected (see Table 4.2) clearly increases the risks for mother-to-infant transmission. Additionally, the disease stage of the infected mother and her viral load are particularly important when considering the risks of mother-to-infant transmission. Infants born to women who are newly infected (primary infection – first 3 months of infection) or who have symptomatic disease or a high viral load are at the greatest risk of becoming vertically infected.

The special vulnerabilities of women, the risks of HIV infection to newborn children, and strategies for preventing mother-to-infant transmission are explored in more detail in Chapters 11 and 12.

IATROGENIC TRANSMISSION

Iatrogenesis refers to the creation of additional problems or complications resulting from medical or nursing interventions, treatments or care. HIV transmission has been documented following exposure as a result of the items described in Figure 4.4. The conundrum of the HIV-infected healthcare worker is explored in more detail in Chapter 15. The number of

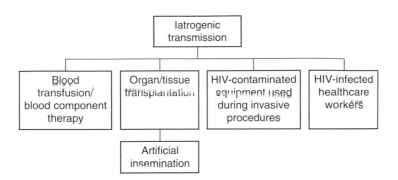

FIGURE 4.4 *Iatrogenic transmission.*

individuals becoming infected via iatrogenic exposure will continue to decline in the industrialized world as the epidemic continues but, although they currently account for only a small percentage of those who have become infected, they continue to haunt the public perception of risk so that it is completely out of proportion to the actual risk.

Risk factors for iatrogenic transmission

Blood and blood products

HIV has been transmitted following transfusion of whole human blood and blood components and the administration of clotting factor concentrates such as Factor VIII, manufactured from pooled plasma and used in the treatment of haemophilia. The routine screening of donor blood for the presence of HIV antibodies (indicating ongoing infection) and the self-exclusion of donors who, on the known means of transmission, may have been exposed to HIV will substantially decrease (but not totally eliminate) infection from blood transfusions. Between the introduction of screening in 1985 and the end of June 2000, only two instances of HIV transmission from transfused blood were reported in the UK. In addition to careful donor selection and HIV screening, viral inactivation processes (e.g. heat treatment, introduced in the UK in 1985) have virtually eliminated the risk of HIV transmission from the use of clotting factor concentrates used for the treatment of haemophilia in the UK.[30]

Donor organs and tissues for transplantation

Donor organs (kidneys, corneas, hearts, etc.) and tissues (e.g. semen used for artificial insemination) are a potential risk and individuals whose previous behaviour or life events have put them at risk of acquiring HIV infection are advised not to donate organs or to carry donor cards. The routine screening of donors for HIV infection will diminish this risk substantially. However, the risk will not disappear completely, as the donor may have only recently become infected and serological tests for HIV infection may be negative. This risk of donated semen can be reduced by the voluntary self-exclusion of donors who may have been exposed to HIV, initially screening donors, and the exclusive use of cryopreserved donor semen, stored for 3–6 months and not used until the donor has been re-tested for HIV infection. The use of fresh semen in artificial insemination programmes will remain a potential risk and is not recommended.

HIV-contaminated equipment used for invasive procedures

Unsterilized equipment contaminated with HIV and used in nursing, medical, surgical or dental invasive procedures is clearly a risk to clients and, in many parts of the world where resources are limited, this may be a significant mode of transmission for HIV.[31] Other unsterilized equipment used for acupuncture, tattooing and body piercing may also present a risk to clients.

HIV-infected healthcare workers

Although there have been many cases of healthcare workers becoming occupationally exposed to, and sometimes infected with, HIV, there have only been a few definite cases of HIV-infected healthcare workers transmitting HIV to patients, or of patient-to-patient transmission of HIV in a healthcare facility.[32,33] Healthcare professionals need to have a real insight into this issue, which is discussed in more detail in Chapters 14 and 15.

Summary

Throughout the world, millions of people are becoming infected with HIV every year as a result of being sexually exposed to this virus. Its success in establishing a near-perpetual global pandemic is owed in no small part to its ability to transmit itself from person to person during one of the most frequent, intimate and private of human behaviours. Added to this are the risk to children from mother-to-infant transmission, the risk to women from unsafe blood transfusions, the risk to those on the margins of society, such as commercial sex workers, men who have sex with men and drug users – all spinning around creating a seemingly unstoppable whirlwind of vulnerability driving national epidemics out of control. It is by having a clear understanding of how this virus is transmitted that nurses and other healthcare professionals can effectively engage in patient education encounters designed to prevent further exposure and infection, based not on myths, but on scientific fact.

Prologue to Chapter 5

We have so far plotted the growth of this global pandemic in Chapter 1, noting the general trend of escalation in most nations. In Chapters 2 and 3, we then explored the causes of AIDS, reviewing both the general biology of viruses and the specifics of retroviruses, the family of viruses to which HIV belongs. In this chapter we clarified the known means of HIV transmission, especially noting that most people become infected as a result of being sexually exposed to this virus. Before we examine the pathological consequences of being infected, especially the deleterious effects HIV infection has on the immune system (**immunopathogenesis**), we need to understand how this system protects us against infectious diseases. That is what is reviewed in the next chapter, in order to prepare for an exploration of immunopathogenesis in Chapter 6.

REFERENCES

1. Anonymous. The Durban Declaration. *International AIDS Society Newsletter* December 2000; **17**(1):14.

2. Gallo RC, Salahuddin SZ, Popovic M et al. Frequent detection and isolation of cytopathic retroviruses (HTLV-III) from patients with AIDS and at risk for AIDS. *Science* 1984; **224**:500–3.

3. Zagury D, Bernard J, Leibowitch J et al. HTLV-III in cells cultured from semen of two patients with AIDS. *Science* 1984; **226**:449.

4. Pudney J, Oneta M, Mayer K et al. Pre-ejaculatory fluid as potential vector for sexual transmission of HIV-1 [Letter]. *Lancet* 1992; **340**:1470.

5. Groopman JE, Salahuddin SZ, Sarngadharan MG et al. HTLV-III in saliva of people with AIDS-related complex and healthy homosexual men at risk for AIDS. *Science* 1984; **226**:447–9.

6. Fujikawa LS, Palestine AG, Nussenblatt RB et al. Isolation of human T-lymphotropic virus type III from the tears of a patient with the acquired immune deficiency syndrome. *Lancet* 1985; **ii**:529–30.

7. Thirty L, Sprecher-Goldberger S, Jonckheer T et al. Isolation of AIDS virus from cell-free breast milk of three healthy virus carriers. *Lancet* 1985; **ii**:891–2.

8. Levy JA, Hollander H, Shimabukura J et al. Isolation of AIDS-associated retroviruses from cerebrospinal fluid and brain of patients with neurological symptoms. *Lancet* 1985; **ii**:586–8.

9. Anonymous. Global AIDS surveillance Part II. *Weekly Epidemiological Record (WER)* December 2000; **48**:386–92.

10. Joint United Nations Programme on AIDS (UNAIDS), World Health Organization (WHO). *Report on the Global HIV/AIDS Epidemic*. Geneva: UNAIDS and WHO, June 2000, UNAIDS/00, 13E, 135 pp. Available from UNAIDS or online at: http://www.unaids.org/

11. Vittinghoff E, Douglas J, Judson F, McKirnan D, MacQueen K, Buchbinder SP. Per-contact risk of human immunodeficiency virus transmission between male sexual partners. *American Journal of Epidemiology* 1999; **150**:306–11.

12. Vernumd SH, Tabereaux PB, Kaslow RA. Epidemiology of HIV sexual transmission. In: Merigan TC, Bartlett JG, Bolognesi D (eds), *Textbook of AIDS Medicine*, 2nd edn. Baltimore: Williams & Wilkins, 1999, 101–9.

13. Rothenberg RB, Scarlett M, del Rio C, Reznik D, O'Daniels C. Oral transmission of HIV. *AIDS* 1998; **12**:2095–105.

14. PHLS AIDS and STD Centre – Communicable Disease Surveillance Centre, and Scottish Centre for Infection & Environmental Health. *AIDS/HIV Quarterly Surveillance Tables – Cumulative UK Data to end September 2002*. October 2002, 56:02/3. Available online at: http://www.phls.co.uk/

15. Mastro TD, de Vincenzi I. Probabilities of sexual HIV-1 transmission. *AIDS* 1999; **13**(Suppl. A):S75–82.

16. Vernazza PL, Eron JJ, Fiscus SA, Cohen MS. Sexual transmission of HIV: infectiousness and prevention. *AIDS* 1999; **13**:155–66.

17. Quinn TC, Wawer MJ, Sewankambo N et al. for the Rakai Project Study Group. Viral load and heterosexual transmission of human immunodeficiency virus type 1. *New England Journal of Medicine* 2000; **343**:921–9.

18. Nelson KE, Rungruengthanakit K, Margolick J et al. High rates of transmission of subtype E human immunodeficiency virus type 1 among heterosexual couples in Northern Thailand: role of sexually transmitted diseases and immune compromise. *Journal of Infectious Diseases* 1999; **180**:337–43.

19. Ghys A. HIV shedding, STD and immunosuppression. *AIDS* 1997; **11**:F-85–93.

20. Wawer MJ, Sewankambo NK, Serwadda D et al. and the Rakai Project Study Group and Ronald H. Gray. Control of sexually transmitted diseases for AIDS prevention in Uganda: a randomised community trial. *Lancet* 1999; **353**:525–35.

21. Clapham PR, Weiss RA. The virus and its target cells. In: Merigan TC, Bartlett JG, Bolognesi D (eds), *Textbook of AIDS Medicine*, 2nd edn. Baltimore: Williams & Wilkins, 1999, 13–21.

22. Weiss H, Quigley MA, Hayes RJ. Male circumcision and risk of HIV infection in sub-Saharan Africa: a systematic review and meta-analysis. *AIDS* 2000; **14**:2361–70.

23. Halperin DT, Bailey RC. Male circumcision and HIV infection: 10 years and counting. *Lancet* 1999; **354**:1813–15.

24. Szabo R, Short RV. How does male circumcision protect against HIV infection? *British Medical Journal* 2000; **320**:1592–4.

25. Holmberg SD. Risk factors for sexual transmission of human immunodeficiency virus. In: Curran J, Essex M, Fauci AS (eds), *AIDS: Etiology, Diagnosis, Treatment and Prevention*, 4th edn. Philadelphia: Lippincott-Raven, 1997, 569–75.

26. Chaisson MA, Stoneburner RL, Hildebrandt DS et al. Heterosexual transmission of HIV-1 associated with the use of smokable freebase cocaine (crack). *AIDS* 1991; **5**:1121–6.

27. Centers for Disease Control. Unexplained immunodeficiency and opportunistic infections in infants – New York, New Jersey, California. *Morbidity & Mortality Weekly Report (MMWR)* 17 December 1982; **31**:665–7.

28. Oleske J, Minnefor A, Cooper R et al. Immune deficiency in children. *Journal of the American Medical Association* 1983; **249**:2345–9.

29. UNAIDS/WHO. *AIDS Epidemic Update* (UNAIDS/02.58E). Geneva: Joint United Nations Programme on HIV/AIDS and the World Health Organization, December 2002. Available online from: http://www.unaids.org

30. PHLS AIDS and STD Centre – Communicable Disease Surveillance Centre, and Scottish Centre for Infection & Environmental Health. AIDS and HIV infection in the United Kingdom: monthly report. *Communicable Disease Report* 29 September 2000; **10**:357–8.

31. Velandia M, Fridkin SK, Cardenas V et al. Transmission of HIV in a dialysis centre. *Lancet* 1995; **345**:1417–22.

32. Centers for Disease Control. Update: Transmission of HIV infection during an invasive dental procedure – Florida. *Morbidity & Mortality Weekly Report (MMWR)* 14 June 1991; **40**:377–81.

33. Lot F, Séguer JC, Fégueux S et al. Probably transmission of HIV from an orthopaedic surgeon to a patient in France. *Annals of Internal Medicine* 1999; **130**:1–6.

CHAPTER 5

Understanding immunology

Introduction

Immunity has evolved in humans over many millennia and affords essential protection against infectious diseases, without which survival would be impossible. The human immunodeficiency virus (HIV) targets key immune system cells for infection, which, over time, results in a gradual impairment of immune functions. This leaves immunocompromised individuals vulnerable to a range of infections and tumours (neoplasia) that thrive in the bleakness of depressed and increasingly ineffective immune responses. An understanding of normal immune mechanisms is necessary for nurses to fully appreciate the link between progressive immune dysfunction, predictable clinical outcomes and treatment options.

Learning outcomes

After studying and reflecting on the material in this chapter, you will be able to:

- describe the components of innate (natural) immunity and discuss their role in protecting people from diseases;
- compare and contrast cell-mediated and humoral adaptive (acquired) immune responses and describe how these two systems co-operate to mount a specific immune response following exposure to specific antigens;
- describe the role of cytokines in facilitating an effective immune response.

BACKGROUND

Immunology is the study of systems, organs, cells and molecules that are involved in the recognition and destruction of foreign (non-self) materials that enter the human body (such as infectious microorganisms and proteins) and their responses to, and inter-reactions with, each other. Immune responses can be divided into **innate** (natural or non-specific) and **adaptive** (acquired) mechanisms.

Innate immunity

We all use many natural, non-specific mechanisms to protect ourselves against infection. We call them non-specific because they are used to protect against a wide range of potential pathogens (microorganisms that cause disease) that our bodies recognize as foreign. Innate mechanisms are not enhanced as a result of previous exposure to the invading pathogen (or any other foreign material) and, consequently, are said to be without **memory**, an essential feature of adaptive immunity.

Innate immunity is geared towards either the **prevention** of pathogenic invasion or **containment** and eventual **resolution** should invasion occur. It encompasses mechanical and chemical barriers, normal bacterial flora and humoral and cell-mediated mechanisms.

Prevention of invasion

A variety of **mechanical barriers** and **surface secretions** are located in various parts of the body and protect from invasion by pathogenic microorganisms. These include the following.

Intact skin
A healthy, intact skin provides a good barrier against infection by pathogens. It is an effective barrier because the outer, horny layer of the skin is principally made of keratin, which most microorganisms cannot digest and which, consequently, protects the living cells of the epidermis from pathogens and toxins. In addition, the dry nature of the skin, covered by a film of salt derived from drying perspiration and its slight acidity (pH 5.5), is either **bacteriostatic** (inhibitory to bacterial growth) or **bactericidal** (killing bacteria) to many microorganisms.

A variety of substances and secretions further enhance the protective action of the skin in preventing infection, including fatty acids, in both perspiration and sebaceous secretions, and lactic acid – both of which are bactericidal and fungicidal. Other skin surface secretions that have important antimicrobial activity include: secretions from sebaceous glands (triglycerides, wax, alcohols); sweat (amino acids, ammonia, uric acid); and substances (steroids and complex polypeptides) produced as a result of the ongoing conversion (cornification) of skin epithelial cells into keratin, forming the hard outer layer of tough horny cells that make up the topmost layer of the epidermis (stratum corneum).

It is unusual, however, for skin to be perfectly intact (especially the skin on the hands of nurses and other healthcare professionals!), as all of us have a variety of small or microscopic abrasions or lesions on our skin. In addition, sweat glands, hair follicles etc. provide an entry for many potential pathogens, for example *Staphylococcus aureus*.

Mucous membranes and ciliated cells
External openings of the body are guarded by mucous membranes. For example, the mouth, nose, urethra, vagina and rectum are all lined with mucous membranes. These membranes secrete sticky mucus, which traps pathogens that enter the body by one of these routes. Some of these membranes, for example those lining the respiratory passages, are associated with cells that have hair-like processes, known as **cilia**, that are able to waft pathogens away from deeper structures, eventually assisting in expelling them from the body, acting like an

escalator. Antiviral and antibacterial substances, including mucopolysaccharides and the antibody immunoglobulin A (IgA) in nasal secretions and saliva, afford additional protection, as does an antibacterial agent (lysozyme) in tears and in mucous secretions of the respiratory, alimentary and genito-urinary tracts.

pH changes

Various substances and secretions in different parts of the body determine its acid, alkaline or neutral basis. On a pH scale, 7 is neutral; above 7, alkalinity increases, and below 7, acidity increases. Some areas of the body have a pH that is hostile to many pathogens. For example, the pH of the skin (pH 5.5) and vagina (pH 4.5) is acid and microorganisms that require an alkaline medium to reproduce may not be successful in establishing infection in this environment. Microorganisms that survive and replicate in blood (pH 7.4) require a slightly alkaline condition. The pH changes in the gastrointestinal tract – where ingested food is first mixed with alkaline saliva in the mouth, then swallowed into the acid environment of the stomach, and eventually passed into the duodenum where the pH is very alkaline – can be either bacteriostatic or bactericidal for many pathogens.

Washing and flushing actions

The washing action of tears, flowing away from the eye, and the flushing action of urine are both effective mechanisms employed in preventing pathogenic invasion.

Resident bacterial population

The normal bacterial flora of the body provides good protection by two mechanisms. First, their growth results in the production of substances (such as antibiotics and lactic acid) that have antimicrobial activity. Second, by competing with potential pathogens for essential nutrients, the growth of normal bacterial flora protects by excluding the growth of other, harmful microorganisms. This is an important consideration in antimicrobial therapy, where antibiotics may destroy normal gut flora, allowing other, antibiotic-resistant pathogens to establish infection. It is important to remember that **commensals** (i.e. the bacteria that make up the normal flora) are both beneficial and harmless in those areas in which they are normally present, but may cause illness if they are transported to other areas of the body where they do not normally reside. For example, *Escherichia coli*, a common gut commensal, is also a frequent cause of genito-urinary tract infection, gaining access to the genito-urinary tract via a urinary catheter.

Containment of invading pathogens

Effective as these non-specific mechanisms are, pathogenic invasion does occur from time to time. The body still has some fairly sophisticated, innate mechanisms available to deal with these pathogens, which, if successful, contain them, limit the damage they may cause and eventually, destroy them. These innate devices include both **humoral** and **cell-mediated** mechanisms (not to be confused with humoral and cell-mediated mechanisms in **adaptive immune responses**, discussed later).

Humoral innate mechanisms

Humoral refers to soluble antimicrobial substances in the tissues and body fluids as opposed to cells. These substances include lysozyme, basic polypeptides, acute phase proteins, interferon and complement enzymes.

Lysozyme

This enzyme is found in most tissue fluids (except cerebrospinal fluid, sweat and urine). It attacks the sugars making up part of the cell wall on Gram-positive (and some Gram-negative) bacteria, causing their lysis (dissolution).

Basic polypeptides

These are antibacterial basic proteins that also attack the microorganism's cell surface. They are derived from tissues and blood cells. Important basic polypeptides include spermine and spermidine – which can kill *Mycobacteria tuberculosis* and some staphylococci – and arginine, protamine and histone.

Acute phase proteins

During the acute phase of infection, **macrophages** (mononuclear phagocytic cells found in tissues and serous cavities, such as the pleura and peritoneum) release small protein messenger molecules (**cytokines**) known as **interleukin type 1 (IL-1)**. IL-1 is termed an endogenous pyrogen because it is responsible for the rise in temperature seen in acute infection. Its role is to stimulate the liver to release acute phase proteins, such as **C-reactive protein**, which binds to the cell walls of some microorganisms and activates the **classical complement pathway** (discussed below). Other acute phase proteins include **fibrinogen** and **serum amyloid A protein**. The serum levels of these protein molecules are greatly increased during acute infection and help to contain the spread of the infecting microorganism and facilitate further immune responses.

Interferon

Interferons are also cytokines (discussed in more detail later in this chapter) and have a powerful broad-spectrum **antiviral effect**. There are two types of interferon: type 1 and type 2. **Type 1 interferons** consist of alpha-interferon (**INFα**) and beta-interferon (**INFβ**), both of which are important cytokines associated with innate immunity. There are over 20 types of INFα released by a variety of cells, such as lymphocytes, monocytes and macrophages. INFβ (of which there is only one type) is principally manufactured by fibroblasts (but can probably be produced by many other cells in the body). Gamma-interferon (**INFγ**) is the only **type 2 interferon**, an essential component of adaptive (acquired) immunity. Unlike type 1 interferons, INFγ can only be produced by and secreted from T-lymphocytes and natural killer (NK) cells. This is also discussed in more detail later in this chapter.

Once cells are infected with viruses, they secrete interferons into the extracellular fluid, where they bind onto specific surface receptors of uninfected neighbouring cells. The interferon-treated cell then makes a variety of enzymes that are toxic to the virus, inhibiting further viral replication and destroying viral nucleic acid. This results in a chain (or palisade) of uninfected cells being thrown around the virus-infected cell, isolating it and containing the infection.

Complement system

Antigens are discussed in some detail later in this chapter. However, because antigens activate the complement system, it is worth briefly defining them here. Antigens are foreign materials that the immune system recognizes as 'non-self'. They are usually small proteins and are commonly composed of elements of invading microorganisms, or they may be foreign tissue cells, for example from a transplanted organ, and are capable of provoking an immune response. The presence of antigens activates the **complement system**, another important element of a non-specific (or innate) immune response.

What is complement? Early in the twentieth century, it was found that antibody-mediated lysis of red cells, as occurs in mismatched blood transfusions, required the presence of a heat-labile substance which, as it complemented the activity of the antibody, was called complement. It is now known that complement consists of around 20 serum proteins, normally in inactive forms. Once activated by the pathways described below, these proteins are powerful components of both innate and adaptive (antibody-mediated) immune responses. When complement is exposed to antigens, this enzyme system is sequentially activated along two different pathways, known as the **classical** (because it was the first described) and **alternative** pathways (Figure 5.1).

The **classical pathway** is activated when complement enzymes encounter and bind to **immune complexes**. A complex is formed by the attachment of an antibody to an antigen. Immune complexes containing IgM or IgG antibodies (discussed later) are especially provocative in activating the classical pathway. Both C-reactive protein (an acute phase

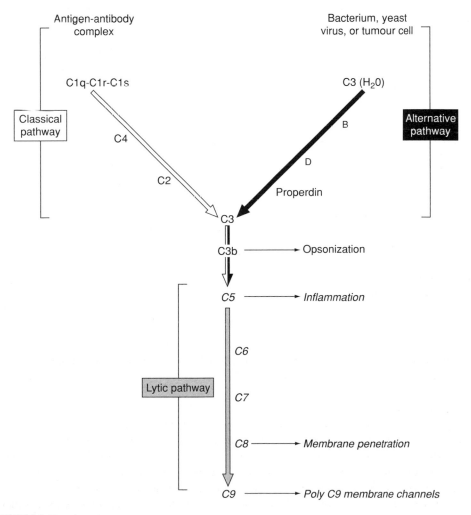

FIGURE 5.1 *Complement system.*

protein discussed above) and protein A (a cell-wall protein found in many strains of *Staphylococcus aureus*) can also activate the classical pathway.

The **alternative pathway** is activated by some immune complexes composed of other classes of antibodies, that is, IgA and IgE (discussed later), but principally by substances found in the cell walls of many bacteria, viruses, yeasts and some tumours and known as **activators**.

Both pathways converge via C3 onto a final pathway called the **lytic pathway**. Once either pathway is activated, inactive complement enzymes are triggered into action in a **sequential cascade**, the end result being the formation of **active complement** (C3b, C5 and C8, C9), which results in important protective consequences.

1. **C3b** attaches to specific receptors on phagocytic cells (a process known as **opsonization**), switching them on and promoting enhanced **phagocytosis**. Phagocytes are cells that engulf particulate matter, such as foreign substances. Examples of phagocytes are certain white blood cells (neutrophils, monocytes) and macrophages, and these are explained in detail later in this chapter.
2. **C5** releases peptides (short chains of amino acids that form the basic elements of protein) that induce **inflammation**, which then destroys immune complexes. Inflammation is generally a protective mechanism that results in an increased local blood supply (hyperaemia) to the area under attack. This is the cause of the classic signs of local inflammation (heat, redness, swelling and pain). With this increased blood supply come cells that are able to engage in phagocytosis.
3. **C8** and **C9** (**membrane attack complex**) cause **cell-wall damage** and **lysis** to many pathogens, such as malaria parasites, trypanosomes and (with the help of lysozymes) some Gram-negative bacteria. They also contribute to tissue damage in the vicinity of immune complex formation by lysing normal tissue cells – the so-called **bystander lysis**.

The net result of activating the complement network is, in summary, **opsonization, cell-wall lysis, enhanced phagocytosis** and destruction of immune complexes by **inflammation**.

Cell-mediated innate mechanisms

There are two principal types of cells associated with innate defences: **phagocytes** and **natural killer cells**.

Phagocytosis

This is a special function of **phagocytes**, cells that engulf and digest microorganisms (phagocytosis) that enter the tissue fluids or bloodstream. There is a wide variety of cells that are phagocytic, but the principal 'professional' phagocytes are **mononuclear** or **polymorphonuclear phagocytes** (Table 5.1).

Mononuclear phagocytes (so called because their cell nuclei are single spheres or ovals) are found in both blood and tissues. In blood, they are referred to as **monocytes**. When monocytes migrate into tissues, they differentiate (change) into **macrophages**. In different tissues, macrophages are referred to by more specific names (Table 5.1).

Macrophages ('big eaters') are long-lived phagocytic cells that are strategically sited throughout the body where they are likely to encounter invading microorganisms, such as in the lungs, liver, spleen sinusoids, medullary sinuses of lymph nodes and the kidney glomeruli. They act as sentries and are usually the first phagocytic cells that invading microorganisms encounter. Although macrophages are capable of cell killing, their function is somewhat different from that of neutrophils. When they have attacked and ingested foreign material, they **secrete several soluble substances**, such as lysozymes, cytokines (IL-1, INFα, INFβ),

TABLE 5.1 Types of phagocytes

Polymorphonuclear leucocytes
Neutrophils (PMNs)
Eosinophils
Mononuclear phagocytes
Peripheral blood monocytes (PBMs)
Promonocytes
Macrophages
Alveolar macrophages
Connective tissue histiocytes
Sinus-lining macrophages in the spleen, bone and thymus
Kupffer cells in the liver
Mesangial phagocytes in the kidneys
Peritoneal macrophages

complement components and coagulation factors (to name but a few!). In acute infections, these substances summon the real killers to the scene of the battle, the **neutrophils**. Macrophages can be activated from a resting state by a variety of stimuli and can also be up-regulated to higher degrees of activation, and function as either **activated** or **hyperactivated** macrophages. Resting macrophages travel around the body scavenging cellular debris and pollutants. However, once stimulated by encounters with invading microorganisms, they become activated and engage in phagocytosis, engulfing, digesting and processing invading microorganisms. If they become hyperactivated, they are capable of killing tumour cells.

Polymorphonuclear phagocytes (called polymorphonuclear because these white blood cells, or leucocytes, have segmented cell nuclei) are also called **granulocytes**, because their cytoplasm contains easily visible granules. They are of three types, distinguished by the colour of their granules after routine haematological staining: **neutrophils**, **eosinophils** and **basophils**. The neutrophils are the principal 'killer phagocytes'. They are short-lived cells that migrate into tissues when stimulated by the presence of invading microorganisms and engulf foreign material, destroying it by intracellular digestion, after which (usually) they themselves die. Killing takes place inside the neutrophil and this is known as intracellular killing. **Eosinophils** are reserved for the extracellular killing of large, multicellular parasites such as worms (helminth infections). **Basophils** are not phagocytic but produce **histamine**, which is an inducer of the inflammatory response. When production is excessive and inappropriate, it causes the symptoms of allergy, as in asthma, hay fever and urticaria.

Cell killing in phagocytosis is achieved in four phases.

1. During the **attachment phase**, the invading microorganism (antigen) is recognized as foreign and becomes 'coated' with **opsonins**, special molecules that become attached to the surface of the antigen. There are two types of opsonins: **antibodies** (IgM, IgG) and certain **complement fragments**, such as C3b. In *The Doctor's Dilemma* (George Bernard Shaw), a famous line reads: 'The phagocytes won't eat the microbes unless the microbes are nicely buttered for them.' Indeed, the word is derived from a Greek word for the preparation of a meal. Opsonins make up the 'butter' that coats the antigen. Because phagocytes have specialized **opsonin receptors** (Fc receptors for antibodies and C3b receptors for activated complement), they will latch onto the opsonins, making and securing their attachment to the underlying antigen.

2. The second phase is the **ingestion phase**, during which the antigen is engulfed into the cytoplasm of the phagocytes together with the portion of outer cell membrane to which it is bound, so that it is enclosed within a pocket or vacuole known as the **phagosome**.

3. The third phase is the **digestion phase**. Within the cytoplasm of the phagocytes are numerous cell membrane-bound vesicles or vacuoles, termed **lysosomes**, containing potentially toxic molecules. Being contained within vacuoles, these molecules do not kill the phagocytic cell. However, when the lysosomes fuse with the phagosome (forming a **phagolysosome**), the engulfed pathogen is exposed to these molecules and in many cases is killed. (In some infections, such as tuberculosis, the pathogen is resistant to these intracellular killing mechanisms and chronic intracellular parasitism is established.)

4. Last is the **disposal phase**. Following digestion, phagocytes ultimately become full of indigestible foreign elements. They can excrete these elements but this involves danger, as powerful killing enzymes will also be secreted that may damage surrounding extracellular structures. Phagocytes can also just 'store' an accumulating collection of 'indigestibles', or, more commonly, simply die after becoming full and become expelled from the body, for example with sputum or as pus from discharging abscesses. Cell death is the most common outcome for phagocytes that have fulfilled their function in protecting us against invading microorganisms.

Antigen-presenting cells

An essential function of phagocytic cells takes place during digestion. These cells will process foreign material, such as microorganisms, and display 'bits' of their antigens on their cell surface. These 'bits' of antigens are known as **antigenic epitopes**. Each antigen molecule may contain several epitopes, and the selection of those for presentation is under genetic control by the **major histocompatibility complex (MHC) system** – see below. Thus individuals vary in the nature of their immune responses to a given infection. The phagocytic cell has now acquired a new look and a new role – to tumble back into the circulation and 'introduce' the antigen on its surface to circulating lymphocytes so that they can mount a specific *adaptive* response to the foreign invader. Because the phagocytic cell has changed its appearance and function, it is now referred to as an **antigen-presenting cell (APC)**. We will pick up the story of how antigen-presenting cells and lymphocytes mount the final devastating attack on the intruding foreigner when we later explore adaptive immunity.

Natural killer cells

Natural killing refers to the process in which cells that have been infected with viruses are destroyed by an extracellular killing mechanism (unlike the intracellular killing described above). Natural killer cells are large granular lymphocytes (LGLs). They are sometimes referred to as **null lymphocytes** (non-T, non-B), as they are a subset of lymphocytes that do not have B-lymphocyte and T-lymphocyte antigen receptors on their cell surface (discussed later). Other than these large granular lymphocytes, it is likely that a variety of other cells can also carry out natural killing. Natural killer cells are activated by **interferons** and other **cytokines** that act in synergy to stimulate the production of more natural killer cells and increase their killing speed. In addition to **detecting and killing cells infected with viruses**, natural killer cells can detect those **cells undergoing neoplastic change and destroy them**, thus protecting us against **cancers**. They are an important part of our normal tumour surveillance systems.

Activated natural killer cells have cytoplasmic granules containing highly toxic molecules, collectively called **granzymes**. They kill by first binding to their targets, then discharging these granzymes into the target cell, where they act on the cellular DNA and re-programme the target cell for self-destruction, that is, **programmed cell death (apoptosis)**. The natural killer cells then detach themselves from the doomed target cell and hunt other virus-infected or tumour cells. Cytotoxic T-lymphocytes (CTLs) (discussed later) kill by the same mechanism.

Other determinants of innate immunity

Other determinants of innate immunity that influence the ability of the individual to withstand infectious disease include the following.

- *Nutrition.* A well-nourished individual is better able to deal with an infectious process than people who suffer from malnutrition (see Chapter 17).
- *Individual differences.* Thanks to heredity, we are all just 'a little bit different'. Although this polymorphism causes problems in transplant surgery, it contributes to the survival of the species by imparting a range of individual susceptibility or resistance to certain infectious diseases, thereby ensuring that no infectious disease will kill all of the population. In this context, there is evidence that a minority of people have genetically determined resistance to the effects of HIV infection.
- *Age.* The very young and the very old are less able to ward off infectious diseases. On the other hand, in some infections, such as hepatitis A and chickenpox, the severity of resultant disease is greater in adults than in children.
- *Gender.* Both men and women are equally susceptible to infections; however, there is a greater incidence and a higher mortality rate from infectious diseases in men. Women may experience a greater incidence of urinary tract infections due to the short female urethra.
- *Species.* Humans are immune to many of the diseases that affect animals, and vice versa. However, many microorganisms can both infect and cause disease in some animals and humans, such as rabies and tuberculosis.
- *Race.* Some races are either more susceptible or more resistant to certain infections than other races, for example Caucasians (white races) are more resistant to tuberculosis than are members of other racial groups.
- *Hormonal factors.* Increased susceptibility to infections is seen in various endocrine diseases, such as diabetes mellitus and hypothyroidism.

All of these components of innate immunity offer good protection against infectious diseases. However, by themselves, they are not adequate for survival in the hostile environment in which humans find themselves. We need much more focused protection and this is afforded by the specific immune response of adaptive (acquired) immunity.

ADAPTIVE IMMUNITY – A SPECIFIC IMMUNE RESPONSE

During the first few months of life, the infant begins to acquire protection against specific pathogens. This type of immunity, known as **adaptive** (or acquired) **immunity**, allows children to mount a **specific immune response** towards each pathogen they encounter as they progress through those first, vulnerable months and years. Indeed, there is increasing evidence that exposure to microorganisms, both harmless and pathogenic, is essential for the correct maturation of the immune system. The increasing incidence of diseases associated with immune dysregulation – asthma, allergy, autoimmune disease, inflammatory bowel disease, vasculitis and even cancer – in the industrially developed nations appears to be a consequence of the deprivation of immunological experience in today's increasingly artificial environment. For the first 3 months of its life, the child is protected from many infections as a result of the passive transfer of maternal antibodies that occurs before birth and which is augmented by the additional antibodies that are transferred from the mother to the child in breast milk. However, these antibodies are short lived and, by the end of 3 months, the child must begin to acquire its own ability to respond effectively to infectious microorganisms.

Adaptive immunity, like innate immunity, involves two different but interrelated and mutually synergistic processes: **cell-mediated immunity** and **humoral immunity**. Both of these processes are governed by **lymphocytes**.

Lymphocytes

The active agents of acquired immunity are specialized leucocytes (white blood cells) known as lymphocytes, of which there are three distinct types: **B-lymphocytes**, **T-lymphocytes** and **natural killer cells** (discussed earlier). T-lymphocytes and B-lymphocytes are often referred to, respectively, as **T-cells** and **B-cells**. All lymphocytes originate from **haemopoietic stem cells** that are manufactured in the bone marrow. Some of these **lymphoid progenitor stem cells**, destined to become B-lymphocytes (B-cells), are known as **B-cell precursors**. The remaining stem cells, destined to become T-lymphocytes, are **T-cell precursors**.

When fully mature and functional, both types of lymphocytes exist to respond to the presence of antigens. Using their special cell-surface receptors, lymphocytes first recognize and then bind to antigenic determinants (**epitopes**; Figure 5.2). This event activates other lymphocytes and stimulates them to differentiate, that is, to change into potent agents that are capable of either destroying or neutralizing the threat from invading microorganisms or other foreign elements. It is this critical role (i.e. the interaction between lymphocytes and antigens) that is the basis of adaptive immune responses.

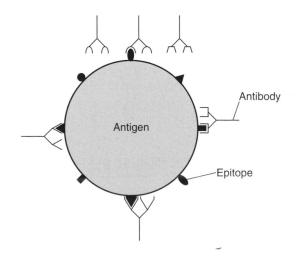

FIGURE 5.2 *Antigen.*

Antigens

Before discussing the two arms of adaptive immunity in more detail, it may be useful to review the **characteristics of antigens**, the substances that provoke the specific immune response in both systems. Antigens are foreign material, such as components of microorganisms (bacteria, viruses) or of foreign tissue cells, that are recognized by the body as different, alien and 'not self'. Antigens are either proteins or sugars. Therefore the first requirement of an antigen is that it must be **foreign**. Another requirement is that, in general, antigens, unless they are going to be attached to a special *carrier molecule*, have to be **large** (having a molecular weight more than 5000 daltons – see Chapter 3). An antigen is usually composed of several antigenic determinants, or epitopes (Figure 5.2). These epitopes must be **topographical**, that is, appear on the surface of the antigen or on the surface of antigen-presenting cells, in order for them to be recognized and interact with the special **antigen receptors** on the surface membrane of lymphocytes.

Antigen receptors

The ability of the immune system to recognize antigens as foreign and bind onto them is contingent upon the antigen making contact and combining with a receptor on the surface of the lymphocyte. These are called **lymphocyte antigen cell-surface receptors**. The diverse molecular patterns of the many different cell-surface receptors on lymphocytes give them the ability to combine with antigenic determinants in potentially unlimited arrangements, providing an infinite number of cell-surface receptors that theoretically recognize an entire range of possible **specific antigens**. In practice, however, the number of epitopes recognized is limited, with each individual having a genetically determined repertoire of epitopes presented on the surfaces of antigen-presenting cells.

The cell-surface receptors on T-lymphocytes – called **T-cell receptors (TCRs)** – are described in the section outlining cell-mediated responses, and the cell-surface receptors on B-lymphocytes – known as **surface antibodies** or **immunoglobulins** – are discussed in association with a description of humoral immunity.

Cell-mediated adaptive immunity

Cell-mediated immune responses involve **T-lymphocytes**, cells that are derived from bone marrow lymphoid progenitor stem cells that also give rise to B-lymphocytes. T-cell precursors migrate to the **thymus gland** for maturation (Figure 5.3). In the thymus gland,

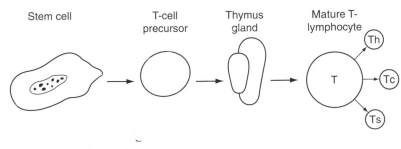

FIGURE 5.3 *The maturation of a T-lymphocyte.*

these T-cell precursors mature and are 'processed' or 'trained' to react uniquely (and differently from the reaction of B-lymphocytes) when they encounter antigens. During maturation, T-lymphocytes acquire special glycoprotein **antigen receptors** on their cell-surface membranes, known as T-cell receptors, that they use to recognize and bind to antigens. Essential T-cell receptor molecules include those known as CD3, CD4 and CD8 (discussed below).

Mature T-cells account for about 70 per cent of the total number of circulating lymphocytes. There are three types of T-lymphocytes, known as **T-cell subsets**, defined in broad functional categories as either **effector** or **regulatory** cells:

- **T-cytotoxic (Tc) CD8⁺ cells** also known as **cytotoxic T-lymphocytes** (CTLs) or killer cells,
- **T-helper (Th) CD4⁺ cells**,
- **T-suppressor (Ts) cells**.

Cytotoxic T-lymphocytes are known as **effector cells** as they have a direct effect on other cells, that is, they kill them. Both T-helper cells and T-suppressor cells regulate the activity of other cells, and consequently they are referred to as **regulatory cells**. T-helper cells enhance or augment immune responses, while T-suppressor cells damp down or suppress immune activity.

Presentation of antigens to T-lymphocytes and the MHC system

For lymphocytes to initiate the deadly sequence of events that culminates in an effective immune response, they must first be introduced or 'presented' to an antigen. It is this presentation that stimulates both B-cells and T-cells to activate and fulfil their unique destinies.

The requirements for efficient antigenic presentation are somewhat different for T-lymphocytes from what they are for B-lymphocytes. Antibodies on the surface of B-lymphocytes (and secreted antibodies) can respond to soluble antigen, that is, they can recognize antigenic determinants on intact (native) antigens. For example, a B-lymphocyte can recognize epitopes on bacteria circulating in the blood plasma and respond. This is a rather 'casual' method of being introduced to an antigen, that is, just meeting it by accident while circulating around in the extracellular fluid compartments of the body.

T-lymphocytes require a more 'formal' introduction to antigens, an introduction that involves two components: MHC system molecules and antigen-presenting cells. This is because T-lymphocytes can only recognize antigenic determinants when they are embedded within a **complex of antigenic fragments** combined with **human cellular molecules** that are produced by host (human) cells. These host cell molecules are known as MHC system molecules (also known as the human leucocyte antigen, or HLA genes). Three classes of MHC molecules (I, II, III) are found on the surface of various host (that is, human) cells. Class I and II MHC molecules are those confined exclusively to the immune system.

The 'presenter' of antigens to T-lymphocytes is known as an antigen-presenting cell (Table 5.2). Examples of antigen-presenting cells include neutrophils and macrophages that capture antigens and process them so that antigen fragments are combined with MHC molecules and expressed on the host cell surface for presentation to T-lymphocytes.

This happens because, when antigens are digested and degraded inside antigen-presenting cells, minute antigen fragments (composed of small protein molecules known as peptides) bond (or associate) inside the cell with MHC molecules. Quite quickly, these **peptide–MHC**

TABLE 5.2 Antigen-presenting cells

APC	Location
Phagocytic cells	
Monocytes	blood
Macrophages	Tissues, spleen and lymph nodes
Kupffer cells	Liver
Lymphocytes	
B-lymphocytes	In lymphoid tissues and wherever
T-lymphocytes	an immune response occurs
Other cell types	
Langerhans cells	Skin
Interdigitating cells	Lymphoid tissue
Follicular dendritic cells	Lymphoid tissue
Astrocytes	Brain
Follicular cells	Thymus
Endothelial cells	Vascular and lymphoid tissue
Fibroblasts	Connective tissue

complexes are displayed on the surface membrane of the host cell, that is, the complexes containing antigenic determinants have become *topographical*. These topographical complexes are then recognized by T-lymphocyte antigen receptors.

Antigen-presenting cells expressing MHC class I molecules and the destruction of viruses

Almost all nucleated cells in the body always express MHC class I molecules and function as antigen-presenting cells. MHC class I molecules bind antigenic peptides produced from *endogenously* produced proteins, such as viral proteins, and present them to receptors on **CD8**$^+$ cytotoxic T-lymphocytes. All cells expressing MHC class I molecules complexed with endogenous antigen peptides will be selected by cytotoxic T-lymphocytes (and other killer cells) for destruction. Because most cells express MHC class I molecules, this allows almost all virus-infected cells in the body to be fatally marked for destruction so that the viral infection can be contained or eliminated.

Antigen-presenting cells expressing MHC class II molecules and the destruction of bacteria

Some antigen-presenting cells are more specialized and are able to express MHC class II molecules. These are responsible for dealing with *exogenous* antigens, such as bacteria, foreign material and other substances found in the **extracellular** environment. These are taken into the antigen-presenting cells by **endocytosis** and processed within them and the resultant peptides combined with MHC class II molecules are displayed on the surface membrane of the antigen-presenting cell, where they are presented to CD4$^+$ T-cell receptors. These cells are not selected for killing, as non-specific killing would destroy many healthy cells. Rather, antigen-presenting cells with MHC class II stimulate T-cell subsets, for example CD4$^+$ T-helper cells, to secrete chemical messengers (**cytokines**) that will summon or activate other immune system cells to destroy the extracellular invaders.

Important antigen-presenting cells that express MHC class II molecules are found in the skin, in mucosa and in lymphoid tissues and include the following.

Langerhans cells and some **squamous epithelial cells** travel from the skin and mucosa through the lymphatic system to adjacent lymph nodes where they mix (or interdigitate) with T-lymphocytes and 'introduce' antigens to them. These antigen-presenting cells are known as **interdigitating cells (IDCs)**.

Also in the lymph nodes, **follicular dendritic cells (FDCs)** and **macrophages**, using complement and antibody, are able to present exogenous antigens to T-lymphocytes. Other important antigen-presenting cells are listed in Table 5.2.[1]

T-cell antigen receptors

The **cell-surface receptors** on T-lymphocytes are characterized by the unique glycoprotein combination of their adhesion molecules, which are classified by **CD** (cluster of differentiation classification system) numbers. The complex of glycoproteins on T-cell receptors includes: **CD3**, which is present on all T-cell receptors and has a constant structure, having an important role in conveying the antigen recognition signal received by the T-cell receptor to the inside of the T-cell, that is, **signal transduction**; **CD4**, which binds to *exogenous* antigen fragments, such as from **bacteria**, presented by MHC class II molecules; **CD8**, which binds to *endogenous* antigen fragments, such as from **viruses**, presented by MHC class I molecules. It is important to remember that CD4 and CD8 are mutually exclusive molecules, that is, cells have either one or the other, not a combination of both types of these molecules.

Cell-mediated response

An antigen-presenting cell, such as a phagocytic cell, engulfs the invading antigen. Once it has been ingested, bits of the antigen become associated with MHC system molecules and this complex of the antigen bound to MHC system molecules is carried to the surface of the cell (becoming topographical) and presented to the T-lymphocyte. This **antigenic presentation** stimulates the T-lymphocyte to change (differentiate) into two major subsets: **helper cells** (expressing **CD4+** T-cell receptors) and **cytotoxic T-lymphocytes** or **killer cells** (expressing **CD8+** T-cell receptors).

Following antigenic presentation, activated T-lymphocytes undergo replication or clonal expansion, resulting in an enlarged antigen-specific population of the appropriate lymphocyte subset. The cells in this clonally expanded population secrete a **cytokine** known as **interleukin-1 (IL-1)**. IL-1 binds to other T-cell receptors, regulating their activation and stimulating the production of other cytokines (discussed below). **Memory cells** are also formed, but the specific immune response to this invasion will now be the responsibility of these quite remarkable T-cell subsets, that is, T-helper (CD4+) and cytotoxic T-lymphocytes (CD8+) cells.

Helper cells (Th CD4+)

Helper cells function by giving help in the form of chemical assistance. The chemical assistance arrives in the form of **cytokines**, which are soluble proteins that interact with specific cell-surface receptors resident on a whole variety of immune system cells. Helper cells control and modulate the development of the immune response by producing and secreting various cytokines. Two types of helper cells are formed when T-lymphocytes have been stimulated by antigenic presentation: helper cells 1 (**Th1**) and helper cells 2 (**Th2**).

These two types of helper cells are distinguished by the different types of cytokines they each produce, that is, their cytokine profile.

Th1/Th2 cells

Th1 cells principally produce **interleukin-2 (IL-2)** and **gamma-interferon (IFNγ)**. Consequently, Th1 cells activate **macrophages** and, equally important, promote **cytotoxic (killer) cell** responses, that is, they facilitate an effective **cell-mediated response**. This results in the destruction of cells harbouring viruses and intracellular bacteria, for example mycobacteria, undergoing neoplastic change or expressing MHC class I molecules, including transplanted tissues or organs.

Th2 cells chiefly produce **IL-4** and **IL-5**. These interleukins further stimulate the **plasma cells** to secrete **circulating antibody** and, consequently, they enhance a **humoral response** (see Figure 5.7). This is discussed in more detail in the section of this chapter that focuses on humoral immunity.

Both Th1 and Th2 produce (in slightly different proportions) other cytokines, namely, tumour necrosis factor (TNF), IL-3 and colony stimulating factor (CSF).

It is important that the right subset of Th cell is switched on during an immune response, such as following infection. If the infecting antigen is an *extracellular* invader, such as bacteria, then a **Th2 response** is best, as it will be humoral defences (i.e. antibodies) that neutralize this threat. Humoral defences are augmented by Th2 cytokines. However, if the antigen is an *intracellular* attacker, for example a virus or intracellular bacterium, then a **Th1 response** is needed, as it is killer cells, such as cytotoxic T-lymphocytes, not antibodies, which are needed to destroy cells infected with viruses. Cytokines released by Th1 cells activate cytotoxic T-lymphocytes.

Some forms of immunopathology, that is, inappropriate immune responses causing tissue damage rather than protection, occur if the wrong type of Th cell is dominant. Thus, for example, a Th1 response elicits protective immunity in tuberculosis but a superimposed Th2 response causes lung damage and cavity formation. Likewise, as mentioned above, a Th1 response is required for the lysis of neoplastically changed cells, and a *Th2 drift* has been observed in various forms of cancer.

Cytokines

Cytokines (literally 'cell energizers') are soluble protein molecules that act as *cell-to-cell messengers*, much like hormones. Over 100 different cytokines have now been identified. These molecules are made by cells of the immune system, such as monocytes, lymphocytes, natural killer cells and macrophages, when they are stimulated to do so. They are secreted in carefully regulated small amounts and are very powerful. Their principal function is to act, via special **cytokine receptors**, on cells (either the cells that produced them or other cells in close proximity) of the immune system and to **stimulate** or **inhibit** the development and growth of immune system cells and **amplify** or **depress** the immune response. In the past, a variety of other names were given to cytokines, depending on their cell of origin, for example **lymphokines, monokines**. These messenger molecules are now known collectively as **cytokines** ('molecules which move between cells'), although some that have been well characterized chemically and functionally and are produced by lymphocytes are, by convention, termed **interleukins** (literally 'between white cells') and distinguished by numbers. Another characteristic of cytokines is that they have **multiple effects** on the growth and differentiation of a **variety of cell types**, often overlapping and sometimes **mutually synergistic** or **antagonistic**. They have **potentially harmful** as well as **beneficial effects** in disease. Table 5.3 describes the activities of some of the better-known cytokines.

TABLE 5.3 Cytokines and their function

Cytokine	Function
Interleukins (IL)	
IL-1 (α and β)	Activates lymphocytes, promotes the release of acute phase proteins from the liver, induces fever and inflammation
IL-2	Made by Th1 CD4⁺ T-cells (and Tc CD8⁺ cells); powerful growth factor for and activator of T-cells, including those cells producing it; stimulates cytotoxicity by NK cells
IL-4	Produced by T-cells (Th2 CD4⁺) and is a powerful growth factor for B-lymphocytes, especially promoting IgG and IgE production from plasma cells
IL-6	Produced by T-cells (Th2 CD4⁺) and stimulates differentiation of B-cells (into plasma cells) and T-cells
IL-10	Produced by T-cells (Th2 CD4⁺) and inhibits the production of IFNγ, suppresses pro-inflammatory cytokines by monocytes/macrophages, enhances B-cell proliferation and antibody secretion
IL-3, IL-5, IL-7, IL-8, IL-9	Other interleukins fully described in 'Further reading' texts listed at the end of this chapter
Interferons (IFN)	
IFNα, IFNβ	Anti-viral activity, regulate other immune system cells, activate NK cells
IFNγ	Immunoregulation, secreted by Th1 cells, activates Tc CD8⁺ killer cells and macrophages, has antiviral activity
Colony stimulating factors (CSF)	
GM-CSF, G-CSF	Stimulates growth of granulocytes, macrophages, neutrophils
M-CSF	Stimulates monocyte and macrophage development and activity
EPO	Produced by the kidneys and regulates red blood corpuscle (erythrocyte) growth
IL-3, IL-7 and SCF	Other CSF cytokines (see 'Further reading')
Tumour necrosis factors (TNF)	
TNFα, TNFβ	Acts on the blood supply to tumours to shrink them, mediates inflammation and healing, promotes release of acute phase proteins, has antiviral and antiparasitic activity, activates phagocytes
	If produced in excess or inappropriately, can cause vascular shock; induces wasting (cachexia) in illnesses such as HIV disease and tuberculosis
Other cytokines	
TGFβ	Transforming growth factors inhibit the activities of other cytokines
Chemotactic factors (also known as **chemokines**)	Attract phagocytic cells to site of infection or tissue damage (see Table 5.4)

Chemokines

Chemokines are a subgroup of cytokines that are principally responsible for the process of chemotaxis, that is, when secreted by immune system cells they act as chemical signals to attract other cells, especially leucocytes, to an area of infection. Because they promote chemotaxis and induce inflammation, these *chemo-attractant* molecules are also known as **chemotactic cytokines**. They also promote tissue repair and play a vital role in **facilitating communication between B-lymphocytes and T-lymphocytes**.

Types of chemokines

There are over 25 different chemokines, all of which are small protein molecules having a mass of no more than 8–10 kilodaltons (kDa) and classified according to their molecular structure. In this structure, chemokines contain two sulphur-containing amino acids, called **cysteines**. They are linked to each other in pairs by a sulphur bridge, that is, a disulphide bond. If pairs of chemokines are separated by an amino acid, they are termed **CXC chemokines** because this group of chemokines have a CXC arrangement (C = cysteine group; X = separated by an amino acid). They are also sometimes referred to as **alpha (α) chemokines**.

When pairs of chemokines are *not* separated by an amino acid, they are termed **CC chemokines** because they have a CC arrangement, that is, the two cysteine groups are paired together. They are also sometimes referred to as **beta (β) chemokines**.

Examples of CXC and CC chemokines that are important within the arena of HIV disease include those in Table 5.4.

TABLE 5.4 Chemokines

CXC chemokines (α chemokines)
SDF-1 (stromal cell-derived factor)
IL-8 (interleukin-8)
GRO (growth-related chemokines)
CC chemokines (β chemokines)
RANTES (regulated-on-activation normal T-cells expressed and secreted)
MIP-1α (macrophage inflammatory protein alpha)
MIP-1β (macrophage inflammatory protein beta)

Chemokine receptors

Each chemokine can bind to a corresponding chemokine receptor on the surface of different cells. Cell-surface receptor sites for α chemokines are referred to as **CXCR** and cell-surface receptor sites for β chemokines are known as **CCR**. These receptors are important in HIV infection in allowing HIV entry into a host cell. They are discussed in more detail in Chapters 6 and 20.

HUMORAL ADAPTIVE IMMUNITY

Stem cells destined to become B-lymphocytes (B-cell precursors) either remain in the bone marrow or migrate to the fetal liver, where they mature into B-lymphocytes. They are known as B-lymphocytes because they were first identified in the part of the hindgut of a bird known as the bursa of Fabricius. Although humans do not have this structure, it is thought that they have similar areas (**bursa-equivalent areas**) composed of similar tissue, such as the fetal liver and the bone marrow, that process or train B-cell precursors. Subsequently, when they develop into fully mature B-lymphocytes, they respond in a specific manner to pathogens and this response forms the basis of antibody-mediated **humoral immunity**. B-lymphocytes account for about 5–15 per cent of the circulating pool of lymphocytes (the remaining 85 per cent being T-lymphocytes and natural killer cells). Figure 5.4 illustrates the development of a mature B-lymphocyte.

During maturation, B-lymphocytes develop **surface receptors** composed of protein

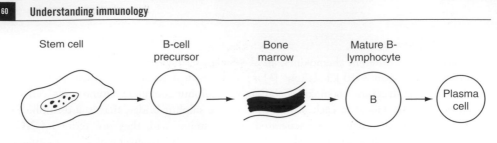

FIGURE 5.4 *The maturation of a B-lymphocyte.*

molecules known as **membrane immunoglobulin (mIg)** or **antibody** (these two terms are synonymous), typically IgM and IgD (discussed later). These membrane antibody receptors are **antigen binding sites**, designed to respond and latch on to specific exogenous antigens that B-lymphocytes encounter.

Just as in cell-mediated responses, humoral immunity is activated by antigenic presentation. Following the capture of the antigen by a B-lymphocyte's cell-surface receptors (membrane antibody), the presence of the antigen stimulates the B-lymphocyte to undergo clonal proliferation and mature into **plasma cells** and **memory cells**. Plasma cells have a specific function, which is to secrete large amounts of **circulating antibody** specific to that particular antigen. The **specificity** of secreted antibody is crucial. For example, if the antigen was derived from *Streptococcus pneumoniae*, antibodies will be secreted from plasma cells that perfectly 'fit' onto that antigen, but these antibodies will not 'fit' onto other antigens, for example they will not 'fit' onto *Staphylococcus aureus*.

The rate of antibody secretion is impressive, in the order of 2000 antibody molecules per second for each plasma cell. This goes on until the plasma cell dies after 4–5 days.

Immunoglobulins (antibodies)

Immunoglobulins are glycoproteins (that is, they contain sugars as well as amino acids), which bind specifically to the antigen that provoked their formation. As mentioned previously, when the two molecules are bound together, this combination of *antibody bound to antigen* is known as an **immune complex** (Figure 5.5).

All antibodies have a four-chain structure and are made up of two identical *light chains* and two identical *heavy chains* (Figure 5.6).

The chains are made out of polypeptides that are bound to each other by disulphide bonds. The light chains are identified by the Greek letters *lambda (λ)* and *kappa (κ)*. There are five types of heavy chains and they are also identified by Greek letters: *gamma (γ)*, *alpha (α)*, *mu (μ)*, *delta (δ)* and *epsilon (ε)*. The heavy chains are found, respectively, in classes of immunoglobulin known as IgG, IgA, IgM, IgD and IgE. The kappa and lambda short chains are found in all five classes.

Some parts of both light chains and heavy chains are made up of amino acid combinations that never vary (the **constant region**). However, the amino acid sequences in other parts of both light and heavy chains in the antibody constantly change, that is, the amino acid sequence differs from molecule to molecule. This part of the antibody fragment is known as the **hypervariable region**.

In the laboratory, antibody molecules can be split into three large pieces by a protein-digesting enzyme (papain). Two of these pieces are exactly the same and contain the **antibody binding site**. They are known as the **Fab fragments**. These fragments consist of the entire light chain and almost half of the heavy chain (linked together by the disulphide

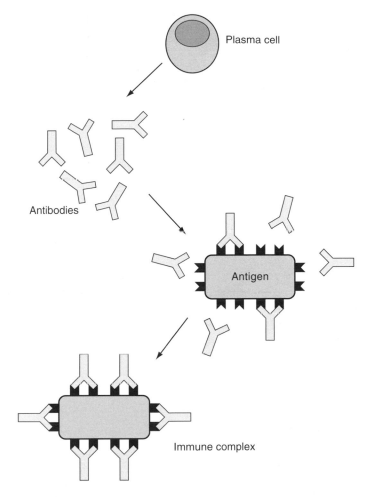

FIGURE 5.5 *Immune complex.*

bonds). **The hypervariable region of the antibody is in the Fab fragment** and this is where the specific lock is made to bind onto a specific antigen. The locks (that is, the complete antibody repertoire) in the hypervariable region are made as a result of constant antibody gene re-arrangement during the growth and development of B-lymphocytes, long before exposure to antigens with the corresponding epitopes. This results in a vast number (thousands) of combinations of molecules that will recognize similar combinations of amino acid molecules on the surface of the thousands of different antigens they may meet throughout the course of our life.

The remaining fragment of the antibody is known as the **Fc fragment** and is important in determining the essential characteristics of the antibody, for example whether or not it can cross the placenta and enter the fetal circulation. The Fc fragment also binds to certain antigens, such as bacteria, and **activates the complement system**. In addition, by Fc binding, the antigen becomes 'buttered' (as in G.B. Shaw's observation, discussed previously), the Fc fragments of certain types of immunoglobulins acting as **opsonins**, sticking to the antigen and attracting phagocytes.

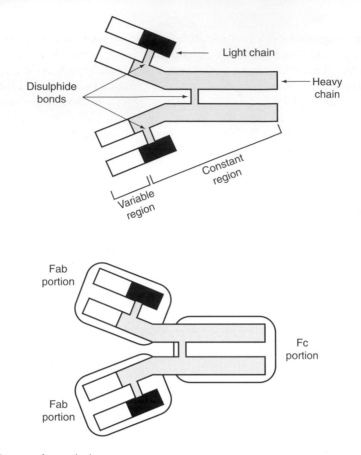

FIGURE 5.6 *Structure of an antibody.*

Antibodies are very diverse and provide **different** and **specific** binding sites to the thousands of different antigenic shapes that they can potentially encounter throughout life. They protect the individual in several ways. First, the antibody attacks the cell wall of the invading pathogen, weakening and eventually destroying it; this is known as **lysis**. Second, and more importantly, when the antibody 'coats' or attaches itself to an antigen, the formation of **immune complexes** activates **complement**. As discussed previously, complement has two important functions: it initiates a **local inflammatory reaction** at the invasion site, which increases the local blood supply, and inflammatory mediators, including **chemokines** and other **cytokines** (discussed earlier), chemically attract neutrophils, monocytes and macrophages to the area under attack. This chemical attraction of phagocytic cells to the invasion site is known as **chemotaxis**. Some microorganisms are destroyed by direct cell wall damage when coated with complement.

We can see that it is critically important for plasma cells to secrete additional **circulating antibody**. As described above, immunoglobulins are classified according to the structure of their heavy chains into IgG, IgM, IgA, IgD and IgE. Immunoglobulins in the IgG and IgA classes are also further divided into subclasses, for example IgG1 and IgG2. The following are a few points about the different classes of immunoglobulins.

IgM

This is a large immunoglobulin (macroglobulin), which appears early in the course of an infectious disease and disappears as the patient recovers. Consequently, its presence in the blood is a **marker of acute infection**. Because this antibody appears early in the infection, IgM is mainly confined to the bloodstream and accounts for about 10 per cent of the total amount of circulating immunoglobulins. As IgM is highly efficient at binding and agglutinating microorganisms, it plays an important role as the first line of defence in bacteraemia (bacterial infection of the blood). Because it can easily cross the placenta from mother to fetus, elevated levels in the neonate indicate intrauterine infection.

IgG (gamma-globulin)

This small antibody accounts for 70 per cent of all the immunoglobulin formed and appears after IgM, during a first or primary response to an antigen. Memory cells for IgG are produced during a primary response, and therefore larger quantities of IgG are produced on further infection (secondary response), appearing earlier in the infection than the IgG produced during a primary response. By contrast, IgM is not associated with memory and the amounts produced and the time scales in primary and secondary antibody responses are very similar. There are four subclasses of this immunoglobulin. Because of its small size, IgG diffuses more easily than other antibodies out of the bloodstream and into the tissue fluids of the body, where it is the principal antibody responsible for neutralizing bacterial toxins, binding to microorganisms, activating complement and promoting phagocytosis. It also readily crosses the placenta, and maternal IgG provides the principal means of defence against infection for the first few months of a baby's life. Because it appears after IgM and memory cells remain in the body for long periods of time (years or a lifetime), **its presence may indicate previous exposure, vaccination or acute infection**.

IgA

This immunoglobulin accounts for up to 13 per cent of the total amount of immunoglobulin formed, but **it accounts for more than 90 per cent of the immunoglobulin found on mucosal surfaces** such as the nose and mouth, and protects the body by blocking and neutralizing antigens that enter by these routes. IgA is found in high levels in seromucous secretions, for example in tears, sweat, saliva, colostrum, urine, and respiratory, gastrointestinal and genito-urinary secretions. This immunoglobulin does not cross the placenta. However, it is present in large quantities in colostrum and breast milk, protecting the infant from infection via breastfeeding. There are two subclasses of this immunoglobulin.

IgD

This class of antibody accounts for less than 1 per cent of the total amount of circulating immunoglobulins and not much is known for certain about its specific function. However, it is found residing on the surface of B-lymphocytes, along with IgM, and they both probably operate as mutually **interacting antigen receptors**, controlling further lymphocyte activation and suppression.[2]

IgE

This antibody accounts for only about 0.002 per cent of immunoglobulin formed. It binds to the surface membranes of mast cells and basophils, causing these cells to release vasoactive substances such as histamine, heparin and serotonin, which are responsible for the common signs and symptoms of **acute allergic reactions**. Mast cells are *fixed* in tissues such as the lungs, whereas basophils are *circulating* mast cells. As elevated levels of IgE are found during parasitic infections, IgE may be important in protecting against this type of infection.

Killer cells and antibody-dependent cell-mediated cytotoxicity

Many cells (natural killer cells, T-lymphocytes, neutrophils, eosinophils) can act as 'killer cells' and are able to kill a whole variety of microorganisms as long as they are first attached to the Fc fragment of antibody. This type of extracellular killing is known as **antibody-dependent cell-mediated cytotoxicity (ADCC)**. It works because, like phagocytes, the killer cells have a special **Fc receptor** that recognizes antigen bound to antibody, i.e. immune complexes.

Memory cells

When provoked by the presence of an antigen, both T-cells and B-cells produce **memory cells**, clones of the stimulated parent cell. These cells remain in circulation and on patrol for months or years. Should the individual encounter the same antigen at any time in the future, the cascade of events that constitute a specific immune response will be accelerated. This is because memory cells 'remember' the characteristics of each specific antigen and respond quickly by rapidly dividing and secreting specific circulating antibody. This is the reason why individuals are vaccinated – to build up a bank of specific memory cells that mediate a rapid and effective secondary response to future infection from specific pathogens that we anticipate may infect us.

Summary of humoral immunity

Humoral immunity is the process whereby B-lymphocytes, provoked by the presence of an antigen, proliferate and undergo change, some changing into memory cells, but most changing into plasma cells. Plasma cells have just one function: to secrete specific antibody that can combine with the antigen, forming immune complexes, activating the complement system and, by different methods, eventually destroying the invading pathogen.

Humoral responses are directly linked to and dependent upon the other arm of acquired immunity, cell-mediated responses. The interactions between humoral and cell-mediated responses are critical and they are summarized in Figure 5.7.

IMMUNE DYSFUNCTION

Survival is impossible without a well-functioning immune system. However, immune dysfunction is clinically well recognized. Some children are born with a **primary immune dysfunction**, such as severe combined immunodeficiency (SCID) or DiGeorge syndrome. In these conditions, fatal flaws in the immune system render the child unable to mount a specific immune response to invading pathogens. Untreated, the child may die of infectious diseases that take the opportunity of establishing themselves in a host who is unable to defend effectively against them – hence these infections are referred to as **opportunistic infections**. However, most individuals are born with a rapidly developing and ultimately a fully functional and effective immune system. As life progresses, events and incidents can

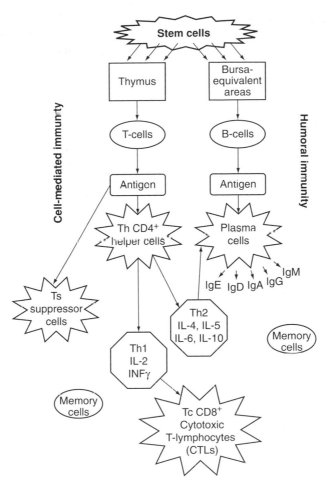

FIGURE 5.7 *Adaptive (acquired) immunity.*

occur that may depress the immune system, either temporarily or permanently. These are the immunodeficiencies, which are secondary to another cause or condition and are therefore called secondary immunodeficiency. They can be caused by the following.

Drugs

The administration of corticosteroids, immunosuppressants and most anti-cancer drugs will depress the immune system. During this period, the patient is at increased risk of opportunistic infections, a fact well known to nurses as evidenced by their careful monitoring of patients while on this type of treatment.

Malignant conditions

Hodgkin's disease, leukaemia and other malignancies can cause a severe immunodeficiency.

Protein depletion conditions

Antibodies are made up of protein molecules. Any condition in which there is an inadequate supply of protein in the body leads to an immunodeficient state. This can be seen in conditions such as the nephrotic syndrome, in which there is a renal loss of protein (especially IgG), and in starvation, where inadequate protein renders the individual (often a child) prone to common infections such as measles, which may then be rapidly fatal.

Radiation

Radiation can depress the bone marrow, affecting its ability to produce the stem cells which eventually become fully mature lymphocytes. Any type of radiation can be harmful, including ultraviolet radiation from the sun (or sun-tanning lamps).

Stress

Both the nervous and endocrine systems (which interact with each other) have a powerful influence on the immune response. The blood supply to lymphatic tissue is innervated by the **sympathetic nervous system** (the 'fright, fight, flight' system), which is activated during periods of stress. Lymphocytes have receptors for many hormones released from various endocrine glands as a result of sympathetic nervous system stimulation. These hormones include **steroids, thyroxine** and **catecholamines** (adrenaline and noradrenaline). In addition, **enkephalins, endorphins** and other neurotransmitters and neuropeptides are released as a result of active nervous system stimulation. These substances are released during times of stress, **depressing the immune response** and reducing the ability of patients to recover from infections.

Other conditions

Ageing, debilitation, various infectious and non-infectious diseases, such as sarcoidosis, leprosy and tuberculosis, can all cause immunodeficiency, resulting in the individual becoming vulnerable to opportunistic disease.

Summary

Various immunological mechanisms protect us from infectious diseases. **Innate** mechanisms, associated with **non-specific**, or **natural immunity**, provide protection against the invasion of disease-causing microorganisms and also help contain those pathogens which have breached this first line of defence. A more **specific immune response** complements these innate mechanisms and is provided by factors and processes associated with **adaptive**, or **acquired**, immunity. These factors and processes allow for the production of a specific immune response (both **humoral** and **cell mediated**) to **specific** invading microorganisms. Unlike innate mechanisms, acquired immunity is associated with **memory**, which allows a faster response on re-presentation of the same pathogen. The immune system is dynamic and interrelated with its own **chemical mediators** to facilitate effective and appropriate responses and, as importantly, its own **inhibitors**, to slow down the immune response once the invader is removed. Because of the dynamic nature and close interdependence in this system, damage to any one element will result in wide-reaching detrimental effects throughout the whole system. This has never been more clearly exemplified than in HIV disease, where infection, and then injury, to CD4$^+$ T-lymphocytes results in such catastrophic, global damage to the entire immune system, allowing the onset of life-threatening opportunistic events, i.e. **acquired immunodeficiency syndrome (AIDS)**.

> ## Prologue to Chapter 6
>
> With our understanding of how the competent immune system protects us against infectious diseases, in the following chapter we will be able to explore and make sense of the means by which the human immunodeficiency virus targets and then wreaks havoc on this critical system. In succeeding chapters, we will use this knowledge to understand the multifarious clinical consequences of HIV infection so that we can assess, plan, implement and evaluate the ongoing nursing care of people with HIV disease.

REFERENCES

1. Weir DM, Stewart J. *Immunology*, 8th edn. London: Churchill Livingstone, 1997.
2. Roitt I, Brostoff J, Male D. *Immunology*, 5th edn. London: Mosby, 1998.

FURTHER READING

Hinchliff SM, Montague SE, Watson R. *Physiology for Nursing Practice*, 2nd edn (Section 6 – Protection and Survival). London: Baillière Tindall, 1996. 780 pp, ISBN 0-7020-1638-1.
Sharon J. *Basic Immunology*. Baltimore, MD: Williams & Wilkins, 1998, 303 pp, ISBN 0-683-07729-5.
Sompayrac, Lauren. *How the Immune System Works*. Malden, MA: Blackwell Science, Inc., 1999, 111 pp, ISBN 0-632-04413-6.
Weir DM, Stewart J. *Immunology*, 8th edn. London: Churchill Livingstone, 1997, 362 pp, ISBN 0-443-05452-5.

Cellular pathogenesis and the journey towards AIDS

Introduction

Acquired immunodeficiency syndrome (AIDS) is the end-stage of a long infectious disease process beginning with primary HIV infection. Our understanding of exactly how this virus causes the relentless, progressive and profound immunosuppression seen in HIV disease has been dynamic, changing as a result of continuing clinical experience and advances in scientific knowledge.

This chapter, building on the material explored in Chapters 2 and 3, explains how HIV targets, invades and establishes a productive infection that results in the destruction of critical immune system cells, leading to the severe immunosuppression associated with end-stage disease – a stage known as AIDS.

Reviewing the material in this chapter is a necessary prelude to understanding that journey from infection to AIDS or, more precisely, the natural history of HIV disease, which is explained in the following chapter.

Learning outcomes

After studying and reflecting on the material in this chapter, you will be able to:

- discuss the mechanisms that HIV uses to infect immune system cells, including the role of viral attachment sites and host cell surface receptors;
- compare and contrast HIV variants associated with syncytium induction and cellular tropism;
- outline the stages associated with HIV replication, including reverse transcription, proviral integration and virion assembly.

A NEW CONCEPT OF THE NATURAL HISTORY OF HIV DISEASE

There has been a tremendous paradigm shift in our understanding of the natural history of HIV infection during the last 10 years, away from an earlier model that described a chronic, latent viral infection, to our present concept of a steady-state model in which viral latency is non-existent. We now know that in the natural course of infection there is a continuous, rapid and high rate of viral replication, with up to 10 billion (10^{10}) virions being produced daily in some people, from the very moment of infection onwards; never ceasing, never slowing, always in competition with a tiring immune system that is attempting to contain the infection.[1] It is this unrelenting viral replication, persistently and progressively destroying immune system cells, that drives the disease process towards the end-points of AIDS and death.[2]

The natural history of HIV disease incorporates three components:

- HIV infection,
- the interaction of continuing high-level viral replication with the immune system (immunopathogenesis), and
- the clinical consequences of a failing immune system (described in detail in the following chapter).

BACKGROUND TO HIV INFECTION

The first step in comprehending HIV infection at a cellular level is to understand the unique mechanisms that HIV uses to infect and replicate within target cells. Before considering this in detail, it is essential to be clear about the 'key and lock' mechanism, that is, the **viral attachment sites** and **cell-surface receptors** that are used by HIV to gain entry into cells.

HIV attachment sites (the 'keys')

As discussed in Chapters 2 and 3, all viruses are externally studded with surface proteins that contain their **attachment sites** (sometimes known as receptor binding sites), structures that they use to dock onto complementary **receptors** on the surface of host cells targeted for infection – a 'key and lock' mechanism. The viral attachment sites, or the 'keys' that HIV uses to dock onto target cells, are located within the surface envelope glycoprotein (gp120 SU – SU stands for **surface**), the 'knob of the spike' protruding from the surface of HIV (Figure 6.1).

Host cell-surface receptors (the 'locks')

A transmembrane glycoprotein molecule called CD4 that naturally resides on the surface of T-lymphocytes and other immune system cells, such as macrophages and Langerhans cells, is the **principal cell-surface receptor** for HIV: it is the 'lock'. This molecule is referred to as CD because, like other T-lymphocyte antigen receptors, it has been described and classified in a system known as the cluster of differentiation. The natural purpose of CD4 is to act as a receptor for antigens in association with (attached to) membrane-bound major histocompatibility complex (MHC) class II molecules (see Chapter 5 to review the MHC system).

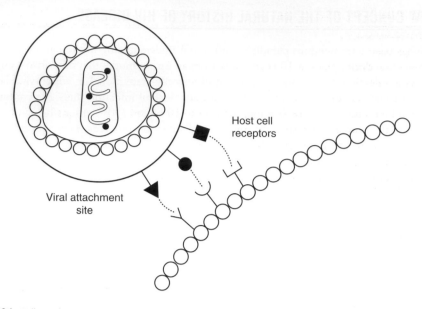

FIGURE 6.1 *Cell attachment sites.*

In macrophages and some other cells with a paucity of CD4 receptors, such as fibroblasts, an Fc receptor site or complement receptor site may be used by HIV for attachment and cell entry (Fc and complement are discussed in Chapter 5).

Small molecules that bind to larger molecules are referred to as **ligands**. For example, a **specific** antigen (being a small molecule) binding to a **specific** antibody (being a larger molecule) is the ligand for that particular antibody, as is a specific hormone, neurotransmitter or chemokine (small molecules) binding to its specific receptor (a larger molecule). The 'natural' ligand for the CD4 receptor is an antigen attached to a MHC class II molecule.

Other host cell-surface receptors (co-receptors)

In 1995/6, medical scientists confirmed a long-held view that, in addition to the CD4 receptor, other complementary cell-surface receptors (**co-receptors**) were necessary for HIV effectively to dock onto and infect CD4-bearing cells[3,4] (Table 6.1). These co-receptors were shown to be **chemokine receptors** (discussed in Chapter 5), specifically **CXCR4** (originally called **fusin**) and **CCR5**. CCR5 is a naturally occurring cell-surface receptor for some CC (*beta*) chemokines, such as **MIP-1α**, **MIP-1β** and **RANTES**, while CXCR4 is a cell-surface receptor for some CXC (*alpha*) chemokines, such as **SDF-1** (see Table 5.4 in Chapter 5). **Not only are these sites designed as receptors for specific chemokine ligands, they also act as co-receptors (in association with CD4 molecules) for HIV.** The discovery of these cell-surface co-receptors for HIV infection was an immensely important scientific advance, as it led to a more complete understanding of HIV immunopathogenesis and may open avenues for the development of new therapeutic and vaccine strategies. Other chemokine co-receptors that may be associated with effective HIV attachment to cell-surface membranes have now been identified and include CCR2b, CCR3, CCR8, US28, BONZO/STRL-33 and BOB/GPR-15.[5]

TABLE 6.1 Primary cellular targets for HIV[7]

- CD4[+] T-lymphocytes
- B-lymphocytes
- Natural killer (NK) lymphocytes
- Endothelial cells
- Haematopoietic stem cells
- CD4[+] blood monocytes and tissue macrophages (tissue histiocytes), including microglial cells in brain
- Epithelial CD4[+] dendritic cells (Langerhans cells)
- Follicular dendritic cells in germinal centres of lymph nodes
- M-cells in Peyer's patches in gut
- Cerebroside cells in nervous tissue (brain) and gastrointestinal epithelial cells

HIV-1 variants

To conclude this background to our understanding of how HIV docks onto those cells that it targets for infection, it is important to realize that there are two principal **variants** (also called isolates, phenotypes, or sometimes strains) of HIV-1. These two variants are related to their **cellular tropism**, that is, the types of target cells they are attracted to, *and* their ability or inability to form aggregations of **uninfected** target cells. These aggregations (or clumps) of target cells are known as **syncytia** and their formation results in a process that culminates in their destruction. Consequently, these two main variants of HIV-1 are referred to as **syncytium-inducing (SI)** and **non-syncytium-inducing (NSI)** variants.

SI and NSI viruses

A syncytium is a clump of non-infected, dysfunctional (not functioning) CD4[+] T-lymphocytes that cluster around a CD4[+] T-lymphocyte infected with an SI variant of HIV-1. This happens because, when an SI variant of HIV-1 infects a CD4[+] T-cell, it leaves excess amounts of viral gp120 on the surface of that cell. Because CD4[+] T-cells have a high affinity for gp120, a mass of uninfected CD4[+] T-cells binds to the infected cell. The result is a fusion of uninfected cells with an infected CD4[+] T-cell, resulting in the formation of a syncytium, that is, a large cell with numerous nuclei. The formation of syncytia facilitates the transfer of viral material between the infected and non-infected cells. Ultimately, the original cell is destroyed by the reticulo-endothelial system, as are the now newly infected cells bound to it in syncytia, killed by the so-called innocent bystander effect. This phenomenon occurs *in vitro* (in laboratory experiments) and almost certainly also occurs *in vivo* (within the body). In general, SI variants are more aggressive and cytopathic (cell killing) than NSI HIV-1 variants, replicating faster and promoting a more rapid progression from infection to end-stage disease.[6]

Variants associated with cellular tropism

The principal receptor for HIV-1 and HIV-2 (and SIV) is the CD4[+] transmembrane glycoprotein molecule.[7] Consequently, the primary cellular targets for HIV infection are those cells that express this molecule on the surface of their cell membranes (see Table 6.1). Although CD4[+] T-lymphocytes and monocyte-derived macrophages are the main cells infected by HIV, two different variants of HIV-1 target slightly different host cells for infection.[8] This affinity, or the attraction that specific viral variants have for specific host cells, is known as **cellular tropism**.

M-tropic and T-tropic viruses

Depending upon its cellular tropism, HIV can be classified into two variants: **M-tropic** or **T-tropic**. Both variants will infect CD4$^+$ T-lymphocytes, but those variants that, in addition, preferentially seek out, infect and replicate in macrophages and monocytes are known as M-tropic variants, whereas T-tropic variants are fairly restricted in their preference to infect CD4$^+$ T-lymphocytes and not macrophages or monocytes.[9]

Two important features are associated with cellular tropism. **M-tropic** variants do not usually form syncytia *in vitro*, that is, they are generally **NSI** variants. Additionally, they preferentially use the **CCR5** co-receptor to gain entry into CD4$^+$ cells.

In contrast, most **T-tropic** variants form syncytia (**SI**) and preferentially use the **CXCR4** co-receptor to gain entry into and infect CD4$^+$ T-lymphocytes.[9]

R5 and X4 viruses

HIV-1 variants that use the CCR5 co-receptor are now often referred to as **R5 viruses**, while those variants that use CXCR4 are termed **X4 viruses**.[10,11]

Summary

Our current concept of how HIV docks onto and infects host cells incorporates an image of the viral attachment sites in the gp120 of HIV resembling a closed fist with two or three fingers extended. HIV needs to find host cells that have at least two of the complementary receptors for these three 'fingers', that is, the host cell needs to have CD4$^+$, CCR5 and/or CXCR4 receptors. While all variants of HIV use CD4$^+$ as the principal viral receptors, M-tropic (NSI) variants (R5 viruses) preferentially use CCR5 as a complementary co-receptor, while T-tropic (SI) variants (X4 viruses) select cells expressing CXCR4 and use that as their complementary co-receptor.

ESTABLISHING A PRODUCTIVE INFECTION

Following exposure to HIV, several events occur that culminate in the establishment of productive infection and continuous viral replication, ultimately leading to a failing immune system and the onset of opportunistic diseases. There are seven stages involved in viral replication (Figure 6.2).

Stage 1. Exposure

As discussed in Chapter 4, HIV is transmitted principally through penetrative (vaginal or anal) sexual intercourse (either heterosexual or homosexual), from the percutaneous introduction of HIV-contaminated blood or blood products, or vertically from an HIV-infected mother to her child (mother-to-child transmission). However, most adolescents and adults throughout the world who have become infected with HIV have done so following sexual exposure to these viruses.

Following sexual exposure, HIV enters the body through the mucous membranes lining the genital tract (and/or rectum) and is attracted to local macrophages and epidermal dendritic cells (Langerhans cells) that reside in these membranes (discussed in more detail in Chapter 5).[12]

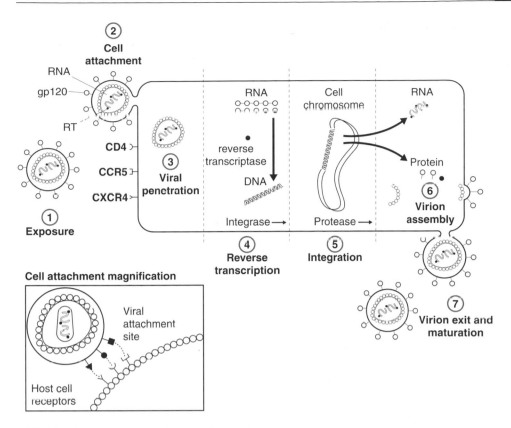

FIGURE 6.2 *Infection, integration and virus production in host cell.*

Stage 2. Cell attachment (gp120 binding)

The CD4 glycoprotein cell receptors ('locks') residing on the surfaces of these local macrophages and dendritic cells act as powerful magnets to cell-free HIV. Using viral attachment sites ('keys') located on the surface envelope glycoprotein (gp120) of the mature virion, HIV becomes **attached** to the host cell (this is called **gp120 binding**). Following sexual (mucosal) exposure, initial infection is principally established by **M-tropic HIV variants** (the variants that preferentially infect macrophages and epidermal dendritic cells). In fact, M-tropic variants dominate in most primary infections, regardless of the route of exposure. As described above, in order to infect a host cell, this variant of HIV (**R5 virus**) needs simultaneously to dock onto two host cell receptors: the **CD4 glycoprotein surface receptor** and the **CCR5 chemokine receptor**.

Stage 3. Viral envelope–cell membrane fusion and penetration

The binding of HIV gp120 to the CD4 and CCR5 (or CXCR4) host cell receptors produces conformational changes in both the viral envelope glycoproteins (gp120 and gp41) and the host cell receptors. These conformational changes involve a rearrangement of the molecules that make up the viral envelope glycoproteins in a specialized domain or area of gp120 known as the **V3 loop** and in the host cell receptors. This triggers a merger of the viral lipid envelope and host cell membranes, which 'melt' into each other. This merging or coherence is known as viral envelope–cell membrane **fusion** and it occurs at the cell surface immediately after binding, allowing the core of the virion to penetrate into the cytoplasm of the host cell, where it begins its replication cycle.[13] It is the **core of the virion** that is inserted into the host cell, that is, the matrix (p17) and capsid proteins (p24), the nucleocapsid proteins (p7 and p9), the two molecules of single-stranded RNA, and multiple copies of the viral enzymes, specifically reverse transcriptase, RNase H, integrase and protease. The outer lipid bilayer and envelope glycoproteins (gp41, gp120) remain behind, fused to the cell surface, and do not penetrate into the host cell.

Stage 4. Uncoating and reverse transcription

After the infecting virion core has been 'internalized', enzymes in the host cell dissolve the core protein. This partial uncoating (or unzipping) of the core releases the viral RNA and viral enzymes into the cytoplasm of the host cell in preparation for viral replication.

When the cell is then activated, all of the viral enzymes, including reverse transcriptase (RT), are also activated and **reverse transcription** takes place. This process involves copying the signal-stranded viral RNA into a genetically identical newly manufactured double strand of DNA. It is referred to as *reverse* transcription because it is the exact opposite of the way in which genetic information is generally transferred within cells when DNA is transcribed into RNA. Retroviruses (*retro* for 'backwards') do the opposite: retroviral RNA is transcribed into DNA, the 'reverse' of normal 'forward transcription'.

Reverse transcriptase

The RT enzyme in HIV is a special protein compound (known as a heterodimer) that is formed by the combination of two quite different polypeptide subunits (p66 and p51) in HIV. The larger subunit (p66) contains two important regions (domains) that are essential in reverse transcription: a **DNA polymerase** domain and a **ribonuclease H (RNase H)** domain. DNA polymerase is an enzyme that facilitates DNA to use itself as a template to replicate, that is, to produce additional identical copies of itself. RNase H is an enzyme that digests single-stranded RNA molecules.

Reverse transcription

Three catalytic steps are involved in this quite unusual metamorphosis that is unique to retroviruses in which RT catalyses the synthesis of a linear double-stranded DNA copy (the **provirus**) of the original viral RNA.

- **Step 1**. The genome of HIV contains two molecules of positively charged single-stranded RNA (**+ssRNA**). Using one of these molecules as a template (a pattern or model), RT produces a DNA copy of it, that is, a molecule of negatively charged single-stranded complementary DNA (**–cDNA**).
- **Step 2**. Once the –cDNA copy has been made, RT, using its enzyme **RNase H**, then degrades (destroys) the original RNA molecule (the template) and the remaining second molecule of single-stranded RNA.
- **Step 3**. RT, using its **DNA polymerase** facility, now recopies the first molecule of –cDNA, producing a second identical molecule of **positively** charged +cDNA. This is then used to form a **double-stranded DNA duplex** (+DNA and –DNA) that is an exact

replica of the original viral RNA. This double-stranded DNA copy of the viral genome is known as the **provirus**.

Stage 5. Integrating the proviral DNA into the nucleus of the host cell

The double-stranded proviral DNA becomes attached to proteins within the cytoplasm of the host cell, forming a **pre-integration complex** (PIC) that is transported to the cell's nucleus, into which it is imported into the nucleus through pores in the nuclear membrane. Inside the nucleus, another viral enzyme, **integrase**, inserts the double-stranded proviral DNA at random into the DNA of the host cell chromosomes. Integrase does this by performing a complicated series of DNA cutting and joining reactions. Once this has happened, the proviral DNA has become integrated into the human DNA, becoming *immortalized* into that person's genes, and the host cell has been converted into a 'factory' for manufacturing more viruses. **HIV infection has occurred at this stage**.

Stage 6. Virion assembly

In time, when that particular 'resting' cell is activated, viral replication is initiated. A variety of stimuli activate different types of resting cells, for example cytokines, new infections and cell division. During replication, proviral DNA in the host cell's nucleus starts to produce a RNA template, which is called **messenger RNA (mRNA)**. This is the first step in 'forward transcription' (as opposed to 'reverse transcription'). The mRNA enters the cytoplasm of the infected cell and, using cellular mechanisms in the host cell, immediately starts to **encode** (give instructions for production) new HIV regulatory proteins: *tat, rev* and *nef*. These regulatory proteins are important for continuing the viral replication process. Other structural and enzymatic proteins are also encoded from the mRNA, such as *gag, pol, env, vif, vpu* and *vpr* (their exact functions are described in more detail in Chapter 3). All of these genes in turn encode for other viral proteins. For example, the products of the *gag* and *pol* genes make up the core of the new mature virion. The *gag* gene encodes for the core proteins (p7, p9, p17 and p24). These are first produced as a single, large multi-protein molecule which, during the maturation process, will require cleaving (cutting or splitting) by the viral enzyme **protease**. Meanwhile, the *pol* gene encodes for the viral enzymes (reverse transcriptase, integrase, protease). Simultaneously, the *env* gene is busy encoding for the surface-coat envelope glycoproteins, first producing a large glycoprotein precursor (gp160) that is cleaved by a cellular protease (not to be confused with viral protease) to yield the finished products that make up the transmembrane (gp41) and surface glycoprotein (gp120) apparatus

Stage 7. Virion exit

Using the split proteins, the viral RNA is 'repackaged' as a new virion is reassembled. This new virion then moves towards the cell membrane, pushing against it and finally exiting the host cell by either cell lysis or 'budding' out of the cell membrane. The half-life of this processing of HIV into mature virions is about 90 minutes, and each infected cell can produce an average of 250 new virions by budding before it fails and dies.

   This ongoing productive infection of immune system cells by HIV results in billions of new virions being released every day, swarming throughout the body, intent only on further massive viral replication that inevitably leads to cell death and fatal damage to the immune system.

MECHANISMS OF HIV CELL KILLING

Although the mechanisms HIV uses to kill CD4⁺ T-cells are not completely understood, medical scientists have identified several phenomena to explain the probable means by which HIV kills cells in the immune system (Figure 6.3).

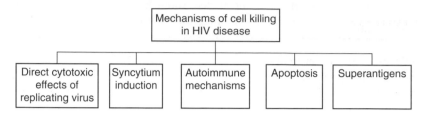

FIGURE 6.3 *Mechanisms of cell killing in HIV disease.*

Viral replication

HIV, replicating in CD4⁺ T-cells, is one cause of cell death. The infected cell dies as a result of attack by CD8⁺ T-cells (cytotoxic killer cells), which detect that they are infected with a virus. In addition, the production of new virions inside the host cell will eventually cause that cell to die as a result of the damage caused by tiny holes punched out of its cell wall by budding virions.

Syncytium induction

Some (but not all) types of HIV will cause the formation of **syncytia**, masses of merged cells. Syncytia develop after a single cell becomes infected with an **SI** form of HIV. This cell then produces viral proteins, including gp120, which the host cell (that is, the infected cell) displays on its cell surface. Because CD4⁺ T-cells have a high affinity for gp120, a mass of **uninfected** helper cells binds to the infected cell. The original cell is destroyed and the uninfected cells bound to it in syncytia are killed by a so-called innocent bystander effect. SI forms of HIV are more cytotoxic than **NSI** forms of HIV. All infected individuals have a mixture of both forms.

Autoimmune mechanisms

Free viral gp120, that is, extra fragments of HIV envelope glycoprotein that are not attached to the intact virion, is found freely circulating in the plasma following HIV infection and will bind to uninfected CD4⁺ T-cells. Although the CD4⁺ T-cell is not infected, it will appear to the killer cells of the immune system to be so, because it has this extra fragment of gp120 attached to its cell surface, and it will be destroyed.

Apoptosis

Apoptosis (pronounced ap"o-to'sis) refers to **programmed cell death** (suicide), a normal phenomenon that occurs in the thymus gland to eliminate abnormal (auto-reactive) T-cells that would otherwise attack the body's own tissue, causing autoimmune disease. HIV infection primes T-lymphocytes (even those not infected with HIV) to commit cellular suicide when they are stimulated by foreign proteins, rather than dividing as they should.[14] This untimely and inappropriate induction of apoptosis not only affects helper cells, but also appears to involve uninfected **CD8⁺ cytotoxic killer cells**.[15] These are the cells which, when functioning effectively, kill those very cells that are infected with viruses.

SUPERANTIGENS

Superantigens are special antigens that react and bind with all T-lymphocytes which have a particular T-cell receptor (**Vβ subset**) and stimulate a much larger number of cells than do conventional antigens.[16] HIV can exert a 'superantigen-like effect' by activating T-cell subsets and making them more susceptible to viral infection. Additionally, superantigens occurring in opportunistic pathogens may also stimulate HIV replication.[17]

MUTATION AND GENETIC DIVERSITY

Many newly forming viruses will mutate. **Mutation**, a common phenomenon among all viruses (especially RNA viruses), refers to errors in replication, usually where there has been a wrong removal or insertion of nucleotides (deletion or insertion mutants) in manufacturing the new viral RNA. Mutations occur because of transcription errors associated with the viral enzymes, especially reverse transcriptase. The mutation rate of HIV during replication is astonishing. Perhaps for every 100 viral particles produced, only one will be a complete and infectious virus.

There are three possible outcomes for the remaining mutations: they are simply defective and die, or they confer no biological advantage and they survive amongst a group of genetically diverse viral variants (quasispecies), or they do confer a biological advantage and evolve to become the dominant quasispecies.

Because of the rapid generation time of the virus, HIV is able to harness this error-prone replication to evolve constantly as environmental pressures change in the host, for example due to drugs, vaccines or illness. The continuing evolution of HIV has extremely important implications for advances in antiretroviral treatment and, incidentally, for the future development of an effective biological vaccine for primary prevention.

THE CONCEPT OF 'HIV DISEASE'

During the course of infection, HIV exists as a mixture of **active** and **inactive** virus in different cells throughout the body. Cells infected with inactive virus (latently infected cells) can be activated in the future and start to produce more virus. These cells, with a half-life of perhaps 40–60 years, are sometimes known as the **latent reservoirs** for HIV, as the virus can survive in them despite intensive antiretroviral therapy, and reinitiate aggressive viral replication once therapy ceases. Cells infected with viruses that are active and replicating are constantly generating new viruses, and these cells are known as **virus-producing cells**. There are always some cells infected with viruses that are active and replicating, budding out and seeking other CD4⁺ T-cells to infect. Consequently, following infection, **there is never a** period of microbiological latency; the virus is always working, replicating, infecting and destroying more and more cells. Although there are usually long periods of **clinical latency**, that is, intervals during which individuals are asymptomatic, the gradual deterioration of the immune system, taking place day by day, month by month, year by year, has led to the evolution of a concept of **HIV disease** as a model of HIV pathogenesis. By definition, HIV disease begins on the day of infection and continues throughout the person's life. This allows for a more rational staging system (which is described in the next chapter) and moves away from the imprecise language (e.g. HIV positive, AIDS-related complex, AIDS, AIDS-related etc.) used in the earlier years of the epidemic.

Summary

Having reviewed this chapter, we have a good understanding of how HIV infects those cells it targets for invasion. We have seen how HIV, using viral attachment sites, docks onto a collection of receptors on the surface of the host cell, infecting it and then hijacking that cell's chemistry to build and establish a productive assembly line that will manufacture new viruses. These new viruses will bud from the infected cell and, when mature, they will find and infect more cells and perpetuate this mortal lesion that will ultimately lead to end-stage disease – AIDS.

In addition to understanding the basic biology of HIV, we are now also familiar with the diverse types of HIV and understand the attraction some variants have for specific host cell receptors and the variations in lethality among these seemingly ever-changing intracellular parasites.

Finally, we have noted the mechanisms that HIV uses to cause cell death, reviewed the importance of viral mutation and genetic diversity, and been introduced to a new concept of immunopathogenesis – the concept of a chronic, unrelenting and ultimately progressive condition now known as HIV disease.

We can also appreciate that the most devastating immunological defect in patients with HIV disease is the absolute reduction in CD4⁺ T-lymphocytes (helper cells) over time. Without the 'help' of these critical immune system cells, the entire intricate pattern of our immune responses becomes dysfunctional, unable to protect us effectively against those microorganisms that can cause disease in immunocompromised individuals.

Prologue to Chapter 7

With the knowledge we have from studying the initial chapters, we can now more competently explore the clinical consequences of HIV infection in the next chapter, setting the scene for a wider discussion of the nursing care needs of HIV-infected patients.

REFERENCES

1. Coffin JM. HIV viral dynamics. *AIDS* 1996; **10**(Suppl. 3):S75–S84.
2. Mellors JW, Rinaldo CR Jr, Gupta P, White RM, Tood JA, Kingsley LA. Prognosis in HIV-1 infection predicted by the quantity of virus in plasma. *Science* 1996; **272**:1167–70.

3. Feng Y, Broder CC, Kennedy PE, Berger EA. HIV-1 entry cofactor: functional cDNA cloning of a seven-transmembrane G protein-coupled receptor. *Science* 1996; **272**:872–7.

4. Dragic T, Litwin V, Allaway GP et al. HIV-1 entry into CD4 cells is mediated by the chemokine receptors CC-CKR-5. *Nature* 1996; **381**:667–73.

5. Clapham PR, Weiss RA. Spoilt for choice of co receptors. *Nature* 1997; **388**:230–1.

6. Tersmette M, Lange JMA, de Goede REY et al. Association between biological properties of human immunodeficiency virus variants and risk for AIDS and AIDS mortality. *Lancet* 1989; 1:983–5.

7. Clapham PR, Weiss RA. The virus and its target cells. In: Merigan TC Jr, Bartlett JG, Bolognesi D (eds), *Textbook of AIDS Medicine*, 2nd edn. Baltimore: Williams & Wilkins, 1999, 13–21.

8. Fauci AS. The human immunodeficiency virus: infectivity and mechanisms of pathogenesis. *Science* 1988; **239**:617–22.

9. Luzuriaga K, Sullivan JL. Viral and immunopathogenesis of vertical HIV-1 infection. In: Pizzo PA, Wilfert CM (eds), *Pediatric AIDS: The Challenge of HIV Infection in Infants, Children, and Adolescents*, 3rd edn. Baltimore: Williams & Wilkins, 1998, 89–104.

10. Cairns JS, D'Souza MP. Chemokines and HIV-1 second receptors: the therapeutic connection. *Nature Medicine* 1998; **4**:563.

11. Littman DR. Chemokine receptors: keys to AIDS pathogenesis? *Cell* 1998; **93**:677.

12. Graham BS. Infection with HIV-1. *British Medical Journal* 1998; **317**:1297–301.

13. Coffin JM. Retrovirology: an overview. In: Wormser GP (ed.), *AIDS and Other Manifestations of HIV Infection*, 3rd edn. Philadelphia: Lippincott-Raven Publishers, 1998, 41–121.

14. Greene WC. AIDS and the immune system. *Scientific American* 1993; **269**:99–105.

15. Weiss RA. How does HIV cause AIDS? *Science* 1993; **260**:1273–9.

16. Roitt I. *Essential Immunology* 8th edn. Oxford: Blackwell Scientific Publications, 1994, 99–102.

17. D'Souza MP, Fauci AS. Immunopathogenesis. In: Merigan TC Jr, Bartlett JG, Bolognesi D (eds), *Textbook of AIDS Medicine*, 2nd edn. Baltimore: Williams & Wilkins, 1999, 59–85.

INTERNET RESOURCES

- To review an animated version of HIV replication, visit Roche Pharmaceuticals' *HIV Focus* website on:
  http://www.roche-hiv.com

- For further information and to review the latest developments in our understanding of the pathogenesis of HIV disease go to the site map *Aidsmap* on:
  http://www.aidsmap.com

CHAPTER

The clinical spectrum of HIV disease

A succession of disasters came on him so swiftly and with such
unexpected violence that it is hard to say when exactly I recognised that
my friend was in deep trouble.

Brideshead Revisited, *Evelyn Waugh*

Introduction

The continuing damage to the immune system caused by HIV infection (reviewed in the previous chapter) will eventually result in dire clinical outcomes for most HIV-infected individuals. In many parts of the industrially developed world, the introduction of highly active antiretroviral therapy (HAART) towards the end of the last decade, and the earlier introduction of specific prophylaxis for commonly occurring opportunistic infections, have modified the pattern of clinical outcomes in those people able to access these therapies. This has had a dramatic and positive impact on the health and quality of life of people living with HIV infection. However, these interventions are not available to everyone; some patients cannot tolerate or adhere adequately to therapy, and many do not continue to respond beneficially to HAART over time.

In this chapter we explore the spectrum of clinical outcomes associated with HIV infection and the standard approaches used for the prevention and management of the most frequently occurring opportunistic events during symptomatic disease. This will allow us to understand the diverse healthcare needs of patients with HIV disease and facilitate our skills in developing relevant nursing interventions. Antiretroviral therapy and important aspects of developing appropriate nursing care plans are discussed in later chapters.

Learning outcomes

After studying and reflecting on the material in this chapter, you will be able to:

- associate progressive immune system damage caused by continuing HIV replication with diverse clinical outcomes;
- describe the prevention and management of opportunistic events occurring during symptomatic HIV disease;
- discuss appropriate classification and clinical staging systems for HIV disease, applicable to countries in both the industrially developed and developing worlds.

THE NATURAL HISTORY OF HIV DISEASE

During the last two decades, there have been tremendous advances in scientific knowledge of the effects of HIV infection on human health. This has given healthcare providers a comprehensive understanding of the immunopathological changes and the resultant clinical events that can be expected to occur during a continuum from initial infection through to end-stage disease and death. This anticipated course of events **occurring in the absence of specific antiretroviral therapy** makes up the **natural history** of HIV disease. This can be divided into three distinct stages: primary infection, clinical latency and symptomatic disease (Figure 7.1).[1] These three stages are encompassed within the current *Classification System for HIV Infection and Expanded Surveillance Case Definition for AIDS among Adults and Adolescents*, published in 1993 by the Centers for Disease Control and Prevention (CDC).[2]

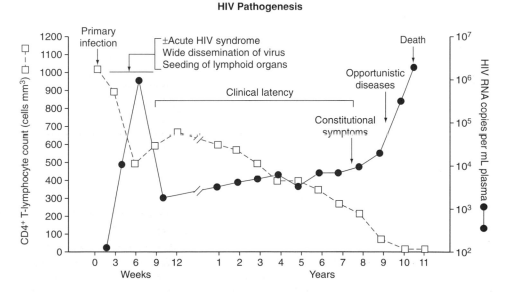

FIGURE 7.1 *The typical course of HIV infection. (D'Souza MP, Fauci AS. Immunopathogenesis. In: Textbook of AIDS Medicine, 2nd edn, Merigan TC, Bartlett JG, Bolognesi D (eds). Baltimore: Williams & Wilkins, 1999, 59–85. Reprinted by permission of Lippincott, Williams & Wilkins.)*

STAGE 1. PRIMARY HIV INFECTION (CDC CATEGORY A)

Primary infection refers to the first few months following infection. During this time, the virus quickly starts to replicate and there is an early burst of viraemia, i.e. a high level of virus in the blood, with the virus rapidly spreading widely throughout the body (Figure 7.1). Initially, there is a **good immune response** with a vigorous CD4[+] T-lymphocyte (helper cell) **humoral reaction** that results in the production of HIV-specific neutralizing antibodies, and a strong **cell-mediated response** produced by CD8[+] T-lymphocytes (cytotoxic killer cells). However, many viruses escape immune surveillance and destruction by frequently mutating, keeping 'one step ahead' of the immune defences. Additionally, although the immune system mounts an effective attack on HIV, it cannot keep up with the unrelenting ability of this virus to continue high-level replication over the many years of infection. Ultimately, the immune system tires, then fails, and AIDS-defining illnesses develop.

During primary infection, HIV in the blood will start to be filtered by the follicular dendritic cells (FDCs) in the lymph nodes, reducing both the viral load and replication in the peripheral blood, but infecting more CD4[+] T-helper cells in the reticuloendothelial system, for example helper cells in the spleen, adenoid glands, tonsils and lymph nodes (the sites where most of these cells reside).

Clinical conditions occurring during primary HIV infections

Within the clinical category of primary HIV infection (CDC Category A), infected individuals may experience three conditions (Table 7.1).

TABLE 7.1 Primary HIV infection: CDC Clinical Category A

- Asymptomatic HIV infection
- Acute retroviral seroconversion syndrome
- Persistent generalized lymphadenopathy (PGL)

Asymptomatic HIV infection

Many people remain completely **asymptomatic** and, unless tested for some other reason, they will be unaware that they are infected. However, they remain infected and infectious to others.

Others may develop a (usually) self-limited illness and then recover (acute retroviral seroconversion syndrome) during primary infection, whereas some may develop multiple swollen lymph glands (persistent generalized lymphadenopathy, PGL).

Acute retroviral seroconversion syndrome

In primary HIV infection, peak levels of plasma viraemia occurring anywhere between 2 and 12 weeks following initial infection are associated with a rapid but temporary depletion of both CD4[+] and CD8[+] T-lymphocytes (lymphopenia)[2] (see Figure 7.1) and, during this period, between 50 and 70 per cent of infected people may develop an acute clinical illness known as acute retroviral seroconversion syndrome (Table 7.2). This syndrome is also known as acute (primary) HIV infection (PHI). Generally, most clinical manifestations of this condition are self-limiting and most people will make an uneventful recovery within 2–4 weeks. However, the development of significant illness during this acute syndrome,

TABLE 7.2 Common clinical manifestations of acute retroviral seroconversion syndrome[2-6]

- Fatigue (may persist for months)
- Fever >38 °C (sometimes associated with night sweats)
- Rash (erythematous maculopapular)
- Lymphadenopathy (especially involving axillary, occipital and cervical nodes; commonly persistent and generalized)
- Joint and/or muscle pains (myalgia and/or arthralgia)
- Headache (retro-orbital pain exacerbated by eye movements)
- Pharyngitis
- Diarrhoea
- Oral or oesophageal thrush (candidiasis)
- Anogenital and/or oropharyngeal ulceration
- Neurological illnesses (encephalopathy, meningitis, neuropathy)
- Nausea and vomiting; weight loss; loss of appetite (anorexia)

specifically signs and symptoms lasting more than 14 days and/or a more severe decrease in the level of lymphocytes (lymphopenia), is associated with a more rapid progression to end-stage disease (AIDS) compared with individuals who experience a more short-lived illness as a result of primary infection.[2,3] During the acute phase of this syndrome, symptoms are treated and antiretroviral therapy (HAART) may be prescribed.[4,5]

Persistent generalized lymphadenopathy

Some individuals infected with HIV develop a persistent and generalized lymphadenopathy (known in France as lymphadenopathy syndrome, LAS). PGL is defined as palpable lymph node enlargement (more than 1 cm) at two or more extra-inguinal sites, persisting for more than 3 months in the absence of an identifiable cause other than HIV infection. Axillary and cervical lymph nodes are commonly involved in this condition. PGL can persist in some individuals for many years without any progression to clinical illness and it does not affect the patient's clinical prognosis. This diagnostic term is generally reserved for those individuals in whom lymphadenopathy is the principal manifestation of HIV infection.

Resolution of primary HIV infection

During primary HIV infection, HIV replication is established in the lymphoid tissue, the central nervous system and the genital tract (where high levels of viral shedding can facilitate sexual transmission to others). In most people, within approximately 3 months following infection, most signs and symptoms of the acute retroviral seroconversion syndrome have resolved, the level of CD4[+] T-lymphocytes increases but does not return to baseline values, CD8[+] T-lymphocyte levels normalize and there is a relative stabilization of the viral load. This signifies the end of primary infection and the onset of clinical latency.

Serology during primary HIV infection

Seroconversion takes place during primary infection. This means that serial blood samples for HIV-1 antibodies (IgM and IgG) and p24 antigen become positive within the first few weeks or months of infection in almost all infected individuals. When serological results are equivocal, HIV DNA or RNA polymerase chain reaction (PCR) may also be used to confirm infection. If tests confirm HIV infection, additional tests for plasma viral RNA (viral load) and CD4$^+$ T-lymphocyte counts will be needed. If antiretroviral drugs are being considered for use during primary HIV infection, drug susceptibility tests (genotypic assays) are recommended.[7,8]

STAGE 2. CLINICAL LATENCY (CDC CATEGORY A)

As we have seen above, when the patient recovers from primary infection, the plasma viraemia declines and the CD4$^+$ T-lymphocyte cell count recovers somewhat (see Figure 7.1). Even without antiretroviral therapy, most infected people will generally experience many years of clinical latency, during which time they are relatively asymptomatic. However, during this period, there continues to be a slow and progressive loss of CD4$^+$ T-lymphocytes with a corresponding increase in viral load. As the CD4$^+$ T-lymphocyte count falls below 350 cells/μL (mm^3), HIV plasma viraemia accelerates, further depressing the CD4$^+$ T-cell count, and individuals are at risk of developing symptomatic disease. HAART is often recommended when the CD4$^+$ T-cell count falls below 350 cells/μL (mm^3) and is always recommended if the CD4$^+$ T-cell count falls below 200 cells/μL (mm^3).[9-11]

STAGE 3. SYMPTOMATIC DISEASE

The inevitable outcome of a continuing deterioration of the immune system, as evidenced by a progressive decline in the numbers of peripherally circulating CD4$^+$ T-cells, and an accelerating level of viral activity, demonstrated by an unrelenting increase in the plasma HIV-1 viral load, is clinically apparent disease (see Figure 7.1). This stage of HIV disease can be divided into **early** and **late** symptomatic disease.

Early symptomatic disease (CDC Category B)

Many individuals develop a variety of indicators of ill-health due to HIV infection *without* developing major opportunistic infections or secondary cancers. The often severe constitutional symptoms and signs seen in this stage of HIV disease are a manifestation of the clinical conditions associated with early symptomatic disease (Table 7.3). Individuals at this stage may often appear chronically ill or even cachectic (severely debilitated and emaciated) and may be affected by a variety of minor opportunistic infections.

Bacillary angiomatosis

This condition is caused by an infection with a species of rickettsiae known as *Bartonella*. The two specific microorganisms implicated are *B. henselae* and *B. quintana*. These are rod-shaped Gram-negative bacteria that are transmitted to humans as a result of contact with cats (and cat fleas). HIV-infected people with low CD4$^+$ T-cell counts are particularly vulnerable to developing various cutaneous (skin) and systematic manifestations of infection. The most common type of skin lesion involves a reddish purple berry-like papule with a scaly collar around it, which bleeds profusely if traumatized. There may be just a few lesions or multiple lesions. Other cutaneous lesions occur, including subcutaneous nodules and indurated, hyperpigmented plaques. Additionally, systematic lesions can occur throughout the body, in bone (osteomyelitis), muscle, mucous membranes and the liver (peliosis hepatitis). Patients

TABLE 7.3 CDC Category B conditions – early symptomatic disease

1. Bacillary angiomatosis
2. Candidiasis, oropharyngeal (thrush)
3. Candidiasis, vulvovaginal; persistent, frequent, or poorly responsive to therapy
4. Cervical dysplasia (moderate or severe)/cervical carcinoma-in-situ
5. Constitutional symptoms, such as fever (38 °C) or diarrhoea lasting more than 1 month
6. Hairy leucoplakia, oral
7. Herpes zoster (shingles), involving at least two distinct episodes or more than one dermatome
8. Idiopathic thrombocytopenic purpura
9. Listeriosis
10. Pelvic inflammatory disease, particularly if complicated by tubo-ovarian abscess
11. Peripheral neuropathy
12. Other conditions

usually have fever, are bacteraemic and may be seriously ill. *B. henselae* also causes **cat scratch fever**, a potentially serious infection in immunocompromised individuals.

Treatment

The treatment for bacillary angiomatosis and cat scratch fever is usually with oral erythromycin, azithromycin or a tetracycline derivative such as doxycline. These drugs may need to be given for 2 months or longer. In some cases, intravenous antibiotic therapy may be needed.

Prevention

Prevention of infection involves taking precautions when in contact with cats, especially young cats and kittens (Table 7.4). Because *B. quintana* infection has been associated with homeless people who have a low socio-economic status and a history of recent infestation with head and body lice and who have had no contact with cats, the prevention and treatment of head and body lice may be helpful in limiting the spread of *B. quintana* infection.[12,13]

TABLE 7.4 General precautions for contact with cats

■ Have pet cats tested for prior exposure to *Bartonella henselae*
■ Keep pet cats inside and do not adopt or handle stray cats
■ Avoid contact with younger cats (under 1 year of age), as they are more likely to be infected with *B. henselae* than older cats
■ Make sure cats are kept free of fleas
■ Cover all wounds and abrasions with a waterproof dressing before handling cats; never allow a cat to lick an open wound
■ Wash hands thoroughly after handling and petting cats and wash any bites or scratches immediately with soap and water
■ Use gloves to empty litter trays, keep trays clean and empty litter daily – if possible, have litter trays emptied by a person who is not infected with HIV
■ Wash hands thoroughly after removing gloves used for contact with litter trays
■ De-clawing of cats is unnecessary, but avoid rough playing with cats

Candidiasis (thrush)

This condition is caused by a fungal infection with the yeast *Candida albicans*, although other strains of *Candida*, such as *Torulopsis glabrata*, may be implicated as a cause of candidiasis in immunocompromised people.

Oropharyngeal candidiasis is common in early symptomatic disease as specific immune defence mechanisms become impaired as a result of advancing HIV disease and the associated decline in CD4+ T-cells. Patients often complain of an altered taste sensation, burning pain in the mouth and difficulty in swallowing (dysphagia). There are different types of oropharyngeal candidiasis and an examination of the mouth and throat commonly reveals painless white spots on the tongue, gums, buccal membranes or throat. In some types of candidiasis, plaques of dead tissue and yeast (which are easily removed) or red patches are present. In more chronic forms of oropharyngeal candidiasis, a condition known as angular cheilitis may develop, which causes painful white or red cracks (fissuring) at the corner of the mouth; in another form of candidiasis, chronic plaques (leucoplakias) of different sizes and shapes (and which cannot be scraped away) are seen throughout the mouth and throat.

Women with **vulvovaginal candidiasis** notice an abnormal creamy-white vaginal discharge and may complain of vaginal or vulvar itching (pruritus) or a burning pain during micturition (dysuria) and/or pain during sexual intercourse (dyspareunia).

Treatment

Both oropharyngeal and vulvovaginal candidiasis generally respond well to either topical or systemic antifungal preparations (Table 7.5); however, recurrence is common. The imidazole group of drugs interact with some antiretroviral drugs (Table 7.6) and nurses and physicians need to be alert to this.

All of the topical vaginal antifungal agents listed in Table 7.5 are supplied as oil-based creams, ointments or pessaries and these can damage latex condoms and diaphragms. While

TABLE 7.5 Drugs used for the treatment of candidiasis

Local antifungal agents
- Amphotericin B (lozenges and oral suspension)
- Nystatin (oral suspension and pastilles) (Nystan®)

Topical vaginal antifungal agents
- Clotrimazole cream (Canesten®)
- Econazole nitrate cream (Ecostatin®, Gyno-Pevaryl®, Pevaryl®)
- Miconazole nitrate cream (Gyno-Daktarin®)
- Fenticonazole nitrate pessaries (Lomexin®)
- Ketoconazole cream (Nizoral®)
- Nystatin cream and ointment (Nystan®)

Systemic antifungal agents (imidazole group of drugs)
- Ketoconazole (Nizoral®)
- Itraconazole (Sporanox®)
- Fluconazole (Diflucan®)

Other systemic antifungal agents
- Amphotericin B
- Flucytosine (Ancotil®)

TABLE 7.6 Drug interactions: imidazole and antiretroviral drugs

- Ketoconazole inhibits metabolism of **indinavir**
- Itraconazole increases plasma concentration of **indinavir**
- Fluconazole increases plasma concentrations of **zidovudine**
- Ketoconazole (and perhaps other imidazoles) increases plasma concentrations of **saquinavir**
- Nevirapine reduces plasma concentration of ketoconazole
- **Ritonavir** increases plasma concentration of ketoconazole (and other imidazoles)
- **Amprenavir** may increase plasma concentrations of itraconazole

using these vaginal medications, women should use a polyurethane condom (Femidom®, Pasante®) or their male partner should use a non-latex polyurethane condom (Durex Avanti®) for insertive sexual intercourse to prevent infection or pregnancy.

The most up-to-date information on drug doses, interactions and side effects is found in the current edition of the *British National Formulary*, which is published every 6 months and which is also accessible online (see 'Internet resources' at the end of this chapter).

First-line treatment is often ketoconazole, which is effective, well absorbed orally, the cheapest systemic drug available and side effects are rare. However, absorption is dependent upon gastric acidity. Acid beverages, such as cola drinks (pH 2.5), may be used to improve the absorption of ketoconazole if acid production is reduced, as is common in some patients with HIV disease, or in those who have to take antacid medications. Fluconazole is more expensive but better absorbed and has fewer side effects. All of these drugs are very effective, but resistance can occur, resulting in a serious clinical management problem.

Cervical dysplasia and cervical carcinoma

It has been recognized for some time that abnormal cervical cytology is more common among immunosuppressed HIV-infected women and is also associated with the presence of **human papillomavirus (HPV)**. The prevention and treatment of women with cervical dysplasia and cervical carcinoma-in-situ are described in more detail in Chapter 11, where the impact of HIV infection on women is discussed.

Constitutional symptoms

A variety of signs and symptoms associated with a declining level of good health frequently occur during early symptom HIV disease, including fevers, night sweats, weight loss, diarrhoea, various skin conditions, lethargy and general malaise. These conditions are often idiopathic (i.e. not traceable to a specific disease or infection), but they do reflect a progressive deterioration of immune functions.

Hairy oral leucoplakia

This condition occurs almost exclusively in immunosuppressed HIV-infected individuals and is associated with **Epstein–Barr virus (EBV)** infection, a type of human herpesvirus (also known as **human herpesvirus 4** or **HHV4**) . This form of leucoplakia presents as a white, corrugated ('hairy') lesion on the lateral surface of the tongue. The lesions wax and wane in extent and, if painful, treatment with systemic antifungal drugs (see Table 7.5) may be prescribed to reduce or eliminate superinfection with *Candida*. Other drugs used include the antiviral agents desciclovir and ganciclovir.[14]

Herpes zoster (shingles)

This condition is caused by a human herpesvirus known as the **varicella-zoster virus (VZV)** – also known as **human herpesvirus 3** or **HHV3** – and usually affects children, causing chickenpox in some. Following childhood infection, the virus becomes dormant in the spinal or cranial ganglia (a groups of nerve cell bodies). Herpes zoster, or shingles, is seen in adults and it represents a reactivation of VZV caused by immunosuppression secondary to old age, debilitating illnesses, immunosuppressant drugs and HIV infection.

Herpes zoster presents as vesicular eruptions on the back and front of (usually) one side of the trunk. These eruptions consist of clusters of small fluid-filled blisters surrounded by small red areas. The neck and head can also be affected, involving the face. More importantly, if the fifth cranial nerve (trigeminal nerve) becomes infected, the infection is likely to spread to the eye. This can cause inflammation and scarring of the cornea and inflammation of the internal structures of the eye (uveitis) that may result in glaucoma. Neuralgic pain in the skin of the associated dermatomes (the area of skin supplied with afferent nerve fibres by a single posterior spinal root) is common and may be severe. The blisters begin to dry and scab approximately 5 days after they have appeared, and most people will make a full recovery. However, in some, neuralgic pain (post-herpetic neuralgia) may continue for months or longer.

Shingles frequently occurs in HIV-infected people and is more severe in them and in anyone else who is immunosuppressed. However, any adult who was not infected in childhood and then becomes exposed to and infected with VZV (primary infection) may develop potentially life-threatening systemic disease. Primary VZV infection is potentially even more catastrophic in an HIV-infected person.

Treatment

Keeping the affected skin areas clean is important in preventing secondary bacterial infection. Specific antiviral drugs for herpesvirus infection are used (Table 7.7) and most people are treated on an outpatient basis. Intravenous antiviral treatment is generally prescribed for those patients with disseminated disease or visceral organ involvement, or those unable to tolerate oral therapy. Drug-resistant virus may respond to treatment with foscarnet.[15] Locally applied wet compresses are soothing, but analgesia will usually be required. In general, corticosteroids are not used in HIV-infected individuals because of the potential risk of further immunosuppression and VZV disseminations.[14] Heterocyclic antidepressants, such as amitriptyline, or antiepileptics, such as carbamazepine, are sometimes used in the management of post-herpetic neuralgia following recovery from acute shingles.

TABLE 7.7 Anti-herpesvirus agents used to treat patients with varicella-zoster (shingles) and herpes simplex disease

Drug	Administration
Aciclovir (Zovirax®)	Topical preparation, tablets, oral suspension or as an intravenous infusion
Famciclovir (Famvir®)	Tablets
Valaciclovir (Valtrex®)	Tablets
Foscarnet sodium (Foscavir®)	Intravenous infusion
Cidofovir (Vistide®)	Intravenous infusion

Prevention

HIV-infected people who do not have a history of having had childhood chickenpox should avoid contact with anyone with chickenpox or shingles. If exposure occurs, **human varicella-zoster immunoglobulin (VZIG)** is effective in preventing severe primary VZV infection in immunosuppressed individuals who have not been infected previously with VZV if administered within 96 hours from the time of a significant exposure.[ ] If time permits, the VZV immune status of the exposed person should be determined serologically, as VZIG is not needed in people who are VZV positive. However, if there would be a delay in obtaining serology results of more than 4 days from the initial exposure, VZIG should be given to any person with symptomatic HIV disease without a history of chickenpox. VZIG is not usually given to people with asymptomatic HIV disease with relatively normal CD4+ T-cell counts as there is no evidence of severe varicella in these individuals.[16] A live, attenuated VZV vaccine is available in the USA, but is currently not licensed for use in the UK; however, it is available on a named patient basis from the manufacturers. More detailed information is available from the current edition of the UK Departments of Health immunization guidelines.[16]

Progressive cytopenias

A variety of haematologic disorders are associated with early symptomatic HIV disease, resulting in a decrease in the number of red blood corpuscles (erythrocytes), white blood cells (leucocytes) and platelets (thrombocytes). **Anaemia**, common in asymptomatic disease, progressively develops in almost all individuals during symptomatic HIV disease, as does **leucopenia** (CD4+ lymphocytopenia). The incidence of platelet disorders is equally common and a type of **idiopathic thrombocytopenic purpura (ITP)** commonly occurs during early symptomatic HIV disease. Platelets are essential for blood clotting, and in HIV-related ITP there is a decrease in the number of circulating platelets, patients presenting with usually modest mucosal bleeding disorders, such as nose bleeds (epistaxis), melaena (blood in faeces) and gingival (gum) bleeding. They also give a history of ease of bruising. There are multiple causes of HIV-related ITP, including an impairment in the manufacture of blood cells due to direct HIV infection of megakaryocytes (bone marrow cells responsible for platelet formation), cross-reacting antibodies on platelets and the subsequent formation of immune complexes leading to their clearance by the reticuloendothelial system, and lifestyle factors, for example chronic alcohol and other recreational drug use.

Treatment

Spontaneous remissions may occur and HAART may facilitate an increase in platelet counts. **Normal immunoglobulin for intravenous use** is sometimes given to increase the platelet count temporarily, for example prior to surgery or during an acute bleed. Short-term therapy with corticosteroids may be cautiously used and, in severe cases, the spleen may be removed (splenectomy) or irradiated.[17,18]

Listeriosis

Listeriaceae are Gram-positive bacilli found worldwide in the environment and in the intestinal tracts of non-human mammals, birds, arachnids (spiders, scorpions and mites) and crustaceans (e.g. lobsters, crabs, shrimps). Infected humans may be asymptomatic carriers, and the duration of faecal carriage, although generally short, may exceed a year in some people.[19] Generally, only *Listeria monocytogenes* causes disease in humans. Infection usually occurs as a result of eating contaminated diary products, some seafood and raw vegetables, for example cabbage in coleslaw.[20] *L. monocytogenes* can survive and grow at usual refrigerator temperatures of less than 10 °C and survive heat at temperatures up to 60 °C.[20]

In immunocompromised individuals, exposure may result in bloodstream infections (bacteraemia) and meningitis. It may rarely cause endocarditis and ophthalmitis with regional lymph gland involvement (oculoglandular listeriosis).

Treatment
Listerial meningitis is usually treated with intravenous penicillin G for 10–14 days after the abatement of fever (defervescence). Both intravenous penicillin G and intravenous tobramycin are frequently given for listerial endocarditis and primary listeraemia, and erythromycin may be prescribed for oculoglandular listeriosis and listerial dermatitis.

Prevention
People living with HIV infection should be advised to take great care to avoid contact with *L. monocytogenes* by ensuring their food is safe. In the UK, this generally means avoiding unpasteurized diary products, soft ripened cheeses and paté and thoroughly reheating cook-chilled foods and ready-to-eat poultry prior to consumption.[20,21] All raw vegetables need to be thoroughly washed and peeled before consumption. (See Table 7.16 for general advice you may wish to discuss with clients in order to help them avoid enteric bacterial infections.)

Pelvic inflammatory disease
This condition is caused by upper genital track infections, usually polymicrobial in nature but commonly due to *Neisseria gonorrhoea* and *Chlamydia trachomatis*. Studies have shown an increased incidence of pelvic inflammatory disease (PID) in women with early symptomatic HIV disease.[22] HIV-infected women tend to have more severe disease than women not infected with HIV and it is frequently complicated by tubo-ovarian abscess. Chronic endometritis is also more common in HIV-infected women.[22] Women with PID frequently have fever, lower abdominal tenderness, abnormal bleeding, dyspareunia and abnormal cervical or vaginal discharge.

Treatment
Appropriate oral or parenteral (intravenous or intramuscular) antibiotics are given, such as doxycycline, gentamicin, clindamycin, and some cephalosporins, such as cefuroxime and cefotaxime.

Peripheral neuropathy
Damage to the peripheral nerves occurs frequently, affecting up to a third of all people in all stages of HIV disease, but especially in early and late symptomatic disease, causing lower-extremity pain and impairment of the sense of touch (dysesthesia), for example a super-sensitivity to touch. Peripheral neuropathies (PN) of several types in HIV-infected people can be caused by the direct action of HIV on the peripheral nerves, by other HIV-related infections and co-morbidities as a result of medications (especially some antiretroviral agents) used for treating symptomatic HIV disease (Table 7.8), or lifestyle factors such as alcohol and recreational drugs. Patients often complain of numbness, tingling, burning or painful dysaesthesia of the feet and hands. Gait is altered and walking may be affected because of pain.

TABLE 7.8 Drugs associated with the development of peripheral neuropathy

Didanosine[a]

Stavudine[a]

Isoniazid

Vincristine

Dapsone

Pyridoxine hydrochloride (vitamin B$_6$)

Lithium carbonate

Metronidazole

Thalidomide

[a]Increased risk if hydroxyurea added to regimen.

Treatment

If PN is caused by a specific drug, relief may be obtained by withdrawing the offending agent. Otherwise treatment is relatively unsatisfactory and is directed at attempting to relieve symptoms. Analgesia, such as ibuprofen, is often helpful. Treatment with antidepressants, for example amitriptyline and doxepin, or acupuncture is often used but there is little evidence to show that they are efficacious.[23]

Other conditions in early symptomatic disease

In addition to the above conditions, people with early symptomatic HIV disease are prone to a variety of other bacterial, fungal and viral infections. Many individuals may also have enlarged spleens (**splenomegaly**) and most will have serological evidence of past exposure to various viruses, for example **cytomegalovirus** (CMV), **Epstein–Barr virus** (EBV), **herpes simplex virus, hepatitis B virus** (HBV) and **hepatitis C virus** (HCV). **Genital warts** (condyloma acuminata) and **molluscum contagiosum**, presenting as large, multiple molluscum situated in the face, are sometimes seen in patients with early symptomatic disease, and both conditions are relatively unresponsive to conventional treatment. **Testicular atrophy** and **malabsorptive diarrhoea** may also be seen.

Latent infection with **herpes simplex virus** – also known as **human herpesvirus 1 or 2 (HHV(HSV) 1 or 2)** – may reactivate in patients during early symptomatic disease, and healing may be prolonged. In severe reactivations, anti-herpesvirus agents (see Table 7.7) are usually prescribed to reduce the period of viral shedding, reduce pain and accelerate healing.

Dermatophytoses (ringworm infections)

Tinea cruris (Jock itch), a fungal skin disease of surfaces of contact in the scrotal, crural and genital areas, and tinea pedis (athlete's foot) are frequently seen. These can be treated with topical antifungal preparations such as the imidazole antifungals (clotrimazole, econazole, ketoconazole, miconazole, sulconazole) or with terbinafine cream. Undecenoates, such as Mycota® and Monphytol®, are commonly used to treat tinea pedis.

Seborrhoeic dermatitis

Treatment depends on location and severity. Tars are used to depress the proliferation of cells and have antipruritic and antiseptic properties. Salicylic acid is frequently combined with tars for its keratolytic action, that is, it helps remove scales, allowing the tars access to the underlying diseased areas. Seborrhoeic dermatitis of the body can be treated with a combination of tars and salicylic acid, for example Gelcosal®. Seborrhoeic dermatitis of the scalp can be treated with a similar preparation, for example Ionil-T®, and ketoconazole 2 per cent shampoo (Nizoral®). Topical steroids also reduce epidermal cell turnover, and low-dose (0.5 per cent) hydrocortisone cream can be used sparingly to treat small areas, such as the scalp and flexures. Aqueous creams are used, and bath emollients such as Aveeno®, Balneum® and Alpha Keri Bath® may be useful. Quinoderm Cream® (potassium hydroxyquinoline sulphate with benzoyl peroxide) is effective for facial folliculitis.

Diarrhoea

Diarrhoea is seen in most patients with symptomatic disease, during both early and late disease. Idiopathic diarrhoea due to an unknown cause is common during early symptomatic HIV disease, but diarrhoea can be caused by bacterial, protozoal, fungal and viral infections of the gut. Cryptosporidium and microsporidium are important protozoal infections that often cause severe diarrhoea associated with late symptomatic HIV disease (discussed later in this chapter). Other causes of diarrhoea include amoebiasis (caused by the protozoon *Entamoeba histolytica*) and giardiasis (caused by another protozoon, *Giardia lamblia*). These are not uncommon enteric infections in men who have sex with men (MSM), and the diarrhoea seen is generally less severe than that seen in cryptosporidiosis. Amoebiasis is treated with oral metronidazole (Flagyl®), tinidazole (Fasigyn®) or diloxanide furoate (Diloxanide®). Giardiasis is generally treated with metronidazole, tinidazole or mepacrine hydrochloride.

Other opportunistic microorganisms associated with diarrhoea in patients with early and late symptomatic HIV disease include *Shigella, Isospora belli, Helicobacter pylori (Campylo-bacter), Salmonella, Strongyloides stercoralis*, CMV and *Mycobacterium avium* complex (MAC). Kaposi's sarcoma may be an additional cause. Diarrhoea caused by isosporiasis is treated with co-trimoxazole (Septrin®), and metronidazole is sometimes used to treat idiopathic diarrhoea.

Diarrhoea is perhaps one of the most distressing complications of HIV disease, and often one of the most difficult to treat. If the causative agent can be identified, specific therapy may be used but, in all cases, supportive treatment and care are essential (Table 7.9).

Malnutrition/cachexia

The patient should be assessed by a dietician, and appropriate diet, dietary supplements and nutritional interventions implemented. This is discussed in greater detail in Chapter 17.

TABLE 7.9 Supportive treatment for patients with diarrhoea

- Anti-diarrhoeals, e.g. loperamide hydrochloride (Imodium®), diphenoxylate hydrochloride with atropine sulphate (Lomotil®) or codeine phosphate may be useful
- If diarrhoea is severe, an oral fluid and electrolyte replacement preparation, such as Rehidrat® or Dioralyte®, is beneficial
- Where this is not available, Oral Rehydration Salts (**ORS**) (World Health Organization formula) may be used or a home-made Oral Rehydration Therapy (**ORT**) solution can be made up with 8 teaspoons of sugar and 1 teaspoon of salt dissolved in 1 L of boiled water
- Intravenous rehydration may be necessary
- Nutritional assessment and support are needed
- Patients with chronic and severe diarrhoea require nursing assessment and appropriate assistance with activities of daily living

Late symptomatic disease (AIDS) (CDC Category C)

The AIDS-defining conditions associated with late symptomatic disease are described in Table 7.10 and are based on the 1987 and 1993 surveillance case definitions published by the CDC in the USA.[2,24] If these patients are not already receiving antiretroviral therapy, HAART is generally recommended during late symptomatic disease, even if their CD4+ T-cell count is over 200 cells/μL (mm³), irrespective of their plasma viral load level.[9-11] HAART is the most effective way to prevent the serious opportunistic events associated with late symptomatic disease.

TABLE 7.10 Late symptomatic disease (CDC Category C conditions) AIDS[2,24]

1. Lymphocytopenia – CD4+ T-lymphocyte cell count less than 200 cells/μL (mm³)
2. *Pneumocystis carinii* pneumonia
3. Candidiasis (of oesophagus, trachea, bronchi or lungs)
4. Cryptococcosis, extrapulmonary
5. Coccidiodomycosis (disseminated)
6. Toxoplasmosis of the brain
7. Cryptosporidiosis (with diarrhoea lasting for more than 1 month)
8. Isosporiasis (chronic intestinal, lasting for more than 1 month)
9. *Salmonella* septicaemia (salmonellosis)
10. Tuberculosis, pulmonary
11. *Mycobacterium avium* complex or *M. kansasii* disease
12. Cytomegalovirus disease (of an organ other than liver, spleen or lymph nodes) – includes cytomegalovirus retinitis
13. Herpes simplex virus infection (mucocutaneous ulcer persisting for more than 1 month; or bronchitis, pneumonitis or oeosophagitis)
14. Pneumonia, recurrent bacterial
15. Kaposi's sarcoma
16. HIV encephalopathy
17. Lymphoma of the brain (primary)
18. Progressive multifocal leucoencephalopathy (PML)
19. Cervical cancer (invasive)
20. HIV wasting syndrome

Lymphocytopenia

In 1992, the CDC revised the 1987 surveillance case definition for AIDS to include a CD4+ T-lymphocytopenia of less than 200 cells/μL (mm³). Consequently, even if an individual is well and does not have one of the symptomatic conditions listed in Table 7.10, he or she will still be diagnosed as having AIDS, because a T-cell lymphocytopenia of this degree is indicative of severe damage to the immune system and, although currently asymptomatic, the individual is extremely vulnerable to late stage symptomatic disease. These conditions are dominated by opportunistic infections. These infections are called opportunistic because they are caused by microorganisms that the body in health contains quite easily. However, in late symptomatic disease, these potential pathogens take the opportunity of a depressed immune system to flourish and establish overt disease. At this stage, people may be admitted to hospital due to one or more of these opportunistic infections.

Pneumocystis carinii pneumonia

Pneumocystis carinii pneumonia (PCP, also referred to as pneumocystosis) is not only the main presenting disease seen in AIDS in the industrially developed world, it is by far the most frequent cause of death in people with AIDS.[25] However, since the introduction of effective chemoprophylaxis for PCP in 1989, and the availability of HAART in most countries in the industrially developed world since the mid-1990s, the incidence of PCP has decreased.

The organism was first described in 1909 as a multiflagellate protozoon and was initially recognized as a human pathogen shortly after World War II, when it caused a fatal plasma cell pneumonia in severely malnourished refugee children. This microorganism is now known to be a fungus rather than a protozoon.[26–28] *P. carinii* is ubiquitous in nature everywhere in the world, infecting humans and a variety of other mammals, such as rabbits, mice, rats, ferrets and pigs. Because the various strains of *P. carinii* infecting different mammalian species are host specific, transmission of this microorganism from mammals to humans (zoonosis) probably does not occur.[29,30] The form of *P. carinii* that infects humans is probably transmitted from person to person by the respiratory route, and there is epidemiological evidence to show that exposure is universal and occurs in early life, with almost all children (in the USA) having specific antibody to this fungus by the age of 2 years.[31] In most people, infection is contained by normal immune mechanisms but remains latent, able to be reactivated should immunosuppression occur.

In the USA, the first case in an adult of pneumonia caused by *P. carinii* was observed in 1954. Until the present epidemic of HIV infection, PCP was only seen in patients whose immune system had been depressed by either a known primary or secondary cause, for example congenital immunodeficiency disorders, or in patients receiving chemotherapy for cancer or immunosuppressant drugs following transplant surgery. It is an important point for the nurse to note that PCP only occurs in immunocompromised individuals, hence hospital personnel and other patients who are not immunocompromised are not at risk of acquiring this disease.

Patients usually develop signs and symptoms insidiously, often giving a 3–4-week history of dry, non-productive cough, difficult or laboured breathing (dyspnoea), chest pain, fever and chills. Tachypnoea (rapid respirations) and cyanosis (a bluish appearance of the skin and mucous membranes) are usually present when the patient is seen in hospital. Patients frequently complain of not being able to take a deep breath. Some patients have a more fulminate course with a much shorter history and may be in acute respiratory failure and extreme distress.

Diagnosis of *P. carinii* pneumonia

The diagnosis of PCP may be difficult. A range of diagnostic tools (Table 7.11) is used to confirm PCP, and all the usual causes of pneumonia will need to be excluded (including tuberculosis) and sputum will need to be obtained for routine culture and sensitivity.

TABLE 7.11 Investigations for suspected *Pneumocystis carinii* pneumonia

- Chest X-ray
- Sputum induction
- Pulmonary function tests (arterial blood gases)
- Bronchoalveolar lavage (BAL)
- Imaging with standard computed tomography (CT) and high-resolution CT (HRCT)
- Serum level of lactate dehydrogenase (LDH)

Chest X-rays   Chest X-rays usually show alveolar and interstitial infiltrates in both the right and left lung fields (bilateral), and thin-walled cysts (pneumatoceles) may be seen.[32,33] However, these changes may be so mild as to be interpreted as normal in some patients.[32]

Sputum induction   Patients with PCP frequently have a dry, non-productive cough and are unable to produce an adequate specimen of sputum for microscopic examination. Consequently, a deep sputum specimen is induced after the patient has fasted throughout the night. To avoid contamination of the sputum specimen with oral debris, patients are asked to brush the buccal mucosa, tongue and gums with a wet toothbrush and rinse their mouths thoroughly with normal saline. Sputum is then induced by inhalation of 20–30 mL of 3 per cent saline through an ultrasonic nebulizer. Gentle chest percussion to aid expectoration is used when necessary and two sputum specimens are then taken promptly to the laboratory. Examination of sputum obtained in this manner can detect evidence of *P. carinii* infection in over 95 per cent of patients, consequently sparing them from bronchoscopy.[34] Prior to sputum induction, chest X-rays are needed to rule out pleural effusions. Sputum induction is contraindicated in a patient with a pleural effusion, as forceful coughing could fatally worsen the effusion.[35]

Sputum inductions are never carried out in an open ward or bay because of the infection risk to staff and other patients from the explosive coughing associated with this procedure. The infection prevention precautions associated with the procedure are described in Chapter 14, where a strategy for infection control and prevention is discussed.

Pulmonary function tests   Abnormalities of arterial blood gases (associated with hypoxaemia) are common. In one study, a partial pressure of arterial oxygen (PaO_2) lower than 80 mmHg or an alveolar–arterial partial pressure of oxygen difference (gradient) – $(A\text{-}a)DO_2$ – higher than 15 mmHg occurred in more than 80 per cent of patients with PCP.[36]

Bronchoalveolar lavage   If the induced sputum is negative, a bronchoalveolar lavage (BAL) of subsegmental bronchi is performed, a distressing procedure for patients with an already established respiratory impairment. Transbronchial or open lung biopsies, associated with significant complications such as bleeding, are now rarely performed.

Nursing staff need to wear protective clothing (a water-repellent, long-sleeved gown) and disposable rubber latex or good quality plastic vinyl gloves, and use an appropriate personal respiratory protection mask (particulate filter respirator) and eye protection when assisting with bronchoscopy. A 'dedicated' bronchoscope is not necessary. Following bronchoscopy, the bronchoscope is thoroughly cleaned and then immersed in 2 per cent glutaraldehyde for at least 1 hour (preferably 2 hours). This is adequate disinfection and the bronchoscope can then be used for any other patient without fear of transmitting HIV, *Mycobacterium tuberculosis* and non-tuberculous environmental mycobacteria, which are commonly associated with HIV disease.[37] Mycobacterial diseases and associated infection control precautions are discussed more fully in Chapters 8 and 14.

Imaging   Patients may be scanned for diagnostic purposes using standard computed tomography (CT) and high-resolution CT (HRCT).

Treatment of *P. carinii* pneumonia
There are a variety of drugs used in the treatment of acute PCP (Table 7.12) depending on the severity of the illness. The following discussion is based on current

TABLE 7.12 Drugs used in the treatment of acute *Pneumocystis carinii* pneumonia

Drug (non-proprietary title)	Route of administration
Mild to moderate episodes	
Co-trimoxazole (low dose) (trimethoprim-sulphamethoxazole)	By mouth
Atovaquone	By mouth
Dapsone	By mouth
Clindamycin with primaquine	By mouth
Aerosolized pentamidine isetionate	By inhalation
Moderate to severe episodes	
Co-trimoxazole (high dose) (trimethoprim-sulphamethoxazole)	By mouth or intravenous infusion
Pentamidine isetionate	Intravenous infusion
Trimetrexate°	Intravenous infusion
Plus	
Corticosteroids, e.g. oral prednisolone or parenteral methylprednisolone	

°Calcium folinate (calcium leucovorin) given orally or parenterally with trimetrexate.

recommendations[29,30,38–41] but, as these are continually revised, nurses need to check for updated guidelines (see 'Internet resources' at the end of this chapter).

Co-trimoxazole   Also known as **trimethoprim-sulphamethoxazole** (TMP-SMX), or Septrin®, this is the drug of choice for the treatment of PCP. It can be given in low-dose or high-dose regimens, orally or parenterally, depending upon the severity of the illness.

Although generally this drug is associated with fewer side effects than pentamidine, a high percentage of HIV-infected patients develop a drug fever, rash and significant leucopenia when treated with this compound. Co-trimoxazole for intravenous use is diluted in either 0.9 per cent sodium chloride or 5 per cent dextrose and is infused slowly. Care should be taken not to use intramuscular preparations intravenously. When given orally, nausea, vomiting and diarrhoea are not uncommon.

If patients develop a significant hypersensitivity to co-trimoxazole, other drugs will be used (Table 7.12), including pentamidine isetionate.

Pentamidine isetionate   During the first decade of the epidemic, pentamidine was the most common drug used for the treatment of PCP. Although still used, it has now been mostly superseded by co-trimoxazole and other drugs. It is administered intravenously or by inhalation through a special nebulizer. Deep intramuscular administration into the buttocks is now rarely employed, and intravenous administration of pentamidine is the preferred route of administration. However, intravenous infusions are administered under close supervision, as they have been associated with intractable hypotension. Direct bolus intravenous injection should be avoided whenever possible and never given rapidly.

Patients receiving pentamidine therapy should have their urine and blood glucose levels measured daily. Arterial blood pressure should be taken and recorded 4-hourly, unless unstable, when it should be taken more frequently. During intravenous administrations of pentamidine, the blood pressure should be taken every 15 minutes.

Aerosolized pentamidine   The use of aerosolized pentamidine is also used both in treating patients with PCP and as a prophylactic measure. Ultrasonic or jet nebulizers are used to deliver small particles (2–4 mm) of pentamidine into the alveoli. The patient is treated in a sitting position and then lying on each side (to increase upper lobe distribution of the drug). The pressure per square inch (psi) gas flow rate is determined by the nebulizer used, but 6 L/minute is usual. Aerosolized pentamidine should be administered in a room with good external ventilation, and nursing personnel must wear particulate filter respirators while caring for patients during this treatment.

Toxicity of pentamidine   Almost half of all patients receiving **intravenous pentamidine** experience grave systemic side effects, ranging from nephrotoxicity (with elevated creatinine levels), hypoglycaemia (and sometimes hyperglycaemia), disorders of blood clotting (such as thrombocytopenia), skin rashes and pruritus (severe itching), tachycardia and hypotension. The most frequent major adverse reaction to pentamidine is neutropenia, and other adverse reactions include hyponatraemia (salt depletion), abnormal liver function and azotaemia (excess urea and other nitrogenous compounds in the blood).

Intramuscular pentamidine administration is painful and frequently associated with sterile abscesses at the injection site. It is also associated with the same toxicity described for intravenous pentamidine. The use of **aerosolized pentamidine** avoids many of the systemic side effects associated with parenteral administration. There only a few side effects of aerosolized pentamidine, such as cough and bronchospasm, which can be treated with ipratropium bromide (Atrovent®). Aerosolized pentamidine therapy can be given on an outpatient basis and at home with the use of a special nebulizer.

Preventing *P. carinii* pneumonia

Respiratory isolation   Because *P. carinii* is transmitted from person to person by the airborne route,[30,42] it would seem sensible to isolate patients with PCP from other immuno-compromised HIV-infected patients, just as it would seem equally sensible to isolate any patient with an active respiratory infection from other immunologically vulnerable patients. However, the hard evidence to demonstrate the efficacy of isolating patients with PCP as standard practice in order to protect other patients is currently equivocal.

Chemoprophylaxis   HIV-infected adults and adolescents (including pregnant women and those on HAART) should receive chemoprophylaxis against PCP if they have a CD4+ T-lymphocyte count of less then 200 cells/μL (mm^3) or a history of oropharyngeal candidiasis. **Co-trimoxazole** (trimethoprim-sulphamethoxazole) is the preferred prophylactic agent and is usually prescribed as one or two 480 mg tablets daily or 960 mg three times weekly. This also confers protection against toxoplasmosis and some other common respiratory bacterial infections. If co-trimoxazole cannot be tolerated, dapsone, atovaquone or aerosolized pentamidine may be used.[39,40,43] Extrapulmonary pneumocystosis and pulmonary break-through infection with *P. carinii* can occur while patients are on prophylactic aerosolized pentamidine. A nursing assessment for patients on such therapy must incorporate a high index of suspicion for developing infections, and the patient's temperature should be taken on each visit.

Fungal diseases in late symptomatic disease

A variety of fungi often cause serious illness during late symptomatic HIV disease (Table 7.13).

TABLE 7.13 Opportunistic fungal diseases in late symptomatic HIV disease

Fungus	Disease
Candida albicans	Candidiasis (oesophageal)
Cryptococcus neoformans	Cryptococcosis
Coccidioides immitis	Coccidiodomycosis
Histoplasma capsulatum	Histoplasmosis
Aspergillus	Aspergillosis

Candidiasis

Oropharyngeal candidiasis (thrush) is common in early symptomatic disease and, as the immune system becomes further depressed, **oesophageal candidiasis** may occur during late symptomatic disease, with patients experiencing difficulty in swallowing (dysphagia), retrosternal pain on swallowing (odynophagia), and nausea. These symptoms make it difficult for patients to eat and drink and they may become severely malnourished. People who have these symptoms may be admitted to hospital for investigation such as endoscopy and/or intravenous chemotherapy.

Candida albicans is the most common fungal pathogen causing oesophageal disease in lay symptomatic HIV disease, but other fungi, viruses and bacteria may also cause this condition. Candidiasis may also occur in other sites, such as the trachea, bronchi or lungs in late symptomatic disease.

Treatment of oesophageal candidiasis   Topical antifungal agents, such as nystatin or amphotericin, are ineffective for treating oesophageal candidiasis, and oral or intravenous **systemic antifungal agents** (see Table 7.5) are used. Fluconazole, because of its lower toxicity and better absorption profile, is the drug of choice for treating this condition;[44] however, ketoconazole is less expensive and is often used initially.[45] The usual treatment duration is 7–14 days and nurses need to be aware of the important interactions between systemic antifungal agents and antiretroviral drugs (see Table 7.6).

Preventing candidiasis   Because of the cost and the danger to patients of developing resistant fungal strains, long-term chemoprophylaxis with systemic antifungal agents is rarely indicated.

Cryptococcosis

This is an important cause of illness in late symptomatic HIV disease for patients who develop primary infection following the inhalation of *Cryptococcus neoformans*, a ubiquitous unicellular fungus (yeast) found in soil, especially when contaminated with pigeon faeces, and also found in pigeon nests and window ledges soiled with pigeon droppings. Because of defective cell-mediated immune responses, pulmonary infection disseminates widely, especially to the central nervous system. Major clinical illnesses seen in late symptomatic HIV disease include subacute meningitis and meningoencephalitis and pulmonary cryptococcosis. Skin manifestations (cutaneous cryptococcosis) also frequently occur.

Patients with central nervous system involvement may present with a slowly developing meningitis or meningoencephalitis, especially complaining of headache, mild pyrexia and sometimes blurred vision. Other neurological signs and symptoms associated with meningitis may be seen, such as behavioural changes, changes in level of consciousness, and nausea and vomiting. However, a few patients may be relatively asymptomatic. When meningitis is suspected, a lumbar puncture is performed. Cryptococcal meningitis is diagnosed by culturing the organism from cerebrospinal fluid, sputum, urine and blood.[45,46]

Treatment The drugs used for treating this severe infection include amphotericin B, 5-flucytosine and fluconazole.

Preventing primary infection and relapse Fluconazole may be prescribed for preventing infection (primary prevention) in severely immunocompromised patients, although this is currently controversial as prolonged use of fluconazole for primary prevention may result in acquired resistance to this important drug.

Fluconazole (or weekly intravenous amphotericin B) chemoprophylaxis may be prescribed to prevent relapse in those patients who have recovered from cryptococcosis.[45,46]

Coccidiodomycosis

Coccidiodomycosis is another, often fatal, fungal disease that may occur during late symptomatic HIV disease. It is caused by *Coccidioides immitis*, a fungus that lives in desert soil and that is endemic to the south-western area of the USA (California, Arizona, parts of New Mexico and Texas), Central America and Argentina, where most long-term residents are infected. Visitors to these areas can also become infected by inhaling fungal spore-laden dust. Primary infection is often asymptomatic, but some people develop a self-limited illness (called valley fever) resembling influenza or acute bronchitis. HIV-infected and other immunosuppressed individuals may develop both pulmonary and extrapulmonary (disseminated) coccidiodomycosis, including meningitis in late symptomatic HIV disease.

Treatment Systemic antifungal drugs (see Table 7.5) are used to treat this condition, such as itraconazole or fluconazole. Seriously ill patients are usually treated with intravenous fluconazole or intravenous amphotericin B. Prolonged treatment may be necessary.

Other fungal diseases found in late symptomatic HIV disease

Although not AIDS-indicator diseases, both **histoplasmosis** and **aspergillosis** are commonly seen during late symptomatic disease.

Histoplasmosis

This condition is caused by *Histoplasma capsulatum*, a fungus found in bird and bat faeces (and found in caves where bats roost). Patients with either primary or secondary (reactivation) disseminated disease complain of fever and weight loss. Pulmonary disease resembles tuberculosis, and cutaneous manifestations are seen, such as oral lesions and a rash resembling folliculitis or molluscum.[45,46] Central nervous system involvement occurs and a few patients present with an acute hypotensive illness similar to septic shock.[46] The diagnosis is made by culturing the fungus from blood or other clinical specimens, chest X-ray and neurological assessment.

Treatment Itraconazole is the drug of choice for treating histoplasmosis;[45] amphotericin B can also be used. Relapse is common and long-term suppressive therapy with itraconazole is necessary.

Aspergillosis

This is a relatively rare illness, which may occur in late symptomatic HIV disease. It is caused by the spores of some *Aspergillus* species, ubiquitous fungi found mainly on decaying vegetation such as mouldy hay. Infection occurs when the fungal spores are inhaled. Patients usually develop pulmonary disease and sometimes central nervous system disease. The prognosis for patients with disseminated aspergillosis is grave.

Treatment   Therapy consists of either amphotericin B or itraconazole and, if the patient survives, long-term itraconazole suppressive therapy is needed.

Diseases caused by coccidian parasitic protozoa

A variety of parasitic protozoa which are members of the *Coccidia* family cause serious illnesses in late symptomatic HIV disease, including *Toxoplasma gondii*, *Cryptosporidium parvum* and *Isospora belli*.

Cerebral toxoplasmosis

Toxoplasmosis is caused by a small, obligate intracellular protozoan parasite, *Toxoplasma gondii*, which exists as three forms, all of which are potentially infectious to humans. Cats are the definitive (primary) source of *T. gondii*, but birds, some mammals and domestic animals can be infected from contact with cat faeces in the soil and then act as secondary hosts. Humans become infected when exposed to the parasite in cat faeces, for example from litter trays or gardening, or by eating undercooked, infected beef, lamb, pork or venison. Human infection is common and occurs worldwide.

People with competent immune systems who become infected are generally asymptomatic; the infection persists in a latent or quiescent state and does not cause any illness. However, should they become immunocompromised, for example due to HIV infection, malnutrition or other debilitating diseases, *T. gondii* infection can reactivate and cause serious, often life-threatening illnesses. In patients with HIV disease, primary or reactivation of latent *T. gondii* infection can cause a variety of clinical disorders, especially in the lungs, eyes and central nervous system. The most common illness in immunocompromised people with *T. gondii* infection is cerebral toxoplasmosis (**toxoplasmic encephalitis**).

Because infection is widespread throughout the brain, there can be a wide range of signs and symptoms associated with the development of toxoplasmic encephalitis (Table 7.14). The onset of illness is usually subacute and patients frequently present with confusion, headache, aphasia (difficulty with speech), hemiparesis and seizures. Patients often have an elevated temperature and are lethargic. The various signs and symptoms may resemble those seen in space-occupying lesions of the brain or those following stroke. The patient is seriously ill and can deteriorate with alarming speed.

Treatment is initiated following a presumptive diagnosis made on the basis of the clinical presentation and neuroradiologic findings, using CT and magnetic resonance imaging (MRI) scans. These scans typically show multiple, bilateral, contrast ring-enhancing lesions with surrounding oedema throughout the cerebral hemispheres in most patients with toxoplasmic encephalitis.[47] Brain biopsy may be needed in those patients who are unresponsive to treatment.

A variety of anti-*T. gondii* drugs can be used, but a combination of pyrimethamine with sulphadiazine or clindamycin is the treatment of choice.[48] Alternative agents include atovaquone, azithromycin, dapsone, co-trimoxazole, clarithromycin or injectable Fansidar® (pyrimethamine with sulfadoxine) for deeply comatose patients.[49,50] Folinic acid, given as

TABLE 7.14 Clinical presentation: toxoplasmic encephalitis

Fever

Headache

Disorientation and confusion

Seizures

Hemiparesis

Aphasia (difficulty in speaking)

Decrease in all forms of mentation (mental activity)

Lethargy

Coma

Vertigo and ataxia

Visual field loss

Behavioural and personality changes

Delusional behaviour and other psychiatric states

calcium folinate (calcium leucovorin), is generally given (usually orally, but it can also be given parenterally) to all patients receiving pyrimethamine in an attempt to prevent the serious bone marrow toxicity associated with the use of this agent, for example leucopenia, thrombocytopenia and anaemia. Corticosteroids are sometimes given to reduce cerebral oedema and may result in early clinical and radiological improvement. However, this may confuse the presumptive diagnosis and their use is generally discouraged.[49] Anticonvulsant drugs may be needed.

Preventing primary infection or relapse following treatment   All HIV-infected individuals should be tested for immunoglobulin G (IgG) antibody to *T. gondii* soon after the diagnosis of HIV infection in order to detect those with latent infection because they are potentially vulnerable to reactivation as their immune system becomes progressively compromised.[39]

The various sources of toxoplasmic infection should be discussed with all HIV-infected individuals, especially those negative for *T. gondii* IgG antibody. They should be advised not to eat raw or undercooked meat, particularly undercooked pork, lamb, beef or venison. They need to know that they must wash their hands thoroughly after any contact with raw meat, and after gardening or any contact with soil. They must also wash fruits and vegetables well before eating them raw. Precautions for pet cats (see Table 7.4) need to be observed, but people should be advised that they do not need to part with their cats or to have their cats tested for toxoplasmosis.[39,40]

Chemoprophylaxis   Because one in three patients with positive toxoplasma serology who have a CD4+ T-lymphocyte count of less then 100 cells/μL (mm³) will develop toxoplasmic encephalitis within 12 months without prophylaxis, all patients with CD4+ T-cell counts of less than 200 cells/μL (mm³) are commenced on primary chemoprophylaxis with either co-trimoxazole or dapsone with pyrimethamine.[48]

Cryptosporidiosis

Cryptosporidia are parasitic coccidian protozoa that replicate intracellularly in the brush border of the small intestine. Cryptosporidiosis occurs worldwide, most cases being caused by *Cryptosporidium parvum*. This microorganism is transmitted in faeces, from animals to humans (zoonotic spread), direct person-to-person contact, and via water contaminated with cryptosporidium. In immunocompetent people, it generally causes an acute, self-limited illness manifested by a watery diarrhoea and abdominal cramps, and sometimes fever, nausea and vomiting.

In HIV-infected people, cryptosporidiosis can be a catastrophic complication. The severity and duration of symptoms are related to the degree of immunosuppression, and patients with CD4+ T-lymphocyte counts of less then 200 cells/μL (mm³) may have profuse diarrhoea, ranging from three to four bowel movements a day to passing large amounts (10–12 L/day) of watery diarrhoea, becoming hypotensive and showing signs and symptoms of electrolyte imbalance. This wasting, weakening disease attacks not only the small bowel, but also the patient's self-esteem, potentially causing psychological havoc and poor quality of life.

The diagnosis is made by using special techniques of staining smears of stool specimens (three to six samples may be needed) or by biopsy of the small intestines or rectal mucosa if a presumptive diagnosis cannot be made by stool investigations.[51,52]

Treatment   At the present time, there is no specific therapy that is curative for this infection. Antiretroviral therapy (HAART) is associated with an improvement in cell-mediated immune functions and often with clinical improvement, remission of symptoms and, in some patients, clearance of cryptosporidium.[48,52] Supportive treatment for diarrhoea (see Table 7.9) will be needed.

Preventing cryptosporidiosis   The various ways that cryptosporidium can be transmitted should be discussed with HIV-infected people (Table 7.15), and an individualized strategy to avoid exposure and infection can be explored.

TABLE 7.15 Transmission potentials for *Cryptosporidium*

▪ Direct contact with infected adults, diaper-aged children and infected animals (especially farm animals)
▪ Drinking contaminated water
▪ Eating contaminated foods, e.g. raw oysters, and foods washed with contaminated water, such as salads
▪ Coming into contact with contaminated water during recreational activities, e.g. swimming
▪ Sexual practices that result in oral exposure to faeces
▪ Contact with infected young pets (dogs, cats)

HIV-infected people need to take care to wash their hands thoroughly after coming into contact with human or animal faeces, after gardening or any contact with soil, and after handling pets. Contaminated water is the most common means by which cryptosporidia are transmitted. Tap water is usually safe, but outbreaks of cryptosporidium contamination can occur, although they are rare in the UK. All brands of bottled water should not be presumed to be free of cryptosporidium. Boiling water for 1 minute during an outbreak will eliminate the risk for cryptosporidiosis. National brands of carbonated drinks, such as colas, and pasteurized beverages, including fruit juices, are safe. HIV-infected people should be advised not to swallow water while swimming. More detailed information can be found in the current online CDC guidelines (see 'Internet resources' at the end of this chapter) for preventing opportunistic infections in HIV-infected individuals.[39,40]

Preventing transmission of cryptosporidium in hospitals   Standard principles for preventing healthcare-associated infections are sufficient for minimizing the risk of cryptosporidium transmission in hospitals.[39,53,54] Gloves should be worn for any potential contact with faeces or any other body substance, and hands washed thoroughly after glove removal. Because of the risk of becoming exposed to cryptosporidium from contaminated inanimate objects (fomites), HIV-infected people, especially those who are severely immunocompromised, should not share a room with a patient who has cryptosporidiosis.[39]

Isosporiasis

Another coccidian protozoon, *Isospora belli*, is a cause of watery diarrhoea in many parts of the developing world and in some immunosuppressed HIV-infected people in late symptomatic disease. The onset is generally quite sudden and the patient may also experience fever, malaise and abdominal pain. In those with an intact immune system, isosporiasis often resolves spontaneously, but in HIV-infected people, the disease may persist for months or years if not treated.

Treatment for isosporiasis   Co-trimoxazole (Septrin®) is used for treatment and is effective in most individuals. Other drugs such as pyrimethamine, sulfadoxine, metronidazole or furazolidone may be used for patients who are intolerant of co-trimoxazole. Supportive measures for patients with diarrhoea (see Table 7.9) are important in the care of patients with this, often debilitating, illness.

Preventing relapse of isosporiasis   The preventative measures described for preventing crypto-sporidiosis are equally relevant to preventing isosporiasis. Following recovery from this condition, patients will require long-term **maintenance therapy** with co-trimoxazole (or one of the other drugs mentioned above) to prevent recurrences.

Other diseases caused by protozoal parasites

Cyclosporiasis

A coccidian protozoon very similar to *I. belli* is *Cyclospora cayetanensis*, a common cause of travellers' diarrhoea. This sometimes causes diarrhoea and gastrointestinal problems in HIV-infected people. Prevention and treatment are much the same as for isosporiasis.

Microsporidiosis

Microsporidia are an important group of spore-forming protozoan parasites that cause serious illness in HIV-infected people. Two species in particular are associated with illness during symptomatic HIV disease: *Enterocytozoon bieneusi* and *Encephalitozoon intestinalis* (also known as *Septata intestinalis*). When ingested, they uncoil in the lumen of the gastrointestinal tract, harpoon a host cell, and inoculate it with nucleated sporoplasm, following which intracellular division takes place. Mature spores then infect other cells or pass into the environment via faeces, urine or skin and have an oral–faecal route of transmission.

Infection causes a range of serious illnesses in late symptomatic HIV disease, including severe diarrhoea, hepatitis, peritonitis and renal and gall-bladder disease.

Treatment and prevention of microsporidiosis   Specific treatment to eradicate the parasite is unavailable, but albendazole, thalidomide or erythromycin may be used for symptomatic treatment. Patients may experience marked improvement when they are commenced on antiretroviral therapy, with subsequent improved immune functions.[51] The preventative measures described for cryptosporidiosis may be equally helpful in preventing microsporidiosis.

Salmonella septicaemia

The Salmonellae are members of the *Enterobacteriaceae*, a group of Gram-negative bacilli that normally reside in the intestinal tract of animals such as chickens, livestock and domestic pets (including turtles) and are transmitted to humans via the faecal–oral route. They cause a variety of serious illness (salmonellosis), including enteric fevers (such as typhoid fever) and gastroenteritis (for example food poisoning). Severely immunocompromised HIV-infected patients may have recurrent episodes of **bacteraemia** (septicaemia), a systemic condition in which the bacteria have infected the blood. Patients may present with fever, chills, sweats, weight loss and diarrhoea and be acutely ill.

Treatment for Salmonella *septicaemia*   Prolonged antimicrobial treatment is necessary and the antibiotics used include ciprofloxacin, co-trimoxazole and amoxicillin.

Preventing Salmonella *infection*   Everyone should ensure that foodstuffs potentially contaminated with *Salmonella*, such as poultry, meat and eggs, are safely handled and properly cooked, stored and refrigerated. Hands need to be washed thoroughly after handling any raw food, even eggs still in their shells. People with *Salmonella* gastrointestinal infection may continue to excrete organisms in their urine and faeces for varying lengths of time following antibiotic treatment and need to be scrupulous in washing their hands thoroughly after using the toilet. Nurses can use the guidance developed by the CDC (Table 7.16) to advise HIV-infected individuals on various ways in which they can avoid enteric bacterial infections.[39,40] In addition, safer sexual practices should be developed by all immunosuppressed individuals to protect against contact with potentially infected faeces and urine.

Pulmonary tuberculosis

One-third of the world's population is latently infected with *M. tuberculosis*, but most do not develop active pulmonary tuberculosis (TB) as a result of this infection. However, should they become immunocompromised, for example as a result of HIV infection, they may reactivate latent infection and develop active TB. Additionally, HIV-infected people have a much greater chance of progressing to active TB primary infection.[55,56] It is not surprising, therefore, that **TB is the most common opportunistic infection associated with symptomatic HIV disease** throughout the world.[57] Because of its importance, TB is discussed in detail in the following chapter.

Mycobacterium avium complex or *Mycobacterium kansasii* disease

A variety of non-tuberculosis (environmental) mycobacteria can cause both pulmonary and disseminated disease in late symptomatic HIV disease, the most notorious being *M. avium* complex. This generally occurs in end-stage HIV disease and is discussed in detail in the next chapter.

Human herpesvirus disease

In addition to shingles (caused by VZV) occurring in early symptomatic HIV disease, primary infection or reactivation of two other herpesviruses, **cytomegalovirus** (CMV or HHV5) and **herpes simplex virus** (HSV 1, 2 or HHV 1, 2), can cause serious illness in immunosuppressed people during late symptomatic HIV disease.

TABLE 7.16 Prevention of exposure to bacterial enteric infections[39,40]

Food

■ Advise HIV-infected individuals not to eat raw or undercooked eggs (including foods that might contain raw eggs, e.g. some preparations of hollandaise sauce, Caesar and certain other salad dressings, some mayonnaises, egg nog); raw or undercooked poultry, meat, seafood, such as Japanese sushi and especially raw shellfish; unpasteurized dairy products, unpasteurized fruit juices; and raw seed sprouts, e.g. alfalfa sprouts, mung bean sprouts

■ Poultry and meat are safest when adequate cooking is confirmed with a thermometer – internal temperature of 82 °C (180 °F) for poultry and 74 °C (165 °F) for red meats. If a thermometer is not used, the risk of illness can be decreased by only consuming poultry and meat that have no trace of pink colour. However, colour change of the meat, e.g. absence of pink, does not always correlate with internal temperatures.

■ All food produce should be washed thoroughly before being eaten.

■ Nurses should advise HIV-infected individuals to avoid cross-contamination of foods. Uncooked meats and their juices should not come into contact with other foods. Hands, cutting/chopping boards, knives and other utensils should be washed thoroughly after contact with uncooked foods.

■ Although the incidence of listeriosis in the UK is low, it is a serious disease that occurs with unusually high frequency among severely immunosuppressed HIV-infected individuals. HIV-infected people with a very low CD4[+] T-lymphocyte cell count who wish to reduce the risk of acquiring listeriosis as much as possible should be advised to:

  avoid soft cheeses, such as Feta, Brie, Camembert, blue veined Stilton and Danish blue (hard cheeses, processed cheese, cream cheese, cottage cheese or yoghurt need not be avoided);

  cook leftover foods or ready-to-eat foods until steaming hot before eating;

  avoid foods from delicatessen counters (such as prepared salads, meats, cheeses) or heat/reheat these foods until steaming hot before eating;

  avoid refrigerated pâté and other meat spreads (tinned or shelf-stable pâté and meat spreads need not be avoided);

  avoid raw or unpasteurized milk, including goat's milk, or milk-products, or foods that contain unpasteurized milk or milk-products.

Pets

■ When obtaining a new pet, HIV-infected people should avoid animals aged less than 6 months, especially those that have diarrhoea.

■ HIV-infected individuals should avoid contact with any animals that have diarrhoea. They should seek veterinary care for animals with diarrhoeal illness, and a faecal sample from such animals should be examined for *Cryptosporidium*, *Salmonella* and *Campylobacter*.

■ Any contact with pet faeces should be avoided and hands should be thoroughly washed after handling pets, especially before eating.

■ HIV-infected people should avoid all contact with reptiles, such as snakes, lizards, iguanas and turtles, because of the risk for salmonellosis.

Cytomegalovirus disease

CMV infection   As children and young adults, most of us will have been exposed to CMV, a common, airborne-spread group of viruses (salivary gland viruses). CMV infection may also occur transplacentally or during birth, and may also be acquired following blood transfusion (post-perfusion syndrome) or following organ or tissue transplantation.

Infection with CMV produces variable results. Congenitally acquired infection may be asymptomatic or cause abortion, stillbirth, postnatal death or severe central nervous system damage. Most children and adults who acquire this infection are asymptomatic, but a few may develop an acute febrile illness (CMV mononucleosis) or hepatitis. CMV is ubiquitous and 80 per cent of adults have been exposed to this virus group and have developed antibodies.[58] When infected with CMV, individuals will excrete this virus in urine, saliva, cervical secretions, semen, faeces and breast milk for several months. Eventually, the process of cell-mediated immunity contains the infection, the individual developing a latent infection and, in most cases, never being aware that he or she had been infected in the first place.

Like other latent viral infections normally contained by a competent immune system, in HIV disease, CMV infection may be reactivated as cell-mediated immunity becomes progressively compromised and may cause a variety of serious conditions, including chorioretinitis, oesophagitis, colitis, pneumonia and encephalitis. CMV-related diseases, like most other opportunistic diseases, have been less common since the introduction of antiretroviral therapy,[25] but still occur in severely immunosuppressed people.

CMV retinitis   Patients developing CMV retinitis may be asymptomatic or sometimes complain of seeing spots (called floaters) before one or both eyes, flashing lights and/or loss of peripheral vision. This condition is not associated with pain or photophobia.[59] Those who are at high risk of CMV retinitis, for example people with a CD4+ T-lymphocyte count of less then 50 cells/μL (mm³), and those with visual symptoms require routine ophthalmologic screening every 3 months.[60] Without early treatment, permanent and irreversible loss of vision will occur.

Treatment of CMV retinitis   The principal drugs licensed for the treatment of CMV retinitis are ganciclovir, foscarnet sodium and cidofovir (Table 7.17), but others are in development. They do not cure this condition, but can delay the rate of progression of CMV retinitis and subsequent visual loss. Following initial treatment, long-term maintenance anti-CMV therapy is necessary, probably for life.

Other CMV diseases   Patients with CMV-related **colitis** often have debilitating diarrhoea, fever, anorexia weight loss and abdominal pain. Patients with CMV **pneumonitis** complain of shortness of breath, dyspnoea on exertion and a non-productive cough. Finally, CMV neurological disease includes acute **ventriculoencephalitis**, patients presenting with lethargy, confusion and fever, and CMV **polyradiculopathy**, characterized by bowel and bladder incontinence and progressive flaccid lower limb paraplegia. The anti-CMV drugs described in Table 7.17 may all be used for these serious conditions associated with late symptomatic HIV disease.

Preventing CMV infection and disease   Because CMV is shed by infected people in semen, cervical secretions and saliva, safer sexual practices that include the male insertive partner using a good-quality intact latex rubber condom are helpful in preventing exposure and subsequent infection. Good hand hygiene helps prevent infection and is particularly important for HIV-infected people caring for infants and children who are frequently infected with CMV and shedding virus.

Oral ganciclovir is sometimes prescribed for chemoprophylaxis in CMV antibody-positive individuals who are severely immunosuppressed, for example those who have a CD4+ T-lymphocyte count of less then 50 cells/μL (mm³), and various regimens employing ganciclovir, foscarnet sodium and/or cidofovir are used for maintenance therapy to prevent a relapse following successful treatment for CMV disease.[39,40] Intra-ocular ganciclovir implants or repetitive intra-vitreous injections of ganciclovir, foscarnet sodium or cidofovir are also used to prevent relapse of CMV retinitis. Immune reconstitution with HAART is probably the most effective means by which CMV disease and relapse can be prevented.[40]

TABLE 7.17 Treatment of active cytomegalovirus (CMV) disease

Drug	Nursing note
Ganciclovir Cymevene® Intraocular implant Vitrasert®	Administered by intravenous infusion for initial (induction) phase, followed by oral capsules for maintenance therapy. May be given by intra-vitreal injection (directly into the eye); a sustained-release intraocular implant device (Vitrasert®) is also available. Not usually given with zidovudine, as these two drugs together cause a profound myelosuppression. Ensure adequate hydration during administration. Ganciclovir is a vesicant (causes blisters) and needs to be infused intravenously with a good flow rate via a plastic cannula. Not given during pregnancy or for neonatal or congenital CMV disease. Ganciclovir is toxic and nurses need to wear gloves and eye protection when handling and administering intravenous forms of this drug. If solution comes into contact with skin or mucosa, it needs to be washed off immediately with soap and water.
Foscarnet sodium Foscavir®	Administered by intravenous infusion. Causes renal impairment and is contraindicated during pregnancy and during breastfeeding. If given via a peripheral vein, may cause thrombophlebitis. Also causes genital irritation and ulceration due to the high concentration of the drug in urine.
Cidofovir Vistide®	Administered by intravenous infusion over 1 hour. Causes renal impairment and is contraindicated during pregnancy and during breastfeeding. Not recommended for children. Often given with probenecid (administered orally 3 hours before the cidofovir infusion) to raise serum levels and it is essential that prior hydration with intravenous fluids is given in order to minimize potential nephrotoxicity. This is usually accomplished by giving 1 L of sodium chloride 0.9% solution intravenously over 1 hour. If tolerated, an additional 1 L may be given over 1–3 hours, starting at the same time as the cidofovir infusion or immediately afterwards. Cidofovir is toxic and nurses need to wear gloves and eye protection when handling and administering intravenous forms of this drug. If solution comes into contact with skin or mucosa, it needs to be washed off immediately with soap and water.
Additional information	Further information on side effects can be found in the current issue of the *British National Formulary*, available online at: www.BNF.org

Herpes simplex virus infection

There are two types of herpes simplex virus (HSV): HSV-1 usually causes herpes labialis (cold sores), and HSV-2 generally causes genital herpes. Following primary infection, eruptions (small, tense blisters with an erythematous base) occur anywhere on the skin or mucosa, but generally around the mouth, on the lips, on the conjunctiva and cornea and on the genitalia. Healing generally occurs within 8–12 days, but HSV remains dormant in nerve ganglia and recurrent herpetic eruptions occur from time to time, with varying frequency in different individuals. Immunosuppressed HIV-infected people often experience more frequent recurrences of a greater severity than are usually seen in people with an intact immune system, and mucocutaneous lesions are less likely to resolve spontaneously.[61] Chronic mucocutaneous HSV lesions persisting for more than 1 month in HIV-infected people is an AIDS-defining illness.[2] These lesions can occur anywhere, but frequently involve the anogenital area, and bacterial superinfection is common.

HSV can also cause bronchitis, pneumonitis or oesophagitis, all AIDS-defining opportunistic conditions.

Treatment of HSV disease The antiviral drugs described in Table 7.7 are used for treating the often distressing lesions associated with chronic and severe recurrent HSV lesions. Cidofovir and foscarnet sodium are often used to treat aciclovir-resistant HSV disease. The nursing implications for these two agents are described in Table 7.17.

Preventing HSV disease   HIV-infected people should use good-quality, intact rubber latex condoms for every act of penetrative oral, vaginal or anal intercourse to reduce the risk of exposure to HSV and to other sexually transmitted pathogens. They should specifically avoid sexual contact when herpetic lesions (genital or orolabial) are evident.

Chemoprophylaxis with aciclovir for either primary or recurrent HSV infection is rarely used. However, for people who have frequent or severe recurrences, daily suppressive therapy with oral aciclovir, famciclovir or valaciclovir may be prescribed. Oral aciclovir prophylaxis during late pregnancy is controversial, but may be prescribed to prevent neonatal herpes transmission.[39] Like CMV disease, immune reconstitution with HAART is probably the most effective means to reduce the frequency of HSV recurrences.[40]

Pneumonia (recurrent bacterial)

People with HIV-related immunosuppression are at an increased risk of developing bacterial pneumonia. Recurrent episodes of bacterial pneumonia, that is, two or more episodes within a year, are common and this has become an AIDS-defining condition because multiple episodes of pneumonia are more strongly associated with immunosuppression than are single episodes. Although a variety of both Gram-positive and Gram-negative bacteria can cause pneumonia, especially in immunocompromised individuals, most bacterial pneumonia in HIV-infected people is caused by *Streptococcus pneumoniae* and a few other common bacterial pathogens (Table 7.18). Generally, Gram-negative bacterial pneumonia is more acute and immediately life threatening than pneumonia caused by Gram-positive bacteria. Infection usually occurs by inhalation, but sometimes pathogens are carried to the lungs by the bloodstream or they migrate to the lungs from a nearby focus of infection.

TABLE 7.18 Bacterial causes of pneumonia in HIV-infected people[62,63]

Streptococcus pneumoniae (pneumococcus)	Gram-positive
Haemophilus influenzae	Gram-negative
Staphylococcus aureus	Gram-positive
Pseudomonas aeruginosa	Gram-negative
Klebsiella pneumoniae	Gram-negative

Pneumonia usually develops suddenly over the course of a few days to a week, often preceded by an upper respiratory tract infection (URI). Patients will often experience a productive cough, sometimes haemoptysis, fever, chills, shaking, chest pain and dyspnoea. They are frequently seriously ill, requiring admission to hospital for aggressive medical interventions and nursing care. Bacteraemia and meningitis can also occur and, like bacterial pneumonia in HIV-infected individuals, are associated with significant mortality.

Pneumococcal pneumonia   Pneumonia caused by *Streptococcus pneumoniae* (often called the pneumococcus) is the most common type of pneumonia in all populations, including HIV-infected people, especially those who are severely immunocompromised. Benzylpenicillin (Penicillin G) is the standard treatment for hospitalized patients, most of whom will have penicillin-sensitive organisms. It is administered parenterally (i.e. intramuscularly), by slow intravenous injection or by intravenous infusion.

Amoxicillin is also used and oral phenoxymethylpenicillin (Penicillin V) is sometimes prescribed for patients who are not seriously ill. For those patients with penicillin-resistant organisms, second-generation cephalosporins, such as cefuroxime, are used.[62]

Preventing pneumococcal pneumonia   Preventing pneumococcal pneumonia is an important element of an overall strategy for managing patients with HIV disease. Patients receiving co-trimoxazole chemoprophylaxis for PCP or azithromycin or clarithromycin for MAC disease have a reduced incidence of pneumococcal pneumonia. Chemoprophylaxis for those who have very frequent recurrences of serious bacterial respiratory infections is sometimes prescribed, but physicians are cautious about doing this because of the risk for the development of drug-resistant microorganisms and drug toxicity.[39,40]

All patients should be vaccinated with a polyvalent pneumococcal polysaccharide vaccine (Pneumovax II®, Pnu-Imune®) as soon as possible after their HIV infection is diagnosed. The effectiveness of this vaccine is reduced in those with a CD4+ T-lymphocyte count of less then 200 cells/μL (mm³), so the earlier the vaccine is given in HIV infection, the better the chance will be that it will provide good protection.[62,63] Re-vaccination is rarely indicated.

Pneumococcal vaccination is recommended during pregnancy for HIV-infected women who have not been vaccinated during the previous 5 years. However, because the vaccine can cause a transient burst of HIV replication, concern exists about an increased risk for in-utero HIV transmission, and vaccination may be deferred until after antiretroviral therapy has been initiated to avoid perinatal HIV transmission.[39,40] The vaccine is not recommended for use in children under the age of 2 years, and vaccination is contraindicated during any acute infection. The vaccine is administered by subcutaneous or intramuscular injection, preferably into the deltoid muscle or lateral aspect of the mid-thigh. Intradermal injection may cause severe local reaction. The vaccine must not be given intravenously. It is administered as supplied; no dilution or reconstitution is necessary.[64]

Haemophilus influenzae pneumonia   HIV-infected people also have an increased incidence of pneumonia caused by *Haemophilus influenzae*, although it is not as common as pneumococcal pneumonia. *H. influenzae* is a Gram-negative bacterium that, despite its name, is not the cause of viral influenza (the 'flu'). Several strains (or types) of *H. influenzae* exist and those encapsulated strains containing the type b (Hib) polysaccharide capsule are the most virulent, able to cause serious diseases such as meningitis, epiglottitis and bacterial pneumonia, especially in children aged 1 year or younger. However, pneumonia in HIV-infected people is more frequently caused by non-typable strains (which limits the use of Hib vaccination). The signs and symptoms of pneumonia caused by *H. influenzae* are similar to those associated with pneumococcal pneumonia, except that bacteraemia is less common.[62] Blood and sputum cultures and sputum Gram stain microscopy are used to establish the diagnosis and drug sensitivity profile. Penicillin resistance is common, and second-generation or third-generation cephalosporins, doxycycline and co-trimoxazole are often prescribed.

Preventing H. influenzae pneumonia   Conjugate Hib vaccine is recommended in the UK as a component of the primary course of childhood immunization from the age of 2 months and it can be given to HIV-infected children.[64] Because the majority of strains that cause pneumonia are non-typable, and the incidence of type b infection in adults is low, Hib vaccine is not generally recommended for HIV-infected adults in the USA,[63] but is routinely used in some UK centres.[62]

Other bacterial pneumonias   Pneumonia caused by *Staphylococcus aureus* is more likely to be hospital acquired rather than acquired in the community. It is treated with co-trimoxazole (Septrin®) or ciprofloxacin.[63] Pneumonia caused by *Pseudomonas aeruginosa* generally occurs as a serious end-stage event in late symptomatic HIV disease in patients with a CD4+ T-lymphocyte count of less then 50 cells/μL (mm³). The diagnosis is made by blood culture and treatment is with parenteral (deep intramuscular or slow intravenous injection or intravenous infusion) antipseudomonal agents, such as piperacillin, ticarcillin and aztreonam.

Kaposi's sarcoma

Kaposi's sarcoma (KS) was a relatively unusual, vascular tumour, first described by an Austrian-Hungarian dermatologist, Moritz Kaposi, in 1872. In the USA and in Western Europe, KS was mainly seen in elderly men, especially those of Italian or Eastern European Jewish ancestry, and was relatively benign in its clinical course. Patients presented with discoloured patches, plaques or nodular skin lesions, brown, red or blue in colour, usually confined to the lower extremities (especially the ankles and soles of the feet). These lesions are the result of a multi-centric tumour arising from local hyperplasia of a cell of the vascular endothelium. Often, as the patients were in the age group 60–79 years, no specific treatment was indicated. This type of indolent, non-aggressive, non-invasive KS has become known as classic KS.

Another form of KS was known to exist in Equatorial Africa, where it was more common than the other forms of the tumour. Four different types of KS have been described in Africa, one of which is similar to classic KS, the remaining three being more aggressive, rapidly progressive neoplastic conditions, affecting young African men and often fatal within a year. This African form of KS is sometimes referred to as endemic KS.

Prior to 1981, a type of KS similar to the African endemic form was observed in renal patients following kidney transplant and iatrogenic immunosuppression. This too was aggressive, but responded well to the discontinuation of immunosuppression therapy and restoration of the patient to immune competence.

Kaposi's sarcoma in the era of HAART   At the beginning of the AIDS epidemic in the Western world in the late 1970s and early 1980s, KS was a frequent first manifestation of AIDS, for example in New York City between 1981 and 1983, it was the initial AIDS diagnosis in 50 per cent of non-injecting drug-using men who had sex with men.[65] Since those early years, with the advent of the widespread adoption of safer sexual practices and especially the introduction of HAART, the incidence of KS has continued to decline dramatically.

In patients with AIDS, an aggressive form of KS, similar to African endemic KS, was seen in young, previously healthy male homosexuals. This AIDS-associated KS became known as epidemic KS, and patients usually present with asymptomatic, pigmented skin lesions, usually red or violet-coloured nodules or papules that may be on any part of the body. The initial lesions are often multi-focal at the time of diagnosis, often involving visceral organs such as the lungs, liver, spleen and gastrointestinal tract, and rapidly disseminate, usually in an orderly fashion. Lesions frequently appear on the feet and the tip of the nose and can generally be identified in the mouth, especially on the hard palate.[66]

The role of HHV8   It is now known that infection with human herpesvirus type 8 is associated with the development of KS in HIV-infected people.[67,68] There are three major routes of HHV8 transmission: oral (the virus infects oral epithelial cells and infection has been associated with deep kissing in one study), via semen (HHV8 is less frequently detected in semen than in saliva), and through blood via needle sharing.[69-71] People who are co-infected with HIV and HHV8 are at risk of developing KS, and there is evidence that progression to KS may be accelerated in HIV-infected individuals who become infected with HHV8.

Treatment of Kaposi's sarcoma   Improving immune function by suppressing HIV replication with HAART has significantly improved treatment outcomes for patients with KS. Specific treatment approaches are developed for the early stages of KS and for more advanced stages.[65,66,72]

In **early KS**, asymptomatic cutaneous lesions are frequently treated for cosmetic reasons. A variety of approaches is used, including topical cryotherapy (using liquid nitrogen) and interlesional injections of vinblastine sulphate for small (less then 1 cm²) lesions, and radiotherapy for larger, symptomatic lesions. When vinblastine is used, it is diluted with 0.1–0.3 mL of sterile water using a tuberculin syringe. Injections may be painful and may have to be frequently repeated. A hyperpigmented area (brownish spots) frequently remains following treatment.

Patients with **advanced** or **visceral KS** are treated with radiotherapy or systemic chemotherapy. Radiotherapy is used for large skin lesions or lesions in the mouth, and chemotherapy is used in advanced visceral disease. In the UK, a regimen of intravenous bleomycin and vincristine is frequently used for **first-line treatment**, for example both drugs being given by slow intravenous injection every 2 weeks. Slow intravenous injections of hydrocortisone may also be incorporated into the regimen to prevent the hypersensitivity reactions caused by bleomycin.[72]

Regimens using newer anti-neoplastic agents are now being routinely used in the treatment of advanced KS and include paclitaxel (Taxol®) and liposomal anthracyclines such as liposomal doxorubicin HCl (Caelyx®) and liposomal daunorubicin (DaunoXome®). These agents are administered by intravenous infusion and are now being used more commonly as first-line therapy in advanced KS.[65] Oral etoposide (Vepesid®) may also be used.[65] Newer approaches to treatment may include the development of specific anti-HHV8 agents, and a variety of other anti-neoplastic agents are currently undergoing trials.

Because of the complexities of the side effects and drug interactions of the various anti-neoplastic agents used, nurses caring for patients being treated for KS need to ensure they have access to up-to-date drug information, such as the current *British National Formulary*, and other web-based resources, for example www.aidsmap.com (see 'Internet resources' at the end of this chapter).

Preventing Kaposi's sarcoma   People who are co-infected with HIV and HHV8 are at risk of developing KS and there is evidence that progression to KS may be accelerated in HIV-infected individuals who become infected with HHV8.[73-75] Physicians may test patients for HHV8 infection to identify those at risk for KS and suitable for chemoprophylaxis with future antiviral drugs. Immune reconstitution by the use of HAART may delay the onset of KS in co-infected people.[39,40]

Patients who are not infected with HHV8 should be counselled on sexual and injecting-drug-using risk reduction techniques. They need to be advised that deep kissing and sexual intercourse with individuals who have a high risk of being infected with HHV8, such as people who have KS or who are infected with HIV, may lead to they themselves becoming infected with HHV8. Condoms for each and every episode of penetrative sexual intercourse (vaginal, anal and oral) may prevent the acquisition of HHV8 (and other sexually transmitted pathogens). Injecting-drug users should be advised never to share drug injection equipment, even if both users are already infected with HIV, because of the risk of becoming infected with HHV8.[39,40]

HIV encephalopathy

This condition, also known as (UK) HIV-associated dementia or (USA) the AIDS dementia complex (ADC), develops in late symptomatic HIV disease and consists of a collection of various motor, cognitive and behavioural signs and symptoms that characterize it as a subcortical dementia. This is perhaps one of the most distressing conditions associated with HIV disease and is discussed in detail in Chapter 9, where other HIV-associated neurological issues are explored.

Lymphoma of the brain

Primary central nervous system lymphomas also occur in late symptomatic HIV disease in individuals with severe CD4+ T-lymphocytopenia. Patients with this condition have focal central nervous system signs and symptoms related to a space-occupying lesion. Like HIV encephalopathy, this grave condition is discussed in detail in Chapter 9.

Progressive multifocal leucoencephalopathy

Like cerebral toxoplasmosis and primary central nervous system lymphoma, progressive multifocal leucoencephalopathy (PML) is the third most important cause of focal central nervous system disease in late symptomatic HIV disease. PML is caused by primary or reactivation of latent JC virus infection. This is an unusual type of papovavirus that was first isolated in 1971 in a patient with PML and subsequently named the JC virus after his initials. The prognosis is poor and this condition is also reserved for discussion in Chapter 9.

Cervical cancer (invasive)

The incidence of cervical intraepithelial neoplasia in HIV-infected women increases as the CD4+ T-lymphocyte cell count falls and immune function progressively weakens. Cervical cancer in HIV-infected women is more extensive and more difficult to cure than that in women not infected with HIV, and cancer frequently recurs following treatment. This condition is discussed in Chapter 11, where the impact of HIV infection on women is explored.

Wasting syndrome

Involuntary weight loss (wasting) frequently occurs during both early and late symptomatic disease. A 10 per cent loss of body weight in the absence of current infection or any other identifiable cause of weight loss constitutes the clinical syndrome known as the wasting syndrome. This syndrome and other nutritional issues are discussed in Chapter 17.

Summary: HIV disease as a journey

Becoming infected with HIV can be viewed as analogous to buying a one-way ticket on a train that terminates in a station called AIDS (Figure 7.2).

On the journey, the train stops at various stations, i.e. the stages of HIV disease. Once the train gets to one of these stations, it can never turn back. The first station the train arrives at is one known as **Station A**, or primary HIV infection. Here, a range of experiences awaits the passenger, from asymptomatic infection, to persistent generalized lymphadenopathy (PGL), to an acute retroviral seroconversion illness. As the train slowly moves on, it eventually

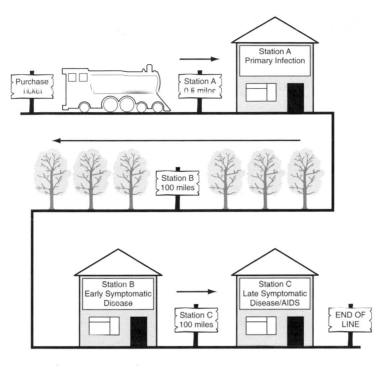

FIGURE 7.2 *The journey from primary HIV infection to AIDS.*

arrives at the second major station, known as **Station B** or early symptomatic disease. By this time, the passenger is tired and worn down from the effects of this long journey. He or she will start to feel unwell and will experience a variety of conditions associated with the stress of the journey. Persevering, the passenger continues the journey and, as the train speeds up, finally arrives at the final destination, **Station C**, also known as late symptomatic disease or **AIDS**. By this time, the passenger is frail, frightened, profoundly unwell and experiencing a range of opportunistic infections and cancers that, without medical and nursing intervention, will ultimately be life threatening.

In assessing the progress of passengers (patients), we can quickly discover where they are on this journey, exactly which station they have arrived at. We are then able to describe more precisely the degree of immune system damage they have incurred on the journey and assist them in making informed decisions in relation to treatment and care. This assessment information is structured within a case definition and classification system, such as the CDC Surveillance Classification System[2] or the system for developing world countries proposed by the World Health Organization (WHO) and the Joint United Nations Programme on AIDS (UNAIDS).[76]

CDC classification system for HIV infection

In the early years of the pandemic, the CDC in the USA developed a case definition for AIDS for surveillance purposes and, since then, it has been revised several times. The current AIDS Surveillance Case Definition for Adolescents and Adults was published in December 1992, to take effect from 1 January 1993 (Table 7.19).[2] The case definition provides a classification

TABLE 7.19 1993 revised classification system for HIV infection and expanded surveillance case definition for AIDS among adults and adolescents[2]

CD4 cell count	Clinical Category A	Clinical Category B	Clinical Category C
1. ≥500 cells/mm³	A1	B1	C1
2. 200–499 cells/mm³	A2	B2	C2
3. <200 cells/mm³	A3	B3	C3

Category A Conditions	Category B Conditions	Category C Conditions
■ No symptoms ■ Acute HIV infection (resolves) ■ Generalized lymphadenopathy	■ Bacillary angiomatosis ■ Oropharyngeal candidiasis ■ Vulvovaginal candidiasis: persistent, frequent, or poorly responsive to therapy ■ Cervical intraepithelial neoplasia II or III ■ Constitutional symptoms: fever, diarrhea >1 month ■ Oral hairy leucoplakia ■ Herpes zoster: multiple episodes or involving >1 dermatome ■ Idiopathic thrombocytopenic purpura ■ Listeriosis ■ Pelvic inflammatory disease: particularly if complicated by tubo-ovarian abscess ■ Peripheral neuropathy	■ Candidiasis of bronchi, trachea, lungs or oesophagus ■ Invasive cervical cancer ■ Coccidioidomycosis, disseminated or extrapulmonary ■ Cryptococcosis, extrapulmonary ■ Cryptosporidiosis (intestinal infection >1 month duration) ■ Cytomegalovirus disease (excluding liver, spleen or lymph nodes) ■ HIV-related encephalopathy ■ Herpes simplex: chronic ulcer >1 month duration, or bronchitis, pneumonitis or oesophagitis ■ Histoplasmosis: disseminated or extrapulmonary ■ Isosporiasis: >1 month duration ■ Kaposi's sarcoma ■ Burkitt's lymphoma ■ Immunoblastic lymphoma ■ Primary lymphoma of the brain ■ *Mycobacterium avium* complex or *M. kansasii*: disseminated or extrapulmonary ■ *M. tuberculosis*: any site ■ *Mycobacterium*: other species or unknown species, disseminated or extrapulmonary ■ *Pneumocystis carinii* pneumonia ■ Recurrent pneumonia ■ Progressive multifocal leucoencephalopathy ■ *Salmonella* septicaemia, recurrent ■ Toxoplasmosis of the brain ■ Wasting syndrome due to HIV

Source: CDC, 1992.[2]

system for grouping patients infected with HIV according to the clinical expression of their disease, but only defines a limited number of specified clinical presentations.

The revised CDC classification system for HIV-infected adolescents and adults categorizes people on the basis of clinical conditions associated with HIV infection and CD4+ T-lymphocyte cell counts. The system is based on three ranges of CD4+ T-lymphocyte counts and three clinical categories and is represented by a matrix of nine mutually exclusive categories (Table 7.20). This system replaces earlier classification systems which included

TABLE 7.20 1993 revised classification system for HIV infection and expanded AIDS surveillance case definition for adolescents and adults

	Clinical categories		
CD4⁺ T-cell categories	(A) Asymptomatic, acute (primary) HIV or PGL	(B) Symptomatic, not (A) or (C) conditions	(C) AIDS-indicator conditions
(1) ≥500/µL	A1	B1	**C1**
(2) 200–499/µL	A2	B2	**C2**
(3) <200/µL AIDS-indicator T-cell count	**A3**	**B3**	**C3**

Bold type, i.e. A3, B3 and C1–3, indicates an AIDS diagnosis.
PGL, persistent generalized lymphadenopathy.

only clinical disease criteria and which were developed before the widespread use of CD4⁺ T-lymphocyte testing.

WHO clinical staging system for HIV infection and AIDS

In 1993, the WHO proposed a clinical staging system for HIV infection and disease, very similar to the CDC 1993 case definition but principally based on clinical criteria. This staging system has been refined (Table 7.21) and may now be used for making antiretroviral treatment decisions in resource-limited settings, with or without laboratory assessments of CD4⁺ T-lymphocyte levels.[76]

TABLE 7.21 WHO staging system for HIV infection and disease in adults and adolescents, 2002[76]

Clinical stage I

1. Asymptomatic
2. Persistent generalized lymphadenopathy

Performance scale 1: asymptomatic, normal activity

Clinical stage II

3. Weight loss <10% of body weight
4. Minor mucocutaneous manifestations (seborrhoeic dermatitis, prurigo, fungal nail infections, recurrent oral ulcerations, angular cheilitis)
5. Herpes zoster within the last 5 years
6. Recurrent upper respiratory tract infections (i.e. bacterial sinusitis)

And/or performance scale 2: symptomatic, normal activity

Clinical stage III

7. Weight loss >10% of body weight
8. Unexplained chronic diarrhoea >1 month
9. Unexplained prolonged fever (intermittent or constant) >1 month
10. Oral candidiasis (thrush)
11. Oral hairy leucoplakia
12. Pulmonary tuberculosis within the past year
13. Severe bacterial infections (i.e. pneumonia, pyomyositis)

And/or performance scale 3: bedridden <50% of the day during the last month

TABLE 7.21 – continued

Clinical stage IV

14. HIV wasting syndrome, as defined by the Centers for Disease Control and Prevention[a]

15. *Pneumocystis carinii* pneumonia

16. Toxoplasmosis of the brain

17. Cryptosporidiosis with diarrhoea >1 month

18. Cryptococcosis, extrapulmonary

19. Cytomegalovirus disease of an organ other than liver, spleen or lymph nodes

20. Herpes simplex virus infection, mucocutaneous >1 month or visceral any duration

21. Progressive multifocal leucoencephalopathy

22. Any disseminated endemic mycosis (i.e. histoplasmosis, coccidioidomycosis)

23. Candidiasis of the oesophagus, trachea, bronchi or lungs

24. Atypical mycobacteriosis, disseminated

25. Non-typhoid *Salmonella* septicaemia

26. Extrapulmonary tuberculosis

27. Lymphoma

28. Kaposi's sarcoma

29. HIV encephalopathy, as defined by the Centers for Disease Control and Prevention[b]

And/or performance scale 4: bedridden >50% of the day during the last month

Note. Both definitive and presumptive diagnoses are acceptable.

[a] HIV wasting syndrome: weight loss of >10% of body weight, plus either unexplained chronic diarrhoea (>1 month) or chronic weakness and unexplained prolonged fever (>1 month).

[b] HIV encephalopathy: clinical findings of disabling cognitive and/or motor dysfunction interfering with activities of daily living, progressive over weeks to months, in the absence of a concurrent illness or condition other than HIV infection which could explain the findings.

Prologue to Chapter 8

Because tuberculosis is the most common opportunistic infection associated with HIV infection, the next chapter explores this, the oldest of human diseases, within the context of symptomatic HIV disease. Subsequent chapters discuss the neurological and nutritional aspects of HIV disease and also the special features of HIV disease in women and children.

REFERENCES

1. D'Souza MP, Fauci AS. Immunopathogenesis. In: Merigan TC, Bartlett JG, Bolognesi D (eds), *Textbook of AIDS Medicine*, 2nd edn. Baltimore: Williams & Wilkins, 1999, 59–85.

2. Centers for Disease Control and Prevention (CDC). 1993 Revised Classification System for HIV Infection and Expanded Surveillance Case Definition for AIDS Among Adolescents and Adults. *Morbidity and Mortality Weekly Report (MMWR)* 18 December 1992; **RR-17**:1–19.

3. Kilby JM, Saag MS. Natural history of HIV-1 disease. In: Merigan TC, Bartlett JG, Bolognesi D (eds), *Textbook of AIDS Medicine*, 2nd edn. Baltimore: Williams & Wilkins, 1999, 49–58.

4. Pedersen C, Lindhardt BO, Jensen BL et al. Clinical course of primary HIV infection: consequences for subsequent course of infection. *British Medical Journal* 1989; **299**:154–7.

5. Mindel A, Tenant-Flowers M. ABC of AIDS: natural history and management of early HIV infection. *British Medical Journal* 2001; **322**:1290–3.

6. Vanhems P, Allard R, Cooper DA et al. Acute HIV-1 disease as a mononucleosis-like illness: is the diagnosis too restrictive? *Clinical Infectious Diseases* 1997; **24**:965.

7. Carr A, Cooper DA. Primary HIV infection. In: Sande MA, Volberding PA (eds), *The Medical Management of AIDS*, 6th edn. Philadelphia: W.B. Saunders Co., 1999, 67–78.

8. Hirsch MS, Brun-Vézinet F, D'Aquila RT et al. Antiretroviral drug resistance testing in adult HIV-1 infection. Recommendations of an International AIDS Society Panel. *Journal of the American Medical Association* 2000; **238**:2417–26.

9. Centers for Disease Control and Prevention. Guidelines for the Use of Antiretroviral Agents in HIV-Infected Adults and Adolescents. February 5, 2001 (includes 23 April 2001 Updates). Living Document available online at: http://www.aidsinfo.nih.gov

10. British HIV Association. Guidelines for the Treatment of HIV-infected Adults with Antiretroviral Therapy. October 2001. Available online at: http://www.aidsmap.com

11. Weller IVD, Williams IG. ABC of AIDS: antiretroviral drugs. *British Medical Journal* 2001; **322**:1410–12.

12. Koehler JE, Sanchez MA, Garrido CS et al. Molecular epidemiology of *Bartonella* infections in patients with bacillary angiomatosis-peliosis. *New England Journal of Medicine* 1997; **337**:1876.

13. Koehler JE. Bacillary angiomatosis and other unusual infections in HIV-infected individuals. In: Sande MA, Volberding PA (eds), *The Medical Management of AIDS*, 6th edn. Philadelphia: W.B. Saunders Co., 1999, 411–28.

14. Greenspan JS, Greenspan D. Oral manifestations of HIV infection and AIDS. In: Merigan TC, Bartlett JG, Bolognesi D (eds), *Textbook of AIDS Medicine*, 2nd edn. Baltimore: Williams & Wilkins, 1999, 521–35.

15. Safrin S, Berger TG, Gilson I et al. Foscarnet therapy in five patients with AIDS and aciclovir-resistant varicella-zoster virus infection. *Annals of Internal Medicine* 1991; **115**:19. As cited in Greenspan JS, Greenspan D. Oral manifestations of HIV infection and AIDS. In: Merigan TC, Bartlett JG, Bolognesi D (eds), *Textbook of AIDS Medicine*, 2nd edn. Baltimore: Williams & Wilkins, 1999, 521–35.

16. UK Departments of Health: Salisbury DM, Begg NT (eds). *1996 Immunisation against Infectious Disease*. London: Stationery Office, p.290. Available from: The Stationery Office Ltd, PO Box 29, Norwich NR3 1GN, UK; e-mail customer.services@theso.co.uk or telephone 0870 600 5522, fax 0870 600 5533.

17. Doweiko JP. Hematologic manifestations of HIV infection. In: Merigan TC, Bartlett JG, Bolognesi D (eds), *Textbook of AIDS Medicine*, 2nd edn. Baltimore: Williams & Wilkins, 1999, 611–27.

18. Hambleton J. Hematologic complications of HIV infection. In: Sande MA, Volberding PA (eds), *The Medical Management of AIDS*, 6th edn. Philadelphia: W.B. Saunders Co., 1999, 265–73.

19. MacGowan AP. Coryneform bacteria and listeria. In: Greenwood D, Slack R, Peutherer J (eds), *Medical Microbiology: A Guide to Microbial Infections: Pathogenesis, Immunity, Laboratory Diagnosis and Control*, 14th edn. London: Churchill Livingstone, 1992, 231–40.

20. Wilson J. *Clinical Microbiology: An Introduction for Healthcare Professionals*, 8th edn. London: Baillière Tindall, 2000, 160–1.

21. Department of Health. ML/CMO (89)3 and Press Release 89/369. *Statement of Advice on Listeria and Food*. London: Department of Health, 1988.

22. Abularach S, Anderson JR. Gynecologic problems. In: Anderson JR (ed.), *A Guide to the Clinical Care of Women with HIV*. US Department of Health and Human Services, 2001, 197–212. Available online at: http://www.hab.hrsa.gov/

23. Shlay JC, Chaloner K, Max MB et al. Acupuncture and amitriptyline for pain due to HIV-related peripheral neuropathy: a randomized controlled trial. *Journal of the American Medical Association* 1998; **280**:1590–5.

24. Centers for Disease Control and Prevention (CDC). Revision of the CDC Surveillance Case Definition for Acquired Immunodeficiency Syndrome. *Morbidity and Mortality Weekly Report (MMWR)* 14 August 1987; **36**:1S.

25. Jones JL, Hanson DL, Dworkin MS et al. Surveillance for AIDS-defining opportunistic illnesses, 1992–1997. *Morbidity and Mortality Weekly Report (MMWR)* 16 April 1999; **48**(SS-2):1–22.

26. Edman JC, Kovacs JA, Masur H et al. Ribosomal RNA sequence shows *Pneumocystis carinii* to be a member of the fungi. *Nature* 1988; **334**:519–22.

27. Pixley FJ, Wakefield AE, Banerji S et al. Mitochondrial gene sequences show fungal homology for *Pneumocystis carinii*. *Molecular Microbiology* 1991; **5**:1347–51.

28. Walzer PD. Editorial review: *Pneumocystis carinii*: recent advances in basic biology and their clinical application. *AIDS* 1993; **7**:1293–305.

29. Huang L, Stansell JD. *Pneumocystis carinii* pneumonia. In: Sande MA, Volberding PA (eds), *The Medical Management of AIDS*, 6th edn. Philadelphia: W.B. Saunders Co., 1999, 305–30.

30. Dubé MP, Sattler FR. *Pneumocystis carinii* pneumonia. In: Merigan TC, Bartlett JG, Bolognesi D (eds), *Textbook of AIDS Medicine*, 2nd edn. Baltimore: Williams & Wilkins, 1999, 191–224.

31. Meuwissen JHE, Tauber I, Leewenbert ADEM et al. Parasitologic and serologic observations of infection with *Pneumocystis* in humans. *Journal of Infectious Diseases* 1977; **136**:43–9.

32. Opravil M, Marincek B, Fuchs WA et al. Shortcomings of chest radiography in detecting *Pneumocystis carinii* pneumonia. *Journal of Acquired Immune Deficiency Syndromes* 1994; **7**:39–45.

33. Sandhu JS, Goodman PC. Pulmonary cysts associated with *Pneumocystis carinii* pneumonia in patients with AIDS. *Radiology* 1989; **173**:33.

34. Leigh TR, Parsons P, Hume C et al. Sputum induction for diagnosis of *Pneumocystis carinii* pneumonia. *Lancet* 1989; **ii**:205–6.

35. Nelson M, Bower M, Smith D, Gazzard BG. Life-threatening complication of sputum induction (correspondence). *Lancet* 1990; **335**:112–13.

36. Katz MH, Baron RB, Grady D. Risk stratification of ambulatory patients suspected of *Pneumocystis* pneumonia. *Archives of Internal Medicine* 1991; **151**:105–10.

37. Ayliffe GAJ, Coates D, Hoffman PN. *Chemical Disinfection in Hospitals*, 2nd edn. London: Public Health Laboratory Service (PHLS), 1993.

38. Alcorn K (ed.). *HIV & AIDS Treatments Directory*, 22nd edn. London: National AIDS Manual (NAM) Publications, December 2002.

39. Centers for Disease Control and Prevention. 1999 USPHS/IDSA guidelines for the prevention of opportunistic infections in persons infected with human

immunodeficiency virus: US Public Health Service (USPHS) and Infectious Diseases Society of America (IDSA). *Morbidity and Mortality Weekly Report (MMWR)* 20 August 1999; **48**(RR-10):1–66.

40. Centers for Disease Control and Prevention. 2001 [draft] USPHS/IDSA guidelines for the prevention of opportunistic infections in persons infected with human immunodeficiency virus: US Public Health Service (USPHS) and Infectious Diseases Society of America (IDSA). Living Document available online from: http://aidsinfo.nih.gov/guidelines/, cited March 2003.

41. Mehta DK (Executive Editor). *British National Formulary (BNF)*, No. 45. London: British Medical Association and the Royal Pharmaceutical Society of Great Britain, 2003.

42. Hughes WT, Bartley DL, Smith BM. A natural source of infection due to *Pneumocystis carinii*. *Journal of Infectious Diseases* 1983; **147**:595.

43. Gazzard B (ed.). *Chelsea & Westminster Hospital AIDS Care Handbook*. London: Mediscript Ltd Medical Publishers, 1999.

44. Dieterich DT, Poles MA, Cappell MS, Lew EA. Gastrointestinal manifestations of HIV disease, including the peritoneum and mesentery. In: Merigan TC, Bartlett JG, Bolognesi D (eds), *Textbook of AIDS Medicine*, 2nd edn. Baltimore: Williams & Wilkins, 1999, 537–65.

45. Cartledge J. Fungal infections. In: Gazzard B (ed.), *Chelsea & Westminster Hospital AIDS Care Handbook*. London: Mediscript Ltd Medical Publishers, 1999, 57–64.

46. Powderly WG. Fungi. In: Merigan TC, Bartlett JG, Bolognesi D (eds), *Textbook of AIDS Medicine*, 2nd edn. Baltimore: Williams & Wilkins, 1999, 357–71.

47. Liesenfeld O, Wang SY, Remington JS. Toxoplasmosis in the setting of AIDS. In: Merigan TC, Bartlett JG, Bolognesi D (eds), *Textbook of AIDS Medicine*, 2nd edn. Baltimore: Williams & Wilkins, 1999, 225–59.

48. Weller IVD, Williams IG. ABC of AIDS: treatment of infections. *British Medical Journal* 2001; **322**:1350–4.

49. Subauste CS, Remington JS. AIDS-associated toxoplasmosis. In: Sande MA, Volberding PA (eds), *The Medical Management of AIDS*, 6th edn. Philadelphia: W.B. Saunders Co., 1999, 379–98.

50. Sadler M. Colonizing tumours of the brain. In: Gazzard B (ed.), *Chelsea & Westminster Hospital AIDS Care Handbook*. London: Mediscript Ltd Medical Publishers, 1999, 161–82.

51. Gazzard B. Weight loss and diarrhoea. In: Gazzard B (ed.), *Chelsea & Westminster Hospital AIDS Care Handbook*. London: Mediscript Ltd Medical Publishers, 1999, 201–14.

52. Soave R, Didier ES. Intestinal parasitic infections: cryptosporidiosis and microsporidiosis. In: Merigan TC, Bartlett JG, Bolognesi D (eds), *Textbook of AIDS Medicine*, 2nd edn. Baltimore: Williams & Wilkins, 1999, 327–55.

53. Pratt RJ, Pellowe C, Loveday HP et al. The Epic Project: developing national evidence-based guidelines for preventing healthcare-associated infections. Phase 1: Guidelines for preventing hospital-acquired infections. *Journal of Hospital Infection* 2001; **47**(Suppl.):S1–82. Available from: http://www.doh.gov.uk/hai/epic.htm

54. Loveday HP, Pellowe C, Harper P, Robinson N, Pratt R. The Epic Project: developing national evidence-based guidelines for preventing healthcare-associated infections. Guidelines for standard principles for the prevention of hospital-acquired infection. *Nursing Times* 2001; **97**:36–7.

55. World Health Organization. *Tuberculosis,* Fact Sheet No. 104, April 2000. Geneva: WHO. Available (Internet): http://www.who.int/

56. Centers for Disease Control and Prevention. *TB Elimination: Now is the Time,* 2001 (cited March 2001). Available online from: www.cdc.gov/nchstp/tb/

57. World Health Organization. *Global Tuberculosis Control. WHO Report 2001.* WHO/CDS/TB/2001.287. Geneva: WHO, 2001, 181 pp. Available online from: http://www.who.int/

58. Tookey P, Peckham CS. Does cytomegalovirus present an occupational risk? *Archives of Diseases in Childhood* 1991; **66**:1009–10.

59. Polis MA, Masur H. Cytomegalovirus infection in patients with HIV infection. In: Merigan TC, Bartlett JG, Bolognesi D (eds), *Textbook of AIDS Medicine,* 2nd edn. Baltimore: Williams & Wilkins, 1999, 373–89.

60. Moyle G. Cytomegalovirus infection. In: Gazzard B (ed.), *Chelsea & Westminster Hospital AIDS Care Handbook.* London: Mediscript Ltd Medical Publishers, 1999, 65–73.

61. Safrin S. Herpes simplex and varicella-zoster virus infections in HIV-infected individuals. In: Merigan TC, Bartlett JG, Bolognesi D (eds), *Textbook of AIDS Medicine,* 2nd edn. Baltimore: Williams & Wilkins, 1999, 391–402.

62. Nelson M. Respiratory disease. In: Gazzard B (ed.), *Chelsea & Westminster Hospital AIDS Care Handbook.* London: Mediscript Ltd Medical Publishers, 1999, 141–50.

63. Bartlett JG. Other HIV-related pneumonias. In: Sande MA, Volberding PA (eds), *The Medical Management of AIDS,* 6th edn. Philadelphia: W.B. Saunders Co., 1999, 331–42.

64. UK Departments of Health: Salisbury DM, Begg NT (eds). *1996 Immunisation against Infectious Disease.* London: Stationery Office, 290 pp. Available from: The Stationery Office Ltd, PO Box 29, Norwich NR3 1GN, UK; e-mail customer.services@theso.co.uk or telephone 0870 600 5522, fax 0870 600 5533.

65. Kaplan LD, Northfelt DW. Malignancies associated with AIDS. In: Sande MA, Volberding PA (eds), *The Medical Management of AIDS,* 6th edn. Philadelphia: W.B. Saunders Co., 1999, 467–96.

66. Miles SA. Kaposi's sarcoma and cloacogenic carcinoma: virus-initiated malignancies. In: Merigan TC, Bartlett JG, Bolognesi D (eds), *Textbook of AIDS Medicine,* 2nd edn. Baltimore: Williams & Wilkins, 1999, 421–36.

67. Chang Y, Cesarman, E, Pessin MS et al. Identification of herpesvirus-like DNA sequences in AIDS-associated Kaposi's sarcoma. *Science* 1994; **266**:1865–9.

68. Su IJ, Hsu YS, Chang YC et al. Herpesvirus-like DNA sequence in Kaposi's sarcoma from AIDS and non-AIDS patients in Taiwan. *Lancet* 1995; **345**:722–3.

69. Pauk J, Huang ML, Brodie SJ et al. Mucosal shedding of human herpesvirus 8. *New England Journal of Medicine* 2000; **343**:1369–77.

70. Cannon MJ, Dollard SC, Smith DK et al. HIV Epidemiology Research Study Group. Blood-borne and sexual transmission of human herpesvirus 8 in women with or at risk for human immunodeficiency virus infection. *New England Journal of Medicine* 2001; **344**:637–43.

71. Whitley D, Smith NA, Mathew S et al. Human herpesvirus 8 seroepidemiology among women and detection in the genital tract of seropositive women. *Journal of Infectious Disease* 1999; **179**:254–6.

72. Bower M, Fife K. HIV-associated malignancy. In: Gazzard B (ed.), *Chelsea & Westminster Hospital AIDS Care Handbook.* London: Mediscript Ltd Medical Publishers, 1999, 93–111.

73. Jacobson LP, Jenkins FJ, Springer G et al. Interaction of human immunodeficiency virus type 1 and human herpesvirus type 8 infections on the incidence of Kaposi's sarcoma. *Journal of Infectious Disease* 2000; **181**:1940–9.
74. Renwick N, Halaby T, Weverling GJ et al. Seroconversion of human herpesvirus 8 during HIV infection is highly predictive of Kaposi's sarcoma. *AIDS* 1998; **12**:2481–8.
75. Martin JN, Ganem DE, Osmond DH et al. Sexual transmission and the natural history of human herpesvirus 8 infection. *New England Journal of Medicine* 1998; **338M**:948–54.
76. World Health Organization. WHO staging system for HIV infection and disease in adults and adolescents. Annex 1 in: *Scaling Up Antiretroviral Therapy in Resource-limited Settings: Guidelines for a Public Health Approach*. Geneva: WHO. Available online at: http://www.who.int/docstore/hiv/scaling/anex1.html

FURTHER READING

Alcorn K (ed.). *HIV & AIDS Treatments Directory*, 20th edn. London: National AIDS Manual (NAM) Publications, August 2001. Updated and published every 6 months and available from: NAM Publications, 16a Clapham Common Southside, London SW4 7AB UK; e-mail: info@nam.org.uk

Anderson JR (ed.). *A Guide to the Clinical Care of Women with HIV*. US Department of Health and Human Services, 2001. Available online at: http://www.hab.hrsa.gov/

Devitta VT Jr, Hellman S, Rosenbert SA. *AIDS. Etiology, Diagnosis, Treatment and Prevention*, 4th edn. Philadelphia: Lippincott-Raven Publishers, 1997, 746 pp, ISBN 0-397-51538-3.

Gazzard B (ed.). *Chelsea & Westminster Hospital AIDS Care Handbook*. London: Mediscript Ltd Medical Publishers, 1999. Available from: Mediscript Ltd Medical Publishers, 1 Mountview Court, 310 Friern Barnet Lane, London N20 0LD, UK.

Mehta DK (Executive Editor). *British National Formulary (BNF)*, current edition. London: British Medical Association and the Royal Pharmaceutical Society of Great Britain. Updated and published every 6 months. Available from: BMJ Books, PO Box 295, London WC1H 9TE, UK, or from their website: www.bmjbookshop.com. The BNF is also available online at: www.BNF.org

Mcrigan TC, Bartlett JG, Bolognesi D (eds). *Textbook of AIDS Medicine*, 2nd edn. Baltimore: Williams & Wilkins, 1999, 1063 pp, ISBN 0-683-30216-7.

Sande MA, Volberding PA (eds). *The Medical Management of AIDS*, 6th edn. Philadelphia: W.B. Saunders Co., 1999, 636 pp, ISBN 0-7216-8102-6.

Weller IVD, Williams IG. *ABC of AIDS*, 5th edn. London: British Medical Association, 2001. Available from: BMJ Books, PO Box 295, London WC1H 9TE, UK, or from their website www.bmjbookshop.com. Also available for downloading from the *British Medical Journal* 2001; **323** (serialized in various issues). Website address for *BMJ*: http://www.bmj.com

Wormser GP. *AIDS and Other Manifestions of HIV Infection*, 3rd edn. Philadelphia: Lippincott-Raven Publishers, 1998, 836 pp, ISBN 0-397-58760-0.

INTERNET RESOURCES

- *A Guide to the Clinical Care of Women with HIV*, Anderson JR (ed.). US Department of Health and Human Services, 2001. Available online at: http://www.hab.hrsa.gov/

- *British National Formulary (BNF)*, published by the British Medical Association and the Royal Pharmaceutical Society of Great Britain, provides up-to-date information in relation to the drugs used in the UK to treat HIV infection and HIV-related illnesses; the online version is updated every 6 months: http://www.BNF.org/

- For a comprehensive guide to drugs used for the prophylaxis and treatment of opportunistic infections and other HIV-related illnesses, see the current edition of the *HIV & AIDS Treatments Directory*, published twice yearly by the National AIDS Manual (email: info@nam.org.uk), and the monthly *AIDS Treatment Update*, available online at: http://www.aidsmap.com

- The latest evidence-based guidelines for preventing opportunistic infections in people infected with HIV produced by the US Public Health Service (USPHS) and Infectious Diseases Society of America (IDSA) are posted online at: http://www.cdc.gov/hiv/pubs/guidelines.htm/

CHAPTER 8

Tuberculosis and HIV disease – a dangerous liaison

Tuberculosis is much more than a medical affliction caused by a specific bacterium. It is by turns a strange, a terrible and a fascinating entity, like the multi-layered mystery of the famous Russian doll. No sooner do we think we understand it, than a new form, as baffling and menacing as ever, appears to confound us.

Frank Ryan[1]

Introduction

Since the beginning of recorded human history, tuberculosis (TB) has always been with us, causing great epidemic plagues during the last millennium that, over the centuries, resulted in more illness and death than those caused by any other infectious disease. Although always simmering away at high endemic levels in the poorer regions of the world, it seemed to us here in the industrially developed world that, by the mid-1900s, TB was coming under control. During the last century, a more complete understanding of the bacterial cause and natural history of TB facilitated the development of effective vaccines, infection control strategies and curative chemotherapy. But then no one reckoned on AIDS . . . HIV came along and gave fresh breath to TB, setting fire to a smouldering global endemic potential and, within just a decade or so, TB once again became a worldwide health emergency, becoming the most common opportunistic disease associated with AIDS. As the global pandemic of HIV disease rapidly escalated, TB became out of control in many countries and the world confronted the spectre of this deadly partnership, TB and HIV infection, working in synergy to threaten the health and life of millions of people.

Learning outcomes

After studying and reflecting on the material in this chapter, you will be able to:

- discuss the history and global epidemiology of TB;
- identify the characteristics of mycobacteria, discuss how they are transmitted and describe the natural history of infection and disease, especially noting the pathogenic synergy that exists between TB and HIV infection;
- describe the clinical presentation of a patient with pulmonary TB and outline the various procedures used to diagnose infection and active disease;
- discuss the principles and the associated nursing implications of antituberculosis chemotherapy for both drug-susceptible and drug-resistant TB;
- describe the role of antituberculosis chemotherapy and BCG vaccination in preventing TB.

THE BEGINNING ...

Tuberculosis has been a misery of humankind since the Neolithic revolution 7000 years BC, and accounts of this disease appear in the earliest surviving literature. TB became established in mainland Europe by 1500 BC and evidence of TB in Britain dates from the time of the Roman Occupation (55 BC to the fifth century AD).[1,2] By the mid-seventeenth century, TB had become one of the great plagues of Europe and in Britain, where one in five deaths in London (recorded in the Bills of Mortality) were due to 'consumption' (TB). Various manifestations of TB have been recorded throughout the ages, including spinal TB, scrofula (enlarged, sometimes discharging, tuberculous lymph glands in the neck), and consumption, i.e. pulmonary TB.[1-3] From the middle of the seventeenth century to the end of the nineteenth century, pulmonary TB gained in epidemic force, becoming known as the white plague, and sweeping through major cities in both Europe and North America (especially London and New York City), infecting half the world's population and, by the beginning of the nineteenth century, killing 7 million people a year.[1-4] During the twentieth century, a dramatic decline in cases was witnessed in North America and Europe, due to a variety of factors. Although good evidence for many of the influences that drove down the incidence of TB over time is lacking, various authorities have attributed this decline to natural selection, improved living conditions and other socio-economic improvements in the earlier part of the century, changing environmental and ecological factors, evolutionary changes in the causative organism, the introduction of an effective vaccine against TB (the BCG vaccination) and, more importantly, advances in chemotherapy (drug treatment) from the mid-1940s onwards.[1,3-6]

THE PUZZLE OF TUBERCULOSIS

The cause of TB was clouded in confusion from antiquity to the beginning of the nineteenth century; a puzzle waiting to be solved – and solved it was, in a series of breathtaking discoveries. The first part of the solution was coming to understand the natural history of TB and this was competently and comprehensively described for the first time in the early nineteenth century by the French physicians Gaspard Laurent Baylea and René Laënnec (both of whom died from the disease). Then, critical for every other step in the solution of this puzzle, was a momentous discovery by the German microbiologist Robert Koch, announced in 1882. After years of scientific enquiry, Koch identified and conclusively demonstrated that a myco-bacterium (now known as *Mycobacterium tuberculosis*) was the bacterial cause of TB. After this great discovery, an Austrian physician, Clemens von Pirquet developed a skin test in 1907 to diagnose infection by *M. tuberculosis* by using a preparation of killed tubercle bacilli, pre-viously developed by Koch and known as old tuberculin. Then a vaccine to prevent disease was developed and first used by the French bacteriologists Albert Léon Calmette and Camille Guérin (the **BCG vaccine**) in 1921. What many then felt was the beginning of the end for this oldest of human plagues occurred just two dozen years later. In 1944, **streptomycin**, the first drug that was truly effective in treating TB, was discovered by the Russian microbiologist Selman Abraham Waksman, working at Rutgers University in New Jersey in the USA.[1,3,5] This was quickly followed by the discovery of other drugs that, along with streptomycin, would prove to be almost miraculous in the treatment of TB. These included **para-aminosalicylic acid (PAS)** in 1946 and **isoniazid (INH)** in 1952. Since then, an impressive repertoire of other drugs has been developed to treat TB, including rifampicin, ethambutol and pyrazinamide. By the late 1950s, the puzzle seemed nearly solved and, by the end of another decade, public health scientists in the World Health Organization (WHO) were planning for the global eradication of one of the most terrible diseases to afflict humankind.

But nobody then could have possibly imagined that already, emerging out of the shadows in the 1970s, was a new infection, destined to become the terrible twin of TB. This was **HIV/AIDS**, and it would spin TB madly out of control throughout the world, so much so that by 1993, TB was declared a **global health emergency**, the first time a disease had ever been so singularly proclaimed by WHO. In a new and deadly twist, TB had entered into a unique and menacing partnership with an even bigger killer – **HIV disease** – and, acting in synergy, they have together become the new scourge of humankind.

EPIDEMIOLOGY – GLOBAL

The WHO estimates that one-third of the world's population (almost 2 billion people) is currently infected with *M. tuberculosis* and, from this pool of people with latent infection, over 8.4 million new cases of active TB (and at least 2 million TB-related deaths) are seen each year (Figure 8.1).[7,8] Without a major global commitment to TB control, this upward trend will continue, and it has been calculated that in 2005, 10.2 million people throughout the world could have active TB, and Africa will be home to more people with active TB (3.4 million) than any other region in the world.[9] The global epidemiological trends in infection, disease and death are staggering (Table 8.1), and TB continues to earn its fearsome reputation as the 'Captain of all of these men of death'.[7,9,10]

On a global scale, HIV disease and TB are among the leading causes of preventable ill-health and death in young people in developing countries, causing approximately 11 million illnesses and more than 5 million deaths each year.[8,9] In addition, it was estimated that, worldwide, at least one-third of the 36.1 million people living with HIV/AIDS at the beginning of 2001 (12 million people) were also infected with *M. tuberculosis*.[11–15]

EPIDEMIOLOGY – INDUSTRIALLY DEVELOPED WORLD

Although more than 75 per cent of people who are infected with *M. tuberculosis* and/or who have active TB disease live in the developing world, TB, going hand in hand with

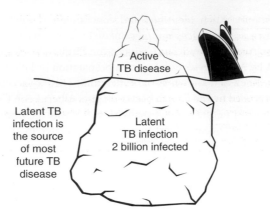

FIGURE 8.1 *The cause of active tuberculosis worldwide. (Source: Centers for Disease Control, July 2001.[8])*

poverty and HIV infection, is re-emerging in industrialized nations as a significant threat to public health.

In the USA, the incidence of individuals with TB continued to decline during the middle of the last century, from more than 84 000 cases in 1953 to a nadir (i.e. the lowest point) of 22 201 cases in 1985. However, there was then a resurgence, and cases began to increase, reaching a new zenith (highest point) of 26 673 cases in 1992. The factors associated with this resurgence (described in Table 8.2) can occur in any country and are a salutary warning of how easily endemic infectious diseases can rapidly evolve into surprising epidemics. Using a variety of aggressive interventions from 1992 onwards, public health professionals were able to reverse this situation and facilitate a resumption of a continuing decline in the annual incidence of TB in the USA, reaching an all-time low of 16 372 by the end of 2000. However, it is suggested that by the end of 2000, approximately 10–15 million people in the USA were latently infected with *M. tuberculosis.*[16–19]

In England and Wales, the incidence of TB also continued to decline, from 46 546 in 1953 to a nadir of 5085 cases in 1987. Since then, there has been a slow but steady increase in the

TABLE 8.1 Global epidemiological trends (2001–2020)[7–9,11–14]

At the beginning of the third millennium …

- Someone in the world is newly infected with *Mycobacterium tuberculosis* **every second**; this will result in **1 billion people** being **newly infected** between 2000 and 2020.
- Between 2000 and 2020, **200 million people** will develop **active tuberculosis (TB)**.
- More than **8.4 million people** become sick with TB (active TB) **each year**, including:

   3 million in South East Asia,

   more than 1.5 million in sub-Saharan Africa,

   well over 250 000 in Eastern Europe.
- Left untreated, each person with active TB will **infect on average between 10 and 15 people** every year.
- Between 2000 and 2020, **35 million people will die from TB** if there is no real improvement in TB control.
- TB **kills** approximately **2 million people** each year.
- TB is rapidly **escalating in Africa** because of the increasing incidence of **HIV/AIDS**.
- **Drug-resistant strains** of *M. tuberculosis* are rapidly spreading throughout the world, including many countries in Western Europe.

TABLE 8.2 Factors associated with the USA resurgence of tuberculosis (TB): 1985–1992[16–19]

- Chronic deterioration of the infrastructure for TB services
- Accelerating epidemic of HIV infection, especially in large cities, which substantially increased the risk for active TB among people with latent TB infection
- Immigration from countries with a high prevalence of people with active TB disease
- Transmission of *Mycobacterium tuberculosis* in congregate settings, such as hospitals and prisons, especially where there were large numbers of immunocompromised people, a situation often referred to as (immunocompromised convergence)
- Increasing incidence of multiple-drug-resistant tuberculosis

number of TB cases reported each year (Figure 8.2).[20,21] However, unlike in the USA, there is no evidence as yet to suggest that HIV infection is responsible for this moderate but continuing trend to increase.

The increase in notifications of TB in the UK is mainly due to TB infection and active TB disease in people who have recently immigrated, or whose families immigrated, into the UK from the Indian subcontinent (India, Pakistan, Bangladesh) or Africa, or have visited these regions, where the prevalence and incidence of active TB are high.[5,22] However, other groups in the UK who continue to be potentially at an increased risk for TB include the elderly, the homeless and anyone who is immunocompromised, including those who are infected with HIV.

THE CAUSE OF TUBERCULOSIS

Tuberculosis in humans is caused by some members of a group of bacteria known as mycobacteria. These small (approximately 0.2–1.0 micrometres (μm) in diameter and

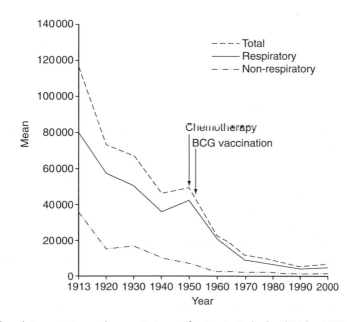

FIGURE 8.2 *Tuberculosis: respiratory and non-respiratory notifications in England and Wales, 1913–2000.*

1.0–10 μm in length) non-sporing, Gram-positive, oxygen-loving (aerophilic) bacilli are slender, curved (often beaded) rods, enveloped by a very thick and complex lipid-rich cell wall, and reproduce slowly by binary fission. As aerobic intracellular microorganisms, mycobacteria require high oxygen tension environments to flourish – the lungs and kidneys being good examples of an attractive oxygen-rich environment.[23] Tuberculosis refers only to disease in humans caused by *M. tuberculosis* (the most common), *M. bovis* (a mycobacterium normally found in cattle) or *M. africaneum* (a type with properties intermediate between those of *M. tuberculosis* and *M. bovis*, principally found in Africa). These three mycobacteria are often grouped together and referred to as the ***Mycobacterium tuberculosis* complex** or, simply, as **tubercle bacilli**. Because mycobacteria resist decolourizing by acid and alcohol after staining in the laboratory with hot carbol fuchsin or other arylmethane dyes, they are commonly referred to as **acid-fast bacilli (AFB)**.

Other environmental, or **non-tuberculous**, mycobacteria (previously called atypical mycobacteria), such as *M. avium* and *M. intracellulare*, can sometimes cause human disease, especially in immunocompromised individuals, and illnesses caused by these mycobacteria are referred to as **mycobacteriosis**, to differentiate them from 'tuberculosis', a term reserved exclusively for disease caused by *M. tuberculosis* complex. ***M. avium-intracellulare* complex** is an important cause of serious illness in HIV-infected people and is discussed in more detail later in this chapter. Another important non-tuberculous mycobacterium (*M. leprae*) is the causative agent of leprosy (Hansen's disease), which causes chronic disease and disability in more than 12 million people worldwide.

TRANSMISSION

M. tuberculosis is usually transmitted from one person to another by the **respiratory route**, that is, by inhalation of tubercle bacilli released from an infected person in small drops of moisture (under 5 mm in diameter) during coughing, sneezing and talking. These airborne droplets of moisture contain just a few viable tubercle bacilli as their nuclei, and as soon as these tiny droplets are released into the air, the water evaporates from the surface of the droplet, making the particle even smaller and concentrating its bacterial content. These microscopic particles are known as **droplet nuclei** and they continue floating in room air for several hours, being wafted through the environment by normal air currents and remaining a potential threat to uninfected susceptible individuals, who can become infected by inhaling them. It has been estimated that human infection requires the inhalation of from 5 to 200 tubercle bacilli.[24]

M. bovis is usually transmitted to town dwellers via contaminated milk from infected cattle, causing lesions in the tonsils, lymph nodes, gastrointestinal tract, bones and joints. However, among those who work with cattle, *M. bovis* is also transmitted by the respiratory route. As bovine TB has been brought under relative control in industrialized countries, it is currently no longer a significant cause of TB in humans in most parts of the developed world.[15] However, a small number of people with TB caused by *M. bovis* infection continue to be reported in the UK each year.[25] Human-to-human transmission of TB due to *M. bovis* is extremely rare, although outbreaks have been reported among HIV-positive and other immunocompromised people.[26,27] In some parts of the developing world, for example in sub-Saharan Africa, *M. bovis* may therefore re-emerge as an important cause of TB in people who are co-infected with HIV.[15]

Although *M. tuberculosis* is unable to penetrate healthy intact skin or mucous membranes, cutaneous transmission (infection through the skin) sometimes occurs, for example following inoculation accidents in medical and laboratory staff, and in pathologists and autopsy room personnel who work with tissues or fluids infected with *M. tuberculosis*.[28] Fomites (inanimate objects, such as bedding and eating utensils) are not involved in the transmission of *M. tuberculosis*.

THE RISK OF INFECTION AND SUBSEQUENT DISEASE

Several factors are related to the risk of both transmission and the probability of an exposed person becoming infected and developing TB following exposure. In addition to the infectiousness of the source patient, the risk of transmission is related to the closeness and intensity of exposure. Anyone sharing the same airspace for a prolonged period, for example family members, patients and healthcare workers, is at more risk of contracting infection than those individuals who are only briefly exposed to the source patient, such as one-time hospital visitors. However, exposure of any length in small, confined, poorly ventilated environments is dangerous. This may include facilities in hospitals and clinics used for cough-inducing procedures, for example physiotherapy, sputum induction, administration of aerosol therapy, bronchoscopy and endotracheal intubations. The likelihood that an exposed person will become infected with and develop TB is related to that person's susceptibility. The factor that is most important in increasing individual susceptibility to primary infection is immunodeficiency, including immunodeficiency secondary to HIV infection. Consequently, HIV-infected individuals, whether they are patients, staff or visitors, should not be exposed to individuals with infectious TB. The infection prevention and control measures that need to be in place to care for patients with TB safely are discussed in more detail in Chapter 14.

THE PATHOGENESIS OF TUBERCULOSIS: INFECTION AND DISEASE

Most people who become infected with *M. tuberculosis* will never develop active TB disease, but they will remain infected. Some of those who become infected will develop active TB, either quite soon after they first become infected (primary infection) or many years later. Consequently, it is useful to think of exposure to *M. tuberculosis* as having various potential outcomes (Figure 8.3).[20]

Tuberculosis infection

A well-understood sequence of events occurs when a person first becomes infected with *M. tuberculosis*.[28-30] During the initial phase of **primary infection**, tubercle bacilli are inhaled by a susceptible person into their distal air spaces, usually in the lower lung fields. When implanted in the alveolus, the tubercle bacilli begin to multiply and, at the same time, are identified, attacked and ingested by scavenging **alveolar macrophages**, the principal phagocytic cells normally resident in the lungs.

Tubercle bacilli are, however, generally resistant to intracellular digestion within most of these non-specifically activated (naïve) macrophages that have never previously encountered them. Although some tubercle bacilli will be destroyed or inhibited following phagocytosis, most will survive and, more importantly, replicate inside the host macrophages. As a result,

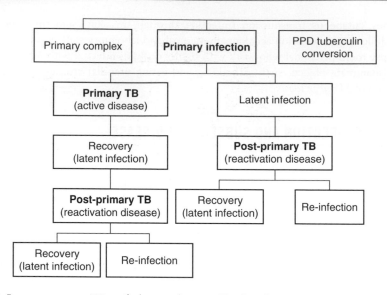

FIGURE 8.3 *Exposure outcomes. PPD, purified protein derivative; TB, tuberculosis.*

tubercle bacilli continue to multiply, their numbers increasing until (usually) the infection is later brought under control by the arrival and deployment of **activated macrophages** and **T-lymphocytes**. Because the tubercle bacilli are multiplying inside naïve macrophages, a humoral immune system response, i.e. B-lymphocytes producing antibodies, is useless. As discussed in Chapter 5, antibodies are only effective against extracellular microorganisms. Tubercle bacilli, replicating in macrophages, are intracellular parasites and only a cell-mediated immune response, facilitated by T-lymphocytes, will eventually arrest this infection.

During the early days of primary infection, most macrophages die as a result of continuing intracellular bacterial growth, and, in dying, release a new generation of tubercle bacilli (and bacterial cellular debris). The newly produced tubercle bacilli proceed to infect more naïve macrophages and the cycle of infection, bacterial replication, host cell death and new infection continues.

This primary focus of infection in the lung tissue, known as the **Ghon focus**, commences as an acute local inflammatory **lesion**, usually in the lower or middle lung field, and then develops into a **granuloma**, a characteristic feature of chronic infection. The granuloma consists of a cluster of activated macrophages around the focus of infection and, in TB, it is called a **tubercle** because Hippocrates noted that it resembled a small potato tuber.

In primary infection, some tubercle bacilli are transported by infected macrophages (acting as antigen-presenting cells) to the regional lymph nodes in the hilum or root of the lungs, where the tubercle bacilli are introduced to the **T-lymphocytes**. The T-lymphocytes become stimulated by this antigenic presentation and differentiate into activated T-cell subsets: **CD4+ T-helper cells** and **CD8+ cytotoxic T-lymphocytes (CTL)**. The CD4+ helper cells in turn differentiate into one of two types: helper cells type 1 (**Th1**) and helper cells type 2 (**Th2**). These cells are discussed in more detail in Chapter 5. The activation of T-lymphocytes in the lymph nodes causes them to become enlarged. The Ghon focus in the lung tissue and the enlarged hilar lymph nodes are together referred to as the **primary complex** (Figure 8.4).

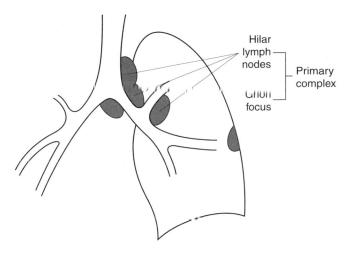

FIGURE 8.4 *Primary complex. (From Crofton J, Horne N, Miller F. Clinical Tuberculosis, 2nd edn, 1999.[27] Reprinted with permission, Macmillan Education Ltd, London.)*

Helper cells (Th1 and Th2 cells) secrete a variety of **lymphokines** (cytokines released by lymphocytes – discussed in more detail in Chapter 5) such as interleukin-2 (**IL-2**) and gamma-interferon (**IFNγ**). IFNγ activates macrophages, enhancing their ability to kill tubercle bacilli engulfed during phagocytosis. Simultaneously, activated macrophages secrete another cytokine known as tumour necrosis factor-alpha (**TNFα**). This cytokine plays a critical role in helping to initiate and maintain the formation of the granuloma (discussed below), a lesion designed to contain and prevent further dissemination of the infection.[23]

This continuing release of cytokines by activated immune system cells, along with the release of bacterial cellular debris from dying infected macrophages and the ongoing inflammatory reaction in the tubercle, produce a powerful chemotactic reaction (**chemotaxis**). This is a biochemical process whereby additional immune system cells, such as T-lymphocytes, monocytes and wandering macrophages, are recruited to the site of primary infection in the alveolus (the Ghon focus), where they surround the tubercle and initiate the formation of an initial granulomatous lesion, a mass of cells known as a **granuloma**.

The granuloma (Figure 8.5) has a core of dead tissue, with a semi-liquid caseous (cheesy) centre surrounded by an outer zone of macrophages and helper T-lymphocytes. More T-lymphocytes and monocytes are positioned on the periphery of the early granuloma, where lymphokines transform monocytes into **activated macrophages**. These cells, known as **epithelioid cells** (because, under the microscope, they look like epithelial cells), surround the maturing granuloma, forming a chain, or **cordon**, many cells thick around it. Many epithelioid cells fuse to form multi-nucleated giant cells (Langhans' giant cells) and strengthen the cordon.

Granuloma formation is a generally successful mechanism for walling off and isolating a site of persistent infection. Because of the acid pH and low oxygen content within the caseous centre of the granuloma, the replication of tubercle bacilli is inhibited and the infection is arrested. This promotes healing and, in time, the granuloma often becomes calcified.

Not all tubercle bacilli within the granuloma are destroyed. Some, known as **persisters**, can survive for many years or decades, causing an outbreak of active disease later in life.[31] However, in most people, cell-mediated immune responses are both efficient and effective

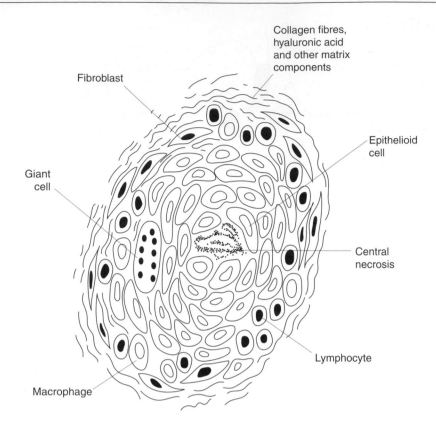

FIGURE 8.5 *Granuloma. (From Yeager H Jr, Azumi N, Underhill CB. Fibrosis: the formation of the granuloma matrix. In: Rom WN, Garay S (eds), Tuberculosis, 1996. Reprinted with permission of Little, Brown & Co. Publishers, Boston, MA, USA.)*

in containing the infection following primary infection, and 90–95 per cent of initial infections go unrecognized, causing no symptoms or health problems, and do not progress to active TB disease. The infection becomes dormant, primary lesions heal and may eventually calcify, and the **tuberculin skin test** becomes positive. As the potential for reactivation remains (because viable tubercle bacilli – 'persisters' – remain in the granuloma), the infection during the period following the healing of the primary lesions is referred to as **latent TB infection**.

In primary infection, some bacilli may escape from the lungs and hilar lymph nodes via the lymphatic system or bloodstream and, in a few individuals, this dissemination may cause serious disease (**primary extrapulmonary tuberculosis**), such as meningitis, renal TB and bone and joint involvement, and may lead to significant mortality in infants and young children (and in immunocompromised adults). In some cases, widespread lesions develop, a condition termed **miliary tuberculosis** because many organs contain millet-seed-sized tubercles (Latin *milium* – a millet seed). People with extrapulmonary forms of TB may also have active pulmonary TB, an important consideration in making infection control decisions. Tubercle bacilli may be seeded in the apices of the lungs during this phase of dissemination, resulting in small nodular scars (**Simon's foci**), which may serve as a breeding ground for later active disease.

Active tuberculosis

In all people, disease progression is related to the number and virulence of infecting bacilli and the competence, or strength, of an individual's immune defences. Clearly, the larger and more virulent the infecting inoculum and the weaker the immune defences, the more likely it will be that a person will go on to develop active disease following infection. In the industrially developed world, for example countries in Northern and Western Europe, Australasia and North America, active disease will develop in 5–10 per cent of individuals who, for a variety of reasons, do not successfully contain their infection in the primary stage. Disease progression is more common in young children (up to the age of 3 years), young adults and immunocompromised individuals. Infants will often rapidly develop active TB, including disseminated disease and tuberculous meningitis, following primary infection. HIV-infected individuals, who have not been infected with M. *tuberculosis* in the past, commonly develop active TB within a few months of primary infection.[32]

Primary and post-primary (reactivation) tuberculosis

Within 3–8 months of primary infection, active disease may develop and this is known as **primary tuberculosis**. Alternatively, the tubercle bacilli can remain dormant for years and then begin multiplying (often in the apical areas of the lungs), eventually causing **post-primary** (or **reactivation**) **tuberculosis**. Approximately half of those individuals who eventually develop TB will develop primary disease within 2 years of infection, the remaining half developing post-primary disease at any time from just over 2 years to many years later. Precipitating factors leading to active disease following primary infection include the onset of diabetes mellitus, corticosteroid therapy, poor nutrition, gradual loss of vigorous immune responses associated with ageing, pregnancy, intercurrent diseases, stress and HIV disease. But in many cases there is no evident cause.

Children over the age of 3 years are relatively resistant to developing TB – the 'safe school age' – the majority of those who are predestined to develop post-primary TB doing so in adolescence or young adulthood. In Europe and North America, TB is more common in young adult females and, in later life, is seen more frequently in men; it is also seen in the elderly, in both sexes and in all races.

An important characteristic of post-primary TB is gross tissue destruction at the site of the lesions, resulting in cavity formation in the lungs. Cavities are very important structures, as tubercle bacilli replicate rapidly within them and gain access to the sputum, leading to infectivity. Such patients are said to have **open tuberculosis**. Cavity formation is due to immunological reactions and is therefore suppressed in immunocompromised people, with implications for infectivity (see below).

Re-infection

Previous primary infection (with or without subsequent active disease) and BCG vaccination (discussed later) give good protection in many countries against active TB due to re-infection, but this protection declines over time. Active TB can be caused by re-infection, especially in immunocompromised individuals, such as those with HIV disease. It is usually difficult to differentiate between active TB caused by reactivation of latent infection or exogenous re-infection, although it is thought that reactivation (post-primary) disease is more common. As a general rule, more people develop active TB as a result of re-infection if they live in regions of the world where the underlying prevalence and incidence of TB are high, such as India and Africa. In the UK and most other countries in the industrially developed world, the prevalence of TB is low and, consequently, relatively more people develop active TB as a result of reactivation of old (latent) infection rather than as a result of re-infection.

CLINICAL PRESENTATION OF PULMONARY TUBERCULOSIS

In the early stages of pulmonary TB, although the individual may be feeling vaguely unwell and tired (**fatigue**), specific health problems may be poorly defined. A low-grade **fever** is common, as are drenching **night sweats**, especially over the top part of the body. Loss of appetite (**anorexia**) and progressive weight loss are eventually experienced, as are respiratory signs and symptoms. Chronic **cough**, a universal symptom in pulmonary TB, gradually becomes more productive of yellow or green mucus, especially in the morning upon awakening. **Haemoptysis** (blood in the sputum) is frequent, especially in advanced disease, **chest pain** and **dyspnoea** (difficult or laboured breathing) can occur at any stage as a result of a pleural effusion or rupture of a lung (spontaneous pneumothorax). A tuberculous cavity may rupture into the pleural space, causing a tuberculous **empyema** and bronchopleural **fistula**. This event is extremely serious and requires urgent medical intervention, including pleural drainage.

As the disease progresses, patients become profoundly ill and progressively debilitated and malnourished, and lose considerable body weight. This generalized state of ill-health and wasting is known as **cachexia**. Without effective treatment, up to one-third of (non-HIV-infected) individuals with chronic TB may survive for many years, with alternating periods of stability and relative well-being and exacerbations of active disease, involving more and more of the lung tissue. However, up to 60 per cent of untreated (or ineffectively treated) individuals with active pulmonary TB will die of this disease, the median survival period following onset of active disease being approximately 2.5 years.

HIV DISEASE AND TUBERCULOSIS

Co-infection with *M. tuberculosis* and HIV compounds the progressive loss of effective cell-mediated responses to both infections because of the dominance of Th2 cytokine activity and the progressive depletion of CD4+ T-lymphocytes. Consequently, the clinical course of both infections is rapidly accelerated. HIV-infected CD4+ T-lymphocytes (helper cells) lose their efficiency in producing **IFNγ**, a critical lymphokine needed to activate macrophages, which, as previously described, are needed to contain the infection. Additionally, activated macrophages secrete the pro-inflammatory cytokines **TNF** and **IL-1**, both of which enhance transactivation and replication of HIV, further damaging immune function and significantly hastening the onset of end-stage HIV disease, i.e. AIDS.[33-35]

HIV-infected individuals who become newly infected with *M. tuberculosis* are at significantly greater risk of progressing to active disease (primary TB) than are those who are not infected with HIV. If a person has latent *M. tuberculosis* infection and then becomes infected with HIV, the progressive loss of immune function caused by HIV infection significantly increases the risk of reactivation (post-primary) TB. In both circumstances, co-infected people are more likely to have a rapid, more severely progressive form of TB and an acceleration of HIV disease. Additionally, people with HIV-related TB are four times more likely to die than those with TB who are not infected with HIV.[36-39]

Tuberculosis is often the initial manifestation of HIV disease, often seen within the first 6 months following HIV infection, and may be the result of either recent exposure and infection or reactivation of latent *M. tuberculosis* infection.[33] A prominent aspect of pulmonary TB is that it is one of the few (and by far the most important) respiratory diseases seen in HIV-infected individuals which, unlike most other opportunistic infections, can be relatively easily transmitted to other susceptible individuals, including those who are not infected with HIV.

In addition, disseminated disease and extrapulmonary TB are much more common in individuals who are infected with HIV, as the associated immunodeficiency facilitates blood-borne spread of tubercle bacilli (bacillaemia) from the primary site of infection in the lungs. The areas most commonly affected during extrapulmonary TB in people who are co-infected with HIV are the lymphatic system, spleen, liver, gastrointestinal and urogenital tracts and bone marrow. However, it is important to remember that most patients with extrapulmonary lesions also have pulmonary TB.

DIAGNOSIS OF TUBERCULOSIS IN PEOPLE INFECTED WITH HIV

Tuberculosis is often seen before an individual is diagnosed as infected with HIV and, consequently, appropriate counselling and serological testing for HIV infection should be considered for all patients with newly diagnosed TB if their history suggests they may have been exposed to HIV. The early diagnosis of TB is essential in reducing the risk of infection to others and preventing transmission in healthcare facilities, i.e. **nosocomial transmission**. Additionally, pulmonary TB in an HIV-infected person is an 'AIDS indicator' disease, so it is essential that HIV disease is diagnosed so that infected people can benefit from specific antiretroviral therapy, in those countries where it is available.

Chest X-ray, sputum microscopy and culture are the principal investigations ordered by the physician to establish a diagnosis of TB, although other investigations may also be needed (Table 8.3).

TABLE 8.3 Investigations for HIV-related tuberculosis

- Medical history, clinical presentation and examination ***
- Chest X-ray **
- Microscopy and/or culture of:

    sputum ****

    bronchoalveolar fluid

    blood

    cerebrospinal fluid

    urine

    pleural fluid

    pleural and lung biopsy specimens

    gastric washings

    pericardial fluid
- Tuberculin (PPD) skin test *
- HIV serology (if positive ↓)

    CD4$^+$ T-lymphocyte count

    HIV viral load measurement

Chest X-rays

Tuberculosis is often difficult to differentiate in chest X-rays from other pulmonary infections commonly seen in individuals with HIV disease. In TB, shadows in the upper zones of the lungs are common, and lesions (infiltrates) above or behind the clavicle are frequently suggestive of a recrudescence in post-primary disease, especially in the older person. In younger adults, lesions may be identified anywhere in the lungs, and pleural effusions (often unilateral) are commonly seen. As TB progresses, the centre of lesions in the lungs becomes necrotic and resembles soft cheese (hence the term caseation). If these lesions erode into a bronchiole or bronchus, the soft caseous material is discharged, resulting in a cavity that is usually clearly seen in a chest X-ray. Cavitations may be extensive and a source of haemoptysis and continuing disease. Serial chest films are usually needed to monitor both disease progression and response to treatment.

Individuals who are immunosuppressed as a result of HIV disease may have a fairly **normal chest X-ray** as their inflammatory reaction is reduced and there is, consequently, less cavitation of pulmonary lesions. Others have very atypical chest X-rays with rapidly changing appearances, and these pose serious interpretational problems.

Sputum microscopy and culture

The principal method used for the rapid diagnosis of pulmonary TB is the microscopic and culture examinations of sputum (not saliva), collected initially when the patient is first seen and then daily (early morning) on 3–5 (or more) consecutive days. If the patient cannot produce a sputum specimen, following fasting (nothing by mouth), early-morning aspiration of gastric contents can be collected, after the patient has coughed and swallowed for 10–15 minutes. This is especially useful (if somewhat distressing) for obtaining specimens from children. Alternatively, fibre-optic bronchoscopy may be employed for bronchoalveolar lavage. If bronchoscopes are used, it is important that the machines used for rinsing these instruments employ sterile distilled water, not tap water, which often contains environmental (non-tuberculous) mycobacteria, for example *M. chelonei, M. avium, M. kansasii*, which may contaminate the specimen.

As mentioned previously, mycobacteria differ from other bacteria in that they are not decolourized by weak acids and/or alcohol after staining by certain dyes. Thus they are often termed acid-fast bacilli or acid-alcohol-fast bacilli (**AFB**). To detect AFB, the most commonly used **microscopic examination of sputum** employs the **Ziehl–Neelsen (ZN) technique**, which is based on the use of hot phenolic solution of fuchsin (carbol fuchsin). Alternatively, or in addition to ZN microscopy, **fluorescence microscopy (FM)**, using phenolic auramine or auramine-rhodamine fluorochrome staining techniques, is now commonly used for rapid scanning of smears under low magnification. Positive FM smears are generally re-checked by ZN microscopy, which has a higher degree of specificity.

Positive and negative sputum smears and cultures

A sputum smear microscopy will be **positive** when there are at least 5000–10 000 AFB present in each 1 mL of sputum.[40,41] In a patient in whom TB is suspected, for example a person ill with signs and symptoms of TB and/or with radiographic changes suggestive of TB on chest X-ray, a single positive sputum smear is presumptive evidence that this patient does have **active pulmonary TB** and is **infectious**. However, not everyone who has active TB will have a positive sputum smear.

There can be several reasons why a patient might have a **negative** sputum smear and still have active pulmonary TB. These include problems with the quality of the sample, processing and interpretation errors in the laboratory when examining the sample, and various administrative errors in reporting the results. More importantly, **patients with moderate to severe immunosuppression, for example as a result of HIV disease**, generally have less or no cavitation and therefore few tubercle bacilli gain access to their sputum and, consequently, even when they have active TB, they may be smear negative. Incidentally, because HIV-infected patients generally have a lower AFB burden in sputum, they are *generally* **less infectious** than non-HIV-infected people with active TB.[42,43] Because not everyone with active TB will have positive smear results, especially if they are immunocompromised, **caution** is needed in interpreting a negative smear.

Definitive microbiological proof is dependent upon **culturing the organisms**, that is, growing and identifying them in culture media, such as Lôwenstein–Jensen (LJ) medium. Because of the slow growth rate of mycobacteria, it takes at least 2–3 weeks to grow cultures of mycobacteria from patients who are smear positive, and even longer (6–8 weeks) for patients who are smear negative.[41] Radiometric culture techniques, for example the BACTEC 460 Radiometric System (Becton Dickinson), and non-radiometric systems, such as the mycobacterial growth indicator tube (MGIT) (Becton Dickinson) and the biphasic BBL-Septi-Chek AFB Culture System (Roche), give sputum culture results much quicker and can also be used for rapid drug-susceptibility testing. These techniques are also used to detect *M. avium-intracellulare* infection in blood.

Other body fluids

For patients who are infected with HIV, blood (and sometimes bone marrow) is frequently cultured for mycobacterial growth. Urine and faeces may also be collected for culturing AFB. If urine specimens are requested, 50 mL of early-morning urine (EMU) are collected on 3 consecutive days; 24-hour urine collections are no longer used for AFB detection.[41] Examination of faeces for AFB is often requested when HIV-infected patients are suspected of having disseminated disease due to non-tuberculous mycobacteria, such as *M. avium-intracellulare*.

Tuberculin skin testing

Although not definitive, and sometimes less useful in HIV-infected people, tuberculin skin testing is helpful in identifying previous exposure to *M. tuberculosis*. This test assesses a person's sensitivity to tuberculin protein: **the greater the size of the tuberculin reaction, the more likely an individual is to have active disease**.[44] The antigen used (tuberculin protein) is known as **purified protein derivative** of tuberculin (**PPD**) and contains heat-treated products of the growth and lysis of tubercle bacilli.

Purified protein derivative is measured in **Tuberculin Units** (**TU**) and comes in various strengths. Care must be taken to ensure that the correct strength, as prescribed, is used. In addition, PPD must be stored in an appropriate refrigerator, between 2 °C and 10 °C, ensuring that it is not frozen and that it is protected from light. It has a shelf-life of approximately 6 months if properly stored. Once an ampoule is opened, it must be used within 1 hour. As PPD can adsorb onto syringe surfaces, it should be drawn up in the syringe immediately prior to injecting, or used within 30 minutes after the syringe is filled.

Two types of PPD skin testing techniques are in common use: the **Mantoux test** (using diluted PPD) and a multiple puncture technique known as the **Heaf test** (for which concentrated, i.e. **undiluted**, PPD is used).

Heaf test

This technique uses a multiple puncture apparatus (known as the Heaf gun) and is useful for mass screening. Special infection control considerations apply to the disinfection of the puncture apparatus, which are described in other publications.[40] Newer Heaf guns use either a disposable head apparatus (Bignall 2000®) or a self-contained single-use device (UniHeaf®). These avoid both the need for disinfection and any risk of cross-infection and are now recommended as the preferred methods for Heaf testing in the UK, especially in schools' BCG vaccination programmes, in which multiple tests are performed in one session.[44]

Concentrated PPD (**100 000 TU/mL**) is used for the Heaf test. This strength is *only* used for Heaf testing. It is supplied in packs of five ampoules of 1.0 mL, each ampoule normally being sufficient for up to about 20 tests.[44]

Following the administration of PPD by the Heaf technique, the test site is inspected any time from 3 to 10 days later (ideally after 7 days) for a reaction to the administration of the PPD. The Heaf reaction is graded 0–4 according to the degree of induration produced (erythema alone is ignored). Heaf grades 0 and 1 are considered negative; grades 2–4 are positive.

The Bignall 2000® Heaf gun can also be used for BCG vaccination (discussed later in this chapter) and a special disposable head apparatus is available specifically for this purpose.

The Mantoux test

The Mantoux test is the technique used in individual testing situations and is the most common test used for assessing TB infection in HIV-infected individuals. It is also the method of choice in epidemiological studies, as the size of the reaction is a direct indicator of the degree of reactivity, whereas the Heaf test is only semi-quantitative. It does, however, call for greater skill in its use. For routine Mantoux testing, the PPD dilution strength used is **100 TU/mL** (supplied in 1.0-mL ampoules). With this strength, the unit dose in each **0.1 mL is 10 TU of PPD** and this is the usual dose used in Mantoux testing in the UK (in the USA, 5 TU of PPD in 0.1 mL of solution is more commonly used). Additionally, a special dilution containing 10 TU/mL (unit dose being 1 TU in each 0.1 mL) is available for use in people in whom TB is suspected, or who are known to be hypersensitive to tuberculin.

The Mantoux test is performed with a 1-mL syringe (tuberculin syringe) and a short-bevel 25 or 26 gauge, 10 mm long intradermal needle. A separate syringe and needle must be used for each person in order to prevent cross-infection. The injection site may be cleaned (if necessary) with alcohol and allowed to dry prior to the injection. The solution of 0.1 mL of the appropriate PPD dilution is injected **intradermally** into the flexor surface of the forearm at the junction of the upper third with the lower two-thirds. The nurse should document which arm is used for the injection (and usually use the left arm in right-handed people) so that there is no confusion 2–3 days later when the results are noted. A correct intradermal injection will cause a small bleb (*peau d'orange*) or lump to be raised, typically of approximately 7 mm in diameter. If a bleb is not raised, the injection was not correctly given. The results (i.e. the diameter of the induration) will be read 48–72 hours later, but can be read up to 96 hours after the test.[44]

For HIV-infected individuals, a **positive** result (both in the UK and in the USA) consists of a transverse induration (i.e. a thickening of the skin, not the area of erythema, or flare) at least **5 mm in diameter**, as measured by a transparent ruler. The larger the size of the induration, the more positive is the result. Any induration less than 5 mm is considered a negative result.[44] However, Mantoux reactivity is affected by regional factors such as the degree of exposure to sensitizing environmental mycobacteria. National guidelines for the interpretation of Mantoux reactivity should therefore be consulted.

Positive and negative PPD test results

A positive result will be found if the person tested has been infected with mycobacteria in the past and has relatively intact cell-mediated immunity. However, it is non-specific and may only indicate previous infection and not active TB disease. The test will also often be positive in people who have been vaccinated in the past with the Bacillus Calmette–Guérin (BCG) vaccine, although this reactivity wanes with time. Infrequently, because of cross-reactivity between mycobacteria antigens, a positive reaction may be seen in individuals who have been exposed to other, non-tuberculous mycobacteria in the environment. A strongly positive result in an adult (Heaf grade greater than 3 or Mantoux response with an induration of at least 15 mm) probably indicates that the person has active TB (or has received BCG vaccination in the past).

Individuals who are infected with HIV may have lost significant cell-mediated immunity by the time they are tested, and often have negative PPD test responses even when infected with *M. tuberculosis*, especially if their CD4+ T-lymphocyte cell count is less than 200 cells/mm³. This is because they are immunocompromised and have developed a diminished capacity to mount a delayed hypersensitivity reaction to the PPD antigen. This condition is known as **anergy** – from the Greek words *an* (negative) plus *ergon* (work) – and individuals with a decreased ability to mount an immune response are said to be **anergic**. This is not an uncommon situation among HIV-infected people and significantly lessens the reliability of tuberculin skin testing as a diagnostic tool for these individuals.

More detailed information and precise instructions for the administration of PPD and the interpretation of the resulting response can be found in the current edition of the UK Departments of Health's 'Green Book' (*Immunisation against Infectious Disease*), which is updated and published approximately every 5 years by the Stationery Office.[44]

Non-tuberculous mycobacteria

There are a variety of non-tuberculous mycobacteria that can cause serious illness in people who are immunocompromised as a result of HIV infection. In the past, these mainly environmental mycobacteria were sometimes referred to as *atypical mycobacteria* to distinguish them from the *M. tuberculosis* complex and *M. leprae*, the cause of Hansen's disease (leprosy). Non-tuberculous mycobacteria are ubiquitous and widely distributed in nature, existing as saprophytes (that is, living off dead or decaying plant or animal matter), principally in soil and water and also in the intestinal tract of animals and birds. Diseases due to these organisms are not usually transmitted from person to person, although this may rarely occur in immunocompromised individuals. Generally, people become infected with these mycobacteria following source exposure to them in the environment, for example in soil, dirt, swimming pools, drinking water, animals, aquaria, fish. The portal of entry following exposure is sometimes via the respiratory system, but more commonly via the gastrointestinal tract. Some mycobacteria that cause cutaneous diseases, such as *M. marinum*, *M. ulcerans* and (rarely) *M. kansasii*, are contracted through abraded skin, especially in swimming pools and from exposure to contaminated aquaria.[23]

These non-tuberculous mycobacteria are much less virulent than *M. tuberculosis* complex, exposure to them is common and infection does not usually cause any illness in individuals who have a competent, normally functioning immune system and who do not have any other serious predisposing illnesses, such as chronic lung disease, cancer, malnutrition or immunosuppressive conditions. In people with HIV disease, infection with these mycobacteria can cause serious illness, including a pulmonary infection resembling TB, and disseminated systematic disease.[45]

The important non-tuberculous mycobacteria commonly associated with patients with HIV disease are listed in Table 8.4. The most commonly involved are two closely related species, *M. avium* and *M. intracellulare*, often grouped together and referred to as **MAC** (*M. avium* complex) or, less frequently, **MAI** (*M. avium-intracellulare*). For reasons that are not understood, most disease caused by non-tuberculous mycobacteria (about 90 per cent of cases), which may be localized or disseminated, in patients with co-existing HIV disease is due to MAC. Occasionally, however, other non-tuberculous mycobacteria can cause disseminated disease in patients with HIV disease, as noted in Table 8.4.[23,45]

TABLE 8.4 Some commonly encountered non-tuberculous mycobacteria

Species	Notes
M. avium	Account for about 90% of
M. intracellulare	pulmonary disease, lymphadenopathy and disseminated disease in HIV disease
M. kansasii	Cause similar localized or disseminated
M. xenopi	disease, but with much less frequency
M. malmoense	Most clinical isolates are of doubtful
M. fortuitum	clinical significance
M. szulgai	
M. chelonae	

Disseminated MAC disease is generally seen in patients with end-stage HIV disease who have a CD4$^+$ T-lymphocyte count less than 100 cells/mm^3. Since the widespread availability of highly active antiretroviral therapy (HAART) in the UK, disseminated MAC disease has become significantly less common.

Common healthcare problems seen in bacteraemic patients with MAC disease include severe fatigue and chronic malaise, anorexia, weight loss (loss of 15–20 per cent of a person's normal weight), fevers and drenching night sweats and diarrhoea.[45,46]

Physicians use the same investigational tools to diagnose MAC disease, and other non-tuberculous mycobacterial diseases, in patients infected with HIV as they use for TB. Blood cultures are especially important in patients with suspected disseminated disease due to MAC. Cultures of bone marrow, lymph nodes, spleen, exudates and abscesses will often show mycobacterial growth, and TB must be excluded before treatment is prescribed.

Other non-tuberculous environmental mycobacteria may cause human disease, especially of soft tissues, skin and surgical wounds, including *M. chelonei*, *M. ulcerans* and *M. marinum*. In addition, post-injection abscesses can be caused by *M. chelonei* and *M. fortuitum*, which may contaminate syringes, needles or injectable material.[23] These are, however, no more commonly seen in patients with HIV disease than in any other members of the community.

NURSING IMPLICATIONS OF CHEMOTHERAPY FOR HIV-RELATED MYCOBACTERIAL DISEASES

The following discussion of chemotherapy is based on recommendations and guidelines available at the time of publication applicable to the treatment and care of people with TB in the UK. These two authoritative references are the **British National Formulary (BNF)** and current treatment guidelines from the **British Thoracic Society**.[47,48] Both are available online, as is the **National AIDS Manual Treatment Directory**,[46] and are easily accessible to nurses and other healthcare practitioners in the UK (see 'Internet resources' at the end of this chapter for website addresses). Worldwide, the authoritative sources of information on therapy are the WHO and the International Union Against Tuberculosis and Lung Diseases, which issues guidelines on management from time to time that are available online (see 'Internet resources'). Additionally, up-to-date guidelines on the management and care of people with HIV-related TB are published by the **Centers for Disease Control and Prevention (CDC)** in the USA and are also available online.[49]

Because concepts of treatment change with continuing innovations in medical science, it is essential that all healthcare practitioners are able to access the most current information on chemotherapy and drug interactions and side effects (see Table 8.5). This is especially important in HIV-related TB, as important interactions exist between the drugs used to treat HIV disease and those used to treat TB, and side effects from antituberculosis drugs occur more frequently.[43]

There are several important **principles** associated with effective treatment regimens for mycobacterial disease.

- Once identified and cultured, the patient's isolate (specific infecting mycobacteria) is tested in the laboratory for susceptibility to a variety of anti-mycobacterial drugs. However, **empirical treatment**, based upon the physician's own previous experience and standard guidelines, usually commences immediately mycobacterial disease is suspected.
- As mycobacteria quickly develop resistance to the drugs used to treat TB and disease due to MAC, single-drug therapy is never used. Multiple drugs are prescribed, using a three-drug or four-drug regimen, all given simultaneously for an extended period of time.
- Tuberculosis is treated in two phases over a 6-month period: an **initial** (or **induction**) **phase** using four drugs for the first 2 months, and then a **continuation phase** using two drugs for at least 4 months.
- For some forms of non-respiratory TB, the duration of treatment may be longer than 6 months, for example treatment for TB-related central nervous system disease such as meningitis may continue for 12–18 months.
- Individuals infected with HIV respond just as well to chemotherapy as those who are not infected with HIV.
- Patient understanding and adherence are critically essential in preventing the emergence of multiple-drug-resistant organisms. In many instances, healthcare workers or other responsible individuals must directly supervise each and every prescribed administration of medication, a practice now referred to as **directly observed therapy** (DOT).
- Non-adherence to prescribed treatment may be related to the untoward **side effects** of the drugs used, and nurses play a critical role in helping patients adjust to these agents and in keeping the physician informed about the occurrence of any side effects.

STANDARD CHEMOTHERAPY REGIMENS IN THE UK FOR TUBERCULOSIS

Standard short-course (6 months) chemotherapy regimens in the UK consist of using four drugs for the first 2 months of therapy (the initial or induction phase) and then two drugs for the remaining 4 months of treatment (the continuation phase). This is also the standard regimen for smear-positive pulmonary TB advocated by the WHO. The drug regimen in the **induction phase** comprises **rifampicin, isoniazid, pyrazinamide** and **ethambutol**. These are known as **first-line** antituberculosis drugs. During the **continuation phase**, patients are treated with **rifampicin** and **isoniazid**.[48] However, all four first-line antituberculosis drugs used in the initial phase may be continued beyond the first 2 months of treatment in patients for whom there has been a culture positive for *M. tuberculosis* but whose full drug-susceptibility result remains outstanding. Although ethambutol is sometimes omitted from the initial phase of treatment for those patients with a low risk of resistance to isoniazid, it is always included in the treatment regimens for patients known or suspected to be infected with HIV, because of the increased possibility that they may be infected with isoniazid-resistant *M. tuberculosis*. If initial pyrazinamide cannot be tolerated, the duration of treatment in adults and children is frequently extended to 9 months. Although routine daily **pyridoxine** (vitamin B_6) to prevent isoniazid-related peripheral neuropathy is not necessary for most patients, it is recommended for patients with HIV-related TB and for others at increased risk of peripheral neuropathy, such as patients with diabetes mellitus, chronic renal failure or malnutrition and for alcoholics.[48]

CHEMOTHERAPY REGIMENS FOR HIV-RELATED TUBERCULOSIS

Guidelines in the UK recommend that individuals with HIV-related TB who have culture-confirmed sensitivity to first-line antituberculosis drugs should be treated with the 6-month regimen described above, i.e. rifampicin, isoniazid, pyrazinamide and ethambutol for the initial phase and rifampicin and isoniazid for the continuation phase (plus vitamin B_6 for the entire 6 months of treatment).[48] HIV-infected and other immunocompromised people commonly have **drug-resistant TB** and these patients require regimens using **reserve antituberculosis drugs** (see Table 8.5) specifically tailored to their resistance pattern (as demonstrated on culture). These reserve, or second-line, drugs are not as effective as first-line drugs and, consequently, need to be taken by the patient for a longer period of time. Additionally, they have more side effects than first-line drugs. This is a particular concern because of the higher incidence of side effects related to antituberculosis drugs experienced by those infected with HIV.[43] Treatment for drug-resistant or multiple-drug-resistant TB may need to be continued for 24 months or longer.

Rifamycins and antiretroviral drugs

Most patients in the UK with HIV disease are on antiretroviral drug regimens that include **protease inhibitors** (PIs), such as saquinavir, indinavir, ritonavir or nelfinavir, and/or may be taking **non-nucleoside reverse transcriptase inhibitors (NNRTIs)**, such as nevirapine, delavirdine and efavirenz. Antiretroviral drugs are discussed in detail in Chapter 20. These drugs interact with a group of drugs known as **rifamycins**, which are used to treat patients with TB and other mycobacterial diseases. Well-known rifamycins include **rifampicin, rifabutin** and **rifapentine**, and also rifampicin-containing antituberculosis compounds, such as, **Rifater®**, **Rifinah®** and **Rimactazid®**. Rifamycins alter the circulating blood levels of PIs and NNRTIs and may also interact with other drugs commonly used in patients with HIV disease, such as **atovaquone** (an antiprotozoal agent), **ketoconazole** (an antifungal drug) and **methadone** (an opioid analgesic frequently used in the treatment of heroin and other opioid dependence). Consequently, rifamycins are often contraindicated for treating TB in patients who are taking PIs or NNRTIs (but not in those patients taking **nucleoside reverse transcriptase inhibitors** (NRTIs), such as zidovudine, didanosine, zalcitabine, stavudine and lamivudine). Recent guidelines from the CDC in the USA recommend that rifabutin (a rifamycin that has the least impact on blood levels of PIs and NNRTIs) is used as a **substitute** for **rifampicin** for patients taking PIs and NNRTIs (unless the patient is taking ritonavir, hard-gel saquinavir, nevirapine, efavirenz), or that a non-rifamycin antituberculosis regimen is utilized, such as one incorporating **streptomycin**.[49]

Chemotherapy for MAC-related disease

As previously discussed, disseminated infection with MAC is commonly seen in patients with advanced HIV disease, causing a variety of serious health problems. As is the case with many non-tuberculosis mycobacteria, the first-line antituberculosis drugs mentioned above are of limited effectiveness against MAC, and the most common drugs used in a regimen to treat disseminated MAC disease are **rifabutin**, **clarithromycin** and **azithromycin**.

TUBERCULOSIS CHEMOTHERAPY: SIDE EFFECTS AND DRUG INTERACTIONS

The nursing implications of the current drugs used in the treatment and/or prophylaxis of both TB and disease due to MAC in patients infected with HIV are described in Table 8.5, including common side effects and important drug interactions.

TABLE 8.5 Drugs used in the treatment of tuberculosis and MAC disease

First-line drugs used in the treatment of tuberculosis	Nursing implications (side effects and drug interactions)
Isoniazid (N.B. Sometimes abbreviated as **INH**) Non-proprietary name: *Isoniazid* (Celltech) *Compounds* Manufacturer's proprietary names: *Rifater®* (Aventis Pharma) [rifampicin, isoniazid, pyrazinamide] *Rifinah®* (Aventis Pharma) [rifampicin, isoniazid] *Rimactazid®* (Swedish Orphan Int AB) [rifampicin, isoniazid]	Unless specifically contraindicated, like rifampicin, isoniazid should always be included in any antituberculous regimen. Usually given orally (as tablets or an elixir) or, very rarely, intravenously or intrathecally. Peripheral neuropathy is the only common side effect. More rarely, hepatitis and psychosis may be associated with isoniazid administration. Insomnia, restlessness and muscle twitching can occur. Concomitant pyridoxine (vitamin B$_6$) administration is often prescribed to reduce the incidence of peripheral neuropathy, especially in HIV-related tuberculosis. Isoniazid may be used for tuberculosis prophylaxis in patients with HIV disease. Prednisolone increases isoniazid levels and isoniazid administration will increase levels of phenytoin, carbamazepine, diazepam and warfarin. Isoniazid may be given during pregnancy. Isoniazid administration reduces serum levels of the antifungal drugs ketoconazole and fluconazole. Isoniazid is combined with other antituberculosis drugs in compounds, e.g. isoniazid with rifampicin and pyrazinamide.

TABLE 8.5 – continued

First-line drugs used in the treatment of tuberculosis	Nursing implications (side effects and drug interactions)
Rifampicin (USA: rifampin) Manufacturer's proprietary names: *Rifadin*® (Aventis Pharma) *Rimactane*® (Swedish Orphan Int AB) *Compounds* Manufacturer's proprietary names: *Rifater*® (Aventis Pharma) [rifampicin, isoniazid, pyrazinamide] *Rifinah*® (Aventis Pharma) [rifampicin, isoniazid] *Rimactazid*® (Swedish Orphan Int AB) [rifampicin, isoniazid]	Like isoniazid, always included in any antituberculosis regimen unless specifically contraindicated, e.g. in patients with jaundice. Because of the interaction between rifampicin and many antiretroviral drugs (discussed above), is commonly contraindicated in patients with HIV-related tuberculosis. Usually given orally but may be given intravenously. Either given 30 minutes before breakfast or immediately prior to going to sleep in the evening. Hepatitis may be associated with treatment during the first 2 months of therapy. On intermittent treatment, six toxicity syndromes have been described following rifampicin therapy: influenza, abdominal symptoms, respiratory symptoms, shock, renal failure and thrombocytopenic purpura (bleeding disorder). Rifampicin may be given during pregnancy. Rifampicin therapy reduces the effectiveness of oral contraceptives. In addition, by its actions on the liver, rifampicin therapy accelerates the metabolism of several drugs, including: phenytoin, corticosteroids, oral coumarin anticoagulants, oral diabetic drugs, digoxin, methadone, morphine, phenobarbitone and dapsone. Rifampicin therapy may decrease levels of zidovudine (AZT) and of the antifungal drugs ketoconazole and fluconazole. Ketoconazole inhibits the absorption of rifampicin. Nurses must warn patients that this drug causes a red-orange discoloration of urine and other secretions, e.g. sweat, saliva and tears. This can cause staining of soft contact lenses and lens implants.
Pyrazinamide Manufacturer's proprietary name: *Zinamide*® (Merck Sharp & Dohme Ltd) *Compounds* Manufacturer's proprietary name: *Rifater*® (Aventis Pharma) [rifampicin, isoniazid, pyrazinamide]	Usually only given during the first 2–3 months of treatment and is always given in tuberculosis meningitis. This drug is contraindicated in patients with liver damage and porphyria. Is given orally; side effects include hepatitis, gastrointestinal disturbances, arthralgias and hyperuricaemia (leading to gout). Pyrazinamide is not usually given during pregnancy as it may be teratogenic.
Ethambutol hydrochloride Non-proprietary name: *Ethambutol* (Genus)	Given with isoniazid, rifampicin and pyrazinamide during the initial phase of treatment. Given orally. Because this drug can cause visual disturbances, e.g. optic neuritis, loss of visual acuity, red/green colour blindness (especially if the daily dosage is >15 mg/kg), it is not given if patients already have poor vision or optic neuritis. Nurses must advise patients to discontinue treatment with this drug immediately if they develop any signs of ocular toxicity and return to clinic for re-evaluation. If a nursing determination is made that an individual patient cannot understand this aspect of the treatment, alternative drugs can be discussed with the prescribing physician. This is especially important in children, who may not be able to tell you that they are having visual problems. Ophthalmic examinations must be performed before, and at intervals during, treatment. This drug can also cause peripheral neuritis, and sometimes rash, pruritus, urticaria, thrombocytopenia. Ethambutol may be given during pregnancy.

TABLE 8.5 – continued

Reserve (second-line) drugs used in the treatment of tuberculosis	Nursing implications (side effects and drug interactions)
Rifabutin Manufacturer's proprietary name: *Mycobutin®* (Pharmacia & Upjohn)	Similar side effects, drug interactions and contraindications to rifampicin. Principally used for treating HIV-related tuberculosis when patients are also receiving certain antiretroviral drugs, e.g. protease inhibitors and non-nucleoside reverse transcriptase inhibitors. Also used for the prophylaxis and treatment of non-tuberculous mycobacterial disease, e.g. MAC.
Cycloserine Manufacturer's proprietary name: *Cycloserine®* (Lilly)	Used in combination with other drugs to treat drug-resistant tuberculosis. Administered orally and blood concentrations monitored (should not exceed 30 mg/L) Neurological side effects common, including headache, dizziness, vertigo, drowsiness, tremor, convulsions, confusion, psychosis and depression. Also causes rashes, anaemia and changes in liver functions; heart failure has been reported with the use of this drug at high doses.
Streptomycin Non-proprietary name: *Streptomycin sulphate* (Medeva)	Belongs to a group of drugs known as aminoglycosides. Not commonly used any more in the UK, except for some cases of multi-drug-resistant tuberculosis. It is given intramuscularly and the standard dose is not more than 1 g/day in adults. The dose is reduced to 500–750 mg in patients weighing <50 kg or those who are >40 years of age. Children are given doses in the range of 15–20 mg/kg daily. This drug causes ototoxicity and can cause deafness, vertigo and gait disturbances. Side effects increase after a cumulative dose of 100 g, and a nursing record of the cumulative dose given must be kept. Monitoring of hearing and balance necessary. Cutaneous hypersensitivity (skin rashes and fever) may occur, usually within 2–3 weeks of initiating treatment with this drug. If fever develops, the drug should be discontinued and the physician consulted. Streptomycin treatment may rarely result in a chronic eczema involving the limbs, often seen after the eighth week of therapy. Anaphylaxis (collapse and cardiac arrest) can occur following injection with streptomycin. Streptomycin is not given to pregnant women because of the risk of fetal ototoxicity. Nurses must wear gloves when preparing and administering streptomycin because of the risk of developing allergic skin reactions to this agent. Injection sites are alternated daily, as it is a painful injection. As streptomycin must be given by injection, ensuring an adequate supply of sterile needles may present problems.
Thiacetazone (also spelt thioacetazone)	Not used in the UK and, in view of its poor therapeutic activity and severe side effects – notably in HIV-infected people, in whom this drug can cause a severe and often fatal cutaneous hypersensitivity reaction known as Stevens–Johnson syndrome – WHO strongly urge its general abandonment. Its only virtue is its very low cost.

TABLE 8.5 – continued

Reserve (second-line) drugs used in the treatment of tuberculosis	Nursing implications (side effects and drug interactions)
Ethionamide and the closely related **Prothionamide**	Rarely used in the UK. Similar to isoniazid (but with a much higher incidence of toxicity) and is given orally. Side effects include severe allergic cutaneous reactions and drug fever, liver damage and severe nausea, diarrhoea and abdominal pain. Nausea may be reduced if this drug is given in the evening, at bedtime. Anti-emetics may need to be prescribed.
Para-aminosalicylic acid (N.B. Sometimes abbreviated as **PAS**)	Replaced by ethambutol as a first-line agent in the 1960s and now rarely used in the UK. Given orally with food as it may cause gastric disturbances, such as diarrhoea, abdominal pain and nausea. Other side effects include goitre, crystalluria and allergic reactions, e.g. rashes, drug fever and haematological disorders.
Azithromycin Manufacturer's proprietary name: *Zithromax*® (Pfizer)	Used in the treatment of MAC. Given orally as tablets or oral suspension Contraindicated in patients with liver impairment. Side effects include anorexia, dyspepsia, taste disturbances, constipation, dizziness, headache, drowsiness, liver and kidney damage and convulsions. Because this drug can cause photosensitivity, patients should be cautioned about exposure to sunlight. Can rarely cause Stevens–Johnson syndrome.
Clarithromycin Manufacturer's proprietary names *Klaricid*® (Abbott)	Given orally (or intravenously) to treat disseminated disease due to MAC. Side effects: as for azithromycin.
Amikacin Manufacturer's proprietary name: *Amikin*® (Bristol-Myers Squibb)	Similar to streptomycin and capreomycin, with a similar profile of side effects, e.g. urticaria and rashes, hearing loss with tinnitus and vertigo, kidney damage and changes in liver function. Monitoring of hearing and balance necessary. Given by intramuscular or slow intravenous injection or by intravenous infusion.
Capreomycin Manufacturer's proprietary name: *Capastat*® (Dista)	Given by deep intramuscular injection. Pain and induration at injection site common. Side effects as for streptomycin and amikacin. Monitoring of hearing and balance necessary.
Clofazimine Manufacturer's proprietary name: *Lamprene*® (Alliance)	Used to treat patients with mycobacterial disease due to MAC (and leprosy). Given orally. Side effects include severe gastrointestinal disturbances and malabsorption and this drug is contraindicated in patients with a history of peptic ulcer disease. Nurses must warn patients that clofazimine may cause a red discoloration of the skin, hair, urine and faeces. Patients should avoid exposure to sunlight while on clofazimine therapy.

MAC, *Mycobacterium avium* complex.

Corticosteroids

Corticosteroids (e.g. prednisolone, dexamethasone) suppress the inflammatory response and are used with caution in the treatment of patients with TB. They are prescribed in some forms of TB to reduce inflammation and subsequent fibrosis which could compromise the function of vital structures, e.g. in tuberculous meningitis (to prevent arteritis and strangulation of cranial nerves by fibrosis of exudates) and in pericardial TB (to prevent constrictive pericarditis). They may also be used in other clinical situations, e.g. pleural and peritoneal effusions, tubercular lesions of the larynx, kidneys and eye, and in patients who are so ill that they may die before anti-mycobacterial drugs can start to work. In addition, physicians may prescribe steroids as part of the management of severe allergic reactions to anti-mycobacterial drugs. Nurses must be familiar with the common side effects associated with steroid administration, including fluid retention, moon-face, reactivation of peptic ulcer disease and, occasionally, confusion and psychosis.

DRUG-RESISTANT TUBERCULOSIS

In many parts of the world, especially in Asia, Africa and the countries of the former USSR, the emergence of a significant increase in cases of drug-resistant TB is alarming. Drug-resistant TB refers to TB in which the tubercle bacilli are **resistant to one or more first-line antituberculosis drugs**. Mycobacteria become resistant to drugs normally used to treat TB chiefly either as a result of poor adherence to therapy, for example when patients stop taking one or more of their drugs, or as a consequence of incompetent or inappropriate prescribing by physicians. Factors leading to drug resistance are listed in Table 8.6.

Primary and secondary drug resistance

There are two types of drug resistance in TB: **initial (primary) drug resistance** and **secondary (acquired) drug resistance**. Initial resistance is the result of being infected with drug-

TABLE 8.6 Factors associated with the development of drug resistance in the treatment of tuberculosis

Inappropriate medical treatment	■ Monotherapy (using just one drug)
	■ Insufficient number of agents in the regimen
	■ Inappropriate drugs in regimen
	■ Suboptimal dosage
	■ Prior inappropriate use of antituberculosis drugs, e.g. 'over-the-counter' availability and inclusion of antituberculosis drugs in cough medicines in developing countries
Inadequate administration or absorption of medication	■ Poor patient adherence to therapy, e.g. erratic drug ingestion
	■ Poor drug absorption
	■ Patient discontinuing one or more of the prescribed agents due to side effects
Drug logistics	■ Drugs are too expensive
	■ Unreliable supply of drugs
	■ Transportation difficulties in accessing drugs from dispensary
	■ Counterfeit drugs in developing countries

resistant tubercle bacilli following exposure to a person with drug-resistant TB. Secondary resistance is acquired by an individual as a result of either poor adherence to therapy or inadequate treatment. Poor adherence is often associated with those who lead chaotic lifestyles or who are socially, economically and educationally deprived, including the homeless, drug users and alcoholics.

Multiple-drug-resistant TB

Multiple-drug resistance is defined as resistance to **both isoniazid and rifampicin**, the two most effective drugs available for the treatment of TB, irrespective of whether or not there is resistance to other drugs.[23] Drug-resistant tubercle bacilli are transmitted in exactly the same way as drug-susceptible organisms. Several studies in the USA have found that HIV-infected individuals had a significantly higher rate of resistance to all first-line antituberculosis drugs.[46] In the UK, HIV infection (independent of ethnic group) increases the chances of single-drug or multiple-drug resistance at least fourfold compared with people not infected with HIV.[50]

The nosocomial transmission of multiple-drug-resistant TB to healthcare workers and to and among HIV-infected patients, in both hospitals and outpatient clinics, is well documented and associated with extraordinarily high case fatality rates.[51,52] Outbreaks have occurred in dedicated HIV services in the USA, the UK and in other European Community countries.[51–55]

It is important to remember that multiple-drug-resistant TB is transmitted in exactly the same manner as drug-susceptible TB, i.e. by AFB smear-positive individuals who are coughing. Patients with **multiple-drug-resistant TB are not more or less infectious than those with drug-susceptible TB**. They are just infectious for a longer period of time.

Prevention of multiple-drug-resistant tuberculosis

Of critical importance in prevention is ensuring that people with drug-susceptible TB are identified and appropriately treated. Several factors are associated with multiple-drug-resistant TB (Table 8.7),[56] and the presence of any one or more of these should alert nurses during assessment to the possibility that an individual may be at increased risk for multiple-drug-resistant TB. Once identified, effective treatment over a prolonged period is needed to render the individual non-infectious and to eradicate the resistant organisms. Treatment strategies usually incorporate ongoing medication supervision to ensure both consistent adherence to the prescribed treatment regimen and completion of therapy. The supervision of therapy is of the utmost importance in order to prevent resistance developing to even more drugs, and the strategy for supervision must be assessed in each instance and resources identified for this strategy.

Table 8.7 Factors associated with an increased risk for multiple-drug-resistant tuberculosis (MDR-TB)[56]

- Previous drug treatment for tuberculosis
- Contact with a case of known MDR-TB
- HIV infected
- Failure of clinical response to treatment
- Prolong sputum smear positive or culture positive while on treatment (sputum smear positive at 4 months or culture positive at 5 months)

PREVENTIVE THERAPY (CHEMOPROPHYLAXIS) FOR TUBERCULOSIS

Because HIV-infected people (and other immunocompromised individuals) who have been in close contact with another person who has been found to have sputum smear-positive pulmonary TB are at an increased risk of developing active TB themselves, they are started on a preventive regimen of antituberculosis drugs, known as **chemoprophylaxis**.[48,56] This involves giving antituberculosis drugs to an uninfected person at high risk of infection. When chemoprophylaxis is given to an already infected person to prevent latent disease progressing to overt disease, it is referred to as **preventive therapy**. Both strategies usually consist of isoniazid for 6 months or isoniazid and rifampicin for 3 months. If the source patient is known to have multiple-drug-resistant TB, the chemoprophylaxis regimens contain at least three antituberculosis drugs chosen on the basis of the drug-susceptibility pattern of the index case.[48] If the drug-susceptibility pattern is not known, the USA CDC suggest giving ofloxacin or ciprofloxacin with pyrazinamide.[49] Chemoprophylaxis for multiple-drug-resistant TB is given for at least 6–12 months and chest X-ray evaluations are carried out every 3 months.[56,57]

Bacillus Calmette–Guérin vaccination

Albert Calmette and Camille Guérin, French physicians at the Pasteur Institute in Paris, developed the BCG vaccine between 1907 and 1921. This is a live vaccine that was developed from a strain of M. *bovis* that was weakened (attenuated) by repeated subculture in the laboratory. The following discussion on the use of BCG is based upon current guidelines from the UK Departments of Health.[44] BCG is an inexpensive vaccine and is available in a freeze-dried preparation in a rubber-capped vial with the diluent in a separate ampoule. Two preparations are available: one for intradermal administration and one for percutaneous use in infants when using the multiple puncture technique only. The vaccine is simple to administer, transport and store and, in general, gives relatively good protection against TB in some circumstances. The vaccine is stored, protected from light, in a refrigerator (between 2 °C and 8 °C and never frozen) and has a shelf-life of approximately 12–18 months.

The vaccination is administered **strictly intradermally** using a separate tuberculin syringe and a 25 or 26 gauge 3/8th inch needle for each patient. The needle must be attached firmly to the syringe with the bevel uppermost.

The recommended site for the injection is at the insertion of the deltoid muscle near the middle of the left upper arm. In girls, for cosmetic reasons, the upper and lateral surface of the thigh is sometimes used, as the resultant scar will be less visible. However, vaccinations should not be given at this site because they are prone to become infected. A correctly given intradermal injection results in a tense, blanched raised bleb (peau d'orange), typically of 7 mm in diameter following a standard injecting dose of 0.1 mL (0.05 mL for infants less than 3 months of age). The vaccine **must not be administered subcutaneously or intramuscularly** and Jet injectors must not be used for BCG immunization.

In **neonates, infants and very young children only**, the percutaneous route (using a modified Heaf gun) may be used as an alternative to the intradermal method. The Heaf gun technique uses several (18–20) needles and a BCG vaccine that has been specifically prepared for percutaneous use. The percutaneous route for BCG immunization is **not recommended** for older children, teenagers and adults.

BCG vaccination has been available for general use in the UK since 1953, when a national immunization programme was initiated, targeted at children aged 13 years. However, the protection afforded by BCG vaccination is variable and is the subject of much controversy. In the UK, conclusive evidence is available which indicates that the BCG vaccination offers a high level of protection, around 80 per cent, against primary TB,[44] while in other countries, BCG may confer less effective protection. Even so, it is probable that BCG vaccination protects newborn children everywhere against the more serious forms of TB, such as meningeal and disseminated disease. For this reason, the WHO continues to recommend BCG vaccination for all newborn children. Because of the geographical variation in efficacy (see below), BCG vaccination is not in general use in the Netherlands and the USA.

BCG vaccination is only given to individuals who have a negative tuberculin skin test, except for babies, who may be given it during the first 3 months of life without first having a tuberculin skin test. In the UK, government guidelines recommend BCG vaccination for school children between the ages of 10 and 13 years, all students, including trainee teachers and student nurses, and all health service staff who may have contact with infectious patients or their specimens. In addition, contacts of AFB smear-positive cases of active TB are vaccinated, unless the contacts are known to be infected with HIV. BCG vaccination may also be offered to new immigrants to the UK from areas of high prevalence of TB (e.g. the Indian subcontinent) or to those travelling to these areas and planning to remain there for an extended period.

It is not safe to give BCG vaccination to people who are infected with HIV. The vaccine is a live attenuated one, but has enough residual virulence to cause severe local lesions or even disseminated BCG infection, sometimes termed **BCG-osis**, which may prove fatal.[58] In addition, immunosuppression may negatively affect the effectiveness of any vaccine, including BCG. Finally, BCG is a powerful activator of T-lymphocytes and it may, by stimulating them, increase HIV replication and subsequent disease progression. Contraindications to BCG vaccination are as in Table 8.8.

In the UK, BCG vaccination is not given to individuals known or suspected to be infected with HIV, including infants born to HIV-infected mothers. HIV-infected contacts of AFB smear-positive cases of TB are referred to specialist physicians for consideration of anti-mycobacterial chemoprophylaxis, rather than being given BCG vaccination. Recommendations in relation to administering BCG vaccinations vary in different parts of the world. The WHO recommends that in countries where TB in children remains a significant problem, BCG should continue to be given to all well children, including those whose mothers are known to be infected with HIV.

TABLE 8.8 Contraindications to BCG vaccination[44]

BCG vaccination should not be given to people:

- who have received BCG vaccine in the past
- who have a positive tuberculin skin test
- who are receiving corticosteroid or other immunosuppressive treatments, including general radiation
- who are suffering from a malignant condition such as lymphoma, leukaemia, Hodgkin's disease or other tumours of the reticuloendothelial system
- in whom the normal immunological mechanism may be impaired, as in hypogammaglobulinaemia
- who are known to be infected with HIV
- who are pregnant
- with pyrexia
- with generalized septic skin conditions (but for patients with eczema, an immunization site should be chosen that is free from skin lesions)

The protective efficacy of BCG vaccination varies in different countries and this is probably related to exposure to local environmental mycobacteria that sensitizes local populations and modifies the protective response to BCG. In addition, it is important to remember that any protection afforded by BCG vaccination in childhood diminishes with time, and young adults remain at risk of developing active TB.

Improved BCG vaccines and new types of vaccines for preventing TB are the subject of much current research.[59]

Preventing nosocomial transmission of tuberculosis in healthcare settings

The most important way to prevent the transmission of *M. tuberculosis* in healthcare settings is quickly to detect, isolate and treat people with active pulmonary (or laryngeal) TB. People with HIV disease respond just as well to antituberculosis treatment as do those who are not infected with HIV. Prompt treatment will quickly render all patients with drug-sensitive TB non-infectious, usually within 2–3 weeks. Consequently, nurses need to have a high degree of suspicion when assessing patients that respiratory signs and symptoms associated with common opportunistic infections in those with HIV disease, such as pneumonia, might also indicate active TB. In this situation, patients in hospital need to be isolated until TB has been eliminated as a source of their symptoms. Specific infection prevention and control practices for preventing nosocomial transmission of *M. tuberculosis* in healthcare facilities are described in more detail in Chapter 14.

Summary

Stephen Joseph remarked that 'Waxing and waning in recent Western consciousness, TB, like the poor whom it seeks out, is always with us.'[60] Second only to HIV disease itself, TB has emerged as a significant and continuing threat to the public health, truly the terrible synergistic twin of the AIDS pandemic. Once again, all nurses are required to increase their competence in developing prevention and care strategies in relation to TB, an often forgotten plague.

REFERENCES

1. Ryan F. *Tuberculosis: The Greatest Story Never Told* (in the USA: *The Forgotten Plague*). Bromsgrove, UK: Swift Publishers, 1992, 446 pp.
2. Evans CC. Historical background. In: Davies PDO (ed.), *Clinical Tuberculosis*, 2nd edn. London: Chapman & Hall Medical, 1998, 3–19.
3. Dormandy T. *The White Death – A History of Tuberculosis*. London: The Hambledon Press, 1999, 1–12.
4. Daniel TM. *Captain of Death: The Story of Tuberculosis*. Rochester, NY: University of Rochester Press, 1997.
5. Davies RPO, Tocque K, Bellis MA, Rimmington T, Davies PDO. Historical decline in tuberculosis in England and Wales: improving social conditions or natural selection? *International Journal of Tuberculosis and Lung Disease* 1999; **3**:1051–4.
6. Grange JM, Gandy M, Farmer P, Zumla A. Historical declines in tuberculosis – nature, nurture and the biosocial model. *International Journal of Tuberculosis and Lung Disease* 2001; **5**:208–12.

7. World Health Organization. *Tuberculosis*, Fact Sheet No. 104, April 2000. Geneva: WHO. Available online from: http://www.who.int/mediacentre/factsheets/who104/en/index.html

8. Centers for Disease Control and Prevention. *TB Elimination: Now is the Time*, 2001 (online publication, cited March 2003). Available online from: www.cdc.gov/nchstp/tb/

9. World Health Organization. *Global Tuberculosis Control*. WHO Report 2001. WHO/CDS/TB/2001.287. Geneva: WHO, 2001, 181 pp. Available online from: http://www.who.int/gtb/publications/globrep01/

10. Bunyan J. *The Life and Death of Mr. Badman*. New York: R.H. Russell, 1900.

11. World Health Organization. *Background – The Burden of HIV-related Disease, and in particular HIV-related TB*. Background statement on TB and HIV. WHO. Geneva: WHO, January 2001. Available online from: http://www.who.int/

12. World Health Organization. *Drug-resistant Strains of TB Increasing Worldwide*. Press Release WHO/19, 24 March 2000. Geneva: WHO, 2000. Available online from: http://www.who.int/inf-pr-2000/en/pr2000-19.html

13. World Health Organization. *HIV Causing Tuberculosis Cases to Double in Africa*. Press Release WHO/21, 23 April 2001. Geneva: WHO, 2001. Available online from: http://www.who.int/inf-pr-2001/en/pr2001-21.html

14. Joint United Nations Programme on AIDS (UNAIDS), World Health Organization (WHO). *AIDS Epidemic Update: December 2000*. Geneva: UNAIDS and WHO, December 2000, UNAIDS/00.44E, 21 pp. Available online from: http://www.unaids.org/

15. Grange JM. The global burden of tuberculosis. In: Porter JDH, Grange JM (eds), *Tuberculosis: An Interdisciplinary Perspective*. London: Imperial College Press, 1999, 3–31.

16. Cantwell MF, Snider DE, Cauthen GM, Onorato IM. Epidemiology of tuberculosis in the United States, 1985 through 1992. *Journal of the American Medical Association* 1994; **272**:535–9.

17. Burwen DR, Block AB, Griffin LD, Ciesielski CA, Stern HA, Onorato IM. National trends in the concurrence of tuberculosis and acquired immunodeficiency syndrome. *Archives of Internal Medicine* 1995; **155**:1281–6.

18. Centers for Disease Control and Prevention. *Reported Tuberculosis in the United States, 1999*. August 2000, 1–95. Available online from: www.cdc.gov/nchstp/tb/

19. Centers for Disease Control and Prevention. World TB Day – March 24, 2001. *Morbidity and Mortality Weekly Report (MMWR)* 23 March 2001; **50**:1. Available online from: www.cdc.gov/nchstp/tb/

20. Communicable Disease Surveillance Centre (CDSC). Increase in tuberculosis continues. *Communicable Disease Report Weekly (CDR Wkly)* [serial online] 2001 [cited 25 January 2001]; **11**(4). Available online from: www.phls.co.uk/

21. Public Health Laboratory Service. *Disease Facts: Tuberculosis*, Table 1: Tuberculosis – respiratory and non-respiratory notifications, England and Wales, 1913–2000. Available online from: http://www.phls.co.uk/

22. Davies PDO. Tuberculosis and migration. In: Davies PDO (ed.), *Clinical Tuberculosis*, 2nd edn. London: Chapman & Hall Medical, 1998, 355–81.

23. Grange JM. *Mycobacteria and Human Disease*, 2nd edn. London: Arnold (Hodder Headline Group), 1996.

24. Dannenberg AM Jr. Immune mechanisms in the pathogenesis of pulmonary tuberculosis. *Review of Infectious Diseases* 1989; **11**(Suppl. 2):S369–78.

25. Communicable Disease Surveillance Centre (CDSC). Enhanced surveillance of *Mycobacterium bovis* disease in humans in England and Wales from January 2001. *Communicable Disease Report Weekly (CDR Wkly)* [serial online] 2001 [cited 05 January 2001]; **11**. Available online from: www.phls.co.uk/

26. Bouvet E, Casalino E, Mendoza-Sassi G et al. A nosocomial outbreak of multidrug-resistant *Mycobacterium bovis* among HIV-infected patients: a case-control study. *AIDS* 1993; **7**:1453–60.

27. Dankner WM, Waecker NJ, Essey MA et al. *Mycobacterium bovis* infection in San Diego: a clinicoepidemiological study of 73 patients and a historical review of a forgotten pathogen. *Medicine* 1993; **72**:11–37.

28. Adler JJ, Rose DN. Transmission and pathogenesis of tuberculosis. In: Rom WN, Garay SM (eds), *Tuberculosis*. Boston, MA: Little, Brown and Company, 1996, 134–6.

29. Grange JM. Immunophysiology and immunopathology of tuberculosis. In: Davies PDO (ed.), *Clinical Tuberculosis*, 2nd edn. London: Chapman & Hall Medical, 1998, 129–52.

30. Crofton J, Horne N, Miller F. *Clinical Tuberculosis*, 2nd edn. London: Macmillan Education Ltd, 1999, 222 pp.

31. Grange JM. The mystery of the mycobacterial persisters. *Tubercle and Lung Disease* 1992; **73**:249–51.

32. Barnes PF, Barrows SA. Tuberculosis in the 1990s. *Annals of Internal Medicine* 1993; **119**:400–10.

33. Garay SM. Tuberculosis and the human immunodeficiency virus infection. In: Rom WN, Garay SM (eds), *Tuberculosis*. Boston, MA: Little, Brown and Company, 1996, 443–65.

34. Centers for Disease Control and Prevention. Prevention and treatment of tuberculosis among patients infected with human immunodeficiency virus: principles of therapy and revised recommendations. *Morbidity & Mortality Weekly Report (MMWR)* 30 October 1998; **47**(RR20):1–51. Available online from: www.cdc.gov/nchstp/tb/

35. Schurmann D, Nightingale SD, Bergmann F, Ruf B. Tuberculosis and HIV infection: a review. *Infection* 1997; **25**:274–80.

36. Perriens JH, Colebunders RL, Karahunga C et al. Increased mortality and tuberculosis treatment failure rate among human immunodeficiency virus (HIV) seropositive compared with HIV seronegative patients with pulmonary tuberculosis treated with 'standard' chemotherapy in Kinshasa, Zaire. *American Review of Respiratory Disease* 1991: **144**:750–5.

37. Nunn P, Brindle R, Carpenter L et al. Cohort study of human immunodeficiency virus infection in patients with tuberculosis in Nairobi, Kenya. *American Review of Respiratory Disease* 1992; **146**:849–54.

38. Kassim S, Sassan-Morokro M, Achah A et al. Two-year follow-up of persons with HIV-1 and HIV-2 associated pulmonary tuberculosis treated with short-course chemotherapy in West Africa. *AIDS* 1995; **9**:1185–91.

39. Stoneburner R, Laroche E, Prevots R et al. Survival in a cohort of human immunodeficiency virus-infected tuberculosis patients in New York City. Implications for the expansion of the AIDS case definition. *Archives of Internal Medicine* 1992; **152**:2033–7.

40. Harries AD, Maher D. *TB/HIV – A Clinical Manual*. Geneva: World Health Organization, 1996, 37–43.

41. Jenkins PA. The microbiology of tuberculosis. In: Davies PDO (ed.), *Clinical Tuberculosis*, 2nd edn. London: Chapman & Hall Medical, 1998, 69–79.

42. Espinal MA, Peréz EN, Baéz J et al. Infectiousness of *Mycobacterium tuberculosis* in HIV-1-infected patients with tuberculosis: a prospective study. *Lancet* 2000; **355**:275–80.

43. Shafer RW, Montoya JG. Tuberculosis. In: Merigan TC, Bartlett JG, Bolognesi D (eds), *Textbook of AIDS Medicine*, 2nd edn. Baltimore, MD: Williams & Wilkins, 1999, 261–84.

44. UK Departments of Health/Salisbury DM, Begg NT (eds). *1996 Immunisation against Infectious Disease*. London: Stationery Office, 1996, 290 pp. Available from: The Stationery Office Ltd., PO Box 29, Norwich NR3 1GN UK; e-mail customer.services@theso.co.uk or telephone 0870 600 5522, fax 0870 600 5533.

45. Young LS. Nontuberculous (atypical) mycobacteria. In: Merigan TC, Bartlett JG, Bolognesi D (eds), *Textbook of AIDS Medicine*, 2nd edn. Baltimore, MD: Williams & Wilkins, 1999, 285–302.

46. Alcorn K (ed.). *HIV & AIDS Treatments Directory*, 19th edn. London: National AIDS Manual (NAM) Publications, December 2000, 259–64. Updated and published every 6 months and available from: NAM Publications, 16a Clapham Common Southside, London SW4 7AB UK; e-mail: info@nam.org.uk and available online at http://www.aidsmap.com

47. Mehta DK (Executive Editor). *British National Formulary (BNF)*, 41st edn. London: British Medical Association and the Royal Pharmaceutical Society of Great Britain, March 2001, 278–82. Updated and published every 6 months and available from: BMJ Books, PO Box 295, London WC1H 9TE UK, or from their website: www.bmjbookshop.com. The current edition of the BNF is also available online at: www.BNF.org

48. Joint Tuberculosis Committee of the British Thoracic Society. Chemotherapy and management of tuberculosis in the United Kingdom: recommendations 1998. *Thorax* 1998; **53**:536–48. Available online from: http://www.brit-thoracic.org.uk/

49. Centers for Disease Control and Prevention (CDC). Prevention and treatment of tuberculosis among patients infected with human immunodeficiency virus: principles of therapy and revised recommendations. *Morbidity and Mortality Weekly Report (MMWR)* 30 October 1998; **47**(RR20):1–51. Available online from: http://www.cdc.gov/epo/mmwr/preview/mmwrhtml/00055357.htm

50. Hayward AC, Bennett DE, Herbert J et al. Risk factors for drug resistance in patients with tuberculosis in England and Wales 1993–94. *Thorax* 1996; **51**(Suppl. 3):S32.

51. Centers for Disease Control and Prevention (CDC). Nosocomial transmission of multidrug-resistant tuberculosis to health-care workers and HIV infected patients in an urban hospital – Florida. *Morbidity and Mortality Weekly Report* 12 October 1990; **39**:718–22.

52. Centers for Disease Control and Prevention (CDC). Nosocomial transmission of multidrug-resistant tuberculosis to health-care workers and HIV infected patients in an urban hospital – Florida 1988–1991. *Morbidity and Mortality Weekly Report* 30 August 1991; **40**:585–91.

53. Daley CL, Small PM, Schecter GF et al. An outbreak of tuberculosis with accelerated progression among persons infected with the human immunodeficiency virus. *New England Journal of Medicine* 1992; **326**:231–5.

54. Di Perri G, Cruciani M, Danzi MC et al. Nosocomial epidemic of active tuberculosis among HIV-infected patients. *Lancet* 1989; **334**:1502–4.

55. Kent RJ, Uttley AHC, Stoker NG, Miller R, Pozniak AL. Transmission of tuberculosis in a British care centre for patients infected with HIV. *British Medical Journal* 1994; **309**:639–40.

56. Joint Tuberculosis Committee of the British Thoracic Society. Control and prevention of tuberculosis in the United Kingdom: Code of Practice 2000. *Thorax* 2000; **55**:887–901. Available online from: http://www.brit-thoracic.org.uk/

57. Centers for Disease Control. National Action Plan to Combat Multidrug-Resistant Tuberculosis; Meeting the Challenge of Multidrug Resistant Tuberculosis. Summary of a conference, Management of Persons Exposed to Multidrug-Resistant Tuberculosis. *Morbidity and Mortality Weekly Report (MMWR)*, 19 June 1992; **41**(RR-11):6.

58. Grange JM. Complications of bacille Calmette–Guérin (BCG) vaccination and immunotherapy and their management. *Communicable Disease and Public Health* 1998; **1**: 84–8.

59. Enserink M. Driving a stake into resurgent TB. *Science* 2001; **239**:234–5.

60. Joseph S. Public Health Policy Forum: Editorial: Tuberculosis, again. *American Journal of Public Health* 1993; **83**:617 8.

FURTHER READING

Centers for Disease Control and Prevention (CDC). Prevention and treatment of tuberculosis among patients infected with human immunodeficiency virus: principles of therapy and revised recommendations. *Morbidity and Mortality Weekly Report* 30 October 1998; **47**(RR-20):1–51. Available online from: http://www.cdc.gov/epo/mmwr/preview/mmwrhtml/00055357.htm

Centers for Disease Control and Prevention (CDC). Treatment of tuberculosis: American Thoracic Society, CDC, Infectious Diseases Society of America Recommendations. *Morbidity and Mortality Weekly Report* 20 June 2003; **52**(RR-11):1–79. Available online from: http://www.cdc.gov/mmwr/preview/mmwrhtml/RR5211A1.htm

Crofton J, Horne N, Miller F. *Clinical Tuberculosis*, 2nd edn. London: Macmillan Education Ltd, 1999, 222 pp, ISBN 0-333-72430-5.

Davies PDO (ed.). *Clinical Tuberculosis*, 2nd edn. London: Chapman & Hall Medical, 1998, 711 pp, ISBN 0-412-80340-2.

Dormandy T. *The White Death – A History of Tuberculosis*. London: The Hambledon Press, 1999, 433 pp, ISBN 1-85285-169-4.

Dubos R, Dubois J. *The White Plague*. New Brunswick, NJ: Rutgers University Press, 1992, 277 pp, ISBN 0-8135-1224-7.

Grange JM. *Mycobacteria and Human Disease*, 2nd edn. London: Arnold (Hodder Headline Group), 1996, 230 pp, ISBN 0-340-64563-6.

Joint Tuberculosis Committee of the British Thoracic Society. Chemotherapy and management of tuberculosis in the United Kingdom: recommendations 1998. *Thorax* 1998; **53**:536–48. Available online from: http://www.brit-thoracic.org.uk/

Joint Tuberculosis Committee of the British Thoracic Society. Control and prevention of tuberculosis in the United Kingdom: Code of Practice 2000. *Thorax* 2000; **55**:887–901. Available online from: http://www.brit-thoracic.org.uk/

Mann T. *The Magic Mountain*. London: Minerva (Mandarin Paperbacks), 1996, 729 pp, ISBN 0-7493-8642-8.

Mayho P. *The Tuberculosis Survival Handbook*. London: XLR8 Graphics Ltd, 1999, 132 pp, ISBN 0-9535139-0-4.

Mehta DK (Executive Editor). *British National Formulary (BNF)*, current edition. London: British Medical Association and the Royal Pharmaceutical Society of Great Britain.

Updated and published every 6 months. Available from: BMJ Books, PO Box 295, London WC1H 9TE UK, or from their website www.bmjbookshop.com. The BNF is also available online at: www.BNF.org

Rom WN, Garay SM. *Tuberculosis*. Boston, MA: Little, Brown and Company, 1996, 1002 pp, ISBN 0-316-75574-5.

Ryan F. *Tuberculosis: The Greatest Story Never Told* (in the USA: *The Forgotten Plague*). Bromsgrove, UK: Swift Publishers, 1992, 446 pp, ISBN 1-874082-00-6.

UK Department of Health/Salisbury DM, Begg NT (eds). *1996 Immunisation against Infectious Disease*. London: Stationery Office, 1996, 290 pp. Available from: The Stationery Office Ltd, PO Box 29, Norwich NR3 1GN, UK; e-mail customer.services@theso.co.uk or telephone 0870 600 5522, fax 0870 600 5533.

INTERNET RESOURCES

- The Joint Tuberculosis Committee of the British Thoracic Society (BTS) develops the most authoritative chemotherapy and management guidelines for the UK and these are updated on a regular basis:
  http://www.brit-thoracic.org.uk/

- The *British National Formulary (BNF)*, published by the British Medical Association and the Royal Pharmaceutical Society of Great Britain, provides up-to-date information in relation to the drugs used in the UK to treat tuberculosis and the online version is updated every 6 months:
  http://www.BNF.org/

- A valuable source of up-to-date treatment information for HIV disease and associated opportunistic diseases, including tuberculosis and MAC disease, is the *HIV & AIDS Treatment Directory*, published by the National AIDS Manual (NAM). The online version is continually updated:
  http://www.aidsmap.com

- The World Health Organization Global Tuberculosis Programme provides a variety of resources related to the global prevention, treatment and control of tuberculosis, including HIV-related tuberculosis:
  http://www.who.int/gtb/

- The International Union against TB and Lung Disease (IUATLD) publishes tuberculosis treatment guidelines and a variety of other resources, including *The International Journal of Tuberculosis and Lung Disease*:
  http://www.iuatld.org/

- The Centers for Disease Control and Prevention (CDC) in Atlanta, Georgia, USA, incorporates the National Center for HIV, STD and TB Prevention, which provides a wealth of information on HIV-related tuberculosis:
  http://www.cdc.gov/nchstp/od/nchstp.html

CHAPTER 9

HIV disease and the nervous system

Introduction

A diverse range of neurologic and neuropsychiatric complications, affecting both the central and peripheral nervous systems, are frequently associated with HIV disease. They are caused by opportunistic infections, neoplastic processes or the primary effect that HIV has on the nervous system. The risk for neurologic and neuropsychiatric disease in an individual is directly linked to the stage of HIV disease and the associated degree of immunosuppression.[1] This chapter explores the various neurologic manifestations linked to each stage of HIV disease that nurses may encounter when assessing and planning individual patient care interventions, and describes important aspects of patient management.

Learning outcomes

After studying and reflecting on the material in this chapter, you will be able to:

- discuss the potential neurologic and neuropsychiatric conditions associated with the different stages of HIV disease;
- identify nursing care issues associated with the management of patients with these conditions.

NEUROLOGIC CONDITIONS DURING THE STAGES OF HIV DISEASE

HIV infects the brain early in the course of HIV infection and, in some individuals, causes neurologic complications.[1] The stages of HIV disease (described in detail in Chapter 7) provide a sensible structure for exploring the neurologic complications that occur during primary HIV infection (asymptomatic), clinical latency and during early and late symptomatic HIV disease.

Primary HIV infection (CDC Category A)

Neurologic complications may be the first manifestation of HIV infection, appearing around the time of or within a few weeks following seroconversion as a component of an acute retroviral syndrome (Table 9.1). Although not affecting every person during primary HIV infection, neurologic conditions of various degrees of severity are not uncommon, but may go unrecognized or unreported.

TABLE 9.1 Neurologic conditions in primary HIV infection

- Headache
- Meningitis
- Encephalopathy
- Neuropathy
- Myelopathy

Headache

Headache is a common neurologic complaint during primary HIV infection, occurring in one-third or more of people, sometimes accompanied by photophobia or other signs of meningeal irritation (Table 9.2).[2]

TABLE 9.2 Meningeal signs

- Fever
- Headache
- Photophobia
- Stiff neck and back
- Vomiting
- Malaise and drowsiness

Aseptic meningitis

Equally as common as headache, although probably under-reported, is aseptic meningitis, a febrile meningeal inflammation due to early central nervous system (CNS) infection with HIV.[3] Patients frequently seek medical attention because of various meningeal signs (Table 9.2).

This type of meningitis is complicated by additional features not generally seen in patients with aseptic meningitis, that is, it is *atypical*. These atypical features include cranial nerve dysfunction, especially involving cranial nerves V, VII and VIII.[4] Involvement of the trigeminal (V) and facial (VII) nerves may evoke facial numbness, palsy and paralysis and trigeminal neuralgia. Involvement of the auditory (VIII) nerve may produce tinnitus, deafness and vertigo.

Investigations for patients with meningeal signs include lumbar puncture, and head computed tomography (CT) or magnetic resonance imaging (MRI) is essential in order to exclude intracerebral abscess caused by *Toxoplasma gondii*, which may present in a similar fashion. Lumbar puncture might be contraindicated due to the risk of a change in the cerebrospinal fluid (CSF) pressure, caused by the sudden withdrawal of fluid from the spinal canal, precipitating herniation of the medulla and cerebellar tonsils into the foramen magnum, a condition known as **coning**, and often associated with fatal results. CSF obtained from lumbar puncture is usually relatively normal, except for an excessive number of lymphocytes (lymphocytic pleocytosis) and an elevated protein count. Bacteria cannot be cultured from the CSF – hence the name *aseptic* meningitis.[4] However, HIV antibodies and HIV p24 antigen may be detected in the CSF at this stage.[5,6]

Treatment and clinical outcome

Treatment is purely symptomatic, and mild analgesics, such as paracetamol or ibuprofen, may be prescribed for headache. This is a self-limiting condition and the majority of affected individuals fully recover within a week or so.

Acute encephalitis

Acute encephalitis is an acute inflammatory disease of the brain due to direct HIV invasion and/or hypersensitivity initiated by HIV infection of the brain. Like acute atypical meningitis, acute encephalitis may occur soon after HIV infection, at the time of seroconversion; however, it is fortunately a much less common condition than meningitis. This condition differs from atypical aseptic meningitis in that there is evidence of cerebral dysfunction (Table 9.3), which is independent of any signs of meningeal inflammation.

TABLE 9.3 Signs of cerebral dysfunction

■ Alterations in level of consciousness
■ Personality change
■ Seizures
■ Paresis
■ Focal neurological signs

Patients with signs of cerebral dysfunction are, like patients with meningeal signs, also investigated by lumbar puncture and CT and/or MRI to exclude cryptococcal meningitis and intracerebral abscess caused by *T. gondii*. Acute encephalitis is a more serious condition than atypical aseptic meningitis and, although recovery can be expected, high-dependency nursing care is required to maintain a therapeutic environment for the patient to recover. The patient's need for nutrition, adequate hydration and to maintain a normal body temperature must be carefully assessed and facilitated. Antipyretics and anticonvulsant medications may be prescribed and antiretroviral drugs may be used.

Other neurologic conditions in primary HIV infection

Other neurologic conditions, such as neuropathies and myopathies, may also be seen at any stage of HIV disease and also occur during primary HIV infection, necessitating a neurological assessment. However, in almost all patients, the neurologic conditions that may accompany primary HIV infection will resolve spontaneously within a short period of time, rarely leaving any long-term sequelae.

Clinical latency (CDC Category A)

Demyelinating polyneuropathies

Serious HIV-related demyelinating polyneuropathies occasionally develop during asymptomatic HIV infection. One type, known as acute inflammatory demyelinating neuropathy is similar to Guillain–Barré syndrome. This is a rapidly developing form of polyneuropathy characterized by progressive muscular weakness in the face, arms and legs, and affecting muscles that control swallowing and breathing. This can lead to paralysis and various disorders of movement, due to stripping away of the insulating myelin that coats and protects the spinal roots and peripheral nerves. It is an autoimmune process in which the body is attacking itself, and patients usually present with signs involving both sides of the body (symmetrical signs). A more chronic form of inflammatory demyelinating polyneuropathy can also occur.

Treatment
As this condition can rapidly evolve over just a matter of hours, and because paralysis may occur and respiratory function may be compromised, patients need to be admitted to hospital as a **medical emergency**. These patients require careful monitoring and support for vital functions, the maintenance of a patent airway, and pulmonary vital capacity measurements to assess the need for respiratory assistance. Plasma exchange is used in the early stages of this condition and is generally considered the treatment of choice in acutely ill patients. This technique is also known as **plasmapheresis** and involves the removal of plasma from the body to filter out immunoglobulins (antibodies) and lymphocytes that may be involved in the autoimmune attack on the nerve's myelin coat, and then transfusing the filtered plasma back into the body. Daily intravenous infusions of immune globulin (γ-globulin) are also effective and may be safer. Corticosteroids are contraindicated and are not used in this condition.[7]

Early symptomatic HIV disease (CDC Category B)

Peripheral neuropathy (PN) is the most common neurologic condition in early symptomatic HIV disease and is also discussed in Chapter 7. PN results from damage to the peripheral nerves arising from a variety of causes (Table 9.4).

TABLE 9.4 Causes of peripheral neuropathy in patients with HIV disease

Damage to the peripheral nerves may result from:
■   direct effect of HIV infection on the peripheral nerves
■   HIV-related opportunistic infections and co-morbidities
■   antiretroviral drugs and other drugs used for the management of opportunistic events
■   Lifestyle factors, e.g. alcohol and other recreational drugs

There is symmetrical involvement of both sensory and motor nerves (**symmetrical sensorimotor neuropathy**) and patients frequently complain of the occurrence of spontaneous pains (dysaesthesia) and pain that is provoked by gentle, light touch or temperature stimulation (hyperaesthesia). People with PN often experience weakness and wasting in the arms and legs, a condition known as **distal atrophy**. Involvement of the spinal nerve roots may produce pain referred to the back of the thigh and leg below the knee, weakness, flaccidity and eventually atrophy of the legs (**radicular syndrome**). Involvement of a peripheral nerve on one side of the body (asymmetric) is characterized by a sensation of numbness, prickling or tingling (paraesthesia), pain and weakness. This condition is known as **mononeuritis multiplex**. Acute PN may present as a facial paralysis and involve only one side of the face (**Bell's palsy**). Treatment with analgesics, antidepressants and alternative forms of therapy, such as acupuncture, are helpful for some, but generally unsatisfactory for most, and many patients are left with a chronic and painful disability unresponsive to treatment.

Late symptomatic HIV disease (CDC Category C)

Most major neurologic and neuropsychiatric complications occur during late symptomatic disease and represent serious clinical conditions with often grave outcomes (Table 9.5).

TABLE 9.5 Neurologic and neuropsychiatric conditions in late symptomatic HIV disease[2]

Central nervous system

1. Opportunistic infections

    Cerebral toxoplasmosis

    Cryptococcal meningitis

    Progressive multifocal leucoencephalopathy (PML)

    Cytomegalovirus (CMV) encephalitis

    Herpes simplex encephalitis

2. Opportunistic neoplasms

    Primary CNS lymphoma

3. Organic mental disorders (acute and chronic)

4. Cerebrovascular disorders

5. Headache (without meningitis)

6. Metabolic and toxic disorders

    Hypoxic encephalopathy

    'Sepsis' encephalopathy

Peripheral nervous system

7. Distal sensory polyneuropathy (DSPN)

8. Toxic axonal neuropathy

9. CMV polyradiculopathy

10. Mononeuritis multiplex

11. Myopathies

1. Opportunistic infections of the central nervous system

Cerebral toxoplasmosis

It is thought that reactivation of latent *T. gondii* infection is responsible for the development of cerebral toxoplasmosis in most patients with late symptomatic HIV disease, rather than newly acquired infection.[2,8] It is the most common cause of space-occupying lesions of the brain occurring in HIV-infected people,[3,9] although the incidence of this condition has decreased over the last decade, principally due to the widespread use of co-trimoxazole (Septrin®) for prophylaxis against pneumonia caused by *Pneumocystis carinii* and which also protects against cerebral toxoplasmosis.[10] Patients experience fever, confusion and headache, along with focal neurologic signs (Table 9.6).[4] This is a serious disease, but most patients will respond well to current therapy. Cerebral toxoplasmosis is discussed in more detail in Chapter 7.

Cryptococcal meningitis

A granulomatous meningitis, with granulomas or cysts developing in the cerebral hemispheres, typically results from this fungal infection of the CNS caused by *Cryptococcus neoformans*. Patients present with a history of headache, fever, nausea and vomiting and photophobia. Some may also experience seizures. This is another serious infectious neurologic complication seen in late symptomatic HIV disease and is discussed in more detail in Chapter 7.

TABLE 9.6 Neurologic signs and symptoms associated with cerebral toxoplasmosis[11]

Focal	Non-focal	Systemic
Hemiparesis	Headache	Fever
Ataxia	Confusion	
Seizures	Lethargy	
Cranial nerve palsies	Coma	
Dysmetria	Psychomotor retardation	
Movement disorder		

Progressive multifocal leucoencephalopathy

Like cerebral toxoplasmosis, progressive multifocal leucoencephalopathy (PML) is another important cause of focal CNS disease in late symptomatic HIV disease. It is caused by either primary infection or (more usually) reactivation of latent JC virus infection, the human papovavirus first successfully cultured in the USA in 1971 from a patient whose initials were JC (not to be confused with Jakob–Creutzfeldt disease). This virus is distributed throughout the world and most people in cities in the Western world have been infected by middle adulthood.[11] Primary infection is asymptomatic in most people, although some will have a mild respiratory illness during which the virus can be transmitted to others by respiratory droplets. The virus then lies dormant in the kidneys and lymphoid tissue in most people[12] and very rarely causes illness in anyone with a healthy, competent immune system. However, latent infection can be reactivated and cause grave illness in people who are immunocompromised, and today, PML is principally seen in late symptomatic HIV disease in patients with profoundly depressed cell-mediated immune responses, typically with CD4+ T-lymphocyte counts of less then 100 cells/mm^3 (μL). In the UK, the incidence of PML in HIV-infected people has increased, as severely immunocompromised people live longer, and now occurs in 4–8 per cent of patients with late symptomatic HIV disease (often being the first AIDS-defining opportunistic infection in these patients).[12]

Progressive multifocal leucoencephalopathy is a subacute or gradual demyelinating CNS disorder that is relentlessly progressive; the duration from onset of symptoms to death is usually 1–9 months. Most patients present with focal neurological signs, including hemiparesis, gait ataxia, aphasia (speech difficulties) and visual disturbances (including hallucinations). There is also significant cognitive decline and other neurologic signs and symptoms may evolve, reflecting the diffuse involvement of the cerebral hemispheres. The diagnosis is made by identifying the virus in the CSF or in brain tissue following biopsy. However, typical clinical, CSF and radiological (especially MRI) findings are generally sufficient to diagnose this condition and avoid brain biopsy.[12] Antiretroviral therapy with zidovudine-containing regimens may be helpful; otherwise, there is no effective treatment for this disastrous late-stage event.

CMV and HSV acute encephalitis

Acute viral encephalitis is an acute inflammatory disease of the brain occurring in late symptomatic HIV disease and caused by reactivation of latent cytomegalovirus (CMV) or herpes simplex virus (HSV) infection. Patients usually have fever and malaise, with or without more extensive meningeal signs (see Table 9.2) and may show signs of cerebral dysfunction (see Table 9.3) and cranial nerve abnormalities.[7] Patients with HSV encephalitis may have repeated seizures early in the course of their disease, and those with CMV encephalitis may have signs and symptoms ranging from acute confusion to a gradual-onset dementia.[13] The antiviral drugs used for HSV and CMV infection are described in Chapter 7

(Tables 7.7 and 7.17). In general, intravenous aciclovir is used to treat HSV encephalitis and intravenous ganciclovir is used in the treatment of CMV encephalitis.

2. Opportunistic neoplasms

Lymphoma and the central nervous system

Lymphomas are cancers arising out of the lymphatic system and caused by uncontrolled multiplication of either T-lymphocytes or, more commonly, B-lymphocytes. These cancerous lymphoma cells can be confined to one or more lymph nodes or can spread away from the lymph nodes (extra-nodal spread) throughout the body to any organ or system, such as the bone marrow. There are different types of **systemic lymphomas**, the most common being Hodgkin's disease, non-Hodgkin's lymphoma (NHL), immunoblastic lymphoma and Burkitt's lymphoma. All of these systemic lymphomas occur at an increased frequency in HIV-infected people, especially NHL.[14,15]

Non-Hodgkin's lymphoma   Non-Hodgkin's lymphoma is usually an aggressive lymphoma, mainly arising from B-lymphocytes (but can sometimes evolve from T-lymphocyte-derived lymphoma cells) and with a tendency for extra-nodal spread, such as to the brain. NHL occurs in patients with both early and late symptomatic HIV disease at an incidence 60 times greater than in people who are not infected with HIV, accounting for at least 3 per cent of AIDS-defining diagnoses in Europe and the USA and ultimately affecting 5–10 per cent of patients during the course of late symptomatic HIV disease.[14,15] More HIV-infected people are now presenting with NHL because combined antiretroviral treatment and chemoprophylaxis for opportunistic infections prolong survival. As people with moderate to severe immunosuppression live longer, they are becoming more vulnerable to these opportunistic cancers, which typically present at the end-stage of HIV disease. Current evidence suggests that the presence of Epstein–Barr virus (EBV), also known as human herpesvirus 4 (HHV4), is associated with transforming healthy lymphocytes in some people into lymphoma cells, that is, it acts as a 'transforming factor'.[14,15] HIV-infected macrophages express cytokines that may also drive polyclonal B-cell proliferation, and human herpesvirus 8 (HHV8), associated with the development of Kaposi's sarcoma, may also be involved in causing NHL.[16]

Primary central nervous system lymphoma

Approximately one out of five HIV-associated lymphomas are primary CNS lymphomas (PCNSL). Primary means that the lymphoma originates in the brain; however, secondary spread to the CNS from systemic NHL can also occur. These space-occupying mass lesions of the brain occur principally in severely immunocompromised people, such as those with CD4+ T-lymphocyte counts of less then 50 cells/mm³ (μL) and, like systematic NHL, it is becoming more common as people with HIV disease live longer at the lower end of a continuum of declining CD4+ T-lymphocytes because of antiretroviral therapy.

Patients with PCNSL often present with a variety of neurologic deficits similar to those of cerebral toxoplasmosis, another cause of space-occupying mass lesions in the brain in patients with late symptomatic HIV disease. They may experience changes in personality, slowing of intellect and movement, hemiparesis, aphasia, headache and seizures. They are usually conscious, although may be confused, lethargic and apathetic.

Diagnostic radiologic investigations include CT and MRI and examination of CSF. *Toxoplasma* serology and other tests to rule out cerebral toxoplasmosis are routine, including lumbar puncture in which the CSF is examined for cytology and HHV4 sequences. Additionally, brain biopsy may be undertaken.

Standard treatment regimens employ high-dose corticosteroids and whole-brain radiotherapy; however, any respite is brief and patients rarely survive beyond 3–5 months following treatment.[15,16] For some severely ill patients, it may be decided to withhold treatment, a decision taken with the patient's own desires paramount. Patients who are not competent enough to discuss this may have expressed their wishes previously in a 'Living Will', which should be respected. Additionally, discussions with the patient's husband or wife, partner, other family member or a person on whom the patient has conferred Power of Attorney are also helpful in this distressing situation.

3. Organic mental disorders

Organic mental disorders (OMDs) are extremely common in patients with AIDS, being seen in upwards of 70 per cent of all patients. They are classified as being either acute or chronic.

Acute organic mental disorders

Delirium is the major acute OMD seen in patients with late symptomatic HIV disease and is characterized by an altered and/or fluctuating level of consciousness. Delirium has an acute onset and is secondary to common underlying conditions seen in patients during late symptomatic HIV disease (Table 9.7).

TABLE 9.7 Some causes of delirium in late symptomatic HIV disease

- CNS opportunistic infections
- Meningitis (e.g. atypical aseptic meningitis)
- HIV encephalopathy
- CNS neoplasms
- Seizure disorders and post-seizure states
- Septicaemia
- Cerebral hypoxia
- Electrolyte imbalance (e.g. hyponatraemia, hyperkalaemia, hyperglycaemia or hypoglycaemia)
- Hypotension resulting from intravenous pentamidine therapy
- Cerebral oedema
- Cerebrovascular infarction or haemorrhage
- Pyrexia
- Brain abscess
- Environmental factors (e.g. isolation, distress, sleep deprivation)
- Various drugs (side effects) and alcohol

Treatment is aimed at correcting the underlying cause of delirium and maintaining a safe environment for the patient to recover. Patients require regular neuropsychiatric nursing assessments, reality orientation and reassurance. Sedatives and analgesics should not be given during this episode as they further depress the cerebral cortex. However, anti-psychotic drugs, such as haloperidol or risperidone, may be prescribed for severe agitation in preference to benzodiazepines.[17] Mania and psychosis can also occur and require specialist nursing interventions.

Chronic organic mental disorders

Chronic OMDs are more frequently encountered in individuals with late symptomatic HIV disease than acute OMD. Dementia is the predominant chronic OMD seen in patients with AIDS and, like acute OMD, has a multifactorial aetiology (Table 9.8).

TABLE 9.8 Some causes of dementia in late symptomatic HIV disease

- HIV-associated dementia (adults) or HIV encephalopathy (children)
- Progressive encephalitis due to other viruses (e.g. CMV, herpes simplex, varicella zoster and JC virus)
- Space-occupying lesions caused by PCNSL or (rarely) Kaposi's sarcoma
- Space-occupying lesions caused by infectious agents (e.g. *Candida albicans*, *Toxoplasma gondii*, *Cryptococcus neoformans*)
- Cerebrovascular accidents

CMV, cytomegalovirus; PCNSL, primary CNS lymphoma.

The most common cause of dementia is the direct effect of HIV infection on either cerebral cortical or subcortical structures of the brain. The resulting dementia has been previously referred to by various terms, including HIV-1 associated cognitive/motor disorder and the AIDS dementia complex (ADC). However, it is now mainly referred to as **HIV-1-associated dementia (HAD)** in adults and **HIV encephalopathy** in children.[18]

Although the incidence of HAD has declined since the introduction of highly active antiretroviral therapy (HAART), it has not declined as much as other AIDS-defining illnesses, and this may reflect the relatively poor penetration into the CNS of many antiretroviral drugs used in HAART regimens.[19] There are no reliable data on the prevalence of HAD in late symptomatic HIV disease in the age of HAART in the UK. However, it is a serious condition with a poor prognosis that develops in people with severely compromised immunity, usually those with a CD4+ T-lymphocyte count of less then 50 cells/mm^3 (μL) and generally in people who have had other AIDS-defining opportunistic illnesses.

This condition is diagnosed by the patient's history and a comprehensive neuro-clinical assessment. Formal neuropsychological testing, such as the HIV Dementia Scale (HDS),[20] and other neuropsychological tests, assessing motor speed and agility and concentration and attention, are frequently used.[2] Neuroimaging, CSF examinations and electroencephalography (EEG) are also used, principally in ruling out other causes of dementia.[2,21]

HIV-1-associated dementia has an insidious onset. There is a progressive loss of cognitive function and a gradual increase in the severity of motor-sensory deficits. Individual presentations can be quite variable, and the degree of brain impairment can range from moderate to severe. Depression commonly accompanies HAD.

HIV frequently affects both motor and sensory nerves in the spinal cord in patients with HAD and produces a **vacuolar myelopathy**. This results in a paraesthesia, weakness and spasticity of the legs. There may be a failure or irregularity of muscular coordination, especially manifested when voluntary muscular movements are attempted (ataxia). Urinary incontinence may develop.

A careful nursing assessment will reveal various indicators of cortical dysfunction (Table 9.9) and disease progression can be documented in a clinical staging system (Table 9.10).[2]

Antiretroviral drugs, especially zidovudine-containing regimens, are used for treating HAD, and other drugs are used in symptom management.[22,23]

Managing the care environment for patients with HAD Adjusting or manipulating the patient's environment in relation to his or her neurocognitive condition, a strategy sometimes referred to as 'milieu management', provides a rational way to provide a safe and reassuring environment for patients experiencing this distressing feature of late symptomatic HIV disease. Milieu management has been well described[17] and the salient features of this model are reflected in Table 9.11.

TABLE 9.9 HIV-associated dementia: indicators of cortical dysfunction

Disorders of intellect

- Memory loss
- Short attention span and impairment in ability to concentrate
- Deterioration in learning abilities and ability to abstract
- Slow and difficult thinking
- Blunting of perception and errors of judgement

Disorders of behaviour

- Social withdrawal
- Disinhibited or embarrassing and anti-social behaviour
- Deterioration in self-care (e.g. lack of attention to personal cleanliness, dress and nutrition)

Disorders of mood

- Labile emotions (easily frustrated, irritable, quickly changing mood)
- Anxiety
- Depression
- Disorders of personality
- Former personality traits accentuated
- Interpersonal relationships altered
- Demanding behaviour and egocentricity

TABLE 9.10 Clinical staging of HIV-associated dementia[2]

Stage	Characteristics
Stage 0 (normal)	Normal mental and motor function
Stage 0.5 (equivocal/subclinical)	Either minimal or equivocal evidence of motor impairment; can work and perform activities of daily living
Stage 1 (mild)	Unequivocal evidence of functional impairment; able to do all but demanding tasks
Stage 2 (moderate)	Cannot work but can perform basic activities of self-care
Stage 3 (severe)	Major intellectual incapacity or motor disability
Stage 4 (end-stage)	Nearly vegetative

TABLE 9.11 Milieu management[17]

- Assess patient's motor function, orientation and memory on a regular basis and adjust the environment to maximize the patient's autonomy and minimize the patient's risks
- Conduct a safety assessment (both for home and institutional care), noting and adjusting all hazards, e.g. electrical, chemical, sharp objects, unstable furniture and carpets and handrails on staircases
- Ensure that hallways, staircases, walkways and rooms are brightly lit and free of clutter
- Provide appropriate reality-orientation cues, e.g. calendars, clocks
- Assess patient's need for supervision (from healthcare professional or family member or friend) and allocate appropriately
- Adopt appropriate communication techniques, e.g.:

  ask simple yes-or-no questions and avoid lengthy explanations, giving short, pragmatic answers;

  because long-term memory is usually intact, sharing remote reminiscences may be soothing; however, because short-term memory is impaired, patients may find immediate recall efforts frustrating;

  speak in a low-pitch, clear, slow and even tone of voice
- Assess well-being of caregivers and family and friends and arrange appropriate support

4. Cerebrovascular disorders

Transient cerebral ischaemic attack or stroke-like events may sometimes occur in late symptomatic HIV disease, but major strokes are rare.[2] CNS bleeding related to emboli from non-bacterial endocarditis, immune thrombocytopenic purpura (ITP) or cerebral arteritis is sometimes seen in patients in late symptomatic HIV disease. The onset of symptoms is usually abrupt, with headache followed by steadily increasing neurological deficits. Hemiparesis is seen in major bleeds located in the hemispheres. Symptoms of cerebellar or brainstem dysfunction (e.g. conjugate eye deviation or ophthalmoplegia, stertorous breathing, pinpoint pupils and coma) occur when the bleed is located in the posterior fossa. Nausea and vomiting, focal or generalized seizures and loss of consciousness are all common. The diagnosis is made with CT scans and MRI. Lumbar puncture is usually contraindicated, as the change in CSF pressure during lumbar puncture may precipitate transtentorial herniation. Treatment is symptomatic, and a rehabilitation plan is developed during the early recovery period.

5. Headache

Headache can be accompanied by many of the neurologic conditions in late symptomatic disease. However, patients sometimes have severe and protracted headache ('HIV headache') for which an underlying cause is not apparent.[1,24] It is suggested that circulating vasoactive cytokines may cause this condition in some patients.[1] Tricyclic antidepressants may be prescribed and some patients may require opiate analgesia.

6. Metabolic and toxic disorders

Patients may develop metabolic or toxic encephalopathies secondary to systemic non-neurologic diseases, such as pneumonias with hypoxia and systemic sepsis.[1] Wernicke's encephalopathy, caused by an inadequate intake or absorption of thiamine coupled with continued carbohydrate ingestion, may also occur as a result of food faddism or alcoholism. Encephalopathy is a serious medical condition and patients may become ataxic, confused, drowsy or stuporous and require intensive nursing care.

7. Distal sensory polyneuropathy

Painful or burning dysaesthesia of the feet and hands (in a 'stocking and glove' distribution) is commonly encountered in symptomatic HIV disease. Pain may be mild to moderate or so severe that it interferes with walking. Antidepressants and analgesics may be prescribed, but, as in other forms of peripheral neuropathy, treatment is often unsatisfactory.

8. Toxic axonal neuropathy

This is another sensory neuropathy caused by the toxic effect of some nucleoside antiretroviral drugs (the 'd' drugs), such as zalcitabine (ddC), didanosine (ddI), and stavudine (d4T). If recognized early, this condition may be slowly reversible when the offending drugs are discontinued.

9. Cytomegalovirus polyradiculopathy

Although rare, this condition is important in late symptomatic HIV disease because it causes a catastrophic polyradiculopathy leading to severe lumbosacral and radicular pain along with bladder and bowel dysfunction, and ascending weakness and sensory loss. It is also important because, being caused by CMV, it can be treated. Early recognition and treatment may arrest and, in some cases, reverse the condition.[2,25] Various anti-CMV drugs that are active against CMV (Table 9.12) are used to treat this serious neurologic complication of HIV disease.

10. Mononeuritis multiplex

Cytomegalovirus infection can damage multiple independent nerves, causing an aggressive and potentially fatal multifocal neuropathy in late systematic HIV disease. Untreated, patients may develop progressive paralysis and eventually die from this condition. Antiviral drugs active against CMV (Table 9.12) are frequently given on an empirical basis if this condition is suspected.

TABLE 9.12 Antiviral drugs active against cytomegalovirus

Drug	Nursing note
Ganciclovir (Cymevene®)	Administered by intravenous infusion May be given in combination with foscarnet sodium This drug is toxic and nurses need to be adequately protected during handling and administration If solution comes into contact with skin or mucosa, it must be washed off immediately with soap and water
Foscarnet sodium (Foscavir®)	Administered by intravenous infusion May be given in combination with ganciclovir
Cidofovir (Vistide®)	Administered by intravenous infusion Usually given in combination with probenecid Prior intravenous hydration with sodium chloride 0.9% required immediately before cidofovir infusion This drug is toxic and nurses need to be adequately protected during handling and administration If solution comes into contact with skin or mucosa, it must be washed off immediately with soap and water

Consult *British National Formulary* for contraindications, side effects, cautions, dose and administration instructions.

11. Myopathies

Myopathy in HIV disease is a slowly progressive condition in which patients develop muscle wasting and proximal weakness. This condition may be caused by the direct action of HIV or, more commonly, the toxic effects of zidovudine, the first antiretroviral drug widely used. Zidovudine toxicity is dose related and current treatment regimens use less toxic doses. Consequently, zidovudine-related myopathy is now less common.

CARING FOR PATIENTS WITH NEUROLOGIC AND NEUROPSYCHIATRIC SYNDROMES

In assessing patients, nurses need to be alert to potential problems associated with neurologic and neuropsychiatric syndromes occurring during HIV disease (Table 9.13) and plan appropriate interventions.

In addition, a functionally orientated nursing neurological evaluation (Table 9.14) is helpful in patient assessment.[26] Following assessment, nursing interventions can be planned that incorporate both general and individualized nursing care objectives.

TABLE 9.13 Potential patient problems associated with neurologic and neuropsychiatric syndrome in HIV disease

Potential problem	Origin of problem
Alterations in maintaining self-care requisites	Nervous system dysfunction
Fever, headache, nausea and vomiting, drowsiness, stiff neck	CNS opportunistic infections and meningeal inflammation
Alterations in level of consciousness, focal neurological signs, seizures, paresis, personality changes	Cerebrovascular accidents and cerebral dysfunction
Pain, weakness and wasting in arms and legs, flaccidity and atrophy of legs, paraesthesia, facial paralysis	Peripheral neuropathy
Paraesthesia, weakness and spasticity of legs, ataxia, urinary incontinence	Vacuolar myelopathy
Erectile failure, diarrhoea, hypotension	Autonomic neuropathy
Muscular weakness, disorders of movement	Polyneuropathy
Impairment of reason, perception, intuition, memory, language and ability to learn	HIV-associated dementia
Delirium, dementia, impaired cognitive function, incontinence	Organic mental disorders
Pressure sores	Incontinence, immobility
Emotional lability	Cerebral dysfunction
Disturbances in gait and sense of balance	Neuropathy, cerebellar dysfunction
Airway obstruction	Unconsciousness

TABLE 9.14 Organization of a functionally oriented nursing neurological evaluation[26]

General category	Functional category	Examples of specific function which may be tested
Consciousness	Arousing (reticular activating system)	Arousability, response to verbal and tactile stimuli
Mentation	Thinking (general cortical function plus specific regional functions)	Educational level, content of conversation, orientation, fund of information, insight, judgement, planning
	Feeling (affective)	Mood and affect, perception and reaction to ability, disability
	Language	Content and quality of speech, ability to name objects, repeat phrases, to read, write and copy
	Remembering	Attention span, recent and remote memory
Motor function	Seeing (cranial nerves II, III, IV, VI)	Acuity, visual fields, extra-ocular movement, pupil size, shape, reactivity, presence or absence of diplopia, nystagmus
	Eating (cranial nerves V, IX, X, XII)	Chewing, swallowing, gag (if swallowing impaired)
	Expressing facially (cranial nerve VII)	Symmetry of smile, frown
	Speaking (cranial nerves VII, IX, X, XII)	Clarity, presence or absence of nasality
	Moving (motor and cerebellar systems)	Muscle tone, mass, strength, presence or absence of involuntary movements. Coordination: heel-to-toe walk, observing during dressing, posture, gait, position
Sensory function	Smelling (cranial nerve I)	Ability to detect odours
	Blinking (cranial nerve V)	Corneal reflex
	Hearing (cranial nerve VIII)	Acuity, presence or absence of unusual sounds
	Feeling (sensory pathways)	Pain: pin prick, touch, stereognosis, temperature (warm, cold)

GENERAL NURSING CARE OBJECTIVES FOR PATIENTS WITH HIV-RELATED NEUROLOGIC AND NEUROPSYCHIATRIC CONDITIONS

The primary objectives of care are to:

- maintain a safe environment in which the patient can recover;
- prevent complications from neurological assault;
- maintain vital functions and patent airways;
- provide support to the patient, family and friends;
- facilitate the patient to regain maximum independence; and
- assist the patient to meet self-care requisites.

Altered level of consciousness

Where serious neurologic disease affects the patient's level of consciousness, additional information to inform a nursing assessment may need to be obtained from a variety of sources, including family, friends and neighbours, as the patient will not be able to provide a reliable history. The assessment must take into consideration any medications or non-prescription drugs the patient may be using. A **Glasgow Coma Scale**[27,28] (Figure 9.1) is initiated to compare changes in the patient's level of consciousness over a given period of time. This scale assesses three aspects of behavioural response that indicate the general functioning or dysfunction of the brain: eye opening, verbal response and motor response.

Eye opening
- Spontaneously – patient opens eyes when nurse approaches bed.
- Opening to speech – patient opens eyes in response to his/her name being spoken either at normal speaking voice or increased volume.
- Opening to pain – patient opens eyes in response to painful stimuli.
- No eye opening – eyes do not open to speech or painful stimuli.

Best verbal response
Response is recorded to simple, direct questions (light touch or painful stimuli may be used).

Best motor response
- The patient's response to commands to raise his or her arm or two fingers is noted. Asking the patient to grasp the nurse's fingers is unreliable, as the grasp reflex may still be present.
- Ability to localize pain is noted when the patient moves a limb in response to painful stimuli.
- Flexion withdrawal to pain occurs when the arm bends at the elbow in response to painful stimuli, for example pressure on the patient's fingernail bed.
- Abnormal flexion is noted and refers to the arm flexing at the elbow and the turning of the hand so that the palm faces downwards or backwards, making a fist (pronation).
- Abnormal extension to pain occurs when the patient straightens the elbow and moves the arm away from the body (abduction), often with internal rotation, in response to painful stimuli to the fingernail bed.

Other responses assessed on the Glasgow Coma Scale include the following.

			Date						
			Time						
GLASGOW COMA SCALE	Eye opening	4. Spontaneously							Eyes closed due to swelling = C
		3. To speech							
		2. To pain							
		1. None							
	Best verbal	5. Oriented							Endotracheal tube or tracheostomy = T
		4. Confused							
		3. Inappropriate							
		2. Incomprehensible							
		1. None							
	Best motor	6. Obeys commands							Usually record best arm response
		5. Localizes to pain							
		4. Flexion/withdrawal to pain							
		3. Abnormal flexion							
		2. Abnormal extension							
		1. None							
Pupils	Right eye	Size							+ = Reacts − = No reaction C = Eyes closed
		Reaction							
	Left eye	Size							
		Reaction							
LIMB MOVEMENT	Arms	Normal power							Record right (R) and left (L) separately if there is a difference between the two sides
		Mild weakness							
		Severe weakness							
		Spastic flexion							
		Extension							
		No response							
	Legs	Normal power							
		Mild weakness							
		Severe weakness							
		Extension							
		No response							

Pupil scale
mm
1 •
2 •
3 •
4 •
5 ●
6 ●
7 ●
8 ●

Blood pressure

Systolic   = ∨
Diastolic   = ∧
Blue   = Lying
Red   = Sitting
            Standing

Pulse = •
  (Red)

Respirations = •
  (Blue)

210
200
190
180
170
160
150
140
130
120
110
100
90
80
70
60
50
40
30
25
20
15
10

42
41
40
39
38
37
36 °C
35
34
33
32
31
30

Temperature = •
  (Blue)

30
25
20
15
10

Comments

FIGURE 9.1 *The Glasgow Coma Scale for the assessment of level of consciousness.*

Pupils

Pupil size is measured by comparing it to the pupil scale on the chart; pupil reaction is measured in response to light, such as a direct beam from an ophthalmoscope or pen light. In health, pupils are of equal size and constrict briskly when stimulated by a direct beam of light.

patients may be detained in hospital under either the Mental Health Act of 1983 or the Public Health (Control of Diseases) Act of 1984 (inclusive of the statutory regulations made by the Secretary of State on 22 March 1986).

Mental Health Act 1983 (Part II)

The following sections of the Mental Health Act 1983 (Part II) can be used, if required, to detain a patient in hospital.

Section 2. A patient may be admitted to hospital for assessment, for a period not exceeding 28 days, either for his or her own health or safety, or with a view to the protection of other persons.

Section 4. A patient may be admitted to hospital for emergency assessment for a period of 72 hours.

Section 5. Under 5(2), a patient who is already an in-patient in hospital may be further detained in hospital for a period of 72 hours. This will allow the consultant in charge to have the patient detained on the ward and will give medical staff an opportunity to decide on further action and, if appropriate, apply for detention under other sections of the Mental Health Act.

Further sections of the Act can be used to detain patients for varying periods of time.

Public Health (Control of Diseases) Act 1984

Statutory regulations made by the Secretary of State (22 March 1986) provide for AIDS being a notifiable disease for the purposes of Sections 35, 38, 43 and 44 of the Act. This Act allows for the provision of compulsory medical examination and for compulsory removal of a patient to hospital, where the interests of the sufferer, his or her family and the public appear to justify that such action should be taken. Section 38 of the Act allows for the compulsory detention in hospital of a patient already in hospital.

Obviously, the detention of any citizen in hospital against his or her will is a serious event, which, fortunately, is rarely required. However, there are circumstances when, either for the good of the patient or for the good of the community, compulsory admission may be appropriate. It may be necessary initially for the patient to be evaluated in a general hospital to rule out treatable neurologic infections such as opportunistic CNS infections. If the patient is suffering from intercurrent psychosis, such as a depressive or hypomanic phase of an existing manic–depressive illness, or if a patient with a chronic psychosis develops HIV disease and requires in-patient care, this care is best delivered in a psychiatric service.

Clearly, nurses have a profound duty to ensure that the legalities of compulsory admission have been properly enacted and to support the patient, family and friends during this frightening period.

Long-stay patients in psychiatric hospitals who are infected with HIV are, of course, able to sexually transmit this infection to other individuals. Sexual activity amongst psychiatric in-patients in long-stay units is probably quite common, perhaps compounded by the effect of chronic psychosis, which may diminish judgement and self-control.[30] Considerable vigilance is required from nursing staff to circumvent this risk. Additionally, the potential risk of violence is always real in individuals who are frightened, confused and have an altered mental state.

Summary

HIV-related neurologic and neuropsychiatric illnesses are common, especially in late symptomatic HIV disease. Both the central and peripheral nervous systems can be involved, causing a continuum of ill-health from progressive mental and physical disability to life-threatening infections and cancers. In this chapter, we have reviewed the impact of HIV infection on the nervous system, relating various neurologic and neuropsychiatric manifestations to specific patient problems. This information enables nurses to assess accurately individual patient needs and plan and implement appropriate nursing support and interventions.

REFERENCES

1. Price RW. Management of neurologic complications of HIV-1 infection and AIDS. In: Sande MA, Volberding PA (eds), *The Medical Management of AIDS*, 6th edn. Philadelphia: W.B. Saunders Company, 1999, 217–40.
2. Price RW. Neurologic complications of HIV-1 infection and AIDS. In: Merigan TC, Bartlett JG, Bolognesi D (eds), *Textbook of AIDS Medicine*, 2nd edn. Baltimore: Williams & Wilkins, 1999, 477–97.
3. Weisberg LA. Neurologic abnormalities in human immunodeficiency virus infection. *Southern Medical Journal* 2001; **94**:266–75.
4. Lechtenberg R, Sher JH. *AIDS in the Nervous System*. New York: Churchill Livingstone, 1988, 53 pp.
5. Hollander H, Stringari S. HIV-related meningitis: clinical course and correlations. *American Journal of Medicine* 1987; **83**:813–16.
6. McArthur JC, Cohen BA, Farzedegan H et al. Cerebrospinal fluid abnormalities in homosexual men with and without neuropsychiatric findings. *Annals of Neurology* 1988; **23**(Suppl.):S34–7.
7. Beers MH, Berkow R (eds). Disorders of the peripheral nervous system. In: *The Merck Manual of Diagnosis and Therapy*, 17th edn. Whitehouse Station, NJ: Merck Research Laboratories, 1999, 1494–5.
8. Grant I, Gold J, Rosemblum M et al. *Toxoplasma gondii* serology in HIV-infected patients: the development of central nervous system toxoplasmosis in AIDS. *AIDS* 1990; **4**:519.
9. Porter SB, Sande MA. Toxoplasmosis of the central nervous system in the acquired immunodeficiency syndrome. *New England Journal of Medicine* 1992; **327**:1643–8.
10. Jones JL, Hanson DL, Dworkin MS et al. Surveillance for AIDS-defining opportunistic illnesses, 1992–1997. *Morbidity and Mortality Weekly Report (MMWR)* 16 April 1999; **48**(SS-2):1–22.
11. Chaisson RE, Griffin DE. Progressive multifocal leukoencephalopathy in AIDS. *Journal of the American Medical Association* 1990; **264**:79–82.
12. Sadler M. Colonizing tumours of the brain. In: Gazzard B (ed.), *Chelsea & Westminster Hospital AIDS Care Handbook*. London: Mediscript Ltd Medical Publishers, 1999, 161–82.
13. Moyle G. Cytomegalovirus infection. In: Gazzard B (ed.), *Chelsea & Westminster Hospital AIDS Care Handbook*. London: Mediscript Ltd Medical Publishers, 1999, 65–73.

14. Karp JE. Overview of AIDS-related lymphomas: a paradigm of AIDS malignancies. In: Merigan TC, Bartlett JG, Bolognesi D (eds), *Textbook of AIDS Medicine*, 2nd edn. Baltimore: Williams & Wilkins, 1999, 437–50.

15. Bower M, Fife K. HIV-associated malignancy. In: Gazzard B (ed.), *Chelsea & Westminster Hospital AIDS Care Handbook*. London: Mediscript Ltd Medical Publishers, 1999, 93–111.

16. Kaplan LD, Northfelt DW. Malignancies associated with AIDS. In: Sande MA, Volberding PA (eds), *The Medical Management of AIDS*, 6th edn. Philadelphia: W.B. Saunders Company, 1999, 467–96.

17. Capaldini L. Psychosocial issues and psychiatric complications of HIV disease. In: Sande MA, Volberding PA (eds), *The Medical Management of AIDS*, 6th edn. Philadelphia: W.B. Saunders Company, 1999, 241–63.

18. Dana Consortium on Therapy for HIV Dementia and Related Cognitive Disorders. Clinical confirmation of the American Academy of Neurology algorithm for HIV-1 associated cognitive/motor disorder. *Neurology* 1996; **47**:1247–53.

19. Dore GJ, Correll PK, Li Y et al. Changes to AIDS dementia complex in the era of highly active antiretroviral therapy. *AIDS* 1999; **13**:1249–53.

20. Power C, Selnes OA, Grim JA, McArthur JC. HIV Demential Scale: a rapid screening test. *Journal of the Acquired Immune Deficiency Syndrome & Retrovirology* 1995; **8**:273–8.

21. Whitaker RE. Neuropsychiatry of HIV-associated dementia. *Psychiatric Times* March 2001; **17**. Available online at: http://www.mhsource.com/pt/p010357.html

22. Whitaker RE. Psychopharmacological treatment issues in HIV disease. *Psychiatric Times* 1999; **16**:24–30.

23. Whitaker RE. Significance of community psychiatry to HIV disease. *Psychiatric Times* 1999; **16**:58–64.

24. Holloway RG, Kieburtz KD. Headache and the human immunodeficiency virus type 1 infection. *Headache* 1995; **35**:245.

25. So YT, Olney RK. Acute lumbosacral polyradiculopathy in acquired immunodeficiency syndrome: experience with 23 patients. *Annals of Neurology* 1994; **35**:53–8.

26. Mitchell PH, Irvin N. Neurological examination: nursing assessment for nursing purposes. *Journal of Neurosurgical Nursing* 1977; **9**:23–8.

27. Teasdale G. Acute impairment of brain function – Part 1. Assessing conscious level. *Nursing Times* 1975; **71**:914–17.

28. Teasdale G, Galbraith S, Clarke K. Acute impairment of brain function – Part 2. Observation record chart. *Nursing Times* 1975; **71**:972–3.

29. Kim MJ, McFArland GK, McLane AM (eds). *Pocket Guide to Nursing Diagnosis*. St Louis, MO: C.V. Mosby, 1984, 326.

30. Fenton TW. AIDS and psychiatry: practical, social and ethical issues – practical problems in the management of AIDS-related psychiatric disorder. *Journal of the Royal Society of Medicine* 1996; **80**:271–4.

FURTHER READING

Pemberton L. The unconscious patient. In: Alexander MF, Fawcett JN, Runciman PJ (eds), *Nursing Practice – Hospital & Home*, 2nd edn. Edinburgh: Churchill Livingstone, 2000, 851–71. (A succinct overview of the nursing care of patients with an altered level of consciousness.)

INTERNET RESOURCES

- For a comprehensive review of HIV-related dementia, see Rupert Whitaker's article 'Neuropsychiatry of HIV-associated dementia' in *Psychiatric Times* 2001; **17**. Available online at:
  http://www.mhsource.com
- The current issue of the National AIDS Manual (NAM) *HIV & AIDS Treatment Directory* in the UK provides a valuable resource and is available from NAM, 16a Clapham Common Southside, London SW4 7AB (Tel. +44 (0)207627 3200). You can also contact NAM online at:
  www.aidsmap.com

CHAPTER

Viral hepatitis and HIV disease

Introduction

People who are vulnerable to infection with HIV are also at an increased risk of being infected with hepatitis (hepatotropic) viruses, as the 'at-risk behaviours' that lead to exposure for these enterically, parenterally and sexually transmitted viruses are similar. It is not surprising, therefore, that both acute and chronic viral hepatitis commonly occurs in people living with HIV disease, adding to their burden of ill-health and increasing the complexity of their treatment. An understanding of the issues associated with HIV and hepatotropic virus co-infection is important in developing sound nursing prevention and care strategies and in the early identification of complications associated with treatment or disease progression.

Learning outcomes

After studying and reflecting on the material in this chapter, you will be able to:

- describe the various hepatotropic viruses that may cause acute or chronic hepatitis in people living with HIV disease;
- discuss the inter-relationship between viral hepatitis and HIV infection;
- outline the clinical management of patients with viral hepatitis;
- identify drug contraindications and increased risks of side effects in co-infected patients;
- advise patients on effective strategies for primary and secondary prevention.

BACKGROUND

Acute viral hepatitis, the characteristic inflammation of the liver, can be caused by many infectious and non-infectious agents, but the most common causes are viruses. Several human herpesviruses have been recognized as causing acute hepatitis, including the Epstein–Barr virus (EBV), cytomegalovirus (CMV) and herpes simplex viruses (HSV1 and HSV2). However, viruses that specifically target the functional cells of the liver (hepatocytes) are the most common cause of acute and chronic viral hepatitis and these are known as hepatotropic viruses (Table 10.1).

TABLE 10.1 Hepatotropic viruses

- Hepatitis A virus (HAV)
- Hepatitis B virus (HBV)
- Hepatitis C virus (HCV)
- Hepatitis D virus (HDV) (Delta)
- Hepatitis E virus (HEV)
- Hepatitis G virus (HGV) (GBV-C)

CLINICAL FEATURES OF ACUTE VIRAL HEPATITIS

Most patients developing acute viral hepatitis have similar clinical features (Table 10.2), although immunosuppressed individuals may have a more severe illness. During the incubation period (also called the prodromal or **pre-icteric phase**) most patients will feel unwell before they develop jaundice (**icteric phase**). Despite worsening jaundice during this phase, symptoms begin to regress and the patient starts to feel better. As the jaundice fades and symptoms resolve, the patient begins to make a recovery (**recovery phase**).

TABLE 10.2 Clinical features of acute viral hepatitis

Pre-icteric phase

Prodromal or incubation phase occurs 2–3 weeks before the onset of jaundice with the development and a progressive worsening of anorexia, malaise, nausea and vomiting, fever, distaste for cigarette smoking (if a smoker). Sometimes urticarial, pruritic hives, maculopapular lesions and/or fleeting, irregular patches of erythema; arthralgias (joint pains) occasionally occur, especially in HBV infection. Myalgias (muscle pains), chills and right upper quadrant abdominal pain may occur.

Icteric phase (jaundice)

Lasts 1–3 weeks

Dark urine and jaundice: eyes show scleral icterus, and faeces may be clay coloured

Temperature usually normal, as are vital signs; however, there may be a bradycardia (slow heart rate) if the patient has severe hyperbilirubinaemia

Serum bilirubin may increase to 20 times normal; hepatic transaminase levels, i.e. aspartate transaminase (AST) and alanine aminotransferase (ALT) may increase to 100 times normal and an increase in alkaline phosphatase (1–3 times normal) may also be seen

Systemic symptoms begin to regress and the patient feels better, despite worsening jaundice

Recovery phase

Jaundice gradually recedes during a 4–8-week recovery phase

These three phases represent the **natural history** of acute viral hepatitis, although there is significant variation in the length of each phase, the severity of illness experienced by the patient and the long-term outcomes in relation to viral carriage and chronic liver disease. The degree of difference in natural history is influenced by both the individual patient's immune competence and health reserves, and the characteristics of the specific infecting hepatotropic virus. For example, the incubation period for acute disease caused by hepatitis A or hepatitis E viruses is significantly shorter than that for acute hepatitis caused by hepatitis B or hepatitis C viruses. A carrier state and the potential for chronic liver disease are only associated in some people following infection with hepatitis B and hepatitis C viruses.

There is evidence to show that co-infection with some hepatotropic viruses (hepatitis C virus) accelerates HIV disease progression and that HIV infection may worsen liver damage or increase the likelihood of chronic infection in people co-infected with some hepatotropic viruses, especially hepatitis B and hepatitis C viruses.[1-5]

CHARACTERISTICS OF HEPATOTROPIC VIRUSES

The hepatotropic viruses are a mixture of viral species from different virus families, showing similarities to and differences from each other and each having a well-known natural history and its own menu of potential health outcomes (Table 10.3). It is important to understand these different viral characteristics, as acute or chronic hepatitis in a person living with HIV disease can vastly complicate his or her medical and nursing management, quality of life and long-term prognosis. Like HIV, infection with any of the hepatotropic viruses can be avoided, and nurses need reliable information to engage effectively in patient education opportunities focused on primary prevention.

Since hepatitis A and hepatitis E viruses are enteric pathogens, transmitted by the faecal–oral route, they will be discussed first, followed by a discussion of hepatitis B, hepatitis C and hepatitis G viruses, which are blood-borne viruses, transmitted parenterally, sexually and from mother to child (vertical transmission).

Hepatitis A

Hepatitis A virus (HAV) is an RNA **enterovirus** that infects cells in the gut and then spreads to the liver via the blood.[6] Following infection, HAV is principally found in the faeces and transmission generally occurs from person to person by the faecal–oral route. HAV can also be transmitted as a result of faecal contamination of food or water (and faecally contaminated water used to wash salads and other raw and unpeeled vegetables and fruits). Shellfish may also be contaminated from filter feeding in water that has been contaminated by human faeces. All of this occurs most commonly where sanitation and hygiene are poor. When these standards improve, as has happened in the developed world, the incidence of infection and the prevalence of natural antibody to this virus fall. In the UK, a high proportion of people (around 70 per cent in some regions) reach the age of 50 years without acquiring natural antibodies to hepatitis A and so remain susceptible to infection. HAV can also be transmitted sexually, for example following some types of sexual foreplay and/or oral–anal sexual activity. Finally, during the incubation period, there is a transient viraemia, when HAV can be found briefly in the serum, and occasionally HAV transmission can occur following exposure to infectious blood or other body fluids.

Hepatitis A has a short incubation period. Following exposure, an infected person excretes virus in the faeces and urine[6] for 2–3 weeks before the onset of symptoms, and for 1–2 weeks thereafter. The disease is generally mild, and complete recovery usually occurs within 4–8 weeks. Progression to chronic hepatitis is rarely, if ever, seen. The severity of the

TABLE 10.3 Summary: characteristics of hepatotropic viruses

	Hepatitis A virus (HAV)	Hepatitis B virus (HBV)	Hepatitis C virus (HCV)	Hepatitis D virus (HDV)	Hepatitis E virus (HEV)	Hepatitis G virus (GBV-C)
Virus group	Enterovirus	Hepadnavirus	Flavivirus	Incomplete	Calicivirus	Flavivirus
Nucleic acid in genome	ssRNA$^+$	dsDNA	ssRNA$^+$	Incomplete RNA^a	ssRNA$^+$	ssRNA$^+$
Serologic diagnosis	IgM anti-HAV	HBsAg^b	Anti-HCV	Anti-HDV	Anti-HEV	GBV-C RNA or antibodies
Incubation period (weeks)	2–4	6–23	2–26	6–9	3–8	Unknown
Transmission						
Faeces	Yes	No	No	No	Yes	No
Blood	Uncommon	Yes	Yes	Yes	Uncommon	Yes
Saliva^c	Uncommon	Yes	Yes	?	Uncommon	?
Sexual	Possible	Yes	Uncommon^d	Yes	Possible	?
Mother to child	No	Yes	Uncommon^d	Yes	No	?
Epidemics	Yes	No	No	No	Yes	No
Chronic infection	No	Yes (5–10%)	Yes (>50%)	Yes	No	Yes
Liver cancer	No	Yes	Yes	Yes	No	?
Prevention						
Passive immunization	Normal immunoglobulin	Hepatitis B immunoglobulin	No	Prevented by preventing HBV infection	No	No
Active immunization^e	Various formaldehyde-inactivated vaccines	Various vaccines containing inactivated HBsAg prepared from yeast cells by recombinant DNA technique	No	Prevented by preventing HBV infection	No	No

^{a}HDV requires the presence of HBV for replication.
^{b}HBsAg = hepatitis B virus surface antigen.
^{c}All body fluids are potentially infectious, though some (e.g. urine) are less infectious.
^{d}HCV: sexual and mother-to-child transmission may be more efficient in patients co-infected with HIV.
^{e}Combined hepatitis A and hepatitis B vaccines are available.

illness ranges from asymptomatic (subclinical) infection (common), through to clinical hepatitis (with or without jaundice) to (rarely) fulminant hepatic failure. In areas of high prevalence, most children have antibodies to HAV by the age of 3 years, and these early childhood infections are generally asymptomatic or very mild. In later life, HAV infection tends to cause clinical disease, with 70–80 per cent of adults developing jaundice, preceded typically by malaise, anorexia, nausea and fever. Patients over 49 years of age, and those with existing liver disease, have a higher risk of both morbidity and mortality.

Following primary infection, immunoglobulin M (IgM) antibodies to HAV appear and are present for 2–6 months before disappearing and being replaced by immunoglobulin G (IgG) HAV antibodies. The presence of specific HAV IgM antibodies is indicative of primary infection, whereas the presence of HAV IgG antibodies indicates previous exposure and immunity from further attacks. Humoral immunity and the formation of antibodies (immunoglobulins) are discussed in detail in Chapter 5.

HAV infection is not associated with a carrier state. Faecal excretion of the virus declines rapidly once clinical symptoms appear and usually ceases within 2 weeks following the onset of clinical hepatitis. HAV infection is prevalent throughout the world and is maintained in the human population through faecal–oral contamination routes.

Hepatitis E

Hepatitis E virus (HEV) is a member of the family of viruses known as *Caliciviridae*. Like other members of this family, such as 'small round structured viruses' (SRSVs) and Norwalk virus, caliciviruses replicate in the gastrointestinal tract and generally cause diarrhoea and vomiting. HEV has an RNA genome and, like HAV, is transmitted enterically (faecal–oral route). It is a major cause of epidemic water-borne hepatitis in many parts of the world, but not in the UK. The incubation period and clinical features are much the same as in HAV infection, except the illness may be more severe, especially in pregnant women, in whom high mortality rates may be seen.

This virus is endemic in tropical and subtropical developing countries, where infection is strongly linked with water contaminated by human faeces. Visitors and tourists to these regions may become infected and develop acute viral hepatitis when they return home.

Hepatitis E virus infection is not associated with a carrier state or progression to chronic liver disease. Hepatitis E is diagnosed by finding HEV antibody (anti-HEV) in the blood.

Preventing hepatitis A and hepatitis E

Good personal hygiene helps to avoid exposure. Nurses in particular must be alert to the potential risk of viral contamination from handling faeces, urine, blood and other body fluids and take appropriate infection prevention precautions, including using gloves and an effective hand-washing technique. These Standard Principles for preventing healthcare-associated infections must be observed for all patients at all times without exception.[7] Food handlers must consistently use effective hand hygiene measures, especially after using the toilet.

Travellers to regions where there is likely to be unreliable sanitation should ensure that they drink bottled or boiled water and avoid ice cubes in drinks unless they are confident they have been made from safe water. They should also refrain from eating raw shellfish and should peel all fruit and vegetables before eating them. Because salad ingredients may have been washed in contaminated water, salads should be avoided in areas where the water supply is unsafe.

Passive immunization, using **human normal immunoglobulin (HNIG),** can be used for temporary and immediate protection against hepatitis A, and active immunization is available using one of several **inactivated HAV vaccines**.[8] Hepatitis A vaccination is safe for HIV-infected people and is recommended if their sexual behaviour or travel plans put them at risk of hepatitis A.[9] Hepatitis A vaccination is particularly recommended for people with chronic hepatitis C because the risk of serious complications, such as fulminant hepatitis, associated with hepatitis A appears to be increased in HCV co-infected individuals.[10,11]

Individuals should be tested for HAV IgG prior to either form of immunization if time allows and if they are over 50 years of age (especially if they have lived overseas) or have a history of jaundice.[9] The reason for this is that if they are positive for HAV IgG, they may not require immunization – depending on the level (titre) of antibody in their blood – as a protective level of HAV IgG demonstrates previous infection and immunity to disease following new HAV infections.

Unfortunately, neither passive nor active immunization products are available to prevent hepatitis E.

Hepatitis B

Hepatitis B virus (HBV) is a **hepadnavirus** and has a DNA genome with at least four distinct, intimately related antigen–antibody (Ag–Ab) systems (Figure 10.1).

- **HBV surface antigen (HBsAg).** This is associated with the viral surface coat and its presence in serum usually provides the first evidence of acute HBV infection. Excess viral coat protein (HBsAg, or Australia antigen) is produced and these extra pieces of HBsAg outnumber the intact hepatitis B virion (the **Dane particle**). HBsAg characteristically appears during the incubation period, usually 1–6 weeks before clinical or biochemical illness develops, and disappears during convalescence. The corresponding antibody (**anti-HBs**) appears only weeks or months after clinical recovery, and usually persists for life. In up to 10 per cent of patients, HBsAg persists after acute infection and anti-HBs does not develop. These patients become asymptomatic carriers of the virus and some will develop chronic hepatitis.
- **HBV core antigen (HBcAg).** This is associated with the viral inner core. Antibody to the core (**anti-HBc**) appears at the onset of clinical illness, with gradually diminishing titres thereafter, usually for years or life.

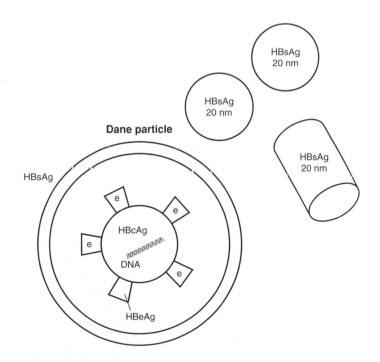

FIGURE 10.1 *Structure of the hepatitis B virus.*

- **HBV 'e' antigen (HBeAg).** This appears to be a peptide derived from the viral core (not to be confused with hepatitis E virus). It is found only in patients with detectable HBsAg in their blood. Its presence reflects more active viral replication and is generally associated with greater infectivity of blood (and other body fluids such as semen) and a greater likelihood of progression to chronic liver disease. In contrast, presence of the corresponding antibody (**anti-HBe**) signals lower infectivity and a better outcome.

HBV infection is diagnosed by identifying HBsAg in blood, and its presence indicates acute primary HBV infection. The corresponding antibody, anti-HBs, appears after recovery and persists for life. Its presence indicates previous infection and immunity from disease following new HBV infections.

During primary infection, an impressive level of virus is found in the blood, for example as high as 500 µg/mL of viral antigen and 10 trillion extra particles of surface antigen (HBsAg) in each millilitre of blood.[12] Following infection, HBV can be found in most body fluids, for example in blood, saliva, seminal fluid, cerebrospinal fluid, breast milk and urine.

HBV transmission

Hepatitis B virus is transmitted parenterally, typically by contaminated blood or blood products in many countries where screening of human blood for transfusion is unreliable or inconsistent. In the UK, all donor blood is screened for HBV infection and transmission rarely, if ever, occurs from blood transfusions or blood products. Injecting drug users frequently become infected with HBV (and other parenterally transmitted viruses, such as HIV and hepatitis C virus) following exposure resulting from sharing blood-contaminated injecting equipment. Occupational exposure to HBV following needle-stick injuries is a recognized risk in healthcare settings.

Non-parenteral spread occurs, including sexual transmission between both heterosexual and homosexual partners. Sexual exposure is the most frequent means of HBV transmission in the UK.

Mother-to-child (vertical) transmission also occurs during pregnancy or birth or, following birth, from breast milk. Breastfeeding is the most frequent mode of transmission in some developing countries, especially in the Far East, where it is an important cause of HBV perpetuation in the population. In the UK, all pregnant women are offered and recommended HBV (and HIV) testing during antenatal care,[13-15] and it is therefore uncommon for HBV to be vertically transmitted in the UK.

The incubation period for hepatitis B ranges from 6 to 23 weeks following exposure to the virus. Approximately 2–10 per cent of those infected as adults will become chronic carriers of HBV. Those carriers in whose serum HBeAg can be detected are the **most infectious** to others, as opposed to carriers in whose serum the **antibody** to this antigen (anti-HBe) is detected, who are generally of low infectivity. Chronic viral carriage is more frequent in those infected as children, and rises to 90 per cent in those infected perinatally. Worldwide, 20–25 per cent of chronic carriers develop progressive liver disease, often leading to cirrhosis and hepatocellular carcinoma.[9]

Hepatitis B is endemic in most countries, and globally remains one of the most serious, persistent viral infections. In South and East Asia up to 20 per cent and in Africa and Central and South America up to 10 per cent of the population may be carriers.[16,17] Although the incidence of overt cases of hepatitis B in the UK is low and shows a trend to decrease,[9] there are estimated to be 1 million cases of acute hepatitis B and 90 000 new cases of chronic hepatitis B in Europe every year.[16,18]

Hepatitis D

The hepatitis D virus (HDV), also called the delta agent, is a unique, defective RNA virus that can replicate only in the presence of HBV, never alone. It occurs as either a co-infection with acute HBV infection or a superinfection in established chronic hepatitis B.

Injecting drug users are at a relatively high risk of acquiring HDV infection in Europe and North America. In other parts of the world, HDV is more commonly acquired following sexual exposure. Mother-to-child transmission also occurs.

Clinically, HDV infection is typically manifested by: unusually severe (fulminant) acute viral hepatitis; acute exacerbation in chronic HBV carriers (superinfection); or a relatively aggressive course of chronic hepatitis B. HDV is diagnosed by detecting antibodies to the virus (anti-HDV) in the blood.

Non-A, non-B hepatitis

Following the introduction of testing blood donors for HBV infection in the 1970s and for HAV infection in the 1980s and excluding those found positive, it was hoped that **post-transfusion viral hepatitis** would virtually disappear. However, it did not and, as people continued to develop hepatitis following blood transfusions or from the use of blood components, it was clear that there must be other, unknown, hepatotropic blood-borne viruses. Viral hepatitis not caused by HAV or HBV infection was referred to as **non-A, non-B hepatitis**. The responsible viruses are transmitted parenterally and sexually (and sometimes vertically, i.e. from a mother to her newborn child), similar to HBV transmission, or enterically, infecting people by the faecal–oral route of transmission, exactly like HAV infection. In 1988, the non-A, non-B virus responsible for the vast majority of cases of post-transfusion hepatitis was identified and termed **hepatitis C virus**. Two years later, in 1990, scientists identified another non-A, non-B hepatotropic virus that was being transmitted enterically, principally in faecally contaminated water in many countries in the developing world (just like HAV), and this virus was named the **hepatitis E virus** (discussed earlier).

Hepatitis C

Hepatitis C virus (HCV) is an RNA virus belong to the flavivirus family. It is endemic worldwide, with high prevalence rates in South and East Asia and Eastern Europe.[18] There are at least six closely related strains (**genotypes**) of HCV, referred to as 1–6, and more than seven **subtypes**, referred to as: a, b and c. The prevalence of different genotypes varies in different geographical locations throughout the world. In the UK, Europe and North America, genotypes 1a, 1b, 2a, 2b and 3a are the most common.

HCV transmission

HCV is predominantly transmitted by blood and blood products. Prior to the introduction of HCV screening of all donor blood in 1990, most infections in Europe and North America occurred following blood transfusions or the use of blood products. This mode of transmission has now been virtually eliminated. Today, the greatest risk of acquiring HCV infection in the industrially developed world is from exposure to HCV-contaminated blood as a result of injecting drug use. Sexual and mother-to-child HCV transmissions do occur, but are not common; however HIV co-infection may increase this risk.[3] There is no evidence that HCV is transmitted by breast milk and, consequently, breastfeeding is considered safe.[19] Healthcare workers are at an increased risk of HCV infection following occupational exposure to blood or blood-contaminated body fluids, especially if the source patient was viraemic, that is, his or her blood was positive for HCV RNA.[20,21] This is discussed in more detail in Chapter 15.

Clinical outcomes

The natural history and clinical course of hepatitis C can be influenced by virus characteristics such as the specific genotype, viral load, co-infection with other viruses, including HIV, geographical location, alcohol use, drug use (including some antiretroviral and antituberculosis drugs), and other unexplained factors.[19]

Acute hepatitis C

Following primary HCV infection, most patients will remain asymptomatic, with only one-third presenting with malaise, weakness, anorexia and sometimes jaundice. However, all patients will sustain some degree of liver cell injury during this period, as demonstrated by blood tests for liver function (Table 10.4). Antibodies to HCV (anti-HCV) will appear in almost all patients within 90 days, but only about 15–25 per cent will be able to clear the virus and make a complete recovery from acute hepatitis C; they will remain anti-HCV positive but will become HCV RNA negative. Most (75–85 per cent) HCV-infected individuals will develop chronic infection with persistent (sometimes intermittent) viraemia and it is this **propensity for chronic infection that is a unique hallmark of hepatitis C.**[19]

TABLE 10.4 Liver function tests

■ Full (complete) blood count (FBC or CBC)

■ Coagulation tests
　　Prothrombin time

■ Biochemical tests
　　Urea and electrolytes

■ Liver function tests (plasma)
　　Aspartate aminotransferase (AST)
　　Alanine aminotransferase (ALT)
　　Alkaline phosphatase
　　Gamma-glutamyl transferase (GGTP)
　　Proteins (total and albumin)

Chronic hepatitis C

Most people with chronic HCV infection are asymptomatic for the first two decades following primary infection. Serological testing will reveal that they are anti-HCV and HCV RNA positive. Some may develop non-specific symptoms during this period, such as malaise and fatigue. Somewhere between 60 per cent and 70 per cent of chronically infected people will have persistent or fluctuating alanine aminotransferase (ALT) elevations indicating **active liver disease**; the remaining 30–40 per cent will have normal ALT levels and will not progress to active liver disease. The course of chronic liver disease is variable and, over a 20–30-year period, 10–20 per cent of people will develop **cirrhosis**. This condition, leading to end-stage liver disease, may develop rapidly in some patients, especially if there is concomitant alcohol use.[19] Between 1 per cent and 5 per cent of people with chronic liver disease, usually those with cirrhosis, will develop **hepatocellular carcinoma (HCC)**.[3,19,21] A variety of other extra-hepatic conditions may also be caused by chronic hepatitis C, including arthritis and glomerulonephritis.[19]

HIV and HCV co-infection

As previously mentioned, although somewhat conflicting, evidence does suggest that HIV-infected people co-infected with HCV, especially HCV genotype 1, may progress to end-stage AIDS more rapidly then those who are not co-infected with HCV.[3-5] However, the evidence seems fairly conclusive that HIV and HCV co-infection can worsen the clinical outcomes of hepatitis C.[1-3,19]

PREVENTING HBV, HDV AND HCV INFECTION

Hepatitis B vaccination is recommended for everyone at risk of exposure, including those with hepatitis C.[7,9-11,21] Additionally, hepatitis A vaccination is strongly recommended for people with chronic hepatitis C because the risk for fulminant hepatitis associated with hepatitis A appears to be increased in HCV co-infected people.[7,8] Both vaccines can be safely given to HIV-infected people; however, the ability of these vaccines to produce a protective response is dependent upon a person's degree of immunodeficiency. Consequently, the sooner a person is immunized against hepatitis A and B following a diagnosis of HIV infection, the better.

Antenatal screening for hepatitis B is important in preventing neonatal HBV infection,[13] and screening all donor blood, plasma, tissues, organs and semen for both HBV and HCV infection will prevent infections in people without behavioural risks for these infections. Additionally, consistently using standard principles for preventing infections in all patients in all circumstances will reduce the risk of nosocomial (healthcare-associated) transmission of blood-borne viruses.[7,21] Safer sexual practices and harm-minimization techniques for injecting drug use (Table 10.5) will help those whose behaviour or lifestyle places them at risk to avoid infection.[10,11,21]

TREATMENT OF CHRONIC HEPATITIS B AND C

The treatment of chronic hepatitis B and hepatitis C is a rapidly changing area of clinical practice. Current drugs licensed for use in chronic viral hepatitis include interferon alfa (and peginterferon alfa 2b), ribavirin and lamivudine.[8]

Chronic hepatitis B

Interferon alfa is given by injection for 3–4 months, after which treatment is assessed. If there is no improvement at this time, interferon alfa is usually discontinued. Lamivudine (3TC, Epivir®, Zeffix®) can be used for those patients for whom interferon alfa either cannot be

TABLE 10.5 Prevention messages for people with high-risk behaviours[10,11,18]

People who use or inject recreational drugs should be advised:

- to stop injecting recreational drugs

- to enter and complete substance-abuse treatment, including relapse-prevention, programmes

- if continuing to inject drugs:

  never to re-use or 'share' syringes, needles, water or drug preparation equipment; if injection equipment has been used by other people, to first clean the equipment with bleach and water, as is recommended for the prevention of HIV transmission

  to use only sterile syringes and needles obtained from a reliable source, e.g. syringe and needle exchange programme or pharmacy (chemist)

  to use a new sterile syringe and needle to prepare and inject drugs

  if possible, to use sterile (boiled) water to prepare drugs; otherwise to use clean water from a reliable source (such as fresh tap water)

  to use a new or disinfected container ('cooker') and a new filter ('cotton') to prepare drugs

  to clean the injection site before injection with a new alcohol swab; and to dispose of syringe and needle safely after one use

  to be vaccinated against hepatitis A and hepatitis B

People who use intranasal recreational drugs ('snorting') should be advised:

- to be aware that this practice has been associated with HCV transmission and

- not to share equipment (e.g. straws) with other users

People considering tattooing or body piercing should be informed of:

- the potential risks of acquiring blood-borne infections that could be transmitted if equipment is not sterile or if effective infection prevention precautions are not followed, such as washing hands, using latex gloves, and cleaning and disinfecting instruments

To reduce the risks for acquiring blood-borne infections, all patients should be advised:

- not to share tooth brushes, razors or other personal care articles

People who are at risk for sexually transmitted diseases should be advised:

- to use safer sexual practices, although the efficiency of sexual transmission of HCV is low

- to use latex condoms correctly and every time for penetrative sexual intercourse to protect themselves and their partners from diseases spread through sexual activity

- that if condoms are not used, to use safer, non-penetrative sexual practices

- to be vaccinated against hepatitis A and hepatitis B

---

used or is not effective. Both of these agents are associated with significant side effects, and nurses need to ensure they consult the latest edition of the *British National Formulary (BNF)* if they are administering these drugs to patients with chronic hepatitis B.[8] Interferon alfa is usually given by subcutaneous injection, but some preparations can be given by intramuscular or intravenous injection.

Chronic hepatitis C

Guidelines from the UK National Institute for Clinical Excellence (NICE) recommend that patients with severe to moderate chronic hepatitis C should be treated with a combination of interferon alfa and ribavirin (Rebetol®) for 6 months. Extension of treatment by a further 6 months is recommended only in those patients infected with HCV of genotype 1 who have responded to treatment during the first 6 months (as judged by clearing of circulating HCV RNA).[8]

HEPATITIS G (GBV-C OR HEPATITIS G VIRUS)

In 1995, novel flaviviruses similar to but distinct from HCV, were identified in the serum of a surgeon (his initials being GB).[22] These three GB viruses are transmitted by blood and have been termed GBV-A, GBV-B and GBV-C. The first two are tamarin (South American monkey) viruses, and only GBV-C can infect humans, although it is unlikely to cause significant liver disease.[23] Although high rates of GBV-C infection have been seen in injecting drug users with chronic hepatitis C, co-infection does not apparently lead to a significant change in clinical presentation, severity of liver disease, hepatitis C viraemia or response to interferon treatment.[24,25]

Recent research has shown that HIV-infected individuals who are co-infected with GBV-C and HIV have significantly longer survival and slower progression to AIDS. Additionally, survival after the development of AIDS has also been found to be better among co-infected patients.[25] The researchers speculated that GBV-C infection may inhibit HIV replication or may be a marker for the presence of other factors that lead to a favourable HIV response.[25] This discovery has potentially important therapeutic implications for the future management of HIV disease.

NURSING ASSESSMENT AND INTERVENTION

The nursing history and ongoing nursing observations will elicit the typical signs and symptoms of acute viral hepatitis (see Table 10.2), and nursing interventions are focused on actual and potential patient problems, including activity intolerance, altered nutrition and potential fluid volume deficit. There is no substantial evidence to suggest that either dietary or activity restrictions have any benefit for patients with acute hepatitis, but alcohol intake is usually restricted in order to minimize liver damage. The patient's appetite usually returns to normal during the icteric phase of acute hepatitis. The use of drugs that are toxic to the liver, such as paracetamol (acetaminophen), some antiretroviral and antituberculosis drugs, should be avoided.

Ongoing evaluation of care and continuing nursing observations will detect signs of complications, especially fulminant hepatitis with encephalopathy (Table 10.6), which is a rare condition, often associated with HBV or HCV infection. Highly skilled nursing care is needed if patients are to survive this catastrophic complication. Patient education initiatives might centre on reducing the risk of infection with other blood-borne viruses, such as safer sexual behaviour and harm-minimization techniques for injecting drugs (see Table 10.5). Patients should be advised to avoid alcoholic drinks during acute and chronic phases of hepatitis.

TABLE 10.6 Fulminant hepatitis with encephalopathy

Onset
Sudden rapid clinical deterioration with the onset of hepatic encephalopathy. Patient becomes lethargic and sleepy, with personality and behavioural changes. Coma may develop within hours. An early sign is asterixis, the irregular flapping of forcibly dorsiflexed, outstretched hands. Bleeding is common, resulting from liver failure and disseminated intravascular coagulation (DIC). An increasing prothrombin time is a grave prognostic indicator.

Prognosis
Meticulous nursing care and competent medical management of each specific complaint are required. Survival in adults is rare, although when it does occur, survivors often make a good recovery, with minimal liver damage.

PREVENTING OCCUPATIONAL EXPOSURE TO HEPATITIS VIRUSES

Using Standard Principles (Universal Precautions) for preventing healthcare-associated infections[7] is sufficient to prevent nosocomial transmission and occupational exposure to hepatitis viruses in healthcare settings. This is discussed in more detail in Chapter 14. Needle-stick and other sharp instrument injuries are extremely serious, as the risk of acquiring HBV and HCV infection from a patient with active disease is far greater than the risk of HIV acquisition. Consequently, great care needs to be taken when handling these devices, and all healthcare workers (including students and trainees) should be vaccinated against hepatitis B infection.[9] In hospitals, patients with viral hepatitis do not require single-room accommodation or any other extraordinary infection prevention precautions.

Summary

Acute and chronic viral hepatitis commonly occurs in people living with HIV disease, potentially worsening individual health status and outcomes and complicating and restricting options for antiretroviral treatment. We have seen that a variety of hepatotropic viruses cause hepatitis, but infection with each of these viruses can be prevented. In this chapter, we have reviewed the various viral causes of hepatitis, how they are transmitted and how transmission can be prevented. We have discussed actual and potential health problems associated with having hepatitis, and the medical management (and the nursing care issues associated with treatment) of patients with HIV disease co-infected with hepatitis viruses. This knowledge will enable us more effectively to assess, plan and evaluate care for patients co-infected with HIV and hepatotropic viruses, and to help ensure that avoidable complications are minimized and patients are supported in regaining their maximum level of health.

REFERENCES

1. Main J, McNair A, Goldin R, Thomas HC. Liver disease and AIDS. In: Merigan TC, Bartlett JG, Bolognesi D (eds), *Textbook of AIDS Medicine*, 2nd edn. Baltimore: Williams & Wilkins, 1999, 567–83.
2. Alcorn K (ed.). *HIV & AIDS Treatments Directory*, 20th edn. London: National AIDS Manual (NAM) Publications, August 2001, 273–86.
3. Berenguer M, Wright TL. Hepatitis C infection. In: Sande MA, Volberding PA (eds), *The Medical Management of AIDS*, 6th edn. Philadelphia: W.B. Saunders Company, 1999, 399–410.
4. Ockenga J, Tillmann HL, Trautwein C et al. Hepatitis B and C in HIV-infected patients: prevalence and prognostic value. *Journal of Hepatology* 1997; **27**:18.
5. Sabin C, Telfer P, Philips AN et al. The association between hepatitis C virus genotype and human immunodeficiency virus disease progression in a cohort of hemophilic men. *Journal of Infectious Disease* 1997; **175**:164.
6. Burns SM. Picornaviruses. In: Greenwood D, Slack RCB, Peutherer JF (eds), *Medical Microbiology: A Guide to Microbial Infections: Pathogenesis, Immunity, Laboratory Diagnosis and Control*, 15th edn. Edinburgh: Churchill Livingstone, 1997, 454–67.
7. Loveday HP, Pellowe C, Harper P, Robinson N, Pratt R. The **epic** Project: developing

national evidence-based guidelines for preventing healthcare associated infections. Guidelines for standard principles for the prevention of hospital-acquired infection. *Nursing Times* 2001; **97**:36–7.

8. Mehta DK (Executive Editor). *British National Formulary (BNF)*, No. 45. London: British Medical Association and the Royal Pharmaceutical Society of Great Britain. March 2003. Available from: BMJ Books, PO Box 295, London WC1H 9TE, UK, or from their website www.bmjbookshop.com. The *BNF* is also available online at: www.BNF.org

9. UK Departments of Health/Salisbury DM, Begg NT (eds). *Immunisation against Infectious Disease*. London. Stationery Office, 1996, 290 pp. Available from: The Stationery Office Ltd, PO Box 29, Norwich NR3 1GN, UK; e-mail customer.services@theso.co.uk or telephone 0870 600 5522, fax 0870 600 5533.

10. Centers for Disease Control and Prevention. 1999 USPHS/IDSA guidelines for the prevention of opportunistic infections in persons infected with human immunodeficiency virus: US Public Health Service (USPHS) and Infectious Diseases Society of America (IDSA). *Morbidity and Mortality Weekly Report (MMWR)* 20 August 1999; **48**(RR-10):1–66.

11. Centers for Disease Control and Prevention. 2002 guidelines for preventing opportunistic infections among HIV-infected persons: recommendations of the US Public Health Service and the Infectious Diseases Society of America. *Morbidity and Mortality Weekly Report (MMWR)* 14 June 2002; **51**(RR-08):1–46. Available online at: http://www.cdc.gov/mmwr/preview/mmwrhtml/rr5108a1.htm

12. Dienstag JL, Wands JR, Isselbacher KJ. Acute hepatitis. In: Wilson JD, Braunwald E, Isselbacher KJ et al. (eds), *Harrison's Principles of Internal Medicine*, 12th edn, International Edition. London: McGraw-Hill, 1991, 1322–37.

13. NHS Executive. Screening of pregnant women for hepatitis B and immunisation of babies at risk. *Health Service Circular, HSC 1998/127*. London: NHS Executive, 1987. Available online from: http://www.doh.gov.uk/coinh.htm

14. NHS Executive. Reducing mother to baby transmission of HIV. *Health Service Circular* HSC 1999/183. London: NHS Executive, 1999. Available online from: http://www.doh.gov.uk/coinh.htm

15. Pratt RJ. Antenatal screening for HIV infection: removing tomorrow's children from harms' way. *Journal of Neonatal Nursing* 2000; **6**:179–84.

16. Roure C. Overview of epidemiology and disease burden of hepatitis B in the European region. *Vaccine* 1995; **13**(Suppl. 1):S18–21.

17. Van Damme P, Tormans G, Beutels P et al. Hepatitis B prevention in Europe: a preliminary economic evaluation. *Vaccine* 1995; **13**(Suppl. 1):S54–7.

18. Brook MG. European guidelines for the management of hepatitis B and C virus infections. *International Journal of STD & AIDS* 2001; **12**(Suppl. 3):48–57.

19. Management of Hepatitis C. National Institutes of Health Consensus Statement Online 1997 March 24–26 [cited 2001 October 30]; **15**:1–41. Available online: http://www.odp.od.nih.gov/consensus/cons/105/105_statement.htm

20. Ramsay ME. Guidance on the investigation and management of occupational exposure to hepatitis C. *Communicable Disease and Public Health* 1999; **2**:258–62.

21. Centers for Disease Control and Prevention. Recommendations for prevention and control of hepatitis C virus (HCV) infection and HCV-related chronic disease. *Morbidity and Mortality Weekly Report (MMWR)* 16 October 1998; **47**(RR-19):1–39. Reprinted March 1999. Available online: http://cisat.isciii.es/mmwr/

22. Simons, JN, Leary TP, Dawson GJ et al. Isolation of novel virus-like sequences associated with human hepatitis. *Nature Medicine* 1995; **1**:564–9.

23. Fried MW, Khudyakov YE, Smallwoood GA et al. Hepatitis G virus co-infection in liver transplantation recipients with chronic hepatitis C and nonviral chronic liver disease. *Hepatology* 1997; **25**:1271–5.

24. Goeser T, Seipp S, Wahl R et al. Clinical presentation of of GB-C virus infection in drug abusers with chronic hepatitis C. *Journal of Hepatology* 1997; **26**:498–502.

25. Tillmann HL, Heiken H, Knapik-Botor A et al. Infection with GB virus C and reduced mortality among HIV-infected patients. *New England Journal of Medicine* 2001; **345**:715–24.

FURTHER READING

Brook MG. European guidelines for the management of hepatitis B and C virus infections. *International Journal of STD & AIDS* 2001; **12**(Suppl. 3):48–57.

Pratt RJ. Continuing professional development – infection control: prevention and control of viral hepatitis. *Nursing Standard* 2003; **17**:43–52.

Ramsay ME. Guidance on the investigation and management of occupational exposure to hepatitis C. *Communicable Disease and Public Health* December 1999; **2**:258–62.

INTERNET RESOURCES

All of these sites have links to other related sites and host a variety of useful resources.

- **British Liver Trust and the Liver Nurses Forum**. The British Liver Trust publishes up-to-date information for patients and services, and encourages and funds liver disease research. It is also the internet home to the Liver Nurses Forum, which facilitates the exchange of information and promotes nurse-led liver disease research:
  http://www.british-liver-trust.org.uk

- **UK National Hepatitis C Resource Centre**. This Department of Health-supported site provides information to people living with hepatitis C, healthcare professionals, and the general public and media. It also provides a peer perspective on personal experiences of HCV-positive individuals regarding day-to-day living, treatment, alternative therapies and support:
  http://www.hep-ccentre.com

- **UK Public Health Laboratory Service (PHLS)**. The PHLS provides user-friendly, accurate and up-to-date information on a comprehensive range of infectious diseases, including acute and chronic viral hepatitis:
  http://www.phls.co.uk

- **National AIDS Treatment Advocacy Project (NATAP)**. This USA-based site provides comprehensive and current information on all aspects of hepatitis and HIV co-infection (along with the entire range of HIV treatment information). It has a free weekly e-mail update service and the website is updated weekly. It also provides recordings of its weekly radio programme on 'Living Well with HIV & Hepatitis' and will provide a free copy (download PDF or will post you a hard copy) of its excellent 'Hepatitis C & Hepatitis C/HIV Co-infection Handbook' (in English or Spanish language):
  http://www.natap.org/

- **HIV and Hepatitis Website**. Another excellent USA-based site provides comprehensive and current information on all aspects of hepatitis and HIV co-infection. It has a free weekly e-mail update service and the website is updated weekly:
  http://www.hivandhepatitis.com
- **American Liver Foundation** The American Liver Foundation is dedicated to the prevention, treatment and cure of hepatitis and other liver disease through research, education and advocacy. This is a mega-website and has useful links to other related sites:
  http://www.liverfoundation.org

The impact of HIV infection on women

In the past, women and children seemed to be on the periphery of the
AIDS epidemic. Today, they are at the centre of our concern. AIDS has
not spared them. On the contrary, the epidemic wave has affected
millions of women and their children, and millions more are threatened.

Dr Michael Merson, Executive Director, Global Programme on AIDS,
World Health Organization

Introduction

All over the world, HIV disease has become a leading cause of death among women. In
many societies, in many cultures, being a woman is a significant risk factor for HIV
infection. As more and more women become infected with HIV, an ever-increasing number
of their children will be born also infected with this virus, eventually being robbed of their
mothers, their childhood and, ultimately, their lives. In many large resource-poor countries,
the uninfected children of HIV-infected parents will be destined to join the world of the
'AIDS orphans'. Women are central to the concept of family: to nurturing, protecting and
caring. They have complex relationships and structures in their daily lives and
sophisticated and subtle responsibilities and commitments. Their demise, consequent to
HIV disease, will increasingly rock the stability of communities in every country where the
incidence of HIV infection and AIDS continues to escalate.

Women have many unique vulnerabilities to HIV infection and a variety of gender-
specific healthcare needs when infected. These vulnerabilities and needs are reviewed in
this chapter, along with a variety of issues and strategies associated with preventing HIV
infection in women.

Learning outcomes

After studying and reflecting on the material in this chapter, you will be able to:

- describe gender-specific risk factors for HIV infection in women;
- outline the potential healthcare problems experienced by women during symptomatic HIV disease;
- identify potential adverse pregnancy outcomes;
- compare and contrast the infection prevention effectiveness of different forms of contraceptives;
- Identify primary prevention strategies that could reduce women's risk of HIV infection.

BACKGROUND

By the beginning of 2003, more than 60 million people throughout the world had been infected with HIV and 20 million had died. Of the 42 million people living with HIV disease at the beginning of 2003, 19.2 million were women and 2 million of them had become newly infected in the previous year. In addition, 3.2 million of their children were living with HIV disease.[1]

Although sex between men is responsible for the majority of HIV infections that have occurred in the UK since the beginning of our national epidemic, there has been an unrelenting year-on-year increase in the number of HIV infections heterosexually acquired since the beginning of the last decade. This has accelerated from 1997 onwards and now exceeds the number of new infections acquired by men having sex with other men.[2] In the UK, the majority of heterosexually acquired infections were acquired abroad, often in Africa, particularly sub-Saharan Africa, and in Asia.[2] Globally, the vast majority of adolescents and adults become infected with HIV as a result of heterosexual exposure. As heterosexually acquired infections continue to increase, more and more women all over the world will seek diagnosis, treatment and care as a result of HIV disease.

GENDER-SPECIFIC RISK FACTORS FOR HIV INFECTION IN WOMEN

As a group, women are more vulnerable than men to becoming exposed to and infected with HIV. There are a variety of reasons for this increased vulnerability, including socio-economic status, biological influences, sexual practices and epidemiological factors. Although these are fairly universal gender-specific factors, the degree to which they influence the vulnerability of women in different communities throughout the world varies, often in relation to the culture in which they live and their unique relationships and circumstances (see also Chapter 23).

Socio-economic status

Women may be both socially and culturally vulnerable to HIV infection, as they are often economically dependent on men. Throughout the world, their status is lower than that of men and they have fewer opportunities for education and to acquire financial independence and personal freedom. This often means that they have little power or control over decisions relating to the sexual behaviour of their partners, such as condom use and safer sex, and over access to primary prevention information. Women are vulnerable to coerced sex, including marital and non-marital rape, sexual abuse in and outside of the family, and/or being forced into the sex industry. In many cultures, women are expected to be passive and submissive in their sexual relationships, which are invariably controlled by men. They lack the skills and confidence to discuss sexual behaviour with their partners and have little bargaining power within their sexual relationships. This sexual subordination of women makes it impossible for them to protect themselves from sexually transmitted infections (STIs), including HIV infection.

In many countries, especially in Western Europe and North America, drug use (both injectable and non-injectable) is a major contributor to HIV infection in women. Most drug use increases the likelihood of entering into more high-risk sexual encounters, either as a result of a drug-induced loss of inhibition or related to selling sex for drugs or for money to support their dependency. Injectable drug use also carries the considerable risk of infection with blood-borne pathogens (including HIV and hepatitis B, D and C viruses) from sharing contaminated injection equipment with other users. Many women who do not use drugs themselves are vulnerable to infection with blood-borne pathogens from their drug-using sexual partners, who, because of their heightened risk of infection, may transmit infections to them.

Biological influences

Men are more efficient at transmitting HIV to women than women are to men, and women are biologically more vulnerable to HIV infection than men.[3,4] As the receptive partner, a woman has a larger mucosal surface exposed during sexual intercourse. In addition, semen contains a higher volume and concentration of virus than vaginal or cervical secretions. The presence of covert (asymptomatic) pelvic inflammatory disease (PID) increases the risk of HIV acquisition on exposure, as does any factor which disrupts the vaginal or cervical epithelium, for example genital ulcerative or inflammatory infections, sexual trauma, chemical damage and hormonal influences. Other factors that have been implicated in increasing the susceptibility of women to HIV infection include cervical ectopy, defloration, dyspareunia (painful coitus), perimenopausal status, and the use of certain methods of contraception[3] (discussed later in this chapter).

Young women are particularly susceptible to infection, as their genital tract is not mature at the time they begin to menstruate. The mucous membrane changes from being a thin, single layer of cells to a thick, multi-layer wall. This transition may not be completed until their late teens or early twenties. The intact but immature genital tract surface in young women is less efficient as a barrier to HIV than the mature genital tract of older women. Finally, in postmenopausal women, the mucous membrane becomes thinner and provides a less efficient barrier to the virus.[5]

Sexual practices and epidemiological factors

In many countries throughout the world, women tend to have sex with, and often marry, men who are older than themselves. Men have usually had more partners (and more opportunities to become infected) than the women with whom they have sex. Consequently, women are becoming infected at an earlier age than men and their age on diagnosis of AIDS is, on average, 10 years younger than that of men.[5] HIV-infected women are more likely to transmit HIV to their uninfected partners if they have vaginal sexual intercourse during menstruation, and anal sex increases the risk of women becoming infected from an HIV-infected male partner. The disease stage and immunological status of the infected male partner influence the risk: the danger to the uninfected female sexual partner is greatest when exposure occurs from men during early primary infection or when the male partner has symptomatic HIV disease. This is when the level of virus in body fluids is at its highest.

Women are also vulnerable to HIV infection from HIV-contaminated blood transfusions. Throughout the world, women are the major recipients of blood transfusions that are used primarily to treat anaemia caused by repeated pregnancies and diseases such as malaria, and to treat the complications of childbirth, such as postpartum haemorrhage. Screening blood for HIV infection is beyond the reach of many in most developing countries, and this places the entire female community at considerable risk.

The feminization of poverty limits the economic options open to women, especially single mothers and young girls, and forces many into the sex industry. Here, it will only be a matter of time before they become exposed to a range of STIs, including HIV infection. A comparatively new phenomenon of international sex tourism has, along with drug use, firmly seeded HIV infection in the South Pacific basin, an area where most of the world's population resides and where national epidemics of HIV infection are now well established and flourishing.

Rape, a common form of violence perpetuated against women by men all over the world, adds to the risk of infection. The more violent the assault, the greater the trauma and the more certain the peril of HIV transmission if the attacker is infected.

HEALTHCARE PROBLEMS IN WOMEN WITH HIV DISEASE

There often seem to be many barriers to early diagnosis and treatment for women, including poor access to healthcare facilities and good-quality treatment. In the industrialized countries of the world, women often do not perceive themselves as being at risk of HIV infection. This low index of suspicion is frequently mirrored in providers of healthcare for women, leading to a delay in establishing a correct diagnosis. A lack of targeted health education may leave many women in different communities unaware of the early symptoms of HIV disease.

Women are, in general, prone to the same opportunistic diseases as men (Chapter 7).[6,7] However, oesophageal candidiasis, cytomegalovirus (CMV) disease and herpes simplex virus (HSV) disease occur more frequently in women than in men, and Kaposi's sarcoma is less common in women.[6] In addition, there are several gynaecological conditions that are now associated with HIV disease in women, including:

- **cervical dysplasia** – from moderate to invasive;
- **vulvovaginal candidiasis** – persistent, frequent or poorly responsive to treatment;
- **pelvic inflammatory diseases** – especially those with tubo-ovarian abscess; and
- **herpes simplex lesion** – lasting more than 1 month.

Cervical dysplasia and invasive cervical cancer

Cervical dysplasia refers to abnormal cell changes in the epithelium of the uterine cervix. These pre-cancerous cellular lesions are associated with progression to cervical intraepithelial neoplasia (CIN). Different types of epithelial cell abnormalities occur, including low-grade and high-grade squamous intraepithelial lesions (SIL), squamous cell carcinoma and glandular cell abnormalities.

In 1993, the Centers for Disease Control and Prevention (CDC) in the USA added invasive cervical cancer to the list of AIDS indicator diseases in the expanded surveillance case definition for AIDS.[8] Several studies have identified an increased prevalence of cervical dysplasia among HIV-infected women.[9,10] In addition, other studies have found that a higher prevalence of cervical dysplasia among HIV-infected women is associated with a greater degree of immunosuppression.[10,11] Finally, HIV infection was shown to adversely affect the clinical course and treatment of cervical dysplasia and cancer.[12,13] Since then, several additional studies have confirmed these earlier findings.[14–16]

Cervical dysplasia is frequently caused by some strains of the human papillomavirus (HPV), especially HPV strains 16, 18, 31, 33, 35 and 39.[6,14,16] HPV is a member of a family of viruses known as *Papovaviridae* (papovaviruses), and nearly 80 different strains of HPV have been identified.[17] HPV infection is a common STI, and other HPV strains can also cause genital and anogenital warts (condyloma acuminata) and anal cancer.[6,7,15,16] HPV infection is common and may be transient or benign in the majority of immunocompetent people, i.e. those with an intact, well-functioning immune system. However, it is more likely to lead to warts and genital and anal cancer in immunosuppressed individuals, including those with HIV disease. Although not all women with cervical dysplasia are infected with HPV, this infection is linked to all grades of CIN.

Cervical dysplasia is usually asymptomatic, but can be detected by gynaecological screening, including Papanicolaou (Pap) smears. In the USA, the CDC recommend that all HIV-infected women should have a complete gynaecologic evaluation, including a Pap smear, as part of their initial evaluation.[18] A Pap smear should then be obtained twice in the first year after diagnosis of HIV infection. If the results are normal, an annual Pap smear is recommended. Those with abnormal smears should be monitored more closely. More frequent Pap smears and colposcopy are indicated during the clinical course of HIV disease in women (Tables 11.1 and 11.2).[14]

TABLE 11.1 Suggested frequency of Pap smears[14]

Clinical scenario	Screening frequency
Normal Pap	1 year
Symptomatic HIV disease and/or CD4$^+$ T-lymphocyte cell count < 200 cells/mm^3 (μL)	6 months
ASCUS/LGSIL (evaluated and followed without treatment)	4–6 months
Following treatment of pre-invasive lesions	3–4 months for first year, then 6 months

ASCUS, atypical squamous cells of undetermined significance; LGSIL, low-grade squamous intraepithelial lesion.

TABLE 11.2 Indications for colposcopy[14]

- Cytologic abnormality (atypia or greater, including ASCUS, AGCUS)
- History of untreated abnormal Pap smear
- Consider periodic colposcopy after treatment of cervical dysplasia
- Consider with evidence of HPV infection
- Consider screening colposcopy with CD4$^+$ T-lymphocyte cell count > 200 cells/mm^3 (μL)

ASCUS, atypical squamous cells of undetermined significance; AGCUS, atypical glandular cells of undetermined significance.

Women with invasive cervical cancer may complain of abdominal pain, vaginal bleeding, discharge and lymphadenopathy. High-grade cervical lesions (CIN 2 or 3 or carcinoma-in-situ) require treatment. A variety of treatment options are available for the various stages of cervical cancer, including local cone excision, cryotherapy and laser therapy. Recurrence in immunosuppressed HIV-infected women is high (more than 50 per cent),[19,20] especially associated with cryotherapy, and topical vaginal 5-fluorouracil (5-FU) cream (Efudix®) may be prescribed to reduce the recurrence rates following standard treatments.[21]

Vulvovaginal candidiasis

Recurrent vulvovaginal candidiasis is a common healthcare problem in women with HIV disease. Although usually caused by *Candida albicans*, other strains of *Candida*, especially *Torulopsis glabrata*, are responsible for perhaps a quarter of all cases of vulvovaginal candidiasis in HIV-infected women.[14,22]

Women with vulvovaginal candidiasis notice an abnormal creamy-white vaginal discharge and may complain of vaginal or vulvar itching (pruritus) or a burning pain and/or pain during sexual intercourse (dyspareunia) and difficult or painful urination (dysuria). There may be five or six recurrences a year, and treatment using a variety of standard antifungal agents (along with their interactions with antiretroviral drugs) is described in Chapter 7 (see Tables 7.5 and 7.6). Topical therapies are often given for at least 7 days, and prophylactic use of topical antifungal agents may be needed during periods when antibiotics are being used.[14] Some protease inhibitors, such as ritonavir and indinavir, exert an anti-*Candida* effect.[14,23] Topical boric acid is often used for treating vulvovaginal candidiasis caused by *T. glabrata*, which is often resistant to the imidazole and triazole group of antifungal drugs.[24] Topical vaginal products containing povidone-iodine, such as Betadine®, are sometimes used to treat vulvovaginal candidiasis (and to treat trichomoniasis and other non-specific or mixed vaginal infections). Vaginal preparations intended to restore normal acidity, such as Aci-Jel®, may prevent the recurrence of vulvovaginal candidiasis (and other vaginal infections) and permit the re-establishment of the normal vaginal flora.[25]

Most topical vaginal antifungal agents, such as clotrimazole, econazole nitrate, miconazole nitrate, fenticonazole nitrate, nystatin and ketoconazole, are supplied as oil-based creams (or ointments) and these can damage latex condoms and diaphragms. In these situations, women should use a polyurethane female condom (Reality®, Femidom®) or their male partners should use a non-latex polyurethane condom (Durex Avanti®) for vaginal sexual intercourse to prevent infection or pregnancy.

Bacterial vaginosis

Bacterial vaginosis is an infection of the vagina caused by anaerobic bacteria such as *Gardnerella vaginalis* and *Mycoplasma hominis*, and is another common cause of vaginal discharge that needs to be identified and appropriately treated. Bacterial vaginosis may occur with vulvovaginal candidiasis (or be mistaken for it by women, especially if they are using over-the-counter antifungal agents).

Metronidazole 0.75 per cent vaginal gel (Zidoval®), or clindamycin 2 per cent cream are the usual topical agents used for treating bacterial vaginosis. Sultrin® is a compound of sulphonamides and is used for treating bacterial vaginosis caused by *Haemophilus vaginalis* only. Oral metronidazole is used for treating trichomoniasis and sometimes for bacterial vaginosis.[25]

Pelvic inflammatory disease

Pelvic inflammatory disease refers to infection of the fallopian tubes (salpingitis), although the term is often used to include infections of the cervix (cervicitis), uterus (endometritis) and ovaries (oophoritis). PID is caused by a variety of pathogenic microorganisms, including *Chlamydia trachomatis* and *Neisseria gonorrhoeae*. Numerous other aerobic and anaerobic microorganisms may also cause PID.[26]

Women with PID present with progressively more severe, usually bilateral, lower abdominal pain. There may also be fever, vaginal discharge and irregular vaginal bleeding. Abscesses may develop in the fallopian tubes, involving the ovary (tubo-ovarian abscess), and the one or both tubes may fill with pus (pyosalpinx). Current CDC recommendations for managing immunosuppressed HIV-infected women with PID are for treatment with various broad-spectrum combination antibiotic regimens given either orally or parenterally.[18]

The sexual contacts of women with PID should be traced and examined, and treated if infected. Symptoms that persist despite adequate treatment may be a result of a progressively worsening immune status. PID is a serious illness and women may require urgent admission to hospital (Table 11.3).[18]

TABLE 11.3 Criteria for hospitalizing women with pelvic inflammatory disease based on observational data and theoretical concerns[18]

- Surgical emergencies (e.g. appendicitis) cannot be excluded
- The patient is pregnant
- The patient does not respond clinically to oral therapy
- The patient is unable to follow or tolerate an outpatient oral antimicrobial regimen
- The patient has severe illness, nausea and vomiting, or high fever
- The patient has a tubo-ovarian abscess

Genital herpes

In immunosuppressed HIV-infected women, genital lesions caused by infection with HSV may persist, disseminate and be more painful than lesions in women who are not infected with HIV. Any genital ulcerative lesion in an HIV-infected person puts her sexual partner(s) at an increased risk of HIV infection. Equally important, herpes lesions in a person who is not infected with HIV will increase her risk of becoming infected if she is sexually exposed to HIV.[27]

There are two distinct serotypes of HSV: HSV-1 and HSV-2. Most cases of genital herpes are caused by HSV-2 infection. Genital lesions are painful vesicles that ulcerate and heal without scarring. The first attack (primary infection) is often severe and the lesions are intensely painful and slow to heal, with consequently a prolonged duration of viral shedding. Systemic signs and symptoms, such as fever, photophobia and headache, are almost always experienced in primary infection. Following this first attack, recurrent episodes of herpes lesions occur at variable frequency. In immunosuppressed HIV-infected women, these recurrences are often frequent, severe and prolonged.

The treatment of HSV disease is described in detail in Chapter 7. A variety of antiviral drugs are used for this, including aciclovir (Zovirax®), famciclovir (Famvir®) and valaciclovir (Valtrex®) (see Table 7.7 in Chapter 7). HIV-infected women frequently require prolonged treatment and higher doses of antiviral drugs than do non-HIV-infected women. High-dose intravenous aciclovir may be required in some women during primary HSV infection or during severe recurrences. Antibiotics may be prescribed if lesions are infected with bacteria.

Daily long-term suppressive therapy with aciclovir is often prescribed to reduce the frequency of recurrences for those women who have six or more recurrences per year.

Resistance to aciclovir is encountered in those women who are severely immuno-suppressed with low T-lymphocyte CD4$^+$ counts and/or who have been on long-term aciclovir prophylaxis. Intravenous foscarnet sodium (Foscavir®) or cidofovir (Vistide®) are used for aciclovir-resistant HSV disease.

Patients receiving intravenous cidofovir require prior hydration with 1 L of sodium chloride 0.9 per cent 1 hour immediately prior to the infusion and, if tolerated, an additional litre may be given over 1–3 hours, starting at the same time as the cidofovir infusion or immediately afterwards.[25] Nurses need to be cautious in handling cidofovir as it is very toxic. If any of the solution comes into contact with skin or mucosa, it needs to be washed off immediately with soap and water.

Pregnancy

Women who become infected with HIV tend to do so early in their reproductive years. Women are often worried about the effects that pregnancy will have on their HIV disease and about the impact that HIV disease will have on their pregnancy. There is good evidence to confidently reassure women that pregnancy by itself does not provoke a more rapid progression of HIV disease to an AIDS-defining illness.[28,29] However, the natural changes in immunity experienced during pregnancy may affect the presentation, seriousness, clinical course and treatment of some common opportunistic infections, and this may have a significant impact on potential pregnancy complications.

Some adverse pregnancy outcomes may occur either as a result of HIV disease itself or, in resource-rich countries, secondary to the treatment of HIV disease and associated health problems, or other as yet unidentified factors. A recent meta-analysis examined the evidence for a relationship between HIV disease and potential adverse pregnancy outcomes and the results are summarized in Table 11.4.[29] This analysis suggested a relationship between HIV

TABLE 11.4 Adverse pregnancy outcomes and relationships to HIV infection[32]

Adverse pregnancy outcome	Relationship to HIV infection
Spontaneous abortion	Limited data, but evidence of possible increased risk
Stillbirth	No association noted in developed countries; evidence of increased risk in developing countries
Perinatal mortality	No association noted in developed countries, but data limited; evidence of increased risk in developing countries
Infant mortality	Limited data in developed countries; evidence of increased risk in developing countries
Intrauterine growth retardation	Evidence of possible increased risk
Low birth weight (< 2500 g)	Evidence of possible increased risk
Preterm delivery	Evidence of possible increased risk, especially with more advanced disease
Pre-eclampsia	No data
Gestational diabetes	No data
Chorioamnionitis	Limited data; more recent studies do not suggest an increased risk; some earlier studies found increased histologic placental inflammation, particularly in those with pre-term deliveries
Oligohydramnios	Minimal data
Fetal malformation	No evidence of increased risk

disease and a possible increased risk for preterm delivery (the most common cause of perinatal morbidity and mortality), low birth weight, intrauterine growth retardation, and some evidence for a possible increased risk of spontaneous abortion. Additionally, for HIV-infected women in countries in the industrially developing world, this analysis suggested a possible increased risk of stillbirth, perinatal mortality and infant mortality during pregnancy.

Finally, an important adverse pregnancy outcome, discussed in more detail in the next chapter, is the potential transmission of HIV and other viral and bacterial pathogens, such as HSV, to the newborn infant. Consequently, women need to consider carefully the potential risks to them and to their newborn child when making a decision to become pregnant. Nurses can help provide accurate information during this period, especially in relationship to contraception.

Contraception

HIV-infected women must have access to information in relation to contraception. Various contraceptive methods are available, having different levels of effectiveness both in preventing pregnancy and in protecting against STIs, including HIV infection.

Male condom

Male condoms are made from either rubber latex (the most common) or polyurethane (Avanti®), both substances being impermeable to sperm and to many infectious microorganisms, including HIV. They are relatively inexpensive, readily available and, in addition to their contraceptive properties, they also protect against STIs, including HIV infection. Although highly effective, they do not always prevent pregnancy or provide total protection against infections. Condom failure is usually due to improper storage and subsequent deterioration or improper usage. Condoms tend to become more effective as men become more experienced in using them. Some people are allergic to latex or (more rarely) polyurethane and cannot use them.

Because of a whole range of beliefs that exist about condoms in many different parts of the world and the influence of various cultural, religious or aesthetic values, many men (and women) do not like using condoms. Additionally, many men feel that condoms decrease male sensitivity, although this may be useful in men who experience premature ejaculation.

Lubrication is generally needed when using male condoms. Oil-based lubricants, such as petroleum jelly, cooking oils, baby and massage oils, lotions and oil-based vaginal preparations can damage latex (but not polyurethane) condoms. Water-based lubricants, such as KY Jelly®, or sexual lubricants specifically marketed as condom compatible are recommended for latex condoms. Most condom failure is likely to be due to incorrect use rather than poor condom quality. Condoms can be ripped or split during use, be torn with fingernails or slip off before withdrawal. Some men find standard size condoms too small or too difficult to put on. Larger size condoms are available and men can practise putting them on by themselves, or with their partner, outside of the stress and urgency of sexual intercourse.

Properly used, the male condom is the best barrier method for preventing pregnancy and for reducing the risk of HIV infection during sexual intercourse. Its main disadvantage is that the use of the male condom ultimately relies on men, and women may be unable to persuade them to use this form of contraception.

Female condom

A female condom (Femidom®, Reality®) made from polyurethane was developed in the UK in the early 1990s and is now marketed throughout the world. As these condoms cannot be used without men knowing, women may not even be in control of this protection, the use of which will often require their partners' permission. Because these condoms are much more expensive then the male condom and are generally unavailable in the developing world, the female condom is unlikely to play a major role in HIV prevention, although it increases the options for some women. Figure 11.1 describes the correct procedure for inserting and positioning this type of condom.

Diaphragm and cervical cap

The diaphragm and cervical cap are reasonably effective in preventing pregnancy. They also have the advantages that their use is controlled by women and they can be inserted well before sexual intercourse. It is not certain what efficacy these methods have in preventing STI and HIV transmission, but it is likely to be limited, as, although they prevent semen from reaching the cervix, they offer no protection against vaginal mucosal exposure to infectious microorganisms in the ejaculate.

Intrauterine contraceptive devices

Intrauterine contraceptive devices (IUD) are quite effective in preventing pregnancy. However, they are associated with producing foreign-body inflammatory reactions and an increased menstrual flow duration. Women who use IUD are also at an increased risk of PID.[30]

In addition to the above, various studies have shown that the risks of HIV transmission (either from an infected woman to a non-infected man or from an infected man to a non-infected women) are significantly increased if the woman is using an IUD.[31,32] Because of these risks, IUD use should be discouraged in women who are at risk of HIV infection or who are already infected with HIV.

Hormonal contraceptives

Various hormonal contraceptives are available, including oral (the 'Pill'), parenteral (injectable and implants) and an IUD with slow-releasing levonorgestrel. All of these are extremely effective at preventing pregnancy. They have the advantages of being used by women on a regular basis and of offering continuous contraception unrelated to episodes of sexual intercourse.

They do not, however, offer HIV-infected women (or non-HIV-infected women) any protection against other STIs (and may increase their susceptibility to many of these infections).[30] Additionally, there is concern that the use of some hormonal contraceptives by HIV-infected women may increase genital tract HIV shedding, making transmission to uninfected sexual partners more likely. Also, in uninfected women, hormonal contraceptives may cause cervical ectopy or other epithelial changes, or changes in local immune responses that may increase the risk of HIV infection on exposure.[30,33,34]

Because of their effectiveness, overall safety, ease of use and wide availability, hormonal contraceptives can be an appropriate contraception option for women, but as they do not protect against STIs, consistent condom use should be advised for HIV-infected women or those at risk of infection.

Spermicides

One of the most commonly used spermicides in Europe and North America during the last several decades is a detergent-like chemical called nonoxynol-9 (N-9), which is effective in preventing pregnancy when used with a diaphragm. It is widely available as gels, creams,

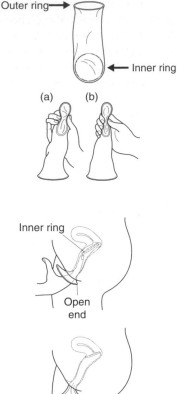

1 OPEN END (outer ring)
The open end covers the area around the opening of the vagina. The inner ring is used for insertion and to help hold the sheath in place.

2. HOW TO HOLD THE SHEATH
(a) Hold inner ring between thumb and middle finger. Put index finger on pouch between other two fingers, or
(b) just squeeze.

3. HOW TO INSERT THE CONDOM
Squeeze inner ring. Insert the sheath as far as it will go. It's in the right place when you can't feel it. Don't worry – it can't go too far, and IT WONT HURT!

4. MAKE SURE PLACEMENT IS CORRECT
Make sure the sheath is not twisted. The outer ring should be outside the vagina.

5. REMOVAL
Remove before standing up. Squeeze and twist the outer ring. Pull out gently. Dispose with waste, not in toilet.

Use more lubricant if:
• the penis does not move freely in and out;
• the outer ring is pushed inside;
• there is noise during sex;
• the female condom comes out of the vagina during sex.

Remove and insert a new female condom if:
• the female condom rips or tears during insertion or use;
• the outer ring is pushed inside;
• the penis enters outside the pouch;
• the female condom bunches inside the vagina;
• you have sex again.

Add lubricant to the inside of the sheath or to the penis. Start with two drops and add more if desired.

FIGURE 11.1 *The correct procedure for inserting a female condom.*

pessaries and foams and can be purchased without a prescription. Because N-9 can inactivate HIV and other viruses and bacteria in laboratory test tube experiments (*in vitro* studies),[35] it was originally thought to be useful in the early years of the pandemic for use as a topical vaginal (and/or anal) microbicide to prevent HIV and other STIs.

However, new clinical trials have now demonstrated that, regardless of results in laboratory experiments, N-9 is not effective in preventing STIs and, because of its local toxicity to mucous membranes, may significantly increase the risk of HIV infection on exposure.[36,37] **Consequently, N-9 is no longer recommended as an effective means of HIV prevention.**[38,39] Newer vaginal microbicides are currently in development but, in the meantime, properly used latex and polyurethane condoms, preferably those not lubricated with N-9, offer the best protection against STIs.

PRIMARY PREVENTION

Primary prevention targeted at both men and women needs to focus on HIV awareness and education, access to effective healthcare, the prevention and control of STIs, safer sex and safer injecting techniques. National AIDS programmes must continue to strive for a comprehensive screening service for blood transfusions. In the meantime, there is an urgent need for continuing research leading to the development of an inexpensive, safe and effective vaginal microbicide that women can use as part of an overall strategy to prevent HIV infection.[40] This would be a potent preventative weapon, the use of which would be under female control. Finally, women will continue to be at risk of HIV infection unless men everywhere help put an end to cultural traditions and socio-economic conditions that lead to women's subordination.

Prologue to Chapter 12

In this chapter, we have examined the special vulnerability of women to HIV infection and identified the HIV-related healthcare problems unique to women and potential adverse outcomes associated with pregnancy. A particularly tragic potential outcome is a pregnant woman infecting her newborn child, causing untold misery to that child and added heartbreak to the mother. In the next chapter, we are going to explore mother-to-child transmission and become familiar with various strategies aimed at preventing this continuing tragedy.

REFERENCES

1. UNAIDS/WHO. *AIDS Epidemic Update* (UNAIDS/02.58E). Geneva: Joint United Nations Programme on HIV/AIDS (UNAIDS) & the World Health Organization (WHO), December 2002, 38 pp. Available from: http://www.unaids.org
2. PHLS. AIDS and HIV infection in the United Kingdom: monthly report. *Community Disease Report Weekly* [serial online] 25 April 2002 [cited 28 April 2002]; **12**(17). Available from:
   http://www.phls.org.uk/publications/CDR%20Weekly/PDF%20files/2002/cdr1702.pdf

3. European Study Group on Heterosexual Transmission of HIV. Comparison of female-to-male and male-to-female transmission of HIV in 563 stable couples. *British Medical Journal* 1992; **304**:809–13.

4. Nicolosi A, Cor`rea Leite ML, Musicco M et al. The efficiency of male-to-female and female-to-male sexual transmission of the human immunodeficiency virus: a study of 730 stable couples. Italian Study Group on HIV Heterosexual Transmission. *Epidemiology* 1994; **5**:570–5.

5. United Nations' Development Programme. Young women: silence, susceptibility, and the HIV epidemic (Editorial). *AIDS and HIV Infection: Fetus to Adolescent* 1994; **5**:1–9.

6. Cotton DJ. AIDS in Women. In: Merigan TC, Bartlett JG, Bolognesi D (eds), *Textbook of AIDS Medicine*, 2nd edn. Baltimore: Williams & Wilkins, 1999, 151–62.

7. Newman MD, Wofsy CB. Women and HIV disease. In: Sande MA, Volberding PA (eds), *The Medical Management of AIDS*, 6th edn. Philadelphia: W.B. Saunders Company, 1999, 537–54.

8. Centers for Disease Control and Prevention. 1993 revised classification system for HIV infection and expanded surveillance case definition for AIDS among adolescents and adults. *Morbidity and Mortality Weekly Report (MMWR)* 18 December 1992; **41**(RR-17):1–19.

9. Laga M, Icenogle JP, Marsella R et al. Genital papillomavirus infection and cervical dysplasia – opportunistic complications of HIV infection. *International Journal of Cancer* 1992; **50**:45–8.

10. Schafer A, Friedmann W, Mielke M et al. The increased frequency of cervical dysplasia – neoplasia in women infected with the human immunodeficiency virus is related to the degree of immunosuppression. *American Journal of Obstetrics and Gynecology* 1991; **164**:593–9.

11. Feingold AR, Vermund SH, Burk RD et al. Cervical cytologic abnormalities and papillomavirus in women infected with human immunodeficiency virus. *Journal of Acquired Immune Deficiency Syndromes* 1990; **3**:896–903.

12. Maiman M, Fruchter RG, Serur E et al. Human immunodeficiency virus infection and cervical neoplasia. *Gynecological Oncology* 1990; **38**:377–82.

13. Klein RS, Adachi A, Fleming I et al. A prospective study of genital neoplasia and human papillomavirus (HPV) in HIV-infected women (abstract). Vol. 1. Presented at the VIII International Conference on AIDS/111 STD World Congress, Amsterdam, The Netherlands, 19–24 July, 1992.

14. Abularach S, Anderson J. Gynecologic problems. In: Anderson JR (ed.), *A Guide to the Clinical Care of Women with HIV*. Rockville, MD: US Department of Health and Human Services, Health Resources and Services Administration, HIV/AIDS Bureau, 2001, 149–96. Available online from: http://www.hab.hrsa.gov/

15. Alcorn K (ed.). *HIV & AIDS Treatment Directory*, 21st edn. London: National AIDS Manual (NAM), February 2002.

16. National AIDS Manual. Human papilloma virus. *National AIDS Manual* [serial online] 2002 May 01 [cited 2002 May 05]. Available from: http://www.aidsmap.com

17. Collier L, Oxford J. *Human Virology*, 2nd edn. Oxford: Oxford University Press, 2000.

18. Centers for Disease Control and Prevention. Sexually transmitted diseases treatment guidelines 2002. *Morbidity and Mortality Weekly Report (MMWR) Recommendations and Reports* 3 May 2002; **51**(RR-06):1–80. Available from: http://www.cdc.gov/mmwr/preview/mmwrhtml/rr5106a1.htm

19. Fruchter R, Maiman M, Sedlis A, Bartley L, Camilien L, Arrastia CD. Multiple recurrences of cervical intraepithelial neoplasia in women with human immunodeficiency virus. *Obstetrics and Gynecology* 1996; **87**:338–44.

20. Holcomb K, Mattews RP, Chjapman JE et al. The efficacy of cervical conization in the treatment of cervical intraepithelial neoplasia in HIV-positive women. *Gynecological Oncology* 1999; **74**:428–31.

21. Maiman M, Watts DH, Andersen J, Clax P, Merino M, Kendall MA. Vaginal 5-fluorouracil for high-grade dysplasia in human immunodeficiency virus infection: a randomized trial. *Obstetrics and Gynecology* 1999; **94**:954–61.

22. Schuman P, Sobel J, Ohmit SE et al. Mucosal candidal colonization and candidiasis in women with or at risk for human immunodeficiency virus infection. HIV Epidemiology Research Study (HERS). *Clinical Infectious Diseases* 1998; **27**:1161–7.

23. Cassone A, DeBernardis F, Torosantucci A, Tacconelli E, Tumbarello M, Cauda R. In vitro and in vivo anticandidal activity of human immunodeficiency virus protease inhibitors. *Journal of Infectious Diseases* 1999; **180**:448–53.

24. Sobel JD, Chaim W. Treatment of *Torulopsis glabrata* vaginitis: retrospective review of boric acid therapy. *Clinical Infectious Diseases* 1997; **24**:649–52.

25. Mehta DK (Executive Editor). *British National Formulary (BNF)*, 44th edn. London: British Medical Association and the Royal Pharmaceutical Society of Great Britain, September 2002. Available from: BMJ Books, PO Box 295, London WC1H 9TE, UK, or from the website www.bmjbookshop.com. The BNF is also available online at: www.BNF.org

26. Bukusi EA, Cohen CR, Stevens CE et al. Effects of human immunodeficiency virus 1 infection on microbial origins of pelvic inflammatory disease and on efficacy of ambulatory oral therapy. *American Journal of Obstetrics and Gynecology* 1999; **181**:1374–81.

27. Heng M, Heng S, Allen S. Co-infection and synergy of human immunodeficiency virus-1 and herpes simplex virus. *Lancet* 1994; **343**:255–8.

28. Alliegro MB, Dorrucci M, Phillips AN et al. Incidence and consequences of pregnancy in women with known duration of HIV infection. Italian Seroconversion Study Group. *Archives of Internal Medicine* 1997; **157**:2585–90.

29. French R, Brocklehurst P. The effects of pregnancy on survival in women infected with HIV: a systematic review of the literature and meta-analysis. *British Journal of Obstetrics and Gynaecology* 1998; **105**:827–35.

30. Anderson JR. HIV and reproduction. In: Anderson JR (ed.), *A Guide to the Clinical Care of Women with HIV*. Washington DC: US Department of Health and Human Services, Health Resources and Services Administration, HIV/AIDS Bureau, 2001, 213–73.

31. Kapiga SH, Shao JF, Lwihula GK, Hunter DJ. Risk factors for HIV infection among women in Dar-es-Salaam, Tanzania. *Journal of Acquired Immune Deficiency Syndromes* 1994; **7**:301–9.

32. Lazzarin A, Saracco, A, Musicco M et al. Man-to-woman sexual transmission of the human immunodeficiency virus. Risk factors related to sexual behaviour, man's infectiousness and woman's susceptibility. *Archives of Internal Medicine* 1991; **151**: 2411–16.

33. Mostad SB. Prevalence and correlates of HIV type 1 shedding in the female genital tract. *AIDS Research and Human Retroviruses* 1998; **14**(Suppl. 1):S11–15.

34. Plummer FA. Heterosexual transmission of human immunodeficiency virus type 1 (HIV): interactions of conventional sexually transmitted diseases, hormonal contraceptives and HIV-1. *AIDS Research and Human Retroviruses* 1998; **14**(Suppl. 1):S5–10.

35. Hicks DR, Martin LS, Getchell JP. Inactivation of HTLV-III/LAV-infected cultures of normal human lymphocytes by nonoxynol-9 in vitro. *Lancet* 1985; **ii**(8469-70):422–3.

36. van Damme L, Ramjee G, Alary M et al. Effectiveness of COL-1492, a nonoxynol-9 vaginal gel, on HIV-1 transmission in female sex workers: a randomised controlled trial. *Lancet* 2002; **360**:971–7. Available online at: www.thelancet.com

37. Roddy RE, Zekeng L, Ryan KA, Tamoufé U, Tweedy KG. Effect of nonoxynol-9 gel on urogenital gonorrhea and chlamydial infection: a randomized controlled trial. *Journal of the American Medical Association* 2002; **287**:1117–22.

38. Centers for Disease Control and Prevention. Notice to readers: CDC Statement on study results of products containing nonoxynol-9. *Morbidity and Mortality Weekly Report (MMWR)* 11 August 2000; **49**:717–18. See also: http://www.cdc.gov/hiv/pubs/mmwr/mmwr11aug00.htm

39. World Health Organization. WHO/CONRAD Technical Consultation on Nonoxynol-9: Summary Report. 9–10 October 2001. Geneva: WHO, 2002, 12 pp. Available online at: http://www.who.int/reproductive-health/rtis/N9_meeting_report.pdf

40. Richardson BA. Nonoxynol-9 as a vaginal microbicide for prevention of sexually transmitted infections: it's time to move on. *Journal of the American Medical Association* 2002; **287**:1171–2.

INTERNET RESOURCES

- For a comprehensive guide to drugs used for the prophylaxis and treatment of opportunistic infections and other HIV-related illnesses, including the special care needs of women, see the current edition of the UK *HIV & AIDS Treatments Directory*, published twice yearly by the National AIDS Manual (email: info@nam.org.uk) and the monthly *AIDS Treatment Update*, available online at: http://www.aidsmap.com

- Anderson JR (ed.). *A Guide to the Clinical Care of Women with HIV*. Rockville, MD: US Department of Health and Human Services, Health Resources and Services Administration, HIV/AIDS Bureau, 2001. This excellent practical text, which comprehensively describes the care and treatment of HIV-infected women, is available free (online, CD and hard copy available.) and is regularly updated. Hard copy can be obtained free of charge by contacting: Womencare, Parklawn Bldg, Rm 11A-33, 5600 Fishers Lane, Rockville, Maryland 20857, USA; Fax: +1-301-443-0791; or e-mail: womencare@hrsa.gov: http://www.hab.hrsa.gov/

- The *British National Formulary (BNF)*, published by the British Medical Association and the Royal Pharmaceutical Society of Great Britain, provides up-to-date information in relation to the drugs used in the UK to treat HIV infection and HIV-related illnesses. The online version is updated every 6 months. Available from: BMJ Books, PO Box 295, London WC1H 9TE, UK, or from the website www.bmjbookshop.com: http://www.BNF.org/

- For continuously updated online guidance on antiretroviral drug regimens for women from the AIDS Information Services (AIDSinfo) of the US Health and Human Services, see:
Perinatal HIV Guidelines Working Group. Recommendations for Use of Antiretroviral Drugs in Pregnant HIV 1 Infected Women for Maternal Health and Interventions to Reduce Perinatal HIV-1 Transmission in the United States, Living Document. Washington, DC: US Public Health Service Task Force, 16 June 2003: http://aidsinfo.nih.gov/guidelines/perinatal/PER_061603.pdf

Preventing mother-to-child HIV transmission

For a child, the risk of becoming infected with HIV is a stark example of the difference between being born in a rich country and being born in a poor country. In countries in the European Union, North America and Australasia, AIDS is a vanishing disease among children. Throughout the developing world, however, the number of new HIV infections in children continues to increase.

Robert Steinbrook, MD[1]

Introduction

As we have seen in the previous chapter, women now account for at least half of the total global number of adults living with HIV/AIDS.[2] Most of these women are of childbearing age and, as more and more women have become infected with HIV, an increasing number of their newborn infants are also at risk of becoming infected from them before, during or soon after childbirth. In the industrially developed world, HIV-infected infants and small children will be destined to a life of chronic infection and an uncertain fate. The majority of HIV-infected children, however, will live in poorly resourced nations in the industrially developing world, where their fate is more certain. These children will live in poverty and will have limited, if any, access to relevant care and specific treatment. They will not have enough nutritious food to eat or clean water to drink and, as their HIV-infected mothers die, they will commonly experience a lack of shelter and safety. Almost all of these children will suffer and die within a few years; half of them dying during their first year of life and the rest before their fifth birthday.[1]

With adequate resources, it is possible to prevent HIV-infected mothers from passing this virus to their infants. In this chapter, we are going to explore various strategies for minimizing the risk of HIV infection to children.

Learning outcomes

After studying and reflecting on the material in this chapter, you will be able to:

- identify the risk of HIV infection to newborn infants;
- outline factors associated with mother-to-child transmission;
- describe various approaches to preventing perinatal HIV transmission;
- discuss the role of antenatal screening for HIV infection.

BACKGROUND

By the beginning of 2003, more then 3.2 million children under the age of 15 years throughout the world were living with HIV/AIDS (Figure 12.1).[2] During the previous year, more than 800 000 children were newly infected with HIV (more than 2250 every day) and more than 1700 children died every day (Figures 12.2 and 12.3).[2] Most HIV-infected children (90 per cent) are born in countries in industrially developing regions, mainly sub-Saharan Africa. However, as national HIV epidemics escalate in South and South East Asia and in Eastern Europe, the number of HIV-infected infants born in these densely populated countries will soon dwarf the current tragedy being experienced today in southern Africa.

In the richer nations of the industrially developed world, comprehensive prevention strategies have dramatically decreased the number of HIV-infected newborn children to the point where it is generally uncommon for children to become infected from their mothers.

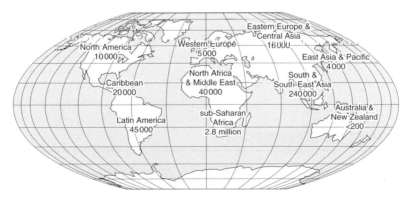

Total: 3.2 million

FIGURE 12.1 *Children (<15 years) estimated to be living with HIV/AIDS as of end 2002. (Courtesy of UNAIDS.)*

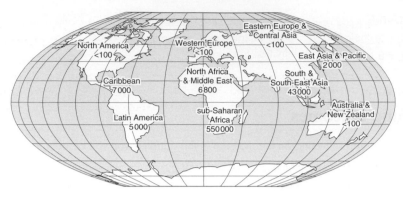

Total: 610000

FIGURE 12.2 *Estimated deaths in children (<15 years) from HIV/AIDS during 2002. (Courtesy of UNAIDS.)*

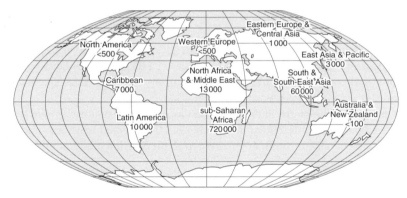

Total: 800000

FIGURE 12.3 *Estimated number of children (<15 years) newly infected with HIV during 2002. (Courtesy of UNAIDS.)*

MOTHER-TO-CHILD TRANSMISSION

Mother-to-child transmission (MTCT), also known as vertical or perinatal transmission, can occur during pregnancy (**in utero**), during birth (**intrapartum**) when the newborn infant comes into contact with infected maternal birth fluids, shortly after birth (**postpartum**) or during the early months of life while being breastfed. Most children (75 per cent) become infected during the **peripartum** period, i.e. during or shortly after delivery.[3]

Risk factors

Several maternal, obstetric and postnatal factors can increase the likelihood of MTCT (Table 12.1), and understanding these risks has led to the development of effective risk-reduction strategies. Women themselves are potentially at risk of initial infection during sexual intercourse with HIV-infected men, from sharing HIV-contaminated injecting equipment, or following treatment with transfusions of unscreened whole human blood or unscreened blood components.

TABLE 12.1 Factors that influence mother-to-child transmission (MTCT)

	Notes
Maternal factors	
Disease stage of mother	Primary HIV infection and symptomatic HIV disease, associated with high levels of HIV in the plasma (viral load) and low numbers of CD4$^+$ T-lymphocytes, are associated with an increased risk for MTCT[4,5]
Plasma and genital tract viral load	High plasma and genital tract viral load is associated with an increased risk for MTCT[4-6]
CD4$^+$ T-lymphocyte number	Low CD4$^+$ T-lymphocyte count and decreased CD4$^+$:CD8$^+$ ratio are both associated with an increased risk for MTCT[5]
Viral characteristics	Different HIV-1 subtypes (clades), e.g. A, C and D, and viral variants (genotype) may influence transmission efficiency and at which stage MTCT may occur[5,7-9]
	Biological growth characteristics of HIV, e.g. macrophage-tropic, non-syncytium-inducing HIV phenotypes may be more efficient at infecting fetal blood mononuclear cells[5,10,11] (see Chapter 3)
Immune response	Individual profile of maternal antibodies and cytokines may affect the risk for MTCT[5,12]
Antiretroviral treatment and prophylaxis	The use of antiretroviral drugs (zidovudine, lamivudine, nevirapine) in treatment regimens for the mother or as chemoprophylaxis for the child has been shown to significantly decrease the risk for MTCT[5]
Vitamin A deficiency	Vitamin A deficiency is associated with an increased risk of pre-term delivery which increases the risk of MTCT[13]
Sexual behaviour	A history of unprotected penetrative sexual intercourse with several partners has been associated with an increased risk for MTCT[5,14]
Sexually transmitted infections	The presence of other sexually transmitted infections increases plasma viraemia (viral load); these infections also increase the number of genital tract inflammatory cells, which stimulates HIV shedding, increasing the risk for MTCT[5,15]
Substance abuse	The use of illicit drugs during pregnancy increases the risk for MTCT[5,16,17]
Cigarette smoking	Cigarette smoking during pregnancy is associated with an increased risk for MTCT[5,18,19]
Obstetric factors	
Gestational age	Pre-term delivery has been shown to increase the risk for MTCT[5,20,21]
Duration of membrane rupture	The risk of MTCT increases linearly with increasing duration of ruptured membranes, with a 2% increase in risk for each hour increment; women with late symptomatic HIV disease (AIDS) have a 31% probability of MTCT after 24 hours of ruptured membranes[22]
Placental disruption–abruption, chorioamnionitis	Chorioamnionitis increases the risk of MTCT[23] and placental abruption causing disruption of the placental–fetal barrier may increase fetal exposure to maternal blood and increases the risk of MTCT[5]
Invasive fetal monitoring	Use of fetal scalp electrodes, fetal scalp sampling, amnioscopy and amniocentesis increases the risk for MTCT[24,25]
Episiotomy, forceps	Use of episiotomy, vacuum extraction or forceps may increase the risk for MTCT by exposing the fetus to maternal blood and genital secretions; however, careful use may shorten duration of labour or ruptured membranes with vaginal delivery and this may decrease the risk of MTCT[5]

TABLE 12.1 – continued

	Notes
	External version should be avoided because of the increased risk for maternal–fetal bleeding
Vaginal vs caesarean delivery	Caesarean delivery performed before the onset of labour and rupture of membranes can reduce the risk of MTCT by 55–88%[26,27]
Postnatal factors	
Breastfeeding	The risk of MTCT from breastfeeding is greatest in early infancy (before 6 months of age) and persists as long as breastfeeding continues[28–30]
	The longer the duration of breastfeeding, the greater the risk of MTCT[31–33]
Blood transfusions	Mothers may initially become infected with HIV as a result of an unscreened blood transfusion during the peripartum period, and during primary HIV infection, when the plasma viral load is high, there is a significantly increased risk for MTCT from breastfeeding

Prevention

There are several options for preventing MTCT (Table 12.2), but the three most important are:

- antiretroviral chemoprophylaxis,
- elective caesarean section delivery, and
- mothers refraining from breastfeeding.

TABLE 12.2 Methods for preventing mother-to-child transmission (MTCT)

Behavioural interventions	Prevent further sexually transmitted infections during pregnancy by reducing the number of sexual partners and
	Reducing the frequency of unprotected sexual intercourse
	Discontinue the use of illicit drugs during pregnancy
	Stop cigarette smoking
Termination of pregnancy	
Therapeutic interventions	Commence mother on antiretroviral therapy, or
	Provide chemoprophylaxis for infant
	Effectively treat any co-existing sexually transmitted infections
	If vitamin A deficient, provide vitamin supplementation
Obstetric interventions	Avoid invasive tests or monitoring during the antenatal and intrapartum period
	Consider the benefits of caesarean delivery
Modification of infant feeding practice	Refrain from breastfeeding, or
	Exclusively breastfeed, and
	Cease breastfeeding as early as possible
	Heat treat expressed breast milk
Blood transfusions	Use only blood and blood components that have been screened for HIV infection

In Western Europe, where these interventions are available, the rate of MTCT fell from an average of 15 per cent to 2 per cent or less by 1999.[34]

Any effective strategy aimed at reducing the risk of MTCT must focus on preventing women from becoming infected in the first place. The special vulnerabilities of women to becoming infected with HIV are extensively discussed in the previous chapter.

All other interventions designed to prevent newborn children becoming infected from their mothers depend upon maternal infection being detected before the child is born. Antenatal screening for HIV infection is an essential element of a comprehensive strategy for preventing women giving birth to HIV-infected children.

European consensus guidelines on the management of HIV infection during pregnancy[35] are available and these are summarized in Table 12.3. UK-specific guidelines[76] are also available and regularly updated, and these can be downloaded from the internet at: http://www.bhiva.org/guidelines.htm. Finally, guidelines from the USA National Institutes for Health[37] are available as a 'Living Document' on the internet at http://www.aidsinfo.nih.gov/guidelines/perinatal/PER_061603.pdf. All three of these guidelines are in general agreement on how best to prevent MTCT of HIV, and nurses, midwives and other healthcare professionals working within this field need to be familiar with their recommendations and advice.

TABLE 12.3 Summary of European Consensus on Management of HIV Infection in Pregnancy[35]

Antenatal screening	All pregnant women and, ideally, those planning a pregnancy are offered and recommended to have an HIV test; HIV testing should also be offered to their sexual partners
Caesarean section (CS) delivery	HIV-infected women should be given the option of delivering their child through a CS performed before labour and before rupture of membranes (usually at 38 weeks' gestation)
Antiretroviral therapy	All HIV-infected women should be offered therapy during pregnancy for their own health, depending on their clinical status and prognostic markers
	Antiretroviral treatment can begin after the first trimester
	Most antiretroviral drugs have not been shown to be associated with an increased risk for birth defects (teratogenicity) except efavirenz, zalcitabine and hydroxyurea, which are contraindicated during pregnancy
Antiretroviral chemoprophylaxis	A three-part zidovudine (ZDN) regimen is used as the standard chemoprophylaxis to prevent MTCT; ZDN is given during pregnancy, during labour and in the neonatal period, commencing at 28–32 weeks' gestation (with elective CS delivery at 38 weeks' gestation)
	If CS delivery is not an option, in addition to ZDN: two doses of nevirapine may be given once labour has been established, *or* lamivudine (3TC) may also be given with ZDN
Breastfeeding	HIV-infected women are strongly advised to refrain from breastfeeding as safe infant-feeding alternatives are available in Europe
	Women who cannot refrain from breastfeeding should be advised to: exclusively breastfeed and not introduce other foods or drinks for 4–6 months breastfeed for as short a time as possible, with rapid cessation
Follow-up of children born to HIV-infected mothers	Long-term follow-up of all children born to HIV-infected mothers should continue, at least until school age

MTCT, mother-to-child transmission.

United Kingdom antenatal screening strategy

Because effective interventions are now available to prevent most infants becoming infected from their mothers, **all pregnant women in the UK are offered and strongly recommended to have an HIV test as an integral part of their antenatal care.**[38] This is known as the *universal offer* and was mandated in 1999 by the UK Departments of Health (DH) to ensure that all women could equally benefit from antenatal HIV testing regardless of the prevalence of infection in the area in which they resided. An appraisal of the UK antenatal screening strategy concluded that it was an essential component of the overall national strategy to reduce to an absolute minimum the number of children becoming infected as a result of MTCT.[39] Additionally, all pregnant women are offered and encouraged to be screened for hepatitis B virus infection.[40]

Pregnant women who present late for antenatal care, especially those from high HIV prevalence areas, should be offered and encouraged to have 'rapid' HIV testing during or close to labour.[35] Although highly sensitive and specific, women testing positive for HIV infection from a 'rapid' HIV test require speedy confirmation with additional tests. Screening and testing are discussed in more detail elsewhere[39] (see also 'Further reading' at the end of this Chapter).

Antiretroviral chemoprophylaxis

HIV is a retrovirus, and the first effective antiretroviral drug introduced into clinical practice in the late 1980s was called azidothymidine (AZT) but is now known as zidovudine (ZDV). Today, many different types of antiretroviral drugs are currently either licensed for use in the European Union or available through expanded access schemes for the treatment of HIV disease. Many more antiretroviral drugs are currently in development and will become available for treating patients in the coming years. These drugs are discussed in detail in Chapter 20. Some antiretroviral drugs are used to prevent MTCT and this is known as chemoprophylaxis.

Three-part ZDV regimen (PACTG 076 ZDV)

Almost a decade ago, an important study known as the Pediatric AIDS Clinical Trials Group Protocol 076 (PACTG 076 ZDV) conclusively demonstrated that a three-part regimen of ZDV could reduce the risk for mother-to-child HIV transmission by nearly 70 per cent.[41] This regimen consisted of (Part 1) oral ZDV initiated at 14–34 weeks' gestation and continued throughout pregnancy, followed by (Part 2) intravenous ZDV during labour and (Part 3) oral (or intravenous) administration of ZDV to the infant for 6 weeks after delivery (Table 12.4). Subsequent epidemiologic studies in the USA and France demonstrated dramatic decreases in perinatal transmission rates to as low as 3–4 per cent following the incorporation of the PACTG 076 ZDV regimen into general clinical practice.[42,43]

TABLE 12.4 Pediatric AIDS Clinical Trials Group (PACTG) 076 zidovudine (ZDV) regimen[41]

Time of ZDV administration	Regimen
Antepartum	Oral administration of 100 mg ZDV five times daily,° initiated at 14–34 weeks' gestation and continued throughout the pregnancy
Intrapartum	During labour, intravenous administration of ZDV in a 1-hour initial dose of 2 mg/kg body weight, followed by a continuous infusion of 1 mg/kg body weight per hour until delivery
Postpartum	Oral administration of ZDV to the newborn (ZDV syrup at 2 mg/kg body weight per dose every 6 hours) for the first 6 weeks of life, beginning at 8–12 hours after birth (note: intravenous dosage for infants who cannot tolerate oral intake is 1.5 mg/kg body weight intravenously every 6 hours)

°Oral ZDV administered as 200 mg three times daily or 300 mg twice daily is currently used in general clinical practice and is an acceptable alternative regimen to 100 mg orally five times daily.

In both Europe and the USA, ZDV monotherapy as per the PACTG 076 ZDV regimen remains the standard prophylaxis for preventing MTCT of HIV.[35,37] However, modifications to this regimen and the use of other drugs, either alone or in combination with ZDV, are increasing.

Alternative chemoprophylaxis regimens

In Europe and the USA, alternative regimens and other antiretroviral drugs are recommended for different clinical scenarios (Table 12.5).[35-37] It is important to remember that as more research data become available, guidance will evolve accordingly, and nurses and other healthcare professionals can access the most current recommendations from the wordwide web (www) (see 'Internet resources' at the end of this chapter).

TABLE 12.5 Alternative chemoprophylaxis regimens for preventing HIV mother-to-child transmission (MTCT) in the USA[37]

Clinical scenario	Recommendation
HIV-infected pregnant women who have not received prior antiretroviral therapy	■ Pregnant women with HIV infection must receive standard clinical, immunologic and virologic evaluation
	■ Recommendations for initiation and choice of antiretroviral therapy should be based on the same parameters used for women who are not pregnant, although the known and unknown risks and benefits of such therapy during pregnancy must be considered and discussed
	■ The three-part ZDV chemoprophylaxis regimen, initiated after the first trimester, should be recommended for all pregnant women with HIV infection, regardless of antenatal HIV RNA copy number, to reduce the risk of MTCT
	■ The combination of ZDV chemoprophylaxis with additional antiretroviral drugs for treatment of of HIV infection is recommended for infected women whose clinical, immunologic or virologic status requires treatment or who have HIV RNA over 1000 copies/mL regardless of clinical or immunologic status
	■ Women who are in the first trimester of pregnancy may consider delaying initiation of therapy until after 10–12 weeks' gestation
HIV-infected women receiving antiretroviral therapy during the current pregnancy	■ HIV-1 infected women receiving antiretroviral therapy in whom pregnancy is identified after the first trimester should continue therapy
	■ ZDV should be a component of the antenatal antiretroviral treatment regimen after the first trimester whenever possible, although this may not always be feasible
	■ Women receiving antiretroviral therapy in whom pregnancy is recognized during the first trimester should be counselled regarding the benefits and potential risks of antiretroviral administration during this period, and continuation of therapy should be considered
	■ If therapy is discontinued during the first trimester, all antiretroviral drugs should be stopped and re-introduced simultaneously to avoid the development of drug resistance
	■ Regardless of the antepartum antiretroviral regimen, ZDV administration is recommended during the intrapartum period and for the newborn
HIV-infected women in labour who have had no prior antiretroviral therapy	■ Several effective regimens are available, including: single-dose nevirapine at the onset of labour followed by a single dose of nevirapine for the newborn at age 48 hours oral ZDV and lamivudine (3TC) during labour, followed by 1 week of oral ZDV/3TC for the newborn intrapartum intravenous ZDV followed by 6 weeks of ZDV for the newborn the two-dose nevirapine regimen combined with intrapartum intravenous ZDV and 6 weeks' ZDV for the newborn

TABLE 12.5 – continued

Clinical scenario	Recommendation
	▪ In the immediate postpartum period, the woman should have appropriate assessments (e.g. CD4⁺ T-lymphocyte cell counts and HIV-1 RNA copy number) to determine whether antiretroviral therapy is recommended for her own health
Infants born to mothers who have received no antiretroviral therapy during pregnancy or intrapartum	▪ The 6-week neonatal ZDV component of the ZDV chemoprophylactic regimen should be discussed with the mother and offered for the newborn
	▪ ZDV should be initiated as soon as possible after delivery, preferably within 6–12 hours of birth
	▪ Some clinicians may choose to use ZDV in combination with other antiretroviral drugs, particularly if the mother is known or suspected to have ZDV-resistant virus; however, the efficacy of this approach for preventing MTCT is unknown, and appropriate dosing regimens for neonates are incompletely defined
	▪ In the immediate postpartum period, the woman should have appropriate assessments (e.g. CD4⁺ T-lymphocyte cell counts and HIV-1 RNA copy number) to determine whether antiretroviral therapy is recommended for her own health
	▪ The infant should undergo early diagnostic testing so that, if HIV-infected, treatment can be initiated as soon as possible

Discussion of treatment options and recommendations should be non-coercive and the final decision regarding the use of antiretroviral drugs is the responsibility of the woman. A decision not to accept treatment with ZDV or other antiretroviral drugs should not result in punitive action or denial of care. Use of ZDV should not be denied to a woman who wishes to minimize exposure of the fetus to other antiretroviral drugs and who therefore chooses to receive only ZDV during pregnancy to reduce the risk of MTCT.

For resource-poor countries where the full PACTG 076 ZDV regimen is unaffordable, the World Health Organization (WHO) recommended a short-course ZDV regimen[44] (Table 12.6) that has been shown to reduce MTCT rates by approximately 50 per cent.[45] Various other ZDV-containing and non-ZDV-containing regimens are used in different countries.[5]

TABLE 12.6 World Health Organization recommendations for short-course zidovudine (ZDV) chemoprophylaxis to reduce mother-to-child transmission for women in developing countries[44]

Time of ZDV administration	Regimen
Antepartum	Oral administration of 300 mg ZDV twice daily, from 36 weeks until labour
Intrapartum	During labour, oral ZDV 300 mg every 3 hours of labour until delivery

Antiretroviral treatment of HIV-infected women

Identifying HIV-infected women during antenatal care is not only important for preventing MTCT, but it also enables women to explore treatment for their own health. Antiretroviral therapy (see Chapter 20) can be offered to infected pregnant women, depending upon their clinical status and prognostic markers, such as their CD4⁺ T-lymphocyte counts and plasma HIV-RNA levels (viral load). In general, antiretroviral therapy is initiated after the first trimester and the treatment regimen almost always includes ZDV.[35-37] Most antiretroviral drugs are considered safe to administer during pregnancy after the first trimester, except efavirenz and zalcitabine. Hydroxyurea is also contraindicated during pregnancy.[35] Nurses can consult a current issue of the *British National Formulary (BNF)*, or the online version (see 'Internet resources' at the end of this chapter), to confirm which drugs are safe to administer during pregnancy.[46]

Elective caesarean section delivery

Evidence for intrapartum transmission is supported from a variety of research findings, including observations that HIV transmission rates are lower in second-born twins compared to first-born twins and following elective caesarean section compared to vaginal delivery.[47,48] HIV has been found in the vaginal and cervical secretions of pregnant women, and also in gastric secretions of infants born to HIV-infected women.[49,50]

Neonates can become infected during vaginal delivery when they are exposed to HIV-contaminated birth fluids, either through ingestion into the gastrointestinal tract or from the close contact their skin and mucous membranes have with these fluids. Ruptured membranes of greater than 4 hours are significantly associated with increased risk of intrapartum transmission to infants born by caesarean section or vaginal delivery, as the neonates have been exposed to infectious material for longer.[51]

Current European and USA recommendations acknowledge that elective caesarean section delivery, carried out before labour at 38 weeks' gestation, significantly reduces the risk of MTCT.[26,27,35-37]

Infant feeding

There are considerable advantages to both mother and infant in breastfeeding, especially during the first 6 months of life. Throughout the world, breastfeeding protects against respiratory infections and diarrhoeal disease, two of the most important causes of childhood mortality, and it has significant economical, social, psychological and family planning advantages. However, in HIV-infected mothers, both cell-free and cell-associated viruses have been consistently identified in colostrum and mature milk, and the transmission of HIV in breast milk, occurring at any point during lactation, has been well documented.[52]

Several factors are involved in or associated with HIV transmission via breast milk. High levels of maternal viraemia (high viral load) will increase the amount of HIV secreted in breast milk and, consequently, increase the amount and duration of HIV exposure to the infant. Vitamin A deficiency in HIV-infected mothers is associated with cracked nipples (and increased vaginal shedding of HIV), which may be an additional source of viral exposure to the infant.[53] Infant prematurity results in an immature neonatal immune system that is unable to mount an effective cell-mediated response to HIV and is associated with an increased risk of viral acquisition from breastfeeding.[53,54]

The actual mechanism of breast-milk transmission is not fully understood. However, neonatal mucous membranes (and skin) cannot effectively prevent HIV infection, and exposure to HIV in breast milk may result in viral infection directly through oral and gastric mucosa.[52] Other conditions that may disrupt the integrity of neonatal oral mucosa, e.g. candidiasis, have been associated with an increased risk of HIV infection from breast milk.[54]

The amount of HIV secreted in breast milk is highest during the first few months following delivery, and 70 per cent of postnatal transmission takes places within the first 4-6 months of life.[55,56]

Avoidance of breastfeeding and the use of breast-milk substitutes will substantially reduce postnatal MTCT of HIV and this strategy is recommended in industrialized countries (including the UK) where safe alternatives to breastfeeding are available. Globally, however, most infants at risk of postnatal MTCT of HIV are breastfed. In many cultures and in many regions of the developing world, it is neither possible nor acceptable for women not to breastfeed their infants.

Exclusive breastfeeding

Studies conducted in South Africa found evidence that women who exclusively breastfed had a lower rate of MTCT than those mothers who also fed their babies other fluids or food together with breastfeeding (mixed infant feeding).[57,58] Potential mechanisms that might explain a reduced risk for MTCT when children are exclusively breastfed include:[59]

- reduction in dietary antigens and enteric pathogens from fluids and food, which may help maintain the integrity of the intestinal mucosal barrier and limit the inflammatory responses to the gut mucosa;
- promotion of beneficial intestinal microflora that may increase resistance to infection and enhance the infant's immune responses;
- the beneficial antimicrobial, anti-inflammatory and immuno-modulating properties of breast milk.

Consequently, if there are no consistently safer alternatives to breastfeeding for HIV-infected mothers, exclusive breastfeeding is the second best option for reducing the risk of MTCT in the postnatal period. However, it must be realized that many mothers in resource-poor countries of the world, suffering malnutrition and poor health themselves, may not produce enough breast milk to be able exclusively to breastfeed their babies, and they will manage the best they can by mixed infant feeding.

Summary

In most countries, the children of HIV-infected mothers will be born into a world where they are immediately disadvantaged. Most will eventually be orphaned, and by 2010, more than 25 million children are expected to lose one or both parents due to HIV disease.[60] The majority of these children will be stigmatized, impoverished and deprived of even their basic needs of food, water, shelter and protection. Their chances of survival will be diminished even further if they have also become infected from their mothers before, during or after birth.

In this chapter we have seen that we have the ability to prevent MTCT of HIV. However, the necessary counselling, testing and treatment needed to do this are hampered by a geographical lottery, where children born in countries with poorly organized and starkly under-resourced prenatal healthcare services will be at most risk. Millions of children have already been infected and thousands more are becoming infected every day.[2]

Prologue to Chapter 13

In the next chapter, we will review the healthcare needs of children living with HIV disease, remaining aware that the care and treatment available depend on where these children live. The impact of national epidemics of HIV disease in industrially developing countries is further discussed in Chapter 23.

REFERENCES

1. Steinbrook, R. Perspective: preventing HIV infection in children. *New England Journal of Medicine* 2002; **346**:1842–3.

2. UNAIDS/WHO. *AIDS Epidemic Update* (UNAIDS/02.58E). Geneva: Joint United Nations Programme on HIV/AIDS (UNAIDS) & the World Health Organization (WHO), December 2002, 38 pp. Available from: http://www.unaids.org/worldaidsday/2002/press/update/epiupdate_en.pdf

3. Mirochnick M, Fenton T, Gagnier P et al. Pharmacokinetics of nevirapine in human immunodeficiency virus type 1-infected pregnant women and their neonates. *Journal of Infectious Diseases* 1998; **178**:368–74.

4. Garcia PM, Kalish LA, Pitt J et al. Maternal levels of plasma human immunodeficiency virus type-1 RNA and the risk of perinatal transmission. *New England Journal of Medicine* 1999; **341**:394–402.

5. Anderson JR. HIV and reproduction. In: Anderson JR (ed.), *A Guide to the Clinical Care of Women with HIV*. Washington DC: US Department of Health and Human Services, Health Resources and Services Administration, HIV/AIDS Bureau, 2001, 213–73.

6. Fang G, Burger H, Anastos K et al. Sequence analysis of the complete HIV-1 pol gene from virions in plasma and genital tract of women: genital tract reservoir and differential drug resistance. HIV Pathology and Treatment Conference. *Abstracts* (Abst 4025), March 13–19, 1998.

7. Dickover R, Garratty E, Plaeger S, Bryson Y. Perinatal transmission of major, minor, and multiple HIV-1 strains in utero and intrapartum. 7th Conference on Retroviruses and Opportunistic Infections. *Abstracts* (Abst 181), January 30–February 2, 2000.

8. Subbarao S, Wright T, Ellerbrock T, Lennox JL, Hart C. Genotypic evidence of local HIV expression in the female genital tract. 5th Conference on Retroviruses and Opportunistic Infections. *Abstracts* (Abst 708), February 1–5, 1998.

9. Renjifo B, Gilbert P, Chaplin B et al. Preferential in-utero transmission of HIV-1 subtype C compared to subtype A or D. 15th International AIDS Conference. *Abstracts* (Abst ThOrD1426), July 7–12, 2002.

10. Palasanthiran P, Ziegler JB, Dwyer DE, Robertson P, Leigh D, Cunningham AL. Early detection of human immunodeficiency virus type 1 infection in Australian infants at risk of perinatal infection and factors affecting transmission. *Pediatric Infectious Disease Journal* 1994; **13**:1083–90.

11. Reinhardt PP, Reinhardt B, Lathey JL, Spector SA. Human cord blood mononuclear cells are preferentially infected by non-syncytium-inducing, macrophase-tropic human immunodeficiency viruse type 1 isolates. *Journal of Clinical Microbiology* 1995; **33**:292–7.

12. Hutto C, Scott GB. Special considerations in children. In: Merigan TC, Bartlett JG, Bolognesi D (eds), *Textbook of AIDS Medicine*, 2nd edn. Baltimore: Williams & Wilkins, 1999, 163–77.

13. Coutsoudis A, Pillay K, Spooner E, Khun L, Coovadia HM. Randomized trial testing the effect of vitamin A supplementation on pregnancy outcomes and early mother-to-child HIV-1 transmission in Durban, South Africa. South African Vitamin A Study Group. *AIDS* 1999; **13**:1517–24.

14. Bulterys M, Landseman S, Burns DN, Robinstein A, Goedert J. Sexual behavior and injection drug use during pregnancy and vertical transmission of HIV-1. *Journal of Acquired Immune Deficiency Syndromes and Human Retrovirology* 1997; **15**:76–82.

15. Plummer FA. Heterosexual transmission of human immunodeficiency virus type 1 (HIV): interactions of conventional sexually transmitted diseases, hormonal

contraception and HIV-1. *AIDS Research and Human Retroviruses* 1998; **14**(Suppl. 1):S5–10.

16. Rodriguez EM, Mofenson LM, Chang BH et al. Association of maternal drug use during pregnancy with maternal HIV culture positivity and perinatal HIV transmission. *AIDS* 1996; **10**:273–82.

17. Lyman WD. Perinatal AIDS: drugs of abuse and transplacental infection. *Advances in Experimental Medicine and Biology* 1993; **335**:211–17.

18. Burns DN, Landesman S, Muenz LR et al. Cigarette smoking, premature rupture of membranes and vertical transmission of HIV01 among women with low CD4 levels. *Journal of Acquired Immune Deficiency Syndromes and Human Retrovirology* 1994; **7**:718–26.

19. Turner BJ, Hauck WW, Fanning R, Markson LE. Cigarette smoking and maternal–child HIV transmission. *Journal of Acquired Immune Deficiency Syndromes and Human Retrovirology* 1997; **14**:327–37.

20. Kuhn L, Abrams EJ, Matheson PB et al. Timing of maternal–infant HIV transmission: associations between intrapartum factors and early polymerase chain reaction results. New York City Perinatal HIV Transmission Collaborative Study Group. *AIDS* 1997; **11**:429–35.

21. Kuhn L, Steketee RW, Weedon J et al. Distinct risk factors for intrauterine and intrapartum human immunodeficiency virus transmission and consequences for disease progression in infected children. New York City Perinatal HIV Transmission Collaborative Study Group. *Journal of Infectious Diseases* 1999; **179**:52–8.

22. Read J, for the International Perinatal HIV Group. Duration of ruptured membranes and vertical transmission of HIV-1: a meta-analysis from fifteen prospective cohort studies. 7th Conference on Retroviruses and Opportunistic Infections. *Abstracts* (Abst 659), January 30–February 2, 2000.

23. Goldenbert RL, Vermund SH, Soepfert AR, Andrews WW. Choriodecidual inflammation. A potentially preventable cause of perinatal HIV-1 transmission? *Lancet* 1998; **352**:1927–30.

24. Maiques V, Garcia-Tejedor A, Perales A, Navarro C. Intrapartum fetal invasive procedures and perinatal transmission of HIV. *European Journal of Obstetrics, Gynecology, and Reproductive Biology* 1999; **87**:63–7.

25. Mandelbrot L, Mayaux MJ, Bongain A et al. Obstetric factors and mother-to-child transmission of human immunodeficiency virus type 1: the French perinatal cohorts. SEROGEST French Pediatric HIV Infection Study Group. *American Journal of Obstetrics and Gynecology* 1996; **175**:661–7.

26. European Mode of Delivery Collaboration. Elective caesarean-section versus vaginal delivery in prevention of vertical HIV-transmission: a randomised clinical trial. *Lancet* 1999; **353**:1035–9.

27. International Perinatal HIV Group. The mode of delivery and the risk of vertical transmission of human immunodeficiency virus type-1. *New England Journal of Medicine* 1999; **340**:977–87.

28. Miotti PG, Taha TE, Kumwenda NI et al. HIV transmission through breastfeeding: a study in Malawi. *Journal of the American Medical Association* 1999; **282**:744–9.

29. Nduati R, John G, MboriNgacha D et al. Effects of breastfeeding and formula feeding on transmission of HIV-1: a randomized clinical trial. *Journal of the American Medical Association* 2000; **283**:1167–74.

30. John GC, Nduati RW, MboriNgacha D et al. Correlates of mother-to-child human

immunodeficiency virus type 1 (HIV-1) transmission: association with maternal plasma HIV-1 RNA load, genital HIV-1 DNA shedding, and breast infections. *Journal of Infectious Diseases* 2001; **183**:206–12.

31. Leroy V, Newell ML, Dabis F et al. International multicentre pooled analysis of late postnatal mother to child transmission of HIV-1 infection. Ghent International Working Group on Mother-to-Children Transmission of HIV. *Lancet* 1998; **352**:597–600.

32. Embree JE, Njenga S, Datta P et al. Risk factors for postnatal mother-to-child transmission of HIV-1. *AIDS* 2000; **14**:2535–41.

33. Read JS, Newell ML, Dabis F, Leroy V. Breastfeeding and late postnatal transmission of HIV-1: an individual patient data meta-analysis (Breastfeeding and HIV International Transmission Study). 15th International AIDS Conference. *Abstracts* (Abst TuOrB1177), July 7–12, 2002.

34. European Collaborate Study. HIV-infected women and vertical transmission in Europe since 1986. *AIDS* 2001; **15**:761–70.

35. Newell ML, Rogers R (eds). Pregnancy and HIV infection: a European Consensus on Management. *AIDS* 2002; **16**(Suppl. 2):S1–18.

36. Lyall EGH, Blott M, de Ruiter A et al. Guidelines for the management of HIV infection in pregnant women and the prevention of mother-to-child transmission. British HIV Association. *HIV Medicine* 2001; **2**:314–330. Available from: http://www.bhiva.org/guidelines.htm

37. National Institutes of Health (Perinatal HIV Guidelines Working Group). Revisions to the February 4, 2002 Public Health Service Task Force Recommendations for the use of antiretroviral drugs in pregnant women infected with HIV-1 for maternal health and for reducing perinatal HIV-1 transmission in the United States August 30, 2002. Available from: http://www.aidsinfo.nih.gov/guidelines/perinatal/Perinatal.pdf

38. NHS Executive. Reducing mother to baby transmission of HIV. *Health Service Circular* 1999 HSC 1999/183. London: National Health Service Executive. Available from: http://www.doh.gov.uk/coinh.htm

39. Pratt RJ. Antenatal screening for HIV infection: removing tomorrow's children from harms' way. *Journal of Neonatal Nursing* 2000; **6**:179–84.

40. NHS Executive. Screening of pregnant women for hepatitis B and immunisation of babies at risk. *Health Service Circular* 1998 HSC 1998/127. London: National Health Service Executive. Available from: http://www.doh.gov.uk/coinh.htm

41. Connor EM, Sperling RS, Gelber R et al. Reduction of maternal–infant transmission of human immunodeficiency virus type 1 with zidovudine treatment. *New England Journal of Medicine* 1994; **331**:1173–80.

42. Simonds RJ, Neesheim S, Matheson P et al. Declining mother-to-child HIV transmission following perinatal zidovudine recommendations, United States (Abstract Tu.C.440). *Volume 1, XIth International Conference on AIDS*, Vancouver, Canada, July 7–12, 1996.

43. Blanche S, Mayaux MJ, Mandelbrot L, Rouzioux C, Delfraissy JF. Acceptability and impact of zidovudine prevention on mother-to-child HIV-1 transmission in France (Abstract). In: *Proceedings from the Fourth Conference on Retroviruses and Opportunistic Infections*. Washington DC, 1997, 176.

44. World Health Organization. Recommendations on the safe and effective use of short-course ZDV for prevention of mother-to-child transmission of HIV. *Weekly Epidemiological Record* 1998 October 9; **73**:313–20.

45. Shaffer N, Chuachoowong R, Mock PA et al. Short-course zidovudine for perinatal HIV-1 transmission in Bangkok, Thailand: a randomized controlled trial. *Lancet* 1999; **353**:773–80.

46. Mehta DK (Executive Editor). *British National Formulary (BNF)*, 44th edn. London: British Medical Association and the Royal Pharmaceutical Society of Great Britain, September 2002. Available from: BMJ Books, PO Box 295, London WC1H 9TE, UK, or from the website www.bmjbookshop.com. The BNF is also available online at: www.BNF.org

47. Goerdert JJ, Duliege AM, Amos CI, Felton S, Biggar RJ and the International Registry of HIV-exposed Twins. Higher risk of HIV-1 infection for first-born twins. *Lancet* 1991; **338**:1471–5.

48. Villari P, Spino C, Chalmers TC, Lau J, Sacks S. Caeserian section to reduce perinatal transmission of human immunodeficiency virus. *On-line Journal of Current Clinical Trials* 1993; **2**:July 8 doc. No. 3.

49. Loussert-Ajaka I, Mandelbrot L, Delmas MC et al. HIV-1 detection in cervicovaginal secretions during pregnancy. *AIDS* 1997; **11**:575–81.

50. Nielson K, Boyer P, Dillon M et al. Presence of human immunodeficiency virus (HIV) type 1 and HIV-1-specific antibodies in cervicovaginal secretions of infected mothers and in the gastric aspirates of their infants. *Journal of Infectious Diseases* 1996; **173**:1001–4.

51. Kuhn L, Abrams EJ, Matheson PB et al. Timing of maternal–infant transmission: associations between intrapartum factors and early polymerase chain reaction results. *AIDS* 1997; **11**:429–35.

52. Nduati R. *HIV and Infant Feeding: A Review of HIV Transmission Through Breastfeeding*. WHO/FRH/NUT 98.3, UNAIDS/98.5. Geneva: WHO, 1998, 1–26.

53. John GC, Nduati RW, Mbori-Ngacha D et al. Genital shedding of human immunodeficiency virus type 1 DNA during pregnancy: association with immunosuppression, abnormal cervical and vaginal discharge and severe vitamin A deficiency. *Journal of Infectious Diseases* 1997; **175**:57–62.

54. Ekpini E, Wikto SZ, Satten GA et al. Late postnatal transmission of HIV-1 in Abidjan, Côte d'Ivoire. *Lancet* 1997; **349**:1054–9.

55. Fantaini J, Yahi C, Delezay O, Tamalet C. HIV transmission across the vaginal epitheliums. *AIDS* 1997; **11**:1663.

56. Simonon A, Lepage P, Karita E et al. An assessment of the timing of mother-to-child transmission of human immunodeficiency virus Type 1 by means of polymerase chain reaction. *Journal of Acquired Immune Deficiency Syndromes* 1994; **7**:952–7.

57. Coutsoudis A, Pillay K, Spooner E, Kuhn L, Coovadia HM. Influence of infant-feeding patterns on early mother-to-child transmission of HIV-1 in Durban, South Africa: a prospective cohort study. South African Vitamin A Study Group. *Lancet* 1999; **354**:471–6.

58. Coutsoudis A, Pillay K, Kuhn L, Spooner E, Tsai WY, Coovadia HM. Method of feeding and transmission of HIV-1 from mothers to children by 15 months of age: prospective cohort study from Durban, South Africa. *AIDS* 2001; **15**:379–87.

59. Smith MM, Kuhn L. Exclusive breast-feeding: does it have the potential to reduce breast-feeding transmission of HIV-1? *Nutritional Review* 2000; **58**:333–40.

60. US Agency for International Development, United Nations Children's Fund, Joint United Nations Programme on HIV/AIDS. *Children on the Brink 2002: A Joint Report on Orphan Estimates and Program Strategies*. Washington DC: TvT Associates/The

Synergy Project, July 2002, 33 pp. Available from:
http://www.synergyaids.com/documents/COB2002.pdf

FURTHER READING

Newell ML, Rogers R. (eds). Pregnancy and HIV Infection: a European Consensus on Management. *AIDS* 2002; **16**(Suppl. 2):S1–18.
Pratt RJ. Antenatal Screening for HIV infection: removing tomorrow's children from harms' way. *Journal of Neonatal Nursing* 2000; **6**:179–84
Pratt RJ, Pellowe C. Breast feeding and HIV transmission: current state of the evidence. *Journal of Neonatal Nursing* 2003; **9**:133–9.

INTERNET RESOURCES

- Anderson JR (ed.). *A Guide to the Clinical Care of Women with HIV*. Rockville, MD: US Department of Health and Human Services, Health Resources and Services Administration, HIV/AIDS Bureau, 2001. This excellent practical text comprehensively describes the care and treatment of HIV-infected women. It is available free (online, CD and hard copy available) and is regularly updated. Hard copy can be obtained free of charge by contacting: Womencare, Parklawn Bldg, Rm 11A-33, 5600 Fishers Lane, Rockville, Maryland 20857, USA; Fax: +1-301-443-0791; or e-mail womencare@hrsa.gov:
  http://www.hab.hrsa.gov/
- The *British National Formulary (BNF)*, published by the British Medical Association and the Royal Pharmaceutical Society of Great Britain, provides up-to-date information in relation to the drugs used in the UK to treat HIV infection and HIV-related illnesses; the online version is updated every 6 months. Available from: BMJ Books, PO Box 295, London WC1H 9TE, UK, or from the website www.bmjbookshop.com:
  http://www.BNF.org/
- Questions and answers on MTCT are available from the UNAIDS website at:
  http://www.unaids.org/publications/documents/mtct/qaweb99.html
- The British HIV Association and European AIDS Clinical Society Guidelines for the Management of HIV Infection in Pregnant Women and the Prevention of MTCT are available online from:
  http://www.bhiva.org/guidelines.htm
- Continuously updated online guidance on the use of antiretroviral drugs in pregnant women infected with HIV-1 for maternal health and for reducing perinatal HIV-1 transmission in the USA are available from the *AIDS Information Services* (AIDSinfo) of the US Health and Human Services and the National Institutes of Health (Perinatal HIV Guidelines Working Group):
  http://aidsinfo.nih.gov/guidelines

Children and HIV disease

All children living with HIV infection must have access to treatment, counselling, education, recreation and social support, and be protected against any form of discrimination.

United Nations Convention on the Rights of the Child[1]

Introduction

In the previous chapter we have seen that it is possible to prevent the vast majority of infants becoming infected with HIV as a result of mother-to-child transmission (MTCT). However, the healthcare structures and resources needed for this are mostly unavailable in Africa, South and South East Asia, Eastern Europe and in many other low-income and middle-income regions of the world. Infants and young children born in countries in these regions will continue to be infected in large numbers during the foreseeable future. Although the numbers of infants becoming infected from MTCT is dramatically declining in most countries in the European Union (EU), North America and Australasia, a low prevalence of infected children will exist for many years to come. All of these HIV-infected infants and young children will require specialist multi-professional care and support throughout their lives.

In this chapter, we review how HIV infection/disease is diagnosed in children and how it is staged according to immunologic and clinical categories. In addition, we explore treatment and immunization schedules and the need for a multidisciplinary approach to caring for children. More detailed information that is beyond the scope of this chapter is available from a variety of standard medical texts on general and paediatric HIV disease (see 'Further reading') and from the 'Internet resources' listed at the end of this chapter.

Learning outcomes

After studying and reflecting on the material in this chapter, you will be able to:

- describe the natural history of HIV disease in children;
- outline a classification system used to stage HIV disease in children;
- discuss antiretroviral treatment in children;
- review issues associated with children adhering to therapy;
- describe the need for childhood immunizations and identify any vaccines that are contraindicated for use in HIV-infected children.

BACKGROUND

As we have seen in the previous chapter, most infants become infected with HIV perinatally as a result of MTCT. In addition, however, young children and adolescents can become infected as a result of receiving unscreened HIV-contaminated transfusions of whole human blood or blood components, from unsterile and HIV-contaminated injection equipment and other medical devices, and from being sexually abused by an HIV-infected person.

There are various differences between children and adults with HIV disease, including the competence of their immune system, disease progression, drug metabolism and clinical outcomes.

NATURAL HISTORY

Because infants and young children have maturing but not fully competent immune systems that mount less effective responses to infection, they become ill and progress to end-stage HIV disease more quickly than do untreated adults and adolescents. Following birth, plasma HIV RNA levels (viral load) increase rapidly in perinatally infected infants and decline only slowly during the first 2 or more years of life. During this period, infants with very high viral loads are at an increased risk for rapid disease progression and death.[2] This is in contrast to HIV-infected adolescents and adults in whom an effective immune response effectively lowers the viral load within several weeks of primary infection (see Chapter 6), which then only slowly increases over several years as the immune system becomes progressively weakened by continuing viral replication and CD4+ T-lymphocyte depletion.

CLASSIFICATION SYSTEM FOR PAEDIATRIC HIV DISEASE

HIV disease in a child under the age of 13 years is staged using the current HIV paediatric classification system developed by the Centers for Disease Control and Prevention (CDC) in the USA.[3] This classifies infected children into **mutually exclusive categories** according to three parameters: **infection, immunologic** and **clinical status**.

A child's classification reflects the **stage** of his or her disease and this has prognostic significance, i.e. it shows where the child is on that continuum from initial infection to end-stage disease. Once classified, an HIV-infected child cannot be re-classified into a less severe category, even if his or her clinical or immunologic status temporarily improves.

Infection status: identifying HIV infection in children

Perinatally exposed infants will usually be tested as early as possible following birth. All children born to HIV-infected mothers will be antibody positive for HIV because of the normal transfer of maternal antibodies across the placenta to the fetus that occurs during pregnancy. However, this does not mean that they are infected; all it means is that they have tested positive for the maternal HIV antibodies they have temporarily inherited from their mother. There is no test available to distinguish between the mother's and the baby's antibodies.[4] Consequently, a standard HIV antibody test for IgG antibodies (anti-HIV IgG antibody) is not a reliable indicator of infection in exposed infants until after the age of 18 months.[5] By this time, most exposed but uninfected infants will have cleared the last traces of maternal anti-HIV IgG antibody, and HIV-infected infants will have started to mount their own antibody response to the virus.

Newborn infants who have been perinatally exposed to HIV are generally tested at or within a few days of birth. Because it is important to identify neonatal HIV infection as early as possible, **antibody tests** are not used during this early period. Instead, HIV infection in infants is diagnosed by different types of **virologic tests**. Three types of virologic tests are in general use in countries in the EU, North America, Australasia and most other industrially developed nations (Table 13.1):

- detection of HIV nucleic acid (DNA or RNA),
- HIV isolation (viral culture), and
- HIV p24 antigen assay.

HIV nucleic acid detection tests are the virologic methods of choice to exclude infection in children less than 18 months of age. Although HIV can be isolated by culture, this test is more complex and expensive to perform and is less well standardized than nucleic acid detection tests.

TABLE 13.1 Virologic tests used to identify HIV infection in infants

Test	Definition
HIV nucleic acid detection tests PCR: proviral DNA	PCR (polymerase chain reaction): a laboratory method that can find the smallest trace of HIV nucleic acid (proviral DNA) within infected circulating mononuclear blood cells and then replicate these molecules repeatedly to amplify (quantify) them so that they can be detected. PCR is used as the principal method for the early diagnosis of paediatric HIV infection, and HIV-exposed infants are usually tested within days of birth.
or Plasma HIV-1 RNA	Plasma HIV-1 RNA test detects HIV RNA and is frequently used for determining the number of copies of HIV RNA per millilitre, i.e. the viral load.
HIV isolation viral culture	This is a laboratory method for growing the virus in a culture medium. The culture is assayed for HIV (p24 antigen) twice weekly for a full 28 days of incubation.[7]
HIV p24 antigen assay	HIV p24 antigen assay can be used to test plasma or serum samples for HIV viral proteins. However, this test is not as sensitive or specific as either the PCR or viral culture.

The laboratory and clinical criteria for diagnosing HIV infection in children are described in Table 13.2.[3,6] It is essential to remember that parents must give consent prior to their child having any type of test for HIV infection. Once a child's infectious status has been confirmed, it is further classified according to his or her immunologic and clinical status.

TABLE 13.2 Diagnosis of HIV infection in children[3,6]

Diagnosis	Criteria – laboratory and clinical

A
HIV infection in a child <18 months who is known to be HIV seropositive or born to an HIV-infected mother and: →
	■ has positive results on two separate determinations (excluding cord blood) from one or more of the following HIV detection tests:
	  HIV culture
	  HIV polymerase chain reaction
	  HIV antigen (p24)
	or
	■ meets the criteria for the acquired immunodeficiency syndrome (AIDS) based on the 1987 AIDS surveillance case definition for children[8]

B **HIV infection** in a child ≥18 months of age born to an HIV-infected mother or any child infected by blood, blood products or other known modes of transmission (e.g. sexual contact) who: →	■ is HIV-antibody positive by repeatedly reactive enzyme immunoassay (EIA) and confirmatory test (e.g. Western blot or immunofluorescence assay (IFA) or ■ meets any of the criteria in A above
C **Not** infected with HIV: a child < 18 months born to an HIV-infected mother who does not meet the criteria for HIV infection (A & B above) but meets the following criteria: ›	**Definitive** ■ at least two negative HIV antibody tests from separate specimens obtained at ≥ 6 months of age or ■ at least two negative HIV virologic tests (as in A above) from separate specimens, both of which were performed at ≥1 month of age and one of which was performed at ≥ 4 months of age and ■ no other laboratory or clinical evidence of HIV infection, i.e. has not had any positive virologic tests, if performed, and has not had an AIDS-defining condition **Presumptive** A child who does not meet the above criteria for definitive 'not infected' status but who has: ■ one negative EIA HIV antibody test performed at ≥6 months of age and **no** positive HIV virologic tests, if performed and ■ one negative HIV virologic test, preferably an HIV nucleic acid (DNA or RNA) detection test, performed at ≥4 months of age and **no** positive HIV virologic tests, if performed or ■ one positive HIV virologic test with at least two subsequent negative virologic tests, preferably an HIV nucleic acid (DNA or RNA) detection test, at least one of which is at ≥4 months of age; or negative HIV antibody test results, at least one of which is at ≥6 months of age and ■ no other laboratory or clinical evidence of HIV infection, i.e. has not had any positive virologic tests, if performed, and has not had an AIDS-defining condition

Immunologic status

Three immunologic categories are used to classify children by the severity of immunosuppression attributable to HIV infection as reflected by their age-specific CD4+ T-lymphocyte cell count (Table 13.3).[3] A depletion in CD4+ cells is a major consequence of

HIV infection, and the level of their progressive decline is used as a marker of immune suppression in both adult and paediatric classification systems. However, it is important to note that normal CD4$^+$ cell counts are higher in infants and young children than in adults and decline over the first few years of life.[9,10] Another important point is that children may develop opportunistic infections at higher CD4$^+$ levels than adults.[11,12]

TABLE 13.3 Immunologic categories based on age-specific CD4$^+$ T-lymphocyte counts and percentage of total lymphocytes[3]

Immunologic category	Age of child <12 months μL (%)	1–5 years μL (%)	6–12 years μL (%)
1. No evidence of suppression	≥ 1500 (≥ 25)	≥ 1000 (≥ 25)	≥ 500 (≥ 25)
2. Evidence of moderate suppression	750–1499 (15–24)	500–999 (15–24)	200–499 (15–24)
3. Severe suppression	<750 (<15)	<500 (<15)	<250 (<15)

Clinical status

HIV-infected or perinatally exposed children are classified into one of four mutually exclusive categories based on their signs, symptoms or diagnoses related to HIV infection (Table 13.4).[3]

Paediatric HIV classification

The infectious status (see Table 13.2), immunologic status (see Table 13.3) and clinical status (see Tables 13.4 and 13.5) of each HIV-infected or perinatally exposed child are cross-tabulated to determine the child's classification (Table 13.6).

MEDICAL MANAGEMENT OF CHILDREN WITH HIV DISEASE

The basic principles of treatment for HIV disease are similar for everyone and consist of using a combination of different types of antiretroviral drugs that interfere with the ability of HIV to replicate. This approach has become known as highly active antiretroviral therapy (HAART). The following brief description is intended to introduce treatment concepts and issues based upon current UK and USA guidelines. However, new drugs and approaches to treatment are continuously being developed, and it is important for nurses, midwives and other healthcare professionals to check the associated websites (see 'Internet resources' at the end of this chapter) for changes or additions to current treatment guidelines.

The medical management of HIV disease in immunologically immature infants and children and in adolescents is complex and dynamic, changing as new research evidence and treatments become available and incorporated into clinical practice guidelines.

Several factors complicate HAART in infants and children. Because of the immaturity of their organ systems, such as the kidneys, spleen and liver, they metabolize and clear antiretroviral and other drugs much less efficiently then do older adolescents and adults and may experience increased drug toxicities. Drug dosages, dosing regimens and drug formulations need to be adjusted for infants and children. Additionally, some perinatally exposed infants may also have been exposed to antiretroviral drugs before, during or after birth and this may influence specific treatment regimens. Finally, consistent adherence to

TABLE 13.4 Clinical categories for children with HIV infection[3]

Category	Examples of conditions associated with category
N Not symptomatic	Children who have no signs or symptoms considered to be the result of HIV infection or who have only one of the conditions listed in Category A
A Mildly symptomatic	Children with two or more of the conditions listed below but none of the conditions listed in Categories B and C: ■ lymphadenopathy ($\geq$ 0.5 cm at more than two sites; bilateral = one site) ■ hepatomegaly ■ splenomegaly ■ dermatitis ■ parotitis ■ recurrent or persistent upper respiratory infection, sinusitis or otitis media
B Moderately symptomatic	Children who have symptomatic conditions other than those listed for Category A or C that are attributed to HIV infection; examples of conditions in this category include but are not limited to: ■ anaemia (<8 g/dL), neutropenia (<1000 mm^3) or thrombocytopenia (<100 000 mm^3) persisting $\geq$30 days ■ bacterial meningitis, pneumonia or sepsis (single episode) ■ candidiasis, oropharyngeal (thrush), persisting (>2 months) in children > 6 months of age ■ cardiomyopathy ■ cytomegalovirus infection, with onset before 1 month of age ■ diarrhoea, recurrent or chronic ■ hepatitis ■ herpes simplex virus (HSV) stomatitis, recurrent (>2 episodes within 1 year) ■ HSV bronchitis, pneumonitis or oesophagitis with onset before 1 month of age ■ herpes zoster (shingles) involving at least two distinct episodes or more than one dermatome ■ leiomyosarcoma ■ lymphoid interstitial pneumonia (LIP) or pulmonary lymphoid hyperplasia complex ■ nephropathy ■ nocardiosis ■ persistent fever (lasting > 1 month) ■ toxoplasmosis, onset before 1 month of age ■ varicella, disseminated (complicated chickenpox)
C Severely symptomatic	Children who have any condition listed in the 1987 surveillance case definition for the acquired immunodeficiency syndrome,[8] with the exception of LIP (see Table 13.5)

therapy, necessary for treatment efficacy and for preventing the emergence of drug-resistant variants of HIV, may be extremely problematic in this age group. However, all of these issues can be factored into an effective HAART strategy that can increase the quality and duration of life for infected children.

Antiretroviral drugs

During the last several years, a variety of antiretroviral drugs have been developed and are now available to treat HIV disease. Newer drugs are in various stages of clinical trials and will probably be available within the next few years. These drugs, and their use in the treatment of adolescents and adults, are discussed in more detail in Chapter 20, and comprehensive information is given on each antiretroviral drug currently licensed for use in countries in the EU and the USA. In addition, the *British National Formulary*,[13] updated and published every 6 months and available online at www.BNF.org provides the most accurate information on all drugs licensed for use in the UK.

TABLE 13.5 AIDS-defining conditions included in Clinical Category 3 for HIV-infected children

Category C: Severely symptomatic[3,8]

■ Serious bacterial infections, multiple or recurrent (i.e. any combination of at least two culture-confirmed infections within a 2-year period), of the following types:
septicaemia
pneumonia
meningitis
bone or joint infection
abscess of an internal organ or body cavity (excluding otitis media, superficial skin or mucosal abscesses, and indwelling catheter-related infections)

■ Candidiasis, oesophageal or pulmonary (trachea, bronchi or lungs)

■ Coccidioidomycosis, disseminated (at a site other than or in addition to lungs, or cervical or hilar lymph nodes)

■ Cryptococcosis, extrapulmonary

■ Cryptosporidiosis or isosporiasis with diarrhoea persisting >1 month

■ Cytomegalovirus disease with onset of symptoms at age >1 month (at a site other than liver, spleen or lymph nodes)

■ Encephalopathy – at least one of the following progressive findings present for at least 2 months in the absence of a concurrent illness other than HIV infection that could explain the finding:
failure to attain, or loss of, developmental milestones or loss of intellectual ability, verified by standard developmental scale or neuropsychological tests
impaired brain growth or acquired microcephaly demonstrated by head circumference measurements, or brain atrophy demonstrated by computerized tomography or magnetic resonance imaging (serial imaging is required for children <2 years of age)
acquired symmetric motor deficit manifested by two or more of the following: paresis, pathologic reflexes, ataxia or gait disturbance

■ Herpes simplex virus infection causing a mucocutaneous ulcer that persists for >1 month; or bronchitis, pneumonitis or oesophagitis for any duration in a child >1 month of age

■ Histoplasmosis, disseminated (at a site other than or in addition to lungs or cervical or hilar lymph nodes)

■ Kaposi's sarcoma

■ Lymphoma of the brain (primary)

■ Lymphoma, small, non-cleaved cell (Burkitt's), or immunoblastic or large cell lymphoma of B-cell or unknown immunologic phenotype

■ *Mycobacterium tuberculosis*, disseminated or extrapulmonary

■ *Mycobacterium*, other species or unidentified species, disseminated (at a site other than or in addition to lungs, skin, or cervical or hilar lymph nodes)

■ *Mycobacterium avium* complex or *Mycobacterium kansasii* disease, disseminated (at a site other than or in addition to lungs, skin or cervical or hilar lymph nodes)

■ *Pneumocystis carinii* pneumonia

■ Progressive multifocal leucoencephalopathy (PML)

■ Toxoplasmosis of the brain with onset at >1 month of age

■ Wasting syndrome in the absence of a concurrent illness other than HIV infection that could explain the following findings:
persistent weight loss >10% of baseline *or*
downward cross of at least two of the following percentile lines on the weight-for-age chart (e.g. 95th, 75th, 50th, 25th, 5th) in a child ≥1 year of age *or*
<5th percentile on weight-for-height chart on two consecutive measurements, ≥30 days apart *plus*
chronic diarrhoea (i.e. at least two loose stools per day for ≥30 days) *or*
documented fever (for ≥30 days, intermittent or constant)

The goal of antiretroviral therapy is to maximally suppress viral replication, preferably to undetectable levels, for as long a time as possible, while preserving and/or restoring immune function. This has been shown to enhance the survival of HIV-infected children and to

TABLE 3.6 Paediatric HIV classification[3]

| | Clinical categories | | | |
	N No signs or symptoms	A Mild signs or symptoms	B Moderate signs or symptoms	C Severe signs or symptoms
Immunologic categories				
1. No evidence of suppression	N1	A1	B1	C1
2. Evidence of moderate suppression	N2	A2	B2	C2
3. Severe suppression	N3	A3	B3	C3

Children whose HIV infection status is not confirmed are classified by using the above grid with a letter 'E' (for perinatally exposed) placed before the appropriate classification code, e.g. 'EN2'.

reduce the incidence of opportunistic infections and other complications of HIV disease.[14,15] HAART regimens always consist of a combination of different types of antiretroviral drugs, and expert guidelines on the most effective combinations have been produced in the UK and USA.[16–18] These guidelines are constantly being updated and republished on the internet (see 'Internet resources' at the end of this chapter).

Currently, the most authoritative treatment guidelines for infants and children with HIV disease are developed by the USA Department of Health and Human Services (DHHS) and these are available online as a continuously updated 'Living Document'.[16] Although treatment needs to be individualized for each patient and recommendations are subject to change, Table 13.7 shows an example of a current regimen strongly recommended by the DHHS for infants and children.[16]

TABLE 13.7 Antiretroviral regimen for initial therapy in children recommended by the USA DHHS (12/2001)[16]

■ One highly active protease inhibitor (PI), such as nelfinavir or ritonavir, *plus*

■ Two nucleoside reverse transcriptase inhibitors (NRTI), such as: zidovudine (ZDV) and didanosine (ddI); *or* zidovudine (ZDV) and lamivudine (3TC); *or* stavudine (d4T) and didanosine (ddI)

Alternative regimens, recommended changes in treatment and more detailed information can be found in the DHHS online guidance at: http://www.aidsinfo.nih.gov/guidelines/ and in Chapter 20.

Starting antiretroviral treatment

Recommendations for when to initiate treatment have been made for different groups of infants and children and these are summarized in Table 13.8. Because HIV-infected infants aged less than 12 months are considered at high risk for disease progression, the DHHS recommends that antiretroviral therapy be initiated as soon as a confirmed diagnosis of HIV infection is established, regardless of the child's clinical or immunologic status or viral load. Therapy is also recommended for all HIV-infected children who have clinical symptoms or evidence of immune suppression. Recommendations for asymptomatically infected children are either to initiate treatment or to monitor closely and start treatment when certain criteria are met, as described in Table 13.8.[16]

Children and their caregivers need to be involved in every aspect of decision-making concerning when to start treatment and the selection of the most appropriate treatment regimen for each child. Antiretroviral drugs for children are generally administered orally as fruit-flavoured solutions, powders, suspensions and syrups. Zidovudine is available as an injection for dilution and use as an intravenous solution and all antiretroviral drugs are available as tablets or capsules. Additionally, medication is sometimes given via a percutaneous endoscopic gastrostomy tube (PEG tube) and these devices may be

TABLE 13.8 Indications for initiation of antiretroviral therapy in children with HIV infection[16]

- Clinical symptoms associated with HIV infection, i.e. clinical categories A, B or C (see Table 13.4)
- Evidence of immune suppression, indicated by CD4+ T-cell absolute number or percentage, i.e. immune category 2 or 3 (see Table 13.3)
- Age <12 months – regardless of clinical, immunologic or virologic status[a]
- For asymptomatic children aged ≥1 year with normal immune status, two options can be considered:
  Option 1: initiate therapy – regardless of age or symptom status
  Option 2: defer treatment in situations in which the risk for clinical disease progression is low and other factors (i.e. concern for the durability of response, safety and adherence) favour postponing treatment; in such cases, the healthcare provider should regularly monitor virologic, immunologic and clinical status; factors to be considered in deciding to initiate therapy include the following:
     high or increasing HIV RNA copy number
     rapidly declining CD4+ T-cell number or percentage to values approaching those indicative of moderate immune suppression, i.e. immune category 2 (see Table 13.3)
     development of clinical symptoms

Indications for initiation of antiretroviral therapy need to take account of issues of adherence. Post-pubertal adolescents should follow the 'Guidelines for the Use of Antiretroviral Agents in Adults and Adolescents' (http://aidsinfo.nih.gov/).[17]

[a]The Working Group recognizes that clinical trial data documenting therapeutic benefit from this approach are not currently available, and information on pharmacokinetics in infants under the age of 3–6 months is limited. This recommendation is based on expert opinion. Issues associated with adherence should be fully assessed and discussed with the HIV-infected infant's caregivers before the decision to initiate therapy is made.

particularly helpful in very young children. Caregivers and children require training and ongoing support to help ensure that medications are given correctly as prescribed. An excellent example of a training programme to support children and their parents and caregivers in teaching children to swallow pills is the protocol developed at St Mary's Hospital NHS Trust in London (Table 13.9).[19]

TABLE 13.9 Pill swallowing protocol (developed by the Family HIV Service at St Mary's Hospital National Health Service Trust London)[19]

The worker who will be carrying out the instructions with the child should be a neutral member of the team who has no prior history with the child. Ask parents not to let the child drink before coming to the clinic so that he or she is slightly thirsty, as the child will have to drink water during the session

Obtaining information

At the appointment, meet with the parents alone initially, in order to explain the procedure and gather information. The following questions are important:

- How well does your child eat?
- Does your child have a good appetite and eat a variety of foods?
- Are meal times difficult, stressful or overly long?
- Can your child swallow meat or other chewy foods?
- Has your child ever had to take pills before?
- Could s/he manage them?
- Has your child ever choked on pills or had any difficulties swallowing them?
- How does your child manage liquid medication?
- How is your child managing at school? (This may highlight difficulties following instructions or learning in general.)
- Does your child have lactose intolerance? (Placebos contain lactose.)
- What have you told your child (if anything) about taking pills?
- Is there anything else we need to know about your child?

TABLE 13.9 – continued

Setting the scene

Parents should be out of the room for the session. To avoid possible disruption later, the child should be encouraged to use the bathroom beforehand. The room used must be free from distractions such as toys or books. A sign on the clinic door will help prevent interruptions.

The worker and child should sit across from each other at a small table. Talk enthusiastically about what the child will learn during the session. This will help establish a rapport. It is important not to hold up the process by chatting about other things. Explain to the child that s/he will be learning how to swallow pills.

It is helpful to mention that the good thing about pills is that you don't taste them when you swallow them and that pill taking will be much quicker than taking liquids. It is important not to let the child know that they will soon be taking a new kind of pill as this may deter them from learning the technique.

The process

Before the first attempt, encourage the child to swallow a mouthful of water. This may help demonstrate any problems the child has with swallowing and the general level of motivation.

Demonstrate the steps to pill swallowing as follows:

- Sit or stand up straight.
- Take a deep breath.
- Breathe out with pursed lips, making an 's' sound.
- Put the pill in the middle of your tongue.
- Keep your head straight.

Keep the range of pill bottles that will be used out of the child's sight. Present the child with the first (smallest) pill, placing two pills on a piece of paper. Let the child choose which pill they want to swallow. Show the child how to swallow the pill by going through the steps as outlined above. Then encourage the child to swallow the pill themselves, reminding them of the steps. You can hold the child's chin gently in order to keep their head straight. A mirror may be useful to help show the child where to place the pill.

Maintain a neutral face and tone of voice throughout, but praise the child for his/her effort, in particular after the pill has been swallowed successfully. Social reinforcement is the primary reward for successful pill swallowing. Rewards such as sweets or toys should not be used unless absolutely necessary.

If the child has difficulties swallowing a pill, encourage the child to repeat the process with another pill of the same size before moving on to the next pill. The child can also teach the worker the correct way to take the pill. Both these moves will help increase their confidence.

If the first or second pill cannot be swallowed on the first attempt, encourage the child to say, 'It's OK, I just need to keep trying'. It is important not to mention this with later pills, as this may reinforce the child getting the pill stuck.

When moving from one pill to the next, it is important not to mention that the child is moving on to taking a bigger pill but the next pill. Any mention of size may increase a child's anxiety. Direct the child to swallow the next pill without asking them if they can do it. Repeat the process as before by using short, repetitive commands, reminding the child of the steps and maintaining a neutral expression throughout.

Repeat the process until the largest pill the child can manage has been swallowed. As the session progresses, decrease the amount of coaching and instruction but continue to praise the child when successful. The worker is more involved when the child is successful than when s/he is unable to complete the task. This will encourage the child to continue.

Limit the session to half an hour – any longer and the child will become tired and frustrated. End the session on a positive note. When the child has demonstrated the technique successfully, ignore them while they are swallowing, only paying attention and praising when they have completed the task. When the child has demonstrated that they can swallow pills successfully, it is no longer necessary to coach them.

And finally . . .

At the end of the session, bring the parents into the room so that the child can show off their new skill. Instruct the parents to sit to one side quietly, withholding comments or praise until the child swallows successfully.

If parents are supportive and keen to be involved, send them home with enough pills of the largest size the child is able to swallow so that they can practice once a day for a week (until the next appointment). Parents should be supplied with written instructions so that they can practise with the child. Parents are advised to stop practising if the child experiences any problems during the practice at home, so that negative experiences are kept to a minimum. Contact details should also be given to parents so that they can ring the clinic if they have any problems or questions.

Supporting adherence to HAART

Therapy for HIV disease is only effective if antiretroviral drugs are consistently taken each and every day exactly as prescribed. Non-adherence is associated with the emergence of drug-resistant viral variants, increase in plasma viral load and treatment failure.[20] Drug resistance is discussed further in Chapter 20 and adherence to therapy for adults is discussed in Chapter 21. There are, however, some unique considerations associated with adherence in infants, young children and adolescents.

Infants and very young children are dependent for drug administration on others who must be trained, assessed as competent and supported. Medicines often have to be mixed with food, and the palatability of drug formulations can be problematic. Many antiretroviral drugs have to be given either with or without food and this can also be difficult when administering drugs to young infants who require frequent feeding. Consistently adhering to a drug regimen can also be complicated by various developmental issues associated with adolescence, such as the need of young people to belong and not to be different from their friends and their sometimes chaotic and unstructured lifestyle.

Comprehensive nursing, social and behavioural assessments of issues that may influence the child's ability to adhere to therapy need to be undertaken before HAART is prescribed (Table 13.10). A variety of strategies have been identified[16] that can support children and their carers to develop consistently good medication adherence patterns, including:

- intensive education of infected children and/or their caregivers regarding the importance of strict adherence to prescribed treatment over several visits before starting treatment;
- using cues and reminders for drug administration;
- development of patient-focused treatment plans to accommodate specific patient needs; and
- mobilizing any available social and community support services.

TABLE 13.10 Pre-treatment assessment (highly active antiretroviral therapy, HAART)

- Ability and willingness of the child to accept and retain the medication
- Ability of the child's caregiver or the adolescent to administer complex drug regimens and availability of resources to support adherence
- Availability and palatability of paediatric formulations
- Feeding patterns and requirements of the child
- Impact of the medication schedule on quality of life, including number of medications, frequency of administration, ability to co-administer with other prescribed medications and the need to take with or without food
- The potential for drug interactions

Immunization and children infected with HIV

Children infected with HIV are at an increased risk from infectious diseases and should be fully immunized as a matter of priority. Vaccine efficacy may be reduced in children who are infected with HIV and they may additionally need passive immune protection from the use of human normal immunoglobulin (HNIG) or specific immunoglobulins, such as human varicella-zoster immunoglobulin (VZIG). If an HIV-infected child is receiving full replacement therapy with intravenous gamma-globulin (i.e. HNIG), an immune response to live virus vaccines (e.g. MMR, polio) may be reduced. Children who are infected with HIV may safely have all of the vaccines listed in Table 13.11 (as can adults), providing that there are no general contraindications to immunizations (Table 13.12).

TABLE 13.11 Immunization schedule (UK) for HIV-infected children[13,21,22]

Vaccine	Age	Notes
■ Adsorbed diphtheria, tetanus and (whole cell) pertussis (DTwP]	1st dose: 2 months 2nd dose: 3 months 3rd dose: 4 months	Primary course
■ Poliomyelitis vaccine (inactivated)		
■ *Haemophilus influenzae* type b (Hib)		
■ Pneumococcal polysaccharide conjugated vaccine (polyvalent – 7 valent)		
■ Meningococcal Group C conjugate vaccine		
■ Measles/mumps/rubella (MMR)	12–15 months	Can be given at any age over 12 months MMR should not be given to children who are severely immunosuppressed
■ *Haemophilus influenzae* type b (Hib)	13 months to 4 years but only if not previously immunized	
■ Polyvalent (23-valent) unconjugated pneumococcal polysaccharide vaccine	After second birthday	
■ Adsorbed diphtheria, tetanus and pertussis [acellular component] (DtaP)	3–5 years	Three years after completion of the primary course
■ Poliomyelitis vaccine (inactivated)		
■ MMR		MMR should not be given to children who are severely immunosuppressed.
■ Adsorbed diphtheria (low dose) and tetanus vaccine for adults and adolescents	13–18 years	
■ Poliomyelitis vaccine (inactivated)		
■ Rubella vaccine (live)	15–18 years or older	For susceptible women of childbearing age

Other vaccines

In addition to those vaccines listed in Table 13.11, HIV-infected children and adolescents can safely be immunized with the following vaccines when clinically indicated: hepatitis A vaccine, hepatitis B vaccine, influenza vaccine, rabies vaccine and capsular polysaccharide typhoid vaccine by injection.

Pneumococcal vaccine

The standard polyvalent (23-valent) unconjugated pneumococcal polysaccharide vaccine for preventing pneumonia caused by *Streptococcus pneumoniae* is not effective in children under the age of 2 years. Consequently, it is now recommended that children at high risk of pneumonia, which includes HIV-infected children, should be immunized with three doses of a conjugated pneumococcal vaccine during their first 4 months (see Table 13.11). Infants not

TABLE 13.12 General contraindications to immunization

Immunization should not proceed in children who:

- have had a severe local or general reaction to a preceding dose (all vaccines)
- are hypersensitive to eggs (influenza vaccine)
- have had previous anaphylactic reaction to eggs (MMR, influenza)
- are suffering from an acute illness and are febrile (all vaccines)
- are suffering from vomiting and diarrhoea (polio)

For further information on specific contraindications, consult the current edition of the *British National Formulary*: www.BNF.org[13]

immunized during this period should receive two doses of the conjugate vaccine at least a month apart if they are aged between 5 and 24 months. After their second birthday, all HIV-infected children should then receive a single dose of polyvalent (23-valent) unconjugated pneumococcal polysaccharide vaccine, as this will provide them with protection against the serotypes of *S. pneumoniae* not covered by the conjugate vaccine.[22]

Poliomyelitis vaccine

In the UK (and the USA), it is recommended that HIV-infected children be vaccinated with the inactivated poliomyelitis vaccine and not given oral live vaccine (OPV).[13]

In industrially developing countries where the incidence of poliomyelitis remains high, the lack of evidence of side effects to OPV supports the World Health Organization (WHO) policy for its continued administration to all children.

BCG vaccine

In the UK, the bacillus Calmette–Guérin (BCG) vaccine is usually given as part of the routine immunization schedule to all children between the ages of 10 and 14 years or during infancy to prevent tuberculosis. However, it is not given to infants or children (or adults) known to be infected with HIV, as serious vaccine dissemination has been reported. In industrially developing countries where the risk of tuberculosis is high, BCG vaccination at birth is still recommended by the WHO, principally to prevent disseminated tuberculosis and tuberculosis meningitis.

Yellow fever vaccine

Yellow fever vaccine is not given to children (or adults) known to be infected with HIV.

Typhoid vaccines

Oral typhoid vaccine is not given to HIV-infected children or adults. Instead, a capsular polysaccharide typhoid vaccine can be given by intramuscular or deep subcutaneous injection.[13]

Consent

Parents must give consent prior to their child being immunized. Mothers who know that they themselves are infected with HIV or who have children being investigated for HIV infection are extremely anxious in relation to the safety of immunizations for their children. Nurses who care for these mothers and their children should have a clear understanding of current immunization recommendations.[21,22]

Summary

In addition to their various medical conditions and treatment requirements, HIV-infected children and their families frequently suffer from being stigmatized and often experience a variety of socio-economic and psychological problems. To meet their needs, they require flexible multidisciplinary models of family-centred care involving doctors, nurses, nutritionists, pharmacists, social workers, counsellors, teachers and community support agencies.

REFERENCES

1. United Nations. *Convention on the Rights of the Child.* Adopted 20 November 1989; entry into force on 02 September 1990, in accordance with UN Article 49. Available from: http://www.unhchr.ch

2. Shearer WT, Quinn TC, LaRussa P et al. Viral load and disease progression in infants infected with human immunodeficiency virus type 1. *New England Journal of Medicine* 1997; **336**:1337–42.

3. Centers for Disease Control and Prevention. 1994 Revised classification system for human immunodeficiency virus infection in children less than 13 years of age. Official authorized addenda: human immunodeficiency virus infection codes and official guidelines for coding and reporting ICD-9-CM. *Morbidity and Mortality Weekly Report (MMWR)* 30 September 1994; **43**(RR-12):1-28. Available from: ftp://ftp.cdc.gov/pub/Publications/mmwr/rr/rr4312.pdf

4. Joint United Nations Programme on HIV/AIDS. *Paediatric HIV Infection and AIDS: UNAIDS Point of View,* September 2002. Available from: http://www.unaids.org/publications/documents/children/JC750-Paediatric-PoV_en.pdf

5. Simpson BJ, Andiman WA. Difficulties in assigning human immunodeficiency virus-1 infection and seroreversion status in a cohort of HIV-exposed children using serologic criteria established by the CDC and Prevention. *Pediatrics* 1994; **93**:840–2.

6. Centers for Disease Control and Prevention. Guidelines for national human immunodeficiency virus case surveillance, including monitoring for human immunodeficiency virus infection and acquired immunodeficiency syndrome. *Morbidity and Mortality Weekly Report (MMWR)* 10 December 1999; **48**(RR-13):29–32. Available from: http://www.cdc.gov/mmwr/PDF/rr/rr4813.pdf

7. Palumbo P, Burchett S. Diagnosis of HIV infection and markers of disease progression in infants and children. In: Pizzo PA, Wilfert CM (eds), *Pediatric AIDS: The Challenge of HIV Infection in Infants, Children, and Adolescents,* 3rd edn. Baltimore: Williams & Wilkins, 1998, 67–87.

8. Centers for Disease Control and Prevention. Current Trends Classification System for human immunodeficiency virus infection in children under 13 years of age. *Morbidity and Mortality Weekly Report (MMWR)* 24 April 1987; **36**:225–30, 235–6. Available from: http://www.cdc.gov/mmwr/preview/mmwrhtml/00033741.htm

9. The European Collaborative Study. Age-related standards for T-lymphocyte subsets based on uninfected children born to human immunodeficiency virus-1 infected women. *Pediatric Infectious Disease Journal* 1992; **11**:1018–26.

10. Denny T, Yogev R, Gelman R et al. Lymphocyte subsets in healthy children during

the first 5 years of life. *Journal of the American Medical Association* 1992; **267**:1484–8.

11. Connor E, Bagarazzi M, McSherry G et al. Clinical and laboratory correlates of *Pneumocystis carinii* pneumonia in children infected with HIV. *Journal of the American Medical Association* 1991; **265**:1693–7.

12. Kovacs A, Frederick T, Church J et al. CD4 T-lymphocyte counts and *Pneumocystis carinii* pneumonia in pediatric HIV infection. *Journal of the American Medical Association* 1991; **265**:1698–703.

13. Mehta DK (Executive Editor). *British National Formulary (BNF)*, 44th edn. London: British Medical Association and the Royal Pharmaceutical Society of Great Britain, September 2002. Available from: BMJ Books, PO Box 295, London WC1H 9TE, UK, or from their website www.bmjbookshop.com. The BNF is also available online at: www.BNF.org

14. Gortmaker S, Hughes M, Oyomopito R et al. Impact of introduction of protease inhibitor therapy on reductions in mortality among children and youth infected with HIV-1. 7th Conference on Retroviruses and Opportunistic Infections, San Francisco, CA, 2000. Abstract 691.

15. DeMartino M, Tovo P-A, Balducci M et al. Reduction in mortality with availability of antiretroviral therapy for children with perinatal HIV-1 infection. *Journal of the American Medical Association* 2000; **284**:190–7.

16. US Department of Health and Human Services. *Guidelines for the Use of Antiretroviral Agents in Pediatric HIV Infection.* Working Group on Antiretroviral Therapy and Medical Management of HIV-infected Children convened by the National Institutes of Health, National Pediatric and Family HIV Resource Center, and the Health Resources and Services Administration. Living Document available online at: http://www.aidsinfo.nih.gov/guidelines/

17. Centers for Disease Control and Prevention. Guidelines for the use of antiretroviral agents in HIV-infected adults and adolescents. *Morbidity and Mortality Weekly Report (MMWR)* 17 May 2002; **51**(RR07):11–82. Living Document available online (dated 04 February 2002) at: http://www.aidsinfo.nih.gov/guidelines/adult/html_adult_02-04-02.html

18. British HIV Association (BHIVA). *Guidelines for the Treatment of HIV-infected Adults with Antiretroviral Therapy*, 2001. Available online at: http://www.bhiva.org/guidelines.htm

19. Collins S, Clayden P. Pill swallowing protocol – Family HIV Service, St Mary's NHS Trust London. In: Paediatric HIV Care, a Report from the HIV i-Base Meeting 'Optimising Options for Paediatric HIV Treatment – a focus on issues for current clinical care', held on Friday 27 October 2000 at London House, Bloomsbury. *HIV Treatment Bulletin* 2001; **12**, Suppl. 1 (Appendix I). Available online from: http://www.i-base.org.uk/publications/paed/index.html

20. Birch C. Implications of poor compliance. *Journal of HIV Therapy* 1998; **3**:63–6.

21. Salisbury D, Begg NT (eds). *Immunisation against Infectious Disease*. London: UK Departments of Health (HMSO), 1996, 290 pp.

22. Department of Health (England). Pneumococcal vaccine for at risk under 2s. *Letter* from the Chief Medical Officer, the Chief Nursing Officer, and the Chief Pharmacist, 4 January 2002. PL/CMO/2002/1. Available from: http://www.doh.gov.uk/cmo/cmo0201.htm

FURTHER READING

Hutto C, Scott GB. Special considerations in children. In: Merigan TC, Bartlett JG, Bolognesi D (eds), *Textbook of AIDS Medicine*, 2nd edn. Baltimore: Williams & Wilkins, 1999, 163 77, ISBN 0 683 30216-7

Pavia AT, Christenson JC. Pediatric AIDS. In: Sande MA, Volberding PA (eds), *The Medical Management of AIDS*, 6th edn. Philadelphia: W.B. Saunders Company, 1999, 525–35, ISBN 0-7216-8102-6.

Pizzo PA, Wilfert CM (eds). *Pediatric AIDS: The Challenge of HIV Infection in Infants, Children, and Adolescents*, 3rd edn. Baltimore: Williams & Wilkins, 1998, 849 pp, ISBN 0-683-303399-6.

INTERNET RESOURCES

- The *British National Formulary (BNF)*, published by the British Medical Association and the Royal Pharmaceutical Society of Great Britain, provides up-to-date information in relation to the drugs used in the UK to treat HIV infection and HIV-related illnesses; the online version is updated every 6 months. Available from: BMJ Books, PO Box 295, London WC1H 9TE, UK, or from their website www.bmjbookshop.com: http://www.BNF.org/

- Continuously updated guidelines on using antiretroviral drugs in children are available online as a Living Document from the US Department of Health and Human Services. *Guidelines for the Use of Antiretroviral Agents in Pediatric HIV Infection*. Working Group on Antiretroviral Therapy and Medical Management of HIV-infected Children convened by the National Institutes of Health, National Pediatric and Family HIV Resource Center, and the Health Resources and Services Administration, December 14, 2001:
http://www.aidsinfo.nih.gov/guidelines

- Information from The National AIDS Manual (NAM), the International HIV/AIDS Alliance and the British HIV Association (BHIVA) covers the entire spectrum of the prevention, care and treatment of adults and children and is available on the premiere UK HIV website:
http://www.aidsmap.com

A strategy for infection control in nursing practice

Introduction

An important component of clinical nursing practice is to protect patients from new infections during periods when they are receiving nursing care in hospitals, clinics or in their homes. It is equally important to ensure that nurses and other healthcare practitioners do not acquire infections from patients as a result of caring for them.

Immunocompromised patients with HIV are at an increased risk of developing a variety of opportunistic infections (see Chapter 7) that could be transmitted to carers or other patients. Additionally, all patients are at an increased risk of acquiring a healthcare-associated infection (HAI) when various medical devices are used in their treatment, such as urinary and central venous catheters. In this and in the following chapter, we explore the infection prevention and control precautions that are used during clinical practice to protect patients and their carers from HAIs and to maintain a safe environment for treatment and care.

Learning outcomes

After studying and reflecting on the material in this chapter, you will be able to:

- discuss the rationale underpinning current recommendations for preventing healthcare-associated infections;
- describe *standard* and *transmission-based* infection prevention and control precautions, and relate these to your own experience of clinical care.

BACKGROUND

Healthcare strategies designed to protect patients and their carers from becoming infected during periods of hospitalization and community and home care have continued to evolve over many decades. Earlier models for preventing infections in hospitals and in the community consisted of either isolating infectious patients in special infectious disease hospitals or using a cubicle system of isolation (individual rooms or cubicles) with barrier nursing in general hospitals.[1] These models evolved into more sophisticated and detailed category-specific and disease-specific isolation precautions.[2]

NEW CONCEPTS IN ISOLATION PRACTICES

In the early 1980s, a profound change in approaches to infection prevention and control practice occurred with the need to care safely for increasing numbers of patients with AIDS. **Blood and Body Fluid Precautions** were developed principally to protect healthcare practitioners from becoming infected with HIV and other blood-borne pathogens, such as hepatitis B virus (HBV). These precautions were used in caring for patients who were known to be or suspected of being infected with HIV. They focused on preventing injuries from needle-sticks and other sharp instruments and on the use of gloves, gowns, masks and eye protection devices to prevent exposure to blood and other body fluids. As national epidemics escalated and the number of patients with AIDS increased, and as the long asymptomatic incubation period of HIV infection and disease became understood, it was apparent by 1985 that an expanded set of Blood and Body Fluid Precautions would need to be 'universally' applied to all patients, regardless of their presumed infection status. This approach became known as **Universal Precautions (UP).**[3]

A few years later, a new system of infection prevention was described and rapidly incorporated into clinical nursing practice.[3] This system was known as **Body Substance Isolation (BSI)** and was an elaboration of UP. BSI focused on the isolation of all moist and potentially infectious body substances (blood, faeces, urine, sputum, saliva, wound drainage, and other body fluids) from all patients, regardless of their presumed infection status, primarily through the use of gloves. Nurses and other healthcare practitioners wore gloves prior to any contact with any mucous membranes and non-intact skin from any patient, and prior to any anticipated contact with moist body substances.[4]

CURRENT ISOLATION PRECAUTIONS

Although there was some evidence to indicate that BSI was effective in reducing the risk of HAIs,[5,6] infection prevention and control strategies continued to evolve and, in 1996, a new isolation guideline was developed by the Centers for Disease Control and Prevention (CDC) in the USA.[7] This synthesized the major features of UP and BSI into a single set of **Standard Precautions** to be used in caring for all patients all the time, regardless of their diagnosis or presumed infection status. It also combined and condensed previous category-specific and disease-specific isolation precautions into three sets of precautions based on routes of transmission. These **transmission-based precautions** were designed to reduce the risk of **airborne**, **droplet** and **contact** transmission and are intended to be used in addition to Standard Precautions.

STANDARD PRINCIPLES FOR PREVENTING HEALTHCARE-ASSOCIATED INFECTIONS

Evidence-based infection prevention and control guidelines for preventing HAIs in England further elaborate current concepts of standard isolation precautions.[8–10] These **Standard Principles** provide guidance that should be applied by all healthcare practitioners to the care of all patients all the time, regardless of their diagnosis or presumed infection status. They include recommendations for hospital hygiene, hand hygiene, the use of personal protective equipment and the use and disposal of needles and other sharp instruments (Table 14.1). They are not detailed procedural protocols, but are designed to be incorporated into local practice guidelines.

TABLE 14.1 Standard Principles for preventing healthcare-associated infections[8,9]

Hand hygiene

- Hands must be decontaminated immediately before each and every episode of direct patient contact
- Hands must be washed if they are visibly or potentially contaminated with dirt or organic material
- Alcohol-based hand rubs may be used to decontaminate hands between caring for different patients and different caring activities for the same patient
- Effective hand hygiene technique ensures thorough hand decontamination and protects skin integrity

Gloves

- Gloves must be worn for invasive procedures, contact with sterile sites and non-intact skin, mucous membranes, and all activities that have been assessed as carrying a risk of exposure to blood, body fluids, secretions and excretions, sharp or contaminated instruments
- Gloves must only be worn once, for one aspect of care and one patient
- Gloves should be disposed of as clinical waste and hands decontaminated following their removal

Aprons and gowns

- Disposable plastic aprons should be worn when there is a risk that clothing or uniform may become exposed to blood, body fluids, secretions and excretions, with the exception of sweat
- Full-body fluid-repellent gowns should be worn where there is a risk of extensive splashing of blood, body fluids, secretions and excretions, with the exception of sweat, onto the skin of healthcare providers

Face mask and eye protection

- Face masks and eye protection should be worn where there is a risk of blood, body fluids, secretions and excretions splashing into the face and eyes

Sharps and needles

- Sharps must not be passed from hand to hand and handling must be kept to a minimum
- Needles must not be bent or broken; needles and syringes must be re-capped/re-sheathed or disassembled by hand prior to disposal
- Used sharps must be discarded at the point of use into a sharps' container (conforming to UN3291 and BS7320 Standards)

Complete guidelines are available on: http://www.doh.gov.uk/hai/epic.htm

Standard infection prevention and control principles are the first tier of isolation precautions designed to reduce the risk of transmission of infectious microorganisms from both recognized and unrecognized sources of infection in healthcare settings. Their correct and consistent use protects patients and healthcare practitioners from exposure to **blood-borne pathogens (BBPs)**, such as HIV and blood-borne hepatitis viruses (discussed in more detail in the following chapter). Standard infection prevention and control principles apply to:

- blood
- *all* body fluids, secretions and excretions (except sweat)
- non-intact skin, and
- mucous membranes

in all healthcare environments, for all patients, all of the time without exception.

TRANSMISSION-BASED PRECAUTIONS

In addition to standard infection prevention precautions, **transmission-based precautions** are used for patients who are suspected or known to be infected with highly transmissible or epidemiologically important pathogenic microorganisms (Tables 14.2 and 14.3). Three types of transmission-based precautions are used: **contact, droplet** and **airborne precautions**.[7] These precautions can be combined for diseases that have multiple routes of transmission or for patients who are suffering from multiple infections.

Contact Precautions

Contact Precautions are used to prevent the transmission of infectious microorganisms by direct or indirect contact. Direct contact refers to skin-to-skin transmission. An example of this might be the hands of a nurse becoming contaminated during caring for a patient who is infected or colonized with an infectious microorganism such as *Clostridium difficile* or *Staphylococcus aureus*. Indirect contact involves contact with a contaminated intermediate object, such as contaminated medical or surgical instruments or dressings.

Contact Precautions include the use of Standard Precautions plus the following.[7]

- **Patient Placement.** Patients are cared for in a single room or in a room or bay with a patient(s) who has active infection with the same microorganism (cohorting). If either facility is unavailable, it is important to seek placement advice from the Infection Control Nurse so that the infected patient is cared for in an area where there is the least likelihood of accidental transmission of the infectious microorganism.
- **Gloves and Hand Decontamination.** In addition to observing the hand decontamination and the glove use advice as described in Standard Principles (see Table 14.1), clean, non-sterile gloves are worn when entering the patient's room and for all aspects of care. Any objects (fomites) in the room are considered potentially contaminated and are only touched when wearing gloves. Gloves are removed prior to leaving the patient's room and the hands are immediately decontaminated by either washing with an appropriate hand-wash preparation or by using an alcoholic hand gel.
- **Gowns.** In addition to the advice for wearing gowns as described in Standard Principles (see Table 14.1), a clean, non-sterile gown is worn when entering the patient's room if the nurse anticipates that his or her clothing will have substantial contact with the patient, environmental surfaces or items in the patient's room or, if the patient is incontinent or has diarrhoea, an ileostomy, colostomy or wound drainage not contained by a dressing.

TABLE 14.2 Clinical syndrome or conditions warranting additional transmission-based infection prevention precautions pending confirmation of diagnosis

Clinical syndrome or condition[a]	Potential pathogens[b]	Empiric precautions
Diarrhoea		
Acute diarrhoea with a likely infectious cause in an incontinent or diapered patient	Enteric pathogens[c]	Contact
Diarrhoea in an adult with history of recent antibiotic use	*Clostridium difficile*	Contact
Meningitis	*Neisseria meningitides*	Droplet
Rash or exanthem, generalized, aetiology unknown		
Petechial/ecchymotic with fever	*N. meningitides*	Droplet
Vesicular	Varicella	Airborne and contact
Maculopapular with coryza and fever	Rubeola (measles)	Airborne
Respiratory infections		
Cough/fever/upper lobe pulmonary infiltrate in an HIV-negative patient or a patient at low risk for HIV infection	*Mycobacterium tuberculosis*	Airborne
Cough/fever/pulmonary infiltrate in any lung location in an HIV-infected patient or a patient at high risk for HIV infection	*Mycobacterium tuberculosis*	Airborne
Paroxysmal or severe persistent cough during periods of pertussis activity	*Bordetella pertussis*	Droplet
Respiratory infections, particularly bronchiolitis and croup, in infants and young children	Respiratory syncytial or parainfluenza virus	Contact
Risk of multi-drug-resistant microorganisms		
History of infection or colonization with multi-drug-resistant organisms	Resistant bacteria	Contact
Skin, wound or urinary tract infection in a patient with a recent hospital or nursing home stay in a facility where multi-drug-resistant organisms are prevalent	Resistant bacteria	Contact
Skin or wound infection		
Abscess or draining wound that cannot be covered	*Staphylococcus aureus* Group A *Streptococcus*	Contact

[a]Patients with the syndromes or conditions listed may present with atypical signs or symptoms (e.g. pertussis in neonates and adults may not have paroxysmal or severe cough). The clinician's index of suspicion should be guided by the prevalence of specific conditions in the community, as well as by clinical judgement.
[b]The organisms listed under the column 'Potential pathogens' are not intended to represent the complete, or even most likely, diagnoses, but rather possible aetiologic agents that require additional precautions beyond Standard Precautions until they can be ruled out.
[c]These pathogens include entero-haemorrhagic *Escherichia coli* 0157:H7, *Shigella*, hepatitis A virus and rotavirus.
Reprinted from Hospital Infection Control Practices Advisory Committee. *Guideline for Isolation Precautions in Hospitals 1996.*[7]

- **Patient Transport.** The patient is transported out of his or her room only if absolutely essential, and Contact Precautions are maintained.
- **Equipment.** Any equipment that cannot be used exclusively for patients requiring Contact Precautions needs to cleaned and disinfected before use by other patients.

No special precautions are needed for dishes, cutlery and other eating utensils that are easily decontaminated by hot water and the detergents used in dishwashers.[7]

TABLE 14.3 Synopsis of types of precautions and patients requiring the precautions

Standard Precautions
Use Standard Precautions for the care of all patients

Airborne Precautions
In addition to Standard Precautions, use Airborne Precautions for patients known or suspected to have serious illnesses transmitted by airborne droplet nuclei. Examples of such illnesses include:
  measles,
  varicella (including disseminated zoster),
  tuberculosis

Droplet Precautions
In addition to Standard Precautions, use Droplet Precautions for patients known or suspected to have serious illnesses transmitted by large-particle droplets. Examples of such illnesses include:
- Invasive *Haemophilus influenzae* type b disease, including meningitis, pneumonia, epiglottitis and sepsis
- Invasive *Neisseria meningitides* disease, including meningitis, pneumonia and sepsis
- Other serious bacterial respiratory infections spread by droplet transmission, including: diphtheria (pharyngeal), Mycoplasma pneumonia, pertussis, pneumonic plague, streptococcal (group A) pharyngitis, pneumonia or scarlet fever in infants and young children
- Serious viral infections spread by droplet transmission, including: adenovirus, influenza, mumps, parvovirus B19, rubella

Contact Precautions
In addition to Standard Precautions, use Contact Precautions for patients known or suspected to have serious illnesses easily tansmitted by direct patient contact or by contact with items in the patient's environment. Examples of such illnesses include:
- Gastrointestinal, respiratory, skin, or wound infections or colonization with multidrug-resistant bacteria judged by the infection control program, based on current state, regional, or national recommendations, to be of special clinical and epidemiologic significance
- Enteric infections with a low infectious dose or prolonged environmental survival, including: *Clostridium difficile*
- For diapered or incontinent patients: enterohemorrhagic *Escherichia coli* 0157:H7, *Shigella*, hepatitis A or, rotavirus; respiratory syncytial virus, parainfluenza virus or enteroviral infections in infants and young children
- Skin infections that are highly contagious or that may occur on dry skin, including: diphtheria (cutaneous), herpes simplex virus (neonatal or mucocutaneous), impetigo, major (non-contained) abscesses, cellulitis or decubiti, pediculosis, scabies, staphylococcal furunculosis in infants and young children, zoster (disseminated or in the immunocompromised host)
- Viral/hemorrhagic conjunctivitis
- Viral hemorrhagic infections (Ebola, Lassa, or Marburg)

Reprinted from Hospital Infection Control Practices Advisory Committee. *Guideline for Isolation Precautions in Hospitals 1996.*[7]

Droplet Precautions

In addition to the use of Standard Principles for preventing infections, Droplet Precautions are used for patients known to be or suspected of being infected with microorganisms that are transmitted by large-particle respiratory droplets (larger than 5 micrometres (μm) in size) that are expelled during coughing, sneezing, talking or the performance of certain investigations and treatment, such as suctioning and bronchoscopy. These large droplets do not remain suspended in air and can only travel short distances, perhaps 1 metre or less.[7] Consequently, droplet transmission requires close contact.

Droplet Precautions include the use of Standard Precautions plus the following.[7]

- **Patient Placement**. Patients are cared for in a single room or in a room or bay with a patient(s) who has active infection with the same microorganism (cohorting). If either facility is unavailable, it is important to seek placement advice from the Infection Control Nurse so that the infected patient is cared for in an area where there is the least likelihood of accidental transmission of the infectious microorganism. In general, a spatial separation of at least 1 metre between infected patients and other patients or visitors needs to be maintained.
- **Face Mask**. A face mask is worn when entering the patient's room, or at least when working within 1 metre of an infected patient.
- **Patient Transport**. The patient is only transported out of his or her room if absolutely essential, and Droplet Precautions are maintained. This is usually best achieved by the patient wearing a mask.

Airborne Precautions

In addition to Standard Principles for preventing infections, Airborne Precautions are used for patients known or suspected to be infected with microorganisms transmitted through the air by **airborne droplet nuclei**, such as *Mycobacteria tuberculosis*. These are small particle residues (5 μm or smaller in size) of evaporated respiratory droplets containing micro-organisms that are suspended in the air and scattered widely by normal air currents within a room or corridor or over long distances.

- **Patient Placement**. Patients with active HIV-related tuberculosis, multi-drug-resistant tuberculosis, measles or varicella are cared for in a respiratory isolation room that has: (a) monitored negative atmospheric pressure in relation to the surrounding areas, (b) 6–12 air changes per hour, and (c) appropriate discharge of air outdoors or via monitored high-efficiency filtration (HEPA) of room air before it is circulated to other areas.[7,11] The door to this room is kept closed and the patient is kept in the room. Cohorting of patients with the same infection is sometimes possible, but expert advice from the Infection Control Nurse is needed before a patient is admitted to a room or bay where other patients are being cared for.
- **Respiratory Protection**. Particulate filter respirators capable of filtering out particles of 5 μm or smaller in size and conforming to European Union Standards (FFP1, 2 or 3 series) are worn when entering the room and during caring for patients in respiratory isolation. Nurses and other healthcare practitioners (and visitors) who are immunosuppressed should not care for patients with active respiratory tuberculosis, measles or varicella, nor should any other person who is susceptible to these infections.

- **Patient Transport.** The patient is only transported out of his or her room if absolutely essential, and Airborne Precautions are maintained. This is usually best achieved by the patient wearing a mask. Patients do not need to wear a particulate filter respirator, as the purpose of the mask is to prevent exhalation of respiratory droplets (not inhalation of droplet nuclei) and an ordinary surgical mask is capable of doing this.

Additional guidance for preventing the transmission of *M. tuberculosis* in healthcare settings is available from the UK Departments of Health[11] and from the CDC.[12]

Summary

Universal Infection Prevention Precautions and Body Substance Isolation have matured into a simpler strategy that uses Standard Precautions for all patients in all settings all the time. In addition, some patients require further transmission-based isolation precautions because of the types of infections they have.

Prologue to Chapter 15

In the next chapter, we are going to explore further how the isolation precautions discussed in this chapter help prevent exposure to and infection with blood-borne pathogens and outline a strategy for managing an exposure incident.

REFERENCES

1. Gage ND, Landon JF, Sider MT. *Communicable Disease*. Philadelphia, PA: FA Davis, 1959.
2. Garner JS, Simmons BP. CDC *Guideline for Isolation Precautions in Hospitals*. Atlanta, GA: US Department of Health and Human Services, Public Health Service, Centers for Disease Control, 1983. HHS publication no. (CDC) 83-8314; *Infection Control* 1983; **4**:245–325, and *American Journal of Infection Control* 1984; **12**:103–63.
3. Centers for Disease Control. Recommendations for preventing transmission of infection with human T-lymphotropic virus type III/lymphadenopathy-associated virus in the workplace. *Morbidity and Mortality Weekly Report (MMWR)* 15 November 1985; **34**(45):681–6, 691–5.
4. Lynch P, Jackson MM, Cummings J, Stamm WE. Rethinking the role of isolation practices in the prevention of nosocomial infections. *Annals of Internal Medicine* 1987; **107**:243–6.
5. Klein BS, Perloff WH, Maki DG. Reduction of nosocomial infection during pediatric intensive care by protective isolation. *New England Journal of Medicine* 1989; **320**:1714–21.
6. Leclair JM, Freeman J, Sullivan BF, Crowley CM, Goldmann DA. Prevention of nosocomial respiratory syncytial virus infections through compliance with gown and glove isolation precautions. *New England Journal of Medicine* 1987; **317**:329–34.
7. Garner JS, Hospital Infection Control Practices Advisory Committee. Guideline for isolation precautions in hospitals. *Infection Control and Hospital Epidemiology* 1996; **17**:53–80. Available on: http://www.cdc.gov/ncidod/hip/isolat/isolat.htm

8. Pratt RJ, Pellowe C, Loveday HP, Robinson N, Smith GW, and the epic Guideline Development Team; Barrett S, Davey P, Harper P, Loveday C, McDougall C, Mulhall A, Privett S, Smales C, Taylor L, Weller B, and Wilcox M. The epic Project: Developing National Evidence-based Guidelines for Preventing Healthcare-associated Infections. Phase 1: Guidelines for Preventing Hospital-acquired Infections. *Journal of Hospital Infection* 2001; **47**(Suppl.):S1–82. Available from: http://www.doh.gov.uk/hai/epic.htm

9. Loveday HP, Pellowe C, Harper P, Robinson N, Pratt R. The **epic** Project: Developing National Evidence-based Guidelines for Preventing Healthcare-associated Infections. Standard Principles for preventing HAIs. *Nursing Times* 2001; **97**:36–7.

10. Pellowe CM, MacRae ED, Loveday HP et al. The scope of guidelines to prevent healthcare-associated infection in primary and community care. *British Journal of Community Nursing* 2002; **7**:374–8. Guidelines available from the National Institute for Clinical Excellence website at: http://www.nice.org.uk/

11. Interdepartmental Working Group on Tuberculosis. *The Prevention and Control of Tuberculosis in the United Kingdom: UK Guidance on the Prevention and Control of Transmission of HIV-related Tuberculosis and Drug-resistant, including Multiple Drug-resistant Tuberculosis*. London: UK Departments of Health, September 1998. Available online at: http://www.doh.gov.uk/tbguide.htm

12. Centers for Disease Control and Prevention. Guidelines for preventing the transmission of tuberculosis in health-care facilities, 1994. *Morbidity and Mortality Weekly Report (MMWR)* 28 October 1994; **43**(RR-13):1–132. Available online at: http://cisat.isciii.es/mmwr/preview/mmwrhtml/00035909.htm

FURTHER READING

Centers for Disease Control and Prevention. Guidelines for preventing the transmission of tuberculosis in health-care facilities, 1994. *Morbidity and Mortality Weekly Report (MMWR)* 28 October 1994; **43**(RR-13):1–132. Available online at: http://cisat.isciii.es/mmwr/preview/mmwrhtml/00035909.htm

Centers for Disease Control and Prevention. Guideline for hand hygiene in health-care settings. *Morbidity and Mortality Weekly Report (MMWR)* 25 October 2002; **51**(RR-16):1–51. Available online at: http://www.cdc.gov/mmwr/preview/mmwrhtml/rr5116a1.htm

Garner JS, Hospital Infection Control Practices Advisory Committee. Guideline for isolation precautions in hospitals. *Infection Control and Hospital Epidemiology* 1996; **17**:53–80. Available online at: http://www.cdc.gov/ncidod/hip/isolat/isolat.htm

Interdepartmental Working Group on Tuberculosis. *The Prevention and Control of Tuberculosis in the United Kingdom: UK Guidance on the Prevention and Control of Transmission of HIV-related Tuberculosis and Drug-resistant, including Multiple Drug-resistant Tuberculosis*. London: UK Departments of Health, September 1998. Available online at: http://www.doh.gov.uk/tbguide.htm

Pratt RJ, Pellowe C, Loveday HP, Robinson N, Smith GW, and the **epic** Guideline Development Team; Barrett S, Davey P, Harper P, Loveday C, McDougall C, Mulhall A, Privett S, Smales C, Taylor L, Weller B, and Wilcox M. The **epic** Project: Developing National Evidence-based Guidelines for Preventing Healthcare-associated Infections.

Phase 1: Guidelines for Preventing Hospital-acquired Infections. *Journal of Hospital Infection* 2001; **47**(Suppl.):S1–82. Available from: http://www.doh.gov.uk/hai/epic.htm

Wilson J. *Infection Control in Clinical Practice*, 2nd edn. London: Baillière Tindall, 2001, ISBN 0-7020-2554-2.

Preventing and managing occupational exposure to blood-borne pathogens

Introduction

There is always a potential risk of serious infection with HIV and other blood-borne pathogens (BBPs) during healthcare activities. Patients are also at risk of healthcare-associated infection if they are exposed to blood from another patient or from infected healthcare providers. The consequences of infection with BBPs can be dire and in many cases lead to chronic infection and illness.

This chapter briefly describes the range and prevalence of BBPs that may be encountered in clinical nursing practice, identifies factors that increase the probability of occupational exposure and defines the risk of transmission and infection following an exposure. It then discusses how exposures and infections may be prevented and identifies a range of current resources that nurses can easily access to keep informed of the latest research and recommendations in this field. Next, using a step-by-step procedure, the management of an exposure is described, including immediate first aid and any available post-exposure prophylaxis (PEP). Finally, there is a brief outline of the issues surrounding nurses and midwives who are chronically infected with a BBP and of how this may affect their own clinical practice.

Learning outcomes

After studying and reflecting on the material in this chapter, you will be able to:

- identify risk factors for occupational exposure to BBPs in healthcare settings;
- describe the exposure characteristics that predispose to infection;
- outline basic principles for preventing occupational exposure and infection;

- adapt a suggested HIV PEP risk assessment protocol to your own clinical practice environment; and
- discuss professional and clinical practice issues that need to be considered by healthcare providers infected with a BBP.

BLOOD-BORNE PATHOGENS

Various BBPs may be encountered during clinical practice, but in general the three most common are **HIV** and two distinct hepatitis viruses – hepatitis B virus (**HBV**) and hepatitis C virus (**HCV**). HIV infection ultimately leads to progressive chronic illness, as described in Chapter 7, and both HBV and HCV acquisition may lead to persistent infection, chronic liver disease, cirrhosis and liver cancer, as discussed in Chapter 10.

This chapter focuses on the risk to nurses, midwives and other healthcare providers of occupational exposure and infection from these three blood-borne viruses. However, other infectious microorganisms (Table 15.1) may be found in blood and other body fluids during both acute and chronic illness and in people with asymptomatic or subclinical infections.

TABLE 15.1 Blood-borne pathogens (BBPs)

Pathogen	Potential clinical outcomes of infection
Hepatitis B virus (HBV)	Acute and chronic hepatitis, primary liver cancer
Hepatitis C virus (HCV)	Acute (rarely) but mainly chronic hepatitis, cirrhosis, primary liver cancer
Human immunodeficiency virus (HIV)	Acquired immunodeficiency syndrome (AIDS)
Human T-cell leukaemia/lymphoma virus type I (HTLV-I)	HTLV-I-associated myelopathy (tropical spastic paraparesis) (HAM/TSP)
Human T-cell leukaemia/lymphoma virus type II (HTLV-II)	Hairy cell leukaemia
Treponema pallidum	Syphilis

PREVALENCE OF BLOOD-BORNE PATHOGENS IN CLINICAL PRACTICE

During the last 25 years, the global pandemic of HIV infection and AIDS has continued to accelerate, with more then 40 million people worldwide now living with HIV disease and at least 15 000 people becoming newly infected each day.[1]

Hepatitis viruses are the cause of some of the most common viral infections throughout the world. HBV has infected a third of the world's population (2 billion people) and an estimated 350 million people have chronic, life-long infections.[2] In addition to the continuing high prevalence of global HBV infection, an estimated 170 million people are chronically infected with HCV, and 3–4 million are becoming newly infected with HCV every year.[3]

The prevalence of infections with these BBPs varies from region to region, country to country and within countries. By comparison with many other European Union (EU) member states, the prevalence of these infections is low in the general population in the UK, but is often higher in patient populations in large metropolitan areas, such as London, Brighton, Manchester and Edinburgh, and in some sub-populations, for example injecting drug users, commercial sex workers and men who have sex with other men. In summary, millions of people throughout the world are infected with HIV, HBV or HCV (and sometimes co-infected with one or more viruses in this dangerous trio).

The first important point to make is that it is never possible to identify reliably all those who are infected with BBPs from their history or from clinical and serological examination. This is because these chronic infections are frequently asymptomatic or subclinical and, even if serologically tested, they may not have yet seroconverted. Consequently, all healthcare providers need to assume that the **blood and body fluids from all patients are potentially infectious and take appropriate precautions at all times with all patients to avoid exposure.**

RISK FACTORS FOR EXPOSURE

Several factors can increase the likelihood that nurses, midwives and other healthcare providers may become exposed to BBPs during clinical practice (Table 15.2). However, the most important risks are the frequency of contact with blood and body fluids in the workplace and the degree to which individuals consistently adhere to infection prevention precautions designed to minimize the risk of exposure to these substances.[4–8]

TABLE 15.2 Factors increasing the risk for blood-borne pathogen (BBP) exposure in nursing practice

- Frequency of contact with blood and body fluids in the workplace
- Extent to which nurses adhere to infection prevention precautions
- Prevalence of BBPs in the general population and population subgroups who access care
- Type of medical or surgical procedures performed
- Circumstances under which these procedures are performed, e.g. emergency or elective
- Type of medical or surgical devices used and the likelihood that these devices could produce parenteral or mucous membrane exposure
- Technical expertise of the nurse
- Length of time a nurse has practised
- Available resources to protect against exposure, e.g. gloves, eye protection

Midwives and nurses working in certain specialist services, for example renal haemodialysis units, accident and emergency (A & E) departments, intensive care units (ICUs), operating theatres, are potentially more likely to come into contact with blood and body fluids than those in general wards or in community and primary care. Emergency procedures are more frequently associated with exposures than are carefully planned elective procedures carried out in a controlled environment. The longer a nurse or midwife has been in practice, the more time they have had to become exposed. Using invasive medical devices, such as vascular access devices, increases the potential for exposure. Finally, the technical expertise of the practitioner is important in avoiding exposure, the inexperienced being the most vulnerable (and requiring the most supervision).

Likelihood of transmission and infection following exposure

There are a variety of exposure-specific and biological factors that influence the likelihood of transmission following exposure (Table 15.3).

TABLE 15.3 Factors increasing the risk for blood-borne pathogen transmission following exposure

■ Type of exposure: percutaneous or mucocutaneous

■ Characteristics of the exposure

■ Type of body fluid exposed to

■ Volume of the inoculum

■ Concentration of virus in inoculum

■ Virus-specific factors

Type and characteristics of exposure

Two general types of exposure occur. **Percutaneous exposure** occurs when the skin is cut or penetrated by a needle or other sharp object, e.g. scalpel blade, trochar, bone spicule. **Mucocutaneous exposure** occurs when the eye(s), inside of the nose or mouth, or an area of non-intact skin is exposed, usually by splashing or spilling incidents. **Percutaneous exposures carry the greatest risk.** In addition, percutaneous exposures that involve **fresh blood and hollow needles** are significantly associated with the greatest risk of viral transmission.

The characteristics of the exposure (e.g. type of wound, depth of injury, type of instrument, amount of blood contamination) may also be associated with the likelihood of infection. Deep injuries, visible blood on sharp devices, and injury from vascular access devices are all associated with a higher risk of viral transmission following percutaneous injury.[9] The type of body fluid is also important, **fresh blood being the single most important risk.**

Biological factors

Various biological factors are important and, in general, the greater the volume of the inoculum, the greater the risk of viral transmission. The concentration of virus (viral load) in the inoculum is also important, and the highest concentration is usually found in blood and bloody body fluids. Different patients have different and variable plasma viral loads at any moment in time, and the higher the viral load in the source patient, the higher the risk of transmission.

Different strains of a particular virus may be more virulent and infectious, for example HBV associated with 'e' antigen. Some strains of HIV may also be drug resistant, limiting the effectiveness of some antiretroviral drugs commonly used for PEP.

Probability of infection following exposure

The estimated likelihood of becoming infected with a BBP following a single percutaneous exposure to blood or bloody body fluids from a patient known to be infected has been calculated (Table 15.4). Although the focus of this chapter is to alert practitioners to identify the potential for occupational transmission of BBPs and develop effective strategies to reduce these events, the reality of the risk needs to be kept in perspective. For example, **most percutaneous exposures to HIV (99.7 per cent) do not result in viral transmission.**[10] Epidemiological studies have indicated that the average risk for HIV transmission after percutaneous exposure to HIV-infected blood in healthcare settings is about 1 per 319 exposures.[9,11,12] However, the risk is likely to be greater if nurses and other healthcare providers are exposed to large volumes of blood from a source patient who has a high HIV RNA viral load.

TABLE 15.4 Probability of infection following percutaneous exposure to blood-borne pathogens[11–15]

Virus	Risk of infection
Hepatitis B virus	HBsAg-positive and HBeAg-negative: 5%
	HBsAg-positive and HBeAg-positive: 19–30%
Hepatitis C virus	1.8–3.3%
Human immunodeficiency virus	0.31%

Percutaneous exposure to blood from a patient with active HBV disease and who is surface antigen (HBsAg) positive and also 'e' antigen positive and who has a high HBV DNA viral load is associated with a high risk of transmission and subsequent infection in susceptible people. At the upper extreme of probability, 1 out of every 3 exposures may result in transmission.[11,13,14] Percutaneous exposure to HCV is associated with a higher risk of infection than HIV exposure, but significantly less than HBV exposure, with approximately 1 out of every 30 HCV exposures resulting in infection.[11,14,15]

Although **mucocutaneous exposures** have been implicated in viral transmission in healthcare settings, the risk of this happening is less well defined, but it is certainly less than the risk following percutaneous exposure. There is no evidence to indicate that contact of intact skin with blood or body fluids presents a risk of BBP transmission. However most nurses, midwives and other healthcare providers do not have intact skin on their hands, especially in the area of their fingernail beds.

Standard Principles for preventing exposure and infection

Accepting that **all blood and body fluids from all individuals are always potentially infectious** and then consistently adhering to current evidence-based guidelines for preventing healthcare-associated infections (HAIs) offers the best protection against exposure and subsequent infection.[4,5] Preventing needle-stick and sharp injuries and other parenteral exposures, along with the judicious use of gloves for procedures in which contact with blood, body fluids or mucous membranes is anticipated, are at the very core of universal infection prevention precautions. As these recommendations have evolved in the UK, they are now referred to as *Standard Principles for Preventing HAI*.[4,5] Standard Principles for preventing exposure and infection, including recommendations from the Health and Safety Commission,[16] are fully described (see Table 14.1) and further elaborated in Chapter 14. Additional guidance on Standard Principles for infection prevention and control is given in the websites for specific references.[5,6]

Specific precautions to reduce the risk of exposure to blood-borne pathogens

Additional, more specific, recommendations pertaining to protection against BBPs in a variety of clinical practice areas, for example in operating theatres, haemodialysis units and ICUs, have been published by the UK Departments of Health and are downloadable from the website.[7,8,17,18]

RISK MANAGEMENT

Healthcare providers carrying out clinical procedures should at all times precisely follow the written infection prevention and control guidelines and policies issued by their employing authority. These policies need to be based on a comprehensive and ongoing assessment of the risk of exposure to BBPs to patients, healthcare providers, other healthcare employees, and visitors.

Before any clinical procedure, the potential risk of exposure to BBPs must be assessed and appropriate precautions then taken to avoid any possibility of exposure. In addition, a periodic risk assessment needs to be conducted in each ward, department and healthcare facility. This assessment is essential for developing a proper **risk management** strategy.

The concept of risk management has always been a key feature of proactive infection prevention and control strategies, as failing to control such risks can have disastrous consequences for healthcare organizations, practitioners and patients. The ongoing cycle of risk management (Figure 15.1) involves a continual evaluation to identify potential risks and assess the methods that are in place to control these. Effective reporting of adverse events, error and 'near misses' is essential to the ongoing identification of risk and developing risk management responses.

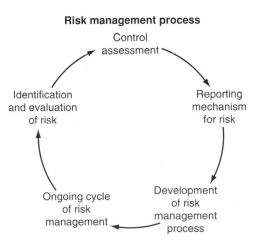

Risk management process

FIGURE 15.1 *Best practice for risk management.*[19] *Risk management is the identification, evaluation and control of potential adverse outcomes that threaten the delivery of appropriate care to patients.*

Management of occupational exposures to blood-borne pathogens

Immediate first aid

Immediately following any exposure incident, the site of the exposure should be washed liberally with soap and water but without scrubbing. There is no evidence that antiseptic/disinfectant skin preparations are more effective than soap and water in this situation and they are probably best avoided, as their effect on local defences is unknown. Free bleeding of the puncture wounds is gently encouraged. Exposed mucous membranes, including conjunctivae, should be irrigated copiously with water before and after removing any contact lenses.[8]

In addition to immediate first aid, medical advice should be sought urgently so that the need for any additional preventative measures can be assessed and serological testing of the source patient and baseline serology of the nurse can be considered. In general, source patients can only be tested with their informed consent. This **consent must not be sought by the exposed healthcare provider**, as this would emotionally charge the interaction. Medical advice is usually accessed through the occupational health services or the A & E department. Every exposure incident needs to be reported to management, documented and thoroughly investigated.

Exposure incidents are psychologically traumatic for nurses and other healthcare providers, and counselling support needs to be available. This is frequently accessed from the occupational health services.

Active and/or passive immunization or post-exposure chemoprophylaxis helps reduce the risk of infection or disease following exposure and is available for some but not all BBPs.

HBV exposure

All nurses, midwives and other healthcare providers (including students) who work in clinical areas where they may have direct contact with blood and other body fluids, or perform exposure-prone procedures (EPPs; see Table 15.6) or who are at risk of injury from blood-stained sharp instruments must be immunized against HBV infection.[17] The vaccine is normally given intramuscularly in the deltoid region, but not in the buttock as this may reduce its efficacy.[20]

Antibody levels (titres) should be checked following vaccination, and a booster is usually given every 5 years if antibody titres fall below 100 miu/mL. Specific hepatitis B immunoglobulin (HBIG) may be used for passive protection in unvaccinated people or those who did not respond to vaccination. Currently, there are no specific anti-hepatitis B antiviral drugs that are recommended to be given following exposure (PEP) to abort infection.

HCV exposure

Unfortunately, there is currently no vaccine or PEP available to prevent infection following exposure to HCV.

HIV exposure

Although there is as yet no vaccine to prevent illness following exposure and infection with HIV, PEP with a combination of antiretroviral drugs is effective in reducing the risk of HIV infection. Current guidelines recommend that if an initial risk assessment indicates that a significant exposure has occurred, the source patient should be tested and PEP recommended.[21,22] A significant exposure usually means being exposed to blood or another high-risk body fluid from a patient or other source either known to be HIV infected or considered to be at high risk of HIV infection, but when the result of an HIV test has not or cannot be obtained, for whatever reason.[21]

The **risk assessment algorithm** in Figure 15.2 was adapted, with permission, from a clinical protocol developed by Borgess Medical Center and West Michigan Air Care in the USA.[23] It provides a logical step-by-step algorithm to assess the degree of risk of a particular exposure to help decide whether or not to commence PEP.

For optimal efficacy, **PEP should commence as soon as possible after the incident** and ideally within an hour. There may be circumstances in which it is appropriate that the exposed healthcare provider is offered the initial doses immediately, pending fuller discussion and risk assessment as soon as practicable. Starter packs of PEP drugs need to be kept in a number of readily accessible and well-advertised places, e.g. occupational health, pharmacy, A & E, specified wards or departments.

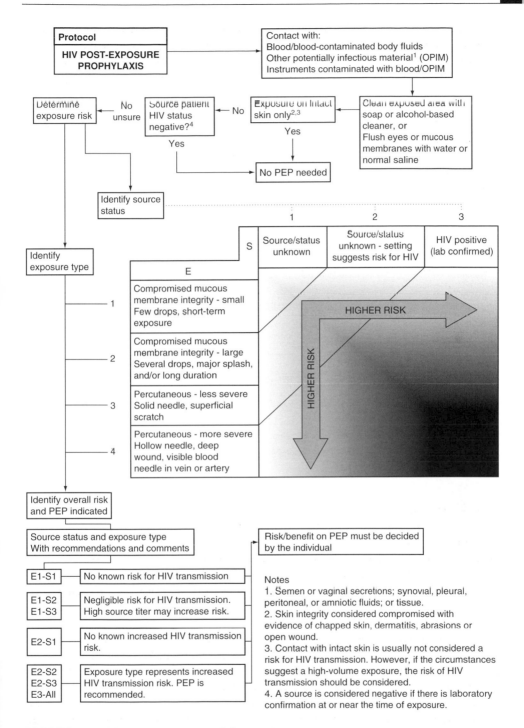

FIGURE 15.2 *Protocol for HIV post-exposure prophylaxis (PEP).*

A combination of antiretroviral drugs is prescribed for 4 weeks (Table 15.5). Pregnancy does not preclude the use of HIV PEP. More detailed information about PEP regimens, antiretroviral drug side effects, drug interactions and other issues associated with PEP can be found in the UK Departments of Health HIV PEP Guidance[21] and the latest guidance from the USA Centers for Disease Control and Prevention,[22] both of which are downloadable from the web (website addresses in Table 15.5).

TABLE 15.5 Examples of post-exposure prophylaxis regimens

UK Departments of Health,[20] July 2000:[a] http://www.doh.gov.uk/eaga/publications.htm

Zidovudine (Retrovir®) 200 mg three times daily or 250 mg twice daily

plus

Lamivudine (Epivir®) 150 mg twice daily

and either

Indinavir (Crixivan®) 800 mg three times daily on an empty stomach

or

Nelfinavir (Viracept®) 750 mg three times daily or 1250 mg twice daily with meals or snacks

USA Centers for Disease Control and Prevention,[21] June 2001:[a]

http://www.cdc.gov/mmwr/preview/mmwrhtml/rr5011a1.htm

■ Basic two-drug regimens

  Lamivudine (Epivir®) 150 mg twice daily

  and either

  Zidovudine (Retrovir®) 600 mg per day in two or three divided doses

  or

  Stavudine (Zerit®) 40 mg (if body weight <60 kg, 30 mg) twice daily

■ Expanded three-drug regimens

The basic two-drug regimen *plus one of the following*:

Indinavir (Crixivan®) 800 mg three times daily on an empty stomach

or

Nelfinavir (Viracept®) 750 mg three times daily or 1250 mg twice daily with meals or snacks

or

Efavirenz (Sustiva®) 600 mg daily at bedtime

or

Abacavir (Ziagen®) 300 mg twice daily

---

[a]Check websites for detailed information and latest recommendations.

Infected nurses, midwives and other healthcare providers

Although the risk of occupational infection with BBPs is low, it has occurred, and nurses, midwives and other healthcare providers have become infected as the result of an exposure incident. Additionally, all healthcare providers are as vulnerable to infection with blood-borne viruses as anyone else in the community as a result of their own social and sexual behaviour and other risk factors, and are more commonly infected in their personal lives rather than during professional practice.

All professional ethical guidelines stress the primacy of the patient's interest, which recognizes that nothing should ever be done by healthcare providers which could put their patients at risk, no matter how low that risk is. Consequently, all nurses and other healthcare providers who believe that they may have been exposed to a BBP, regardless of the circumstances, need to seek competent medical advice and diagnostic serological testing, if appropriate. If found to be infected, they need to remain under the supervision of the occupational health service and specialist medical services, as they will frequently require long-term follow-up.

Nurses and midwives and all other healthcare providers who are infected with a BBP may continue in professional practice. However, depending on their infection status, they may be restricted from performing EPPs (Table 15.6). Specific restrictions for infected healthcare providers are related to the particular infection.

TABLE 15.6 Exposure-prone procedures (EPPs)[8,18]

EPPs are those in which there is a risk that injury to the healthcare provider (HCP) may result in the exposure of the patient's open tissues to the blood of the HCP. These include procedures in which the HCP's gloved hands may be in contact with sharp instruments, needle tips and sharp tissues (spicules of bone or teeth) inside a patient's open body cavity, wound or confined anatomical space where the hands or fingertips may not be completely visible at all times.

Nursing. General nursing procedures do not include EEPs, but the duties of operating theatre nurses, nurses practising in A & E departments and haemodialysis units should be considered individually.

Midwifery. Simple vaginal delivery and the use of scissors to make an episiotomy cut are not exposure prone. Infiltration of local anaesthetic prior to episiotomy, suturing of an episiotomy and attaching sharp scalp electrodes to a baby's head are considered exposure prone.

Operating department assistants/technicians. General duties do not normally include EPPs.

HBV infection

In the UK, nurses, midwives or other healthcare providers who perform EPPs and who test positive for HBV surface antigen (HBsAg-positive) but are 'e' antigen negative (HBeAg-negative) need to have their HBV DNA viral load tested every 12 months. If this does not exceed 10^3 (i.e. 1000) genome equivalents per millilitre, they need not be restricted from performing EPP. If it rises above 10^3 genome equivalents per millilitre, they must cease to perform EPPs.

All nurses, midwives and other healthcare providers who test positive for HBV 'e' antigen (HbeAg-positive) must not perform EPPs, regardless of their viral load.[24]

HCV infection

Nurses, midwives and other healthcare providers in the UK who have been infected with HCV will test positive for HCV antibodies (anti-HCV-positive), but not all of them will have ongoing active infection. This is determined by testing their plasma for HCV RNA. Those found to be HCV-RNA-positive are not allowed to perform EPPs. However, if following antiviral therapy they revert to HCV-RNA-negative and remain so 6 months later, they may be allowed to return to performing EPPs.[25]

HIV infection

HIV-infected nurses, midwives and other healthcare providers must not perform EPPs.[7]

Summary

Although the risk of becoming infected with a BBP during clinical nursing or midwifery practice is low, it is real. Consistently following the guidance described in this chapter and in the associated website references will reduce this risk even further. If an accident does happen, the recommendations for managing an occupational exposure will also reduce the risk of infection. Finally, if infection does occur, nurses need to be aware of potential restrictions on their clinical practice.

REFERENCES AND ASSOCIATED INTERNET RESOURCES

1. UNAIDS. *Report on the Global HIV/AIDS Epidemic 2002*. Geneva: Joint United Nations Programme on HIV/AIDS, 226 pp. Available on: http://www.unaids.org
2. WHO. *Hepatitis B Fact Sheet*, WHO/204. Revised October 2000. Cited online 5 November 2002. Available from: http://www.who.int/inf-fs/en/fact204.html
3. WHO. *Hepatitis C Fact Sheet*, WHO/164. Revised October 2000. Cited online 5 November 2002. Available from: http://www.who.int/inf-fs/en/fact164.html
4. Loveday HP, Pellowe C, Harper P, Robinson N, Pratt R. The **epic** Project: Developing National Evidence-based Guidelines for Preventing Healthcare Associated Infections. Standard principles for preventing HAIs. *Nursing Times* 2001; **97**:36–37.
5. Pratt RJ, Pellowe C, Loveday HP, Robinson N, Smith GW, and the **epic** Guideline Development Team; Barrett S, Davey P, Harper P, Loveday C, McDougall C, Mulhall A, Privett S, Smales C, Taylor L, Weller B, and Wilcox M. The **epic** Project: Developing National Evidence-based Guidelines for Preventing Healthcare-associated Infections. Phase 1: Guidelines for Preventing Hospital-acquired Infections. *Journal of Hospital Infection* 2001; **47**(Suppl.):S1–82. Available on: http://www.doh.gov.uk/hai/epic.htm
6. Garner JS, Hospital Infection Control Practices Advisory Committee. Guideline for isolation precautions in hospitals. *Infection Control and Hospital Epidemiology* 1996; **17**:53–80. Available on: http://www.cdc.gov/ncidod/hip/isolat/isolat.htm
7. Department of Health. General principles of blood-borne virus infection control and exposure prone procedures. In: *HIV-Infected Health Care Workers: A Consultation Paper on Management and Patient Notification*. London: Department of Health Publications, 2002, 15–19. . Available on: http://www.doh.gov.uk/aids.htm
8. UK Health Departments. *Guidance for Clinical Health Care Workers: Protection Against Infection with Blood-borne Viruses*. Recommendations of the Expert Advisory Group on AIDS and the Advisory Group on Hepatitis. London: Department of Health Publications, 1998, 46 pp.
9. Cardo DM, Culver DH, Ciesielski CA. A case-control study of HIV seroconversion in health care workers after percutaneous exposures. *New England Journal of Medicine* 1997; **337**:1485.
10. Gerberding JL. HIV exposure risk assessment and prophylactic treatment. In: Sande MA, Volberding PA (eds), *The Medical Management of AIDS*, 6th edn. Philadelphia: W.B. Saunders Co., 1999, 513–23.
11. Lanphear BP. Trends and patterns in the transmission of bloodborne pathogens to health care workers. *Epidemiologic Reviews* 1994; **16**:437–50.
12. Public Health Laboratory Service AIDS & STD Centre. *Occupational Transmission of HIV*. London: PHLS, 1999, 73 pp.
13. Werner BG, Grady GF. Accidental hepatitis-B-surface-antigen-positive inoculations: use of e antigen to estimate infectivity. *Annals of Internal Medicine* 1982; **97**:367–9.
14. Moloughney BW. Transmission and postexposure management of bloodborne virus infections in the health care setting: where are we now? *Canadian Medical Association*

Journal 2001; **165**:445–51. Available on:
http://www.cmaj.ca/cgi/content/full/165/4/445

15. Centers for Disease Control and Prevention. Recommendations for prevention and control of hepatitis C virus (HCV) infection and HCV-related chronic disease. *Morbidity and Mortality Weekly Report (MMWR)* 16 October, 1998; **47**(RR-19):1–39. Available on: http://www.cdc.gov/mmwr/

16. Health and Safety Commission. *Control of Substances Hazardous to Health Regulations 1999; Approved Codes of Practice.* London: HSE Books, 1999, 75 pp.

17. UK Health Departments. *Protecting Health Care Workers and Patients from Hepatitis B: Recommendations of the Advisory Group on Hepatitis.* HSG(93)40 1993 and Addendum issued under cover of EL(96)77, 1996. London: Department of Health, 1993.

18. Department of Health. *HIV Infected Health Care Workers: A Consultation Paper on Management and Patient Notification.* London: Department of Health Publications, 2002, 72 pp. Available on: http://www.doh.gov.uk/aids.htm

19. O'Neill S. Clinical governance in action. Part 2: Effective risk-management strategies. *Professional Nurse* 2000; **15**:684–5.

20. UK Departments of Health. *Immunisation against Infectious Disease.* London: HMSO, 1996, 95–108.

21. Department of Health. *HIV Post-Exposure Prophylaxis: Guidance from the UK Chief Medical Officers' Expert Advisory Group on AIDS.* London: Department of Health Publications, 2000, 34 pp. Available on: http://www.doh.gov.uk/eaga/publications.htm

22. Centers for Disease Control and Prevention. Updated US Public Health Service Guidelines for the Management of Occupational Exposure to HBV, HCV, and HIV and Recommendations for Postexposure Prophylaxis. *Morbidity and Mortality Weekly Report (MMWR)* 29 June 2001; **50**(RR-11):1–52. Available on: http://www.cdc.gov/mmwr/preview/mmwrhtml/rr5011a1.htm

23. Borgess Medical Center and West Michigan Air Care. *Clinical Protocol: HIV Post-exposure Prophylaxis.* Kalamazoo, MI: Borgess Health Alliance, 2001.

24. NHS Executive. *Hepatitis B Infected Healthcare Workers*, HSC 2000/020. London: Department of Health, 2000, 4 pp. Available on: http://tap.ukwebhost.eds.com/doh/coin4.nsf/

25. Department of Health. *Hepatitis C Infected Health Care Workers*, HSC 2002/010. London: Department of Health, 2002. Available on: http://tap.ukwebhost.eds.com/doh/coin4.nsf and http://www.doh.gov.uk/hepatitisc

FURTHER READING AND INTERNET RESOURCES

All of the recommended further reading and internet resources applicable to this chapter are listed in the above references and Table 15.5.

The individualized care of patients with HIV disease

Robert Pratt and Tim Stephens with Karen Gibson

> The unique role of the nurse is to assist the individual, sick or well, in the performance of those activities contributing to health or its recovery (or to peaceful death) that he would perform unaided if he had the necessary strength, will or knowledge. And to do this in such a way as to help him gain independence as rapidly as possible.
>
> *Virginia Henderson*[1]

Introduction

This chapter is focused on caring for patients admitted to hospital for investigation or treatment of HIV disease and associated opportunistic events as described in previous chapters. The nursing care of people with HIV disease is no different than the nursing care of any other person who has a chronic illness with periods of acute exacerbations. It just sometimes seems different because of the complexity of a variety of external factors associated with this particular infection. These factors include stigma, fear of contagion, judgemental and ill-informed attitudes towards differing sexual orientations and practices, injecting drug use and various social, cultural, ethical and moral issues. They can create an illusion that caring for patients with HIV disease is different and that it requires 'special skills' not possessed by all nurses. Because this mirage can erode personal and professional confidence, a major goal of this chapter is to reassure nurses that, by virtue of their education, clinical experience and professional ethics, they can safely and competently care for all patients, including those with HIV disease. They already have those 'special skills' that are needed, and their involvement in the care and management of patients with HIV disease affords them a further opportunity to continue to positively develop the skills and attitudes that define the best in professional nursing.

Learning outcomes

After studying and reflecting on the material in this chapter, you will be able to:

- identify actual and potential problems patients may experience when they are ill and relate these to your understanding of the pathophysiology of HIV disease discussed in previous chapters;
- describe and use a relevant needs-based, problem-centred approach to systematically assess, plan, implement and evaluate nursing care;
- support colleagues and students in developing confidence and competence in delivering quality nursing care to patients with HIV disease.

BACKGROUND TO STRATEGIC NURSING CARE

Patients admitted for investigation or treatment of HIV-related opportunistic disease may be in a rapidly changing clinical situation and their nursing care must be assessed, planned and evaluated on a frequent basis. This requires a comprehensive understanding by the nurse of the rationale that underpins strategic nursing care.

Strategic nursing care is that care which is carefully planned and implemented by nurses, designed to meet the immediate needs of patients, solve identified actual problems and prevent recognized potential problems from being realized. Because of their training and experience, their comprehensive understanding of the nursing issues involved, and their teaching and management skills, nurses are able to assess and plan the individualized nursing care most appropriate for each patient and to lead and supervise the nursing team implementing this care. Care delivered must be evaluated frequently (often on a shift-by-shift basis) and modified according to the patient's response to nursing interventions. The nurse is ideally placed to act as the patient's advocate and to liaise effectively between the patient and other members of the healthcare team.

Strategic nursing care embraces the concept of a problem-solving approach to the individualized care of each patient. However, it is more than a nursing process style of care. It includes assessment and planning of nursing care on a hospital-wide basis, taking into consideration all the real and possible issues governing the implementation of care, and includes logistical, educational and managerial aspects, which, if not anticipated, may preclude the delivery of individualized, high-quality care.

Needs-based models of nursing, as conceived by Henderson,[2] Roper, Logan and Tierney,[3] and Orem,[4] are valuable tools by which the individualized nursing care of patients with HIV-related illnesses can be planned and implemented efficiently and effectively. These models describe the needs and self-care requisites necessary for normal, healthy living. The use of these models allows for a systematic nursing assessment that will identify actual problems arising from deficits in self-care abilities. It further recognizes potential problems associated with the patient's condition (social, psychological, physical and medical), specific illnesses, hospitalization and medical treatment. Identifying and documenting the needs, self-care requisites, actual and potential problems facilitate the planning of appropriate nursing interventions and allow the effectiveness of these interventions to be evaluated.

Because needs-based models used alone can be potentially de-humanizing, the nursing assessment must also include an examination of how this episode of illness is affecting the *person* (as opposed to the body). A simple set of questions that might be used to structure such an assessment could include the following.

- **Who is this person?** What do they, or did they, do for a living? Where do they live? Who do they live with? What family do they have?
- **What health event brings the person into hospital?** By getting the patient to describe this, the nurse can ascertain the patient's level of understanding and knowledge about their condition. This can help in identifying knowledge deficits the patient may have and in deciding how to individualize patient education.
- **How is this person feeling?** This question is designed to embrace physical, emotional, psychological and spiritual aspects of the person. It allows the patient to talk about themselves and about any hopes or anxieties that they may have, or about anything to do with their current state of mind.
- **How has this event affected the person's usual life-patterns and relationships?** Disruption to health obviously brings with it disruption to normal life. By discussing this, problems as disparate as loss of earnings, loss of ability to engage in leisure activities and loss of intimacy with a partner may all be highlighted.
- **What support does this person have?** This question raises the nurse's awareness of who or what the patient uses to help them cope during times of stress, such as partner, family, friends, religious or spiritual faith. It can also provide a clearer picture of who the patient is socially and which other people may become involved in the patient's care episode. The question can also provide information that will be useful when planning discharge (see Chapter 18).
- **How does this person view their future?** This question raises issues about the meaning of HIV infection to the patient. The patient's experience of living with HIV will probably have a strong effect on how they view their future.

This assessment structure is taken from the Burford Nursing Development Unit Model.[5] The idea behind the model is to allow the nurse to 'connect' with the patient in a way that conventional nursing models do not always allow for. In essence, it aims to help the nurse to see the person in relation to their illness, as opposed to 'a patient with an illness'. In the acute care setting, gaining information to assist with this may often be neglected in favour of physiological assessment. However, when one considers the nature of HIV disease, with its impact on the patient physiologically, psychologically and socially, it would seem vital that a *comprehensive* assessment is carried out. To that end, it is suggested that both these assessments are used together, so that information is gained about the person living with HIV disease (Burford model) as well as about the needs HIV disease generates in that person (needs-based model).

In addition, a wealth of knowledge will exist and be available to nurses to assist them in planning and delivering nursing care. The members of the multidisciplinary team that supports the care of the patient, including the physician, physiotherapist, occupational therapist, pharmacist and dietician, all possess valuable specialist knowledge regarding dimensions of HIV care that the nurse can access and use appropriately when planning, implementing and evaluating a patient's individualized nursing care .

In this chapter, an eclectic needs-based nursing model is used to organize the information provided. Most nurses will already be familiar with this assessment structure, as the list of needs is adapted from Henderson's 'Components of basic nursing' and Roper, Logan and Tierney's 'Activities of daily living'.[2,3] By meeting these needs, it is hoped that the hospitalized patient may return to health or, where this is unachievable, that the effects of illness are minimized.

Fifteen needs are discussed. Each is described as having **potential problems** associated with it. Alongside each of these problems, there is a list of **possible causes**. Neither of these lists is designed to be exhaustive; rather, they are indicative of the conditions and causes that the nurse may most commonly encounter in the ward setting when caring for patients with HIV disease. The intention is to familiarize the nurse with the common conditions associated with HIV disease and the needs that these conditions may engender. Many of the opportunistic diseases listed here are described in more detail in previous chapters.

General **objectives of care** are described for each need. This is followed by a description of relevant **nursing interventions**, introduced by identifying important elements of a **nursing assessment**. In the real world of nursing practice, a more comprehensive assessment of each patient, as previously described, is needed to plan appropriate interventions and care most effectively.

As stated previously, nursing care must be regularly **evaluated** and modified according to the patient's response. A brief description of evaluation (linked to the stated objectives of care) concludes the discussion of each need.

NEEDS

In common with all individuals, patients with HIV-related illnesses have needs that they or others must meet for health to be maintained. The following list itemizes the needs that may be examined during the nursing assessment.

1. The need for adequate respiration.
2. The need for adequate hydration.
3. The need for adequate nutrition.
4. The need for urinary and faecal elimination.
5. The need to control body temperature.
6. The need for movement and mobilization.
7. The need for a safe environment.
8. The need for personal cleansing and dressing.
9. The need for expression and communication.
10. The need for working and playing.
11. The need to maintain psychological equilibrium.
12. The need for adequate rest and sleep.
13. The need to worship according to own faith.
14. The need to express sexuality.
15. The needs associated with dying.

The need for adequate respiration

Potential problems	Possible causes
Dyspnoea, hypoxia, tachypnoea, cyanosis	Pneumonia (caused by *Pneumocystis carinii* or other opportunistic pathogens)
Cough, confusion	Pulmonary tuberculosis Neoplastic involvement caused by Kaposi's sarcoma (KS) or lymphoma Anaemia

Objectives of care

■ To promote optimal respiratory function.
■ To keep the patient well oxygenated.
■ To alleviate associated symptoms, for example cough, dry mouth, anxiety.

Assessment

■ Assess vital signs (blood pressure, pulse, respiratory rate, body temperature, pulse oximetry). Record as baseline and repeat as appropriate. Pulse oximetry may need to be continuous if respiratory function is poor.
■ Assess colour, respiratory effort, chest sounds, sputum production and mental status.
■ Assess peak flow daily to monitor improvement or deterioration in respiratory ability.
■ Obtain sputum specimens for microbiology (culture and sensitivity, acid-fast bacilli, virology, cytology).
■ Be aware of arterial blood gas (ABG) values.
■ Note any history of chronic obstructive pulmonary disease.
■ If pulmonary tuberculosis has not been ruled out as a cause of respiratory signs and symptoms, consider placing the patient in respiratory isolation.

Nursing interventions

Position

The patient should be placed in a position that facilitates good respiratory function. Sitting the patient upright in their bed or in a chair, leaning forward and well supported, is useful as it allows the accessory muscles of respiration to assist respiratory effort. Placing pillows on a patient's table and allowing him or her to lean over may facilitate adequate respiration, especially in the patient who is tiring.

Oxygen

Depending on the patient's clinical condition and ABG values (Table 16.1), the physician may prescribe supplemental oxygen to be administered, or, if pulse oximetry shows the oxygen saturation of a patient falling below 95 per cent, the nurse may need to administer oxygen until the physician is consulted. Oxygen saturation should ideally be maintained at above 95 per cent at rest, but *always* above 90 per cent. Oxygen should be considered a drug and, as such, a prescription for its use should be sought as soon as possible. In general, the lowest concentration of oxygen needed to overcome hypoxaemia will be ordered.

TABLE 16.1 Normal range for arterial blood gases

PaO_2	10.6–13.3 kPa (80–100 mmHg)
$PaCO_2$	4.6–6.9 kPa (35–45 mmHg)
pH	7.35–7.45
Oxygen saturation 94–100%	

Different types of masks will be used, depending on the level of supplemental oxygenation required.

■ A standard (Hudson) face mask is suitable for those patients requiring up to 50 per cent O_2 supplementation. These masks cannot, however, guarantee accuracy of administration.

- For patients requiring high levels of supplemental O_2, or when highly accurate administration is needed, a Ventimask or Venturimask is indicated.
- Nasal catheters and cannulae may be used for patients who require low levels of supplemental oxygenation, although the inspired O_2 concentration can be unpredictable (2 litres per minute of O_2 = approximately 30 per cent O_2 concentration). Patients often prefer these, as they are comfortable and do not interfere with eating, drinking and the wearing of spectacles.

Oxygen therapy should be continuous rather than intermittent, aiming to maintain a constant arterial partial pressure of oxygen (PaO_2) between 10.6 and 13.3 kPa (80–100 mmHg). If oxygen is to be administered for more than 12 hours, humidification is required. This prevents excessive drying of the mouth and solidification of secretions.

Patient safety
The patient may be hypoxic and may be confused due to the limited oxygen supply to the brain. This could compromise patient safety. To minimize the potential risk associated with the effects of hypoxia, the nurse should assess patient safety and be prepared to move the confused patient to an area where they can be easily observed by the nurse, such as an observation bed on the ward. This could be complicated if there is a need to place a patient in respiratory isolation. In this situation, the patient will need to be regularly observed and the necessary safety precautions will need to be implemented to maximize the patient's safety.

There is a potential risk of fire when using oxygen, and non-sparking spanners (wrenches) and other equipment should be used when needed. No lighted flames or cigarette smoking are allowed in a room where oxygen is being administered.

Patient education
Patients should be taught deep-breathing, coughing and relaxation exercises. The use of an incentive spirometer (peak flow) is useful for deep-breathing exercises. Advice from the physiotherapist could assist the nurse when delivering specialist respiratory advice to the patient.

Chest physiotherapy
Extensive chest physiotherapy will be required to assist in establishing and maintaining clear lung fields. Postural drainage is frequently required. Chest physiotherapy must not be conducted in an open ward because of the potential risk of transmitting undiagnosed infectious agents, such as *Mycobacteria tuberculosis* and *Pneumocystis carinii*. The infection prevention considerations are discussed in more detail in Chapter 14.

Continuous positive airway pressure (CPAP)
Continuous positive airway pressure (CPAP) may be required for patients who are maintaining their own airway but who are failing to maintain an O_2 saturation of 95 per cent or above on 60 per cent O_2. This may occur because the patient's condition is deteriorating or because the patient is tiring from the work of breathing. For these patients, it is often prudent to set up the CPAP circuit in advance, ready for use. This should be done *away* from the patient to avoid causing them unnecessary anxiety. The patient on CPAP requires close, and often 1:1, supervision and support.

Endotracheal suction

Patients with severe respiratory embarrassment will require intermittent positive pressure ventilation (IPPV) and will need endotracheal suctioning. Disposable gloves, plastic apron, mask and eye protection are necessary when suctioning patients, as explosive coughing releases a potentially contaminated aerosol spray. Great care must be taken with this procedure, as it is stressful and often painful for patients. Nurses must also be aware of the associated hazards of endotracheal suctioning, such as tracheal mucosal damage, cardiac arrhythmias, atelectasis and hypoxaemia. Like chest physiotherapy, important infection prevention considerations apply when performing endotracheal suction (as discussed in Chapter 14).

Medications

Medications used for the treatment of specific opportunistic events that affect respiration, along with their side effects and drug interactions, are discussed in Chapters 7 and 8.

Reassurance

Patients with respiratory distress will require frequent reassurance from the nurse. Quite naturally, they are often anxious, tending to panic if they feel they cannot breathe. The 'nurse call' system should be placed within easy reach of the patient.

Mouth care

Oxygen, even when humidified, can be drying to mucous membranes, and frequent mouth care will be required. Patients should rinse their mouth out with water every hour.

Nasal care

If nasal cannulae are used, it is useful if the nostrils are lightly coated with a protective ointment such as Vaseline. Oxygen face masks and nasal catheters and cannulae can also cause soreness on the top of the ear with prolonged use. Again, a protective coating of Vaseline is useful.

Evaluation

The patient will be assessed frequently and appropriately to ensure that the objectives of care are being achieved, such as:

- optimal respiratory function, as evidenced by satisfactory ABG and oximetry values;
- alleviation of associated symptoms; and
- anticipation, detection and prompt management of side effects of medications.

Patients need to be closely observed for signs of improvement or deterioration, as they may have another underlying and as yet undetected infection causing respiratory dysfunction. Changes in respiratory status must be reported to the physician immediately.

The need for adequate hydration

Potential problems	Possible causes
Dehydration	Inadequate intake of oral fluids due to: dysphasia secondary to fungal, bacterial or viral oropharyngeal infections or oesophageal KS lesions, respiratory distress, O_2 administration via facemask, lethargy, confusion or coma
	Fluid loss from: diarrhoea, nausea, vomiting, gastrointestinal (GI) suctioning, fever and diaphoresis, rapid (and deep) respiratory rate (hyperpnoea)

Electrolyte imbalance	Diarrhoea, nausea, vomiting, GI suctioning, (more rarely) hyponatraemia secondary to the syndrome of inappropriate anti-diuretic hormone secretion (SIADH)
Renal colic/calculi	Inadequate fluid intake by patients on some antiretroviral drugs, for example indinavir, or patients taking sulphadiazine
Acute renal failure	Nephrotoxicity of drugs used for the treatment of opportunistic infections, such as foscarnet sodium, ganciclovir, famciclovir, amphotericin, cidofovir, high-dose aciclovir

Objectives of care

- To maintain optimal hydration and electrolyte balance.
- To prevent or correct dehydration and electrolyte imbalance.
- To maintain optimal renal function.

Assessment

- Assess the patient's ability to maintain own hydration.
- Identify oropharyngeal infections.
- Assess the patient for the presence of nausea, vomiting, diarrhoea, oral pain/discomfort.
- Assess level of consciousness and cognitive ability.
- Assess drug chart for medications that alter renal function.
- Assess the patient for signs of systemic hypovolaemia.
- Assess skin turgor daily.
- Initiate fluid balance chart for ongoing assessment.
- Be aware of current blood chemistry results.
- Weigh on a regular basis.

Nursing interventions

Fluid balance chart

Where possible, encourage the patient to keep their own record of fluid intake. They will need education and supervised practice in measuring input and output. Toilet (or bedside commodes, bedpans, urinals) and measuring jugs need to be easily accessible to patients to aid compliance with output measurement. Intake and output information needs to be transferred into the nursing notes at regular intervals.

Oral fluids

The patient should be encouraged to drink frequent, small amounts of fluids as tolerated. Fresh cold water should always be left in an accessible place for the patient. If oral intake is poor even with encouragement, the physician may need to prescribe intravenous fluids.

Intravenous rehydration

The physician may prescribe a regimen of intravenous fluids that must be infused at the correct flow rate. Peripheral intravenous insertion sites will need to be inspected regularly by the nurse to ensure they remain patent and free of inflammation and infection. The prevention of serious bloodstream infections in patients with central venous catheters is discussed in detail in Chapters 14 and 17. In England, comprehensive national evidence-based guidelines for preventing infections associated with the use of central venous catheters have been published,[6,7] and nurses need to ensure that this guidance is reflected in both local protocols and routine daily clinical practice.

Electrolyte replacement

The principal electrolyte abnormalities seen in seriously ill patients are decreases in plasma levels of sodium (hyponatraemia) and potassium (hypokalaemia). Excess plasma levels of sodium (hypernatraemia) and potassium (hyperkalaemia) are less frequently encountered. The nurse needs to be aware of the patient's most recent electrolyte values (Table 16.2).

TABLE 16.2 Normal plasma electrolyte parameters

Potassium (K$^+$)	3.8–5.0 mmol/L (mEq/L)
Sodium (Na$^+$)	135–145 mmol/L (mEq/L)
Chloride (Cl$^-$)	100–106 mmol/L (mEq/L)

There are two main causes of electrolyte imbalance in the HIV-infected patient: diarrhoea and vomiting, and neurological conditions that cause the syndrome of inappropriate anti-diuretic hormone secretion (SIADHS). Patients with severe hyponatraemia are at risk of seizures. Patients with a potassium imbalance are at risk from cardiac arrhythmias and may need cardiac monitoring for continuous assessment.

The treatment of hyponatraemia is focused on correcting the underlying cause, water restriction and electrolyte replacement. In general, sodium and potassium depletion is corrected by intravenous infusions of fluids with added electrolytes (potassium, sodium, chloride, bicarbonate). Although potassium and sodium are usually added to intravenous infusions, oral potassium preparations, such as Kloref® or Sando-K®, and/or oral sodium supplementation, such as Slow Sodium®, may be used. Alternatively, oral rehydration salts (ORS), such as Dioralyte® or Rehidrat® (see Chapter 7, Table 7.9), may be used for general electrolyte replacement following diarrhoea. Demeclocycline hydrochloride (Ledermycin®) may be prescribed for use in patients with SIADH to reverse hyponatraemia.

Plasma electrolyte levels need to be carefully monitored and results outside normal parameters reported to the physician immediately.

Urethral catheters

All patients with indwelling urethral catheters require intake and output measurements. Healthcare-associated infections (in hospital, community and primary care) are commonly caused by urinary catheterization, and planned nursing interventions must minimize (not maximize!) this risk of infection. In England, national evidence-based guidelines for preventing these infections have been published,[6,8] and this guidance needs to be incorporated into local protocols and reflected in routine nursing practice.

Mouth care

Patients who are unable to take oral fluids require frequent (2 hourly) mouth care.

Skin care

Dehydrated patients may experience dry skin and may be at increased risk of developing pressure ulcers. They need regular pressure area inspection and care. Emollients, such as Aqueous Cream BP, moisturize the skin and should be applied as appropriate. Emollient bath additives, such as Alpha Keri Bath® or E45® bath oils, may be helpful for some patients.

Patient education

Patients receiving potentially nephrotoxic medications need to be reminded of the importance of drinking adequate volumes of fluids to help maintain normal renal function. Those who are taking indinavir (Crixivan®) as part of their antiretroviral therapy regimen need educational input on the importance of drinking *at least* 1.5 litres of *additional fluids* per day to prevent renal calculi from forming.[9,10] The nurse needs to evaluate the patient's ability to understand any educational input.

Evaluation

The patient will be assessed frequently and appropriately to ensure that the objectives of care are being achieved, such as:

- causes of poor oral intake are addressed and managed;
- fluid loss is adequately replaced by oral and/or intravenous fluids;
- electrolyte imbalance is detected, monitored and reversed;
- risks associated with medications that alter renal function are managed;
- the patient does not display signs of systemic hypovolaemia;
- skin turgor is normal.

The need for adequate nutrition

Potential problems	Probable causes
Involuntary weight loss	Catabolism associated with advanced HIV disease (HIV wasting syndrome) and/or resulting from underlying opportunistic diseases, such as tuberculosis, *Mycobacterium avium–intracellulare* complex disease (MAC), fever, malignancy
Treatment-induced weight loss	Antiretroviral therapy and anorexia caused by other drugs used in the treatment of opportunistic diseases, such as sulphonamides and anti-mycobacterial drugs
Malnutrition	Diarrhoea and malabsorption caused by various opportunistic infections, such as candidiasis, MAC, cryptosporidiosis Diarrhoea may occur without opportunistic pathogens being identified
Reduced food intake	Dysphagia, anorexia, diarrhoea, nausea and vomiting, oesophageal infections and ulcerations, lethargy, loneliness, depression, confusion, immobility, poverty
Loss of lean muscle mass	Metabolic changes associated with advanced HIV disease
Lipodystrophy and other disorders of fat metabolism	Antiretroviral therapy

Objectives of care

- To keep the patient well nourished.
- To prevent further weight loss.
- To enhance weight gain.
- To help the patient develop dietary habits compatible with the antiretroviral treatment regimen.

Assessment

It is important to obtain an accurate baseline weight on admission and to monitor as appropriate. The nursing assessment will include a history of previous dietary patterns, including likes, dislikes and any known food allergies. Information on the current dietary habit of the patient is recorded, including any special diets they may be following and 'alternative' diets such as macrobiotic diets. A comprehensive nutritional assessment is described in the following chapter and will include the following.

■ Appearance – does the patient look thin or wasted?
■ History of recent weight loss – has the patient noticed that clothes have become ill fitting?
■ Normal eating patterns/preferences.
■ Appetite – any oral/oesophageal manifestations that cause difficulties in chewing or swallowing?
■ Presence of nausea and/or vomiting – attempt to identify precipitating factors.
■ Presence of diarrhoea – obtain a history of the problem: is a stool sample required?
■ Medications – any dietary restrictions associated with current antiretroviral and/or tuberculosis treatment regimens? Any gastrointestinal side effects from any drugs being taken?
■ Need for food intake chart?
■ Need to liaise with the dietician?

The dietician should be informed of the patient's admission and, after interviewing the patient, will be able to advise on a suitable nutritional regimen.

Nursing interventions

Oral nutrition

The patient may tolerate small, frequent meals better than the traditional three meals a day. However, as it may be difficult to provide this within the hospital setting, the patient should be encouraged to ask family/friends to bring in favourite foods for them. There are no general restrictions on what the patient may eat, unless advised otherwise by the patient's physician, for example, those patients with elevated serum levels of cholesterol and/or triglycerides may be prescribed a diet low in saturated fatty acids.

Because patients will be immunocompromised, it is essential to recognize the importance of food safety and to advise patients which foods need to be avoided, for example unpasteurized dairy products and some reheated foods (see Chapter 7, Table 7.16).

Patients with respiratory illness may not be able to ingest their food, or may only ingest small amounts at any one time. It is important to allow them to conserve their energy by encouraging them to rest between mouthfuls. If patients are receiving oxygen therapy, the use of nasal cannulae is preferable to masks from a nutritional point of view as they cause less interference with eating.

Nutritional supplements such as Ensure®, Enlive® and Complan® are useful and well tolerated by many patients. Ideally, these drinks should be used to *supplement* meals, rather than replace normal intake. As some nutritional supplements may be lactose based, it is important to assess if they could exacerbate diarrhoea. Ensure® and Elive® are lactose-free preparations.

Patients suffering from nausea and vomiting may be prescribed anti-emetics, such as metoclopramide hydrochloride (Maxolon®), and these are given at least 30 minutes before meals.

Patients may be advised to supplement their diets with a variety of vitamins, minerals and antioxidants, and these are discussed in the following chapter.

Nurses need to be familiar with any dietary requirements associated with different antiretroviral and other drugs the patient may be taking, and to incorporate this information into the nursing care plan (Table 16.3). It is essential that these medications are given at the correct time so that meals do not have to be delayed and normal eating patterns interrupted. If necessary, the dietician and pharmacist can provide further information on the dietary considerations associated with treatment regimens, and nurses need to have access to the current issue of the *British National Formulary (BNF)*[9] in order to ensure they have the up-to-date information on drug administration recommendations. A new edition is published every 6 months and it is also available online (see 'Internet resources' at the end of this chapter). The current *HIV & AIDS Treatments Directory* from the National AIDS Manual (NAM) gives detailed information and advice on all issues associated with antiretroviral therapy, including dietary considerations.[10] Both of these publications are available online

TABLE 16.3 Dietary requirements associated with antiretroviral drugs and some other common medications used for patients with HIV disease

Drugs that require administration on an empty stomach include:

- didanosine (ddI; Videx®) – 1 hour before or 2 hours after food (use cold non-carbonated water or clear apple juice only to swallow tablets; use only cold water for enteric coated tablets); take at least 1 hour apart from indinavir (Crixivan®)
- indinavir (Crixivan®) – 1 hour before food or 2 hours after, unless taken with ritonavir (Norvir®) when food restrictions no longer apply; patients should be advised to drink 1.5 litres of a non-caffeinated drink in addition to their normal fluid intake in order to minimize the risk of renal calculi
- rifampicin (used for the treatment of tuberculosis)

Drugs that should be taken with meals (or within an hour following meals) include:

- zidovudine (ZDV; Retrovir®)
- zalcitabine (ddC; Hivid®)
- nelfinavir (Viracept®)
- saquinavir (Fortovase®, Invirase®) – grapefruit juice may increase absorption
- ritonavir (Norvir®) – liquid formulation may be mixed with a milk-based nutritional supplement but not with water, fizzy drinks or fruit juice; strong flavoured foods and drinks, such as iced fruit juice (e.g. grapefruit or mango juice) or salt and vinegar crisps (potato chips), can be eaten immediately before or after swallowing to disguise the taste
- oral ganciclovir (Cymevene®) (used for maintenance treatment of cytomegalovirus (CMV) retinitis)
- lopinavir with ritonavir (Kaletra®)
- tenofovir (Viread®) (high-fat meal facilitates tenofovir absorption)

Drugs that may be taken with or without food include:

- lamivudine (3TC; Epivir®)
- lamivudine with zidovudine (Combivir®)
- lamivudine with zidovudine and abacavir (Trizvir®)
- stavudine (d4T; Zerit®)
- abacavir (Ziagen®)
- amprenavir (Agenerase®) – but do not take for at least 1 hour following a high-fat meal
- efavirenz (Sustiva®) – if taken with food, drug levels may be increased in some people; avoid taking with a high-fat meal as this may significantly increase absorption (which may increase the risk of side effects), especially during the first few months of therapy
- nevirapine (Viramune®)
- delavirdine (Rescriptor®) – tablets can be dissolved in water or cola and this drug must not be taken within 2 hours from taking indigestion remedies containing antacids, or from taking didanosine (ddI; Videx®)
- hydroxyurea (Hydrea®)

(see 'Internet resources' at the end of this chapter). NAM is the pre-eminent provider of patient information booklets/leaflets and other resources in the UK (usually free of cost or at subsidized rates for those affected by HIV infection), and patients can be referred to their website to access up-to-date, absolutely reliable and easily understandable information and tips on all aspects of living with HIV disease, including nutritional and dietary advice.

Enteral and intravenous nutrition

In addition to or in place of oral nutrition, enteral and intravenous nutrition may be required and these interventions are discussed in the following chapter.

Medications

A variety of drugs may be prescribed to increase appetite and/or to prevent nausea, vomiting and diarrhoea, and these, along with their common side effects, are described in the following chapter.

Evaluation

The patient will be assessed frequently and appropriately to ensure that objectives of care are being achieved, such as:

- the patient is showing a weight gain or at least a cessation of weight loss: although weight loss and malnutrition are often progressive during late symptomatic disease, good nutritional support may improve the patient's quality of life and delay further wasting.

The need for urinary and faecal elimination

Potential problems	Possible causes
Diarrhoea	GI opportunistic infections, such as cryptosporidiosis, microsporidiosis, cytomegalovirus (CMV) disease, amoebiasis, isosporiasis GI-related malignancy (e.g. sarcoma, lymphoma) Treatment related (e.g. antibiotics, antiretroviral drugs) Direct effect of HIV infection on the GI system Irritable bowel syndrome (IBS)
Hyponatraemia	Severe diarrhoea
Oliguria	Dehydration, renal failure (which may be treatment related)
Haematuria	Treatment-induced renal calculi following indinavir (Crixivam®) therapy
Constipation	Reduced mobility, poor fibre and fluid intake Treatment related
Incontinence	Neurological disease, confusion, loss of mobility, terminal illness

Objectives of care

- To assist the patient in preventing and/or managing the effects of diarrhoea, constipation and incontinence.
- To prevent or correct dehydration.
- To prevent the nosocomial transmission of enteric pathogens in healthcare settings.

Assessment

- The presence of diarrhoea, constipation, oliguria, haematuria, incontinence, dehydration and recent weight loss is identified.

- The patient is weighed on admission and during regular intervals and their temperature, pulse, respiratory rate and blood pressure are taken and recorded.
- If the patient is taking indinavir (Crixivan®), urine is tested for occult blood as this drug may cause kidney stones.
- The patient's medication regimen, usual nutrition, hydration and mobility patterns are reviewed, as are their usual urinary and defaecation habits.
- The frequency, consistency and colour of bowel movements are documented and fluid intake and output recorded.
- If an assessment reveals diarrhoea, fever and abdominal cramping, the physician is alerted so that early stool samples can be obtained and sent for laboratory investigation to identify gastrointestinal parasitic, bacterial or viral infections.
- Serum electrolyte levels are monitored in patients with severe diarrhoea to identify early imbalances, such as hyponatraemia.
- If the patient has abdominal pain or cramping, the abdomen is examined and any rigidity or abdominal guarding is reported urgently to the physician.
- Jaundice, if present, is identified and urine is tested for bilirubin if indicated.
- If the patient has a history of incontinence and/or restricted mobility, pressure areas are inspected, along with the condition of the skin in the ano-genital area.

Nursing interventions

Diarrhoea

Diarrhoea is by far the most common GI problem in patients with HIV disease, and chronic diarrhoea is distressing, disabling and debilitating. The cause can generally be identified by history and assessment and is infective or treatment related in the majority of cases. However, IBS commonly causes diarrhoea (alternating with constipation) in many people with HIV disease in the absence of gut infection. Electrolyte loss (especially sodium) may occur during severe episodes of diarrhoea. Table 7.9 (in Chapter 7) describes general measures that are needed to support patients experiencing moderate-to-severe diarrhoea.

Patients with diarrhoea should be nursed in a single room which has private toilet facilities. If the patient is not ambulatory, a bedside commode is preferable to using a bedpan in bed. If used, bedpans may be carefully emptied (to avoid splashing) in the patient's toilet, or the contents disposed of in the bedpan washer.

As an adjunct to rehydration during episodes of acute uncomplicated diarrhoea, the physician may prescribe anti-motility drugs, such as co-phenotrope (Lomotil®) or loperamide hydrochloride (Imodium®) to slow down and decrease the frequency of bowel movements. Anti-spasmodic drugs, such as mebeverine hydrochloride (Colofac®), may be prescribed for patients with IBS.

Patients with diarrhoea need to be advised on using correct hand hygiene measures following defaecation, such as effective hand washing and the use of alcohol-based hand rubs. Nurses and other healthcare providers must adhere to standard infection prevention principles, including decontaminating the hands immediately before each and every episode of direct patient contact/care and after any activity or contact that potentially results in the hands becoming contaminated.[6,11] This will help prevent the transmission of any enteric pathogens to others. Infection prevention measures are discussed in more detail in Chapter 14.

Hydration

Patients with severe diarrhoea may become quickly dehydrated and must be encouraged to drink adequate amounts of fluids to replace those lost due to diarrhoea (see Table 7.9 in Chapter 7). Intravenous rehydration may be necessary in some patients.

Constipation

Constipation can generally be prevented by a balanced diet with adequate fibre and fluid intake. If constipation is present or develops, the use of bulk-forming, stimulant or osmotic laxatives, such as unprocessed wheat bran or ispaghula husk (Fybogel®), senna (Senokot®) or magnesium salts (Magnesium Hydroxide Mixture BP), can relieve this uncomfortable condition. Faecal softeners, such as arachis oil (Fletcher's Arachis Oil Retention Enema®), may be useful to lubricate and soften impacted faeces and promote a bowel movement. An oral emulsion of liquid paraffin is rarely used anymore because it may cause anal seepage of paraffin and consequent anal irritation, along with other side effects. Laxatives can be administered orally, as rectal suppositories and as enemas, and nurses should consult the current issue of the BNF[9] (see 'Internet resources' at the end of this chapter) or the manufacturer's recommendations for information on their correct use.

Incontinence

In male patients, urinary incontinence may be managed by leaving a urinal carefully placed between the patient's legs. Alternatively, an external latex penile sheath, such as the Texas Catheter® (Tyco Healthcare), may be used.

The use of indwelling urethral catheters should be avoided if at all possible because they frequently cause urinary tract infections. However, in seriously ill patients, and in female patients, their use may be unavoidable. If used, current national evidence-based guidelines for preventing infections associated with urethral catheters need to be followed.[6,8]

Patients with faecal incontinence should be nursed on clean, dry incontinence pads, which are placed on a linen drawsheet over a plastic sheet. All patients who are incontinent must be checked hourly. The dietician may be consulted in order to assess if a change in the patient's diet may assist in controlling faecal incontinence.

Skin care

The skin must be kept clean and dry. It is essential that facilities are made available for patients to wash their hands after using the toilet. If the patient is incontinent, barrier creams and ointments may be useful in preventing excoriation of the skin, such as Drapolene®, Sudocrem® or Vaseline. These may also be helpful in preventing soreness in patients with frequent diarrhoea. It is important to clean the area where the cream has been and to re-apply it daily or as necessary.

Dusting powders (talc, starch) should not be applied to moist areas, such as the ano-genital region, because they can cake and abrade the skin. Although talcum powder is a lubricant, it does not absorb moisture.[9]

Patients who are incontinent are at an increased risk of developing pressure ulcers. Pressure area care, including turning the patient on alternate sides, should be undertaken on a regular basis, such as every 2 hours. It is useful to re-assess the patient daily using a validated scoring system such as the Norton or Waterlow risk assessment scoring scales (see Figures 16.1 and 16.2).[12-14] Pressure area care is discussed in more detail later in this chapter.

Infection prevention

Nurses need to wear disposable gloves (natural rubber latex or gloves manufactured from synthetic substances, such as nitrile or vinyl, but not polythene) of the correct size and plastic aprons when disposing of urine or faeces and when caring for faecally incontinent patients. Contaminated linen is preferably double-bagged in a soluble plastic bag, which is then placed in a red nylon linen bag, sealed and sent to the laundry. Careful hand decontamination, prior to and after caring for patients, is exceptionally important with patients who have enteric infections. Wearing gloves does not decrease the need for good hand hygiene techniques.[6,11]

Evaluation

The patient will be assessed frequently and appropriately to ensure that objectives of care are being achieved, such as:

- GI complications of HIV disease are prevented or identified and effectively managed and patients are helped to return to regular patterns of urinary and faecal elimination;
- for those with severe diarrhoea or incontinence, skin excoriation and pressure area breakdown are prevented and nursing interventions minimize the psychological effects of severe diarrhoea and/or incontinence;
- patients are adequately hydrated and tolerate a balanced diet;
- any risk for the nosocomial transmission of enteric pathogens has been minimized.

The need to control body temperature

Potential problem	Possible causes
Fever and night sweats	HIV infection
	Opporunistic infections, including tuberculosis
	Lymphoma
	Drug allergy

Objectives of care

- Identify new infections or other causes of fever.
- Assist in maintaining normal body temperature (36–37.7 °C).
- Keep the patient well hydrated.
- Alleviate discomfort caused by fever.

Assessment

- Assess vital signs and body temperature twice daily and, if the patient is febrile, record body temperature 4 hourly.
- Assess for neurological signs and symptoms, such as headache, neck stiffness, photophobia and other body system signs and symptoms, for example rash, nausea and vomiting, abdominal pain, dysuria, cough, sore throat, ear ache.
- Review the current medication regimen, especially noting newly introduced antiretroviral drugs, such as abacavir (Ziagen®).
- Assess the source of pyrexia and collect required laboratory specimens, such as stool, urine and sputum samples, throat swabs and assist in collecting blood specimens for culture and sensitivity.
- Assess history of rigors, sweating and night sweats.

Nursing interventions

Fever associated with an infection is a protective response that enhances the body's defence mechanisms. The body's temperature normally fluctuates between 36 °C and 37.7 °C over a 24-hour period (circadian cycle), being lowest very early in the morning and highest during late afternoon and early evening. Fever occurs when the body temperature is elevated above the normal daily variation or, more precisely, when the temperature, as measured by an oral thermometer, is 37.8 °C (100 °F) or higher or, when measured rectally, is 38.2 °C (100.8 °F) or higher. The hypothalamus in the brain is the control centre for body temperature and fever results when this centre resets the hypothalamic thermostat upwards. Fevers may show particular patterns, such as peaking each day and then returning to normal, or be intermittent, when the temperature varies but does not return to normal. Some people, such as young children and the elderly, may actually show a drop in temperature below normal as a response to severe infection. Because immunocompromised patients have decreased inflammatory responses, low-grade pyrexia is regarded as significant in patients with HIV disease.

Medication

The physician may prescribe antipyretic medication to reduce body temperature, such as paracetamol BP (acetaminophen USP), aspirin or other non-steroidal anti-inflammatory drugs (NSAIDs), for example ibuprofen (Brufen®). Paracetamol is probably the most effective and has the lowest profile of GI side effects. Antipyretics should be administered as ordered, but generally on a regular basis, as intermittent administration may cause unnecessary diaphoresis (sweating), which is uncomfortable. It is useful to record on the temperature chart each time an antipyretic is given so that variations in temperature can be assessed correctly.

Because fevers associated with infections enhance host defence mechanisms, many physicians believe that they are beneficial and, in older children and adults, fevers should not be treated with antipyretic drugs. All agree, however, that fevers should be treated in younger children because of the risk of associated seizures, and in adults with underlying cardiac or pulmonary insufficiency because fever increases the demand for oxygen (for example, for every 1 °C increase over 37 °C, oxygen consumption increases by 13 per cent). It is also important to remember that fever may cause mental status changes in patients with dementia, and **hyperpyrexia** (body temperature over 41 °C) may cause delirium and death.

Nutrition and hydration

As prolonged fever increases metabolic processes, catabolism and fluid loss, patients with fever should be encouraged to eat a light, nutritious diet and drink adequate amounts of fluids. Cool drinks must be easily available, and glucose drinks, such as Lucozade® or squash, may be beneficial to some patients, although they may exacerbate diarrhoea in others. Intravenous rehydration may be needed in very ill patients. Those with long-term fevers and associated catabolism, for example fever associated with lymphoma or tuberculosis, should have a referral made to the dietician.

Comfort

The patient should be kept clean and comfortable and bed clothes and linen should be light, dry and clean. If hyperpyrexia occurs, a fan and/or sponging with tepid water may prove useful, but care must be taken not to induce chilling, as shivering (or, worse, rigors) may result and this will raise body temperature.

Evaluation

The patient will be assessed frequently and appropriately to ensure that objectives of care are being achieved, such as:

- pyrexia and intermittent fevers are detected promptly and the cause of the fever identified by careful assessment and examination;
- hyperpyrexia is effectively managed;
- relevant laboratory specimens are collected and sent for investigation;
- medication is administered as ordered by the physician;
- the patient remains nourished, well hydrated and comfortable.

The need for movement and mobilization

Potential problems	Possible causes
Muscle atrophy, pressure ulcers, deep vein thrombosis	Catabolism, restricted mobility, weakness and bed rest
Ataxia, motor dysfunction, spasticity, sensory disturbances, pain associated with mobilizing	HIV disease, HIV-related neurologic conditions, antiretroviral therapy

Objectives of care

- To prevent the formation of pressure ulcers and deep vein thrombosis.
- To minimize muscle wasting.
- To achieve full mobilization and independence within the limits of the patient's abilities.

Assessment

- Assess the patient's level of independence and ability to mobilize, along with any signs of muscle wasting, pressure ulcers or venous thrombosis. If a neurologic condition is present, the patient will be re-assessed daily.
- If confined to bed, evaluate the patient's ability to move around, sit up and turn on alternate sides.
- Identify any required aids for mobilizing or moving around in bed.
- Determine the level of assistance that is required to ensure safe mobilization/transfer.
- Assess for co-factors that increase the risk of muscle atrophy.
- Evaluate the impact of any neurologic dysfunction on the patient's ability to mobilize.
- Conduct a risk assessment to identify factors that may contribute to pressure ulcers.
- Review current medication regimens and identify any drugs that may contribute to the patient's difficulty in mobilizing.

Nursing interventions

Peripheral neuropathy

HIV-related peripheral neuropathy (PN), usually caused by the direct effect of HIV infection on the peripheral nerves or certain antiretroviral drugs and/or other drugs used for the management of opportunistic infections, commonly occurs during symptomatic HIV disease. Patients with PN experience pain and paraesthesia in their feet, legs or hands. This condition, discussed in detail in Chapter 9, is frequently refractory to treatment and, although a variety of analgesics and the tricyclic antidepressant drugs amitriptyline or nortriptyline may be prescribed, the associated pain may be difficult to alleviate. PN is a common cause of immobility in patients with HIV disease.

Helpful interventions for some but not all patients with PN might include encouraging them to wear soft shoes, such as 'trainers', using light compression stockings or bandages, for example Tubigrip®, foot massage and cool or iced compresses on the feet or hands. Bed cradles to protect the feet from the pressure of bed linen may also be helpful and, although there is no good-quality evidence of efficacy, some patients with PN find acupuncture helpful.

Cumulative muscle atrophy and neurologic dysfunction

Repeated periods of inactivity caused by recurring illness and hospital admissions may lead to progressive and ultimately profound muscle loss, a condition known as cumulative muscle atrophy (CMA). Other health problems, such as various destructive metabolic processes that break down and excrete body proteins, fats and sugars (catabolism), often occurring in late symptomatic HIV disease, and fever, anaemia, malnutrition and tiredness all accelerate the development of CMA, another frequent cause of immobility.

Finally, various HIV-related neurologic dysfunctions, such as ataxia and motor 'slowing', may be present and will further impair the patient's ability to mobilize. Physiotherapy and pressure area care are needed for all patients experiencing impaired mobility.

Physiotherapy

Patients who are able to mobilize safely and independently need to be encouraged to do so. If they need assistance, time needs to be incorporated into daily care plans for this.

Those on bed rest or who are chair-fast require regular active and passive lower limb exercises to help prevent deep vein thrombosis and lower limb atrophy. These patients should be assessed by a physiotherapist who can develop an individualized exercise programme for them and teach them exercises they can do in bed. In addition, a pull-rope attached to the end of the bed or a trapeze bar on a bed frame may prove useful in helping patients move in bed.

Pressure area care

Pressure ulcers, previously known as pressure or bed sores or decubitus ulcers, are generally preventable by competent nursing care. Any patient who is experiencing impaired mobility, especially those on bed rest or those spending prolonged periods in a chair (chair-fast patients), are potentially at risk of developing pressure ulcers. These ulcers frequently occur on well-known pressure points where the weight of the body compresses skin and associated tissues overlying bony prominences (Table 16.4).[3] Several factors contribute to the development of pressure ulcers (Table 16.5) and all patients admitted to hospital should be assessed for their risk for developing them.

TABLE 16.4 Pressure sites

- Ischial tuberosity
- Sacrum
- Heel
- Side of foot
- Knee
- Iliac crest
- Spinous processes
- Scapula
- Shoulder
- Elbow
- Occiput

From Roper N, Logan WW, Tierney AJ. *The Elements of Nursing*, 4th edn. London: Churchill Livingstone, 1996.

There are several well-validated tools in use to identify those patients at risk. The earliest and still the most widely used is the risk assessment tool developed by Norton and colleagues.[12] This tool uses a scoring scale (as illustrated in Figure 16.1): patients with a total score of 14 or less are assessed as prone to develop pressure ulcers, and patients with a total score below 12 are assessed as more likely than not to develop pressure ulcers.

TABLE 16.5 Factors contributing to pressure ulcers

- Pressure
  Compression of tissue
  Shearing force
  Friction
- Moisture on skin
- Heat
- Poor general nutrition
- Lack of spontaneous body movements
- Age
- Medical diagnosis

Norton's scoring scale		
Patient's name:	Date:	

Physical condition:
 Good   4
 Fair   3
 Poor   2 Score: _____
 V.bad   1

Mental condition:
 Alert   4
 Apathetic   3
 Confused   2 Score: _____
 Stuporous   1

Activity:
 Ambulant   4
 Walk/help   3
 Chairbound 2 Score: _____
 Bedfast   1

Mobility:
 Full   4
 Sl.limited   3
 V.limited   2 Score: _____
 Immobile   1

Incontinent:
 Not   4
 Occasionally 3
 Usually/ur.   2 Score: _____
 Doubly   1

* * * Total score:

FIGURE 16.1 *Norton's scoring scale for pressure ulcer risk.*

Another risk assessment method widely used in the UK is the pressure scoring system developed by Waterlow (as shown in Table 16.6).[13,14] Total scores indicate whether patients are 'at risk' (10+), 'high risk' (15+), or 'very high risk' (20+) of developing pressure ulcers.

Both of these tools are easy to use, but their accuracy is dependent upon subjective judgements made by the assessor. Nurses need to assess all patients admitted to hospital or ill in the community for their risk for developing pressure ulcers, using whatever risk assessment tool has been adopted in their own healthcare facility or service. The risk for the development of pressure ulcers is assessed on admission and weekly thereafter, or whenever there is any significant change in the patient's condition and/or circumstances of care. For those assessed as at risk, a 'Relief of pressure' chart (as illustrated in Figure 16.2) should be commenced.

TABLE 16.6 Waterlow pressure sore prevention/treatment policy[13,14]

Build/weight for height	*	Skin type Visual risk areas	*	Sex Age	*	Special risks	*
Average	0	Healthy	0	Male	1	**Tissue malnutrition**	*
Above average	1	Tissue paper	1	Female	2	e.g.	
Obese	2	Dry	1	14–49	1	terminal cachexia	8
Below average	3	Oedematous	1	50–64	2	cardiac failure	5
		Clammy (temp)	1	65–74	3	peripheral vascular	5
		Discoloured	2	75–80	4	disease	
		Broken/spot	3	81+ 1	5	anaemia	2
						smoking	1
Continence	*	Mobility	*	Appetite	*		
Complete/catheterized	0	Fully	0	Average	0	**Neurological deficit**	*
Occasional incontinence	1	Restless/fidgety	1	Poor	1	e.g.	
Catheterized/incontinent	2	Apathetic	2	N.G	2	diabetes, MS, CVA	4–6
of faeces		Restricted	3	tube/fluids only		motor/sensory	
Double incontinence	3	Inert traction	4	NBM/anorexic	3	paraplegia	
		Chairbound	5				
						Major surgery/trauma	*
						Orthopaedic	5
						Below waist spinal	5
						On table >2 hours	
						Medication	*
						Cytotoxics	4
						High-dose steroids	
						Anti-inflammation	

Score: 10+, at risk; 15+, high risk; 20+, very high risk.
Ring scores in table, add total, several scores per category can be used.
N.G., nasogastric; NBM, nothing by mouth; MS, multiple sclerosis; CVA, cerebrovascular accident.

Preventing pressure ulcers

Patients assessed as at risk for developing pressure ulcers require regular repositioning for pressure area relief. The optimal frequency for regular repositioning has not been established. It is best assessed for each individual patient judged to be at risk in relation to the condition of the skin after 1 hour in a constant position. Consequently, nurses may judge that a particular patient may require repositioning every 2 hours, every hour or even more frequently than every hour.[15] The massage of pressure areas with various body lotions and creams is no longer recommended and should not be done because of the risk of damage to the skin.[16] Because it is the weight of the body on pressure points that causes pressure ulcers, the relief of pressure is at the centre of all care strategies designed to prevent them. **Carefully repositioning the patient at regular intervals is the single most effective measure for preventing pressure ulcers**. Using pressure-reducing/relieving aids, such as pressure-reducing cushions, bed cradles and natural sheepskin fleeces (when in chairs), can also help prevent pressure ulcers. In addition, various pressure-reducing/relieving beds are now available, which are useful for preventing pressure ulcers in those at most risk.[15] Air, rubber or foam rings are no longer recommended.[15,17]

Relief of pressure chart				
Date	Time	Position of patient	Relief of pressure achieved by	Nurse's signature
12/11	0800	Lying on back	Turned on left side	C. Jones
''	1000	LYING ON LEFT SIDE	TURNED ON RIGHTSIDE	E. KARN
ʌ	1200	Lying on right side	Turned on to back	J. Baird
ʋ	1400	Lying on back	Turned on left side	A. Hilton

FIGURE 16.2 *Relief of pressure chart.*

Nurses must be skilful in moving and repositioning patients in order to prevent shearing force to pressure points. The skin needs to be kept clean, and excessive moisture and friction need to be minimized. Dehydration, malnutrition and anaemia are all factors that may lead to the development of pressure ulcers and, when possible, these must be corrected.

Evaluation

The patient will be assessed frequently and appropriately to ensure that objectives of care are being achieved, such as:

- there is effective nursing care to promote mobilization and independence and avoid pressure ulcers, venous thrombosis and excessive muscle wasting;
- underlying causes of pressure ulcers, venous thrombosis and muscle atrophy are alleviated, if possible;
- where pressure ulcers are present, further tissue damage is prevented and there is effective wound care to promote healing;
- pain resulting from peripheral neuropathy is effectively managed.

The need for a safe environment

Potential problems	Possible causes
Increased risk for healthcare-associated infections	Immunodeficiency-associated infections Neutropenia, secondary to HIV disease or associated drug therapy Medical devices, e.g. indwelling urethral catheters, peripheral intravenous or central venous catheters
Accidents	Weakness Confusion secondary to neurological conditions, infections, change in environment and routine Impaired vision secondary to cytomegalovirus retinopathy Hospital environment and equipment
Fire	Oxygen therapy Cigarette smoking

Objectives of care

- Provide a safe environment for care and recovery.
- Minimize the risk of confusion due to a change in environment and routine.
- Prevent healthcare-associated infections.
- Minimize the risk of accidents and fire.

Assessment

- Assess the patient's mental status and orientation and determine his or her ability to understand and co-operate with nursing care.
- Assess the patient's level of independence/dependence and ability to mobilize safely.
- Review the patient's medication regimen, identifying any drugs that may cause confusion or other side effects that may put the patient at an increased risk for accidents or healthcare-associated infections.
- Review the patient's physical condition, noting any history of visual impairment, vertigo, seizures, syncope (fainting) or falls, and assess the level of weakness and debilitation, if present.
- Be aware of the patient's laboratory assessments that may indicate an increased risk for accidents or infections, such as the presence of anaemia, neutropenia.
- Identify any environmental hazards present that may predispose to accidents, such as medical devices, oxygen, hospital equipment, bed height.
- Assess the risks for healthcare-associated infections.
- Assess the patient's ability to understand and co-operate in measures designed to prevent fire.

Nursing interventions

Infection prevention

In addition to the ever-present risk of clinical disease developing from previously acquired latent infections (opportunistic infections), all immunocompromised patients are at further risk for new infections when they are admitted to hospital or are receiving clinical care from community or primary care services. These infections are known as **healthcare-associated infections (HAIs)** and, during the last two decades, they occurred in 9 per cent of patients admitted to hospitals in England[18,19] and probably occurred at the same rate in most hospitals in other UK countries and in most countries in the European Union (EU) and North America. The risk for HAI increases if invasive medical devices are used, such as indwelling urethral catheters or peripheral intravenous or central venous catheters.

There is good evidence from outbreak situations to show that the contaminated hands of healthcare workers are frequently responsible for transmitting infections to patients. **Effective hand decontamination immediately before each and every episode of direct patient contact/care and after any activity or contact that potentially results in the hands becoming contaminated** is the single most important measure that nurses and other healthcare professionals can take to reduce the incidence of HAI.[6,11] National evidence-based guidelines in England describe **Standard Principles** for preventing healthcare-associated infections[6,11] and define key points for effective hand hygiene that all nurses and other healthcare professionals need to observe (Table 16.7). It is not always necessary to *wash* hands to achieve effective decontamination, and the introduction of alcohol-based hand rubs offers a practical and acceptable alternative to hand washing when the hands are not grossly soiled.[11,20]

TABLE 16.7 Key points for hand hygiene[6,11]

- Hands must be decontaminated immediately before each and every episode of direct patient contact
- Hands must be washed if they are visibly or potentially contaminated with dirt or organic material
- Alcohol-based hand rub may be used to decontaminate hands between caring for different patients and different caring activities for the same patient
- Effective technique ensures thorough hand decontamination and protects skin integrity

Disposable gloves are worn whenever there is a potential for exposure to blood, body fluids, secretions and excretions and for all contact with instruments contaminated with blood or other body fluids, and with non-intact skin or mucous membranes during general care and invasive procedures.[6,11] Because gloves can leak, hands need to be decontaminated after gloves have been removed.

A clean hospital environment is also important in preventing HAI, and national guidelines clearly require that both the environment and the equipment used within the environment are clean, that statutory regulations are met and that staff involved in hospital hygiene are aware of their important role in helping to prevent HAI.[6,11]

These same guidelines also describe evidence-based interventions that nurses and other healthcare professionals need to adhere to in caring for patients with indwelling urethral catheters and central venous catheters.[6–8] These and other measures are described in more detail in Chapter 14, which focuses on infection prevention and control.

Neutropenic patients

As discussed in Chapter 7, both HIV infection and the antiretroviral, cytotoxic and some antibiotic drugs used to treat HIV disease or its complications are frequently associated with the suppression of blood cell formation (haematopoiesis). This leads to the development of a variety of blood cell deficiencies (cytopenias), including anaemia, neutropenia and thrombocytopenia.

Neutropenia (also known as granulocytopenia or agranulocytosis) is a disorder in which there is a reduction in the number of neutrophils. The normal neutrophil count varies with ethnic background, but the lower limits of normal are generally over 1500 cells/mm³ (µL), but may be lower in some races. Neutrophils, along with basophils and eosinophils, are white blood cells that collectively are known as granulocytes (or polymorphonuclear leucocytes). Neutrophils make up the majority of granulocytes and they are the principal phagocytic cells in the blood, protecting people from bacterial infections. Consequently, a reduction in the number of neutrophils will increase a patient's vulnerability to both new and opportunistic bacterial and fungal infections, and it has been suggested that up to three-quarters of all patients will experience neutropenia during the course of HIV disease.[21,22]

Neutropenia is classified according to the neutrophil count and the corresponding relative risk for infection (Table 16.8). A variety of pyogenic infections occur in patients with

TABLE 16.8 Classifying neutropenia

Neutrophil count	Relative risk for infection
1000–1500/µL	Mild
500–1000/µL	Moderate
Less then 500/µL	Severe°

° see Table 16.9.

profound neutropenia (Table 16.9), and acute, severe neutropenia is often life threatening in immunocompromised patients.

TABLE 16.9 Infections frequently encountered in patients with severe neutropenia

- Cutaneous cellulites
- Liver abscesses
- Furnuculosis
- Pneumonia
- Bloodstream infections (septicaemia)
- Stomatitis
- Gingivitis
- Peri-rectal inflammation
- Colitis
- Sinusitis
- Otitis media

Because patients who have significant reductions in their neutrophil count are at an increased risk of acquiring new bacterial infections (in addition to opportunistic bacterial infections arising from their own bacterial flora), they are generally nursed in a conventional single room. There is evidence to show that this, along with standard infection prevention principles,[6,11] is as effective in preventing new infections in neutropenic patients as was the older system of 'reverse barrier nursing' (protective isolation), which is now rarely employed for patients with HIV disease.[23-25] If patients have invasive medical devices, such as indwelling urethral catheters or peripheral intravenous or central venous catheters, infection prevention guidelines must be scrupulously adhered to.[6-8] Nurses, other healthcare professionals, visitors and patients who are suffering from infections, for example the common cold, should not have contact with patients who are severely neutropenic. All immunocompromised patients must be protected against contact with people who have contagious diseases (such as tuberculosis, varicella, bacterial pneumonia and influenza) when they are in hospital. It is important to explain carefully to patients the rationale underpinning any infection prevention precautions, especially when they are admitted to a single room, which they may find isolating.

Chemoprophylaxis with co-trimoxazole (Septrin®) may be prescribed to prevent *Pneumocystis carinii* pneumonia and to reduce the incidence of bacterial infections, but it is important to remember that this drug is myelosuppressive and may further worsen the underlying neutropenia. Cytokine therapy with haematopoietic growth factors may be used to stimulate the production of neutrophils. These factors include recombinant human granulocyte-colony stimulating factor (**G-CSF**), also known as filgrastim (Neupogen®) or lenograstim (Granocyte®), and recombinant human granulocyte macrophage-colony stimulating factor (**GM-CSF**), also known as molgramostim (Leucomax®). These cytokines are administered by either intravenous infusion or subcutaneous injection and are all associated with significant side effects. Nurses administering these agents need to consult closely the product literature and/or the current edition of the *BNF*[9] (see 'Internet resources' at the end of this chapter) to familiarize themselves with the wide range of side effects and drug interactions associated with these cytokines, and treatment with either should only be prescribed and administered by those experienced in their use.

Preventing accidents

When admitted to hospital, many patients have some degree of confusion and disorientation due to a new and foreign environment. Patients may have underlying HIV-related medical conditions, such as neurological disease and visual impairment, which can cause confusion and disability, and this can increase the risk for accidents. Many drugs can cause confusion, vertigo, unsteady gait or hypotension. In addition, stress, difficulties in mobilization, weakness and any intellectual impairment all compound the risk for accidents.

Patients with a history of syncope, falling or seizures are assessed as being particularly vulnerable to having an accident. If a nursing assessment indicates that seizures may occur, special care is required, ensuring that an airway and suction are available at the bedside and the bed is kept in the low position.

A careful (and ongoing) **nursing assessment** will identify those most at risk of accidents and an **environmental risk assessment** will help nurses and other healthcare professionals modify the care setting to minimize this risk. The following aspects must be taken into account when care is planned in order to maintain a safe environment and prevent accidents.

- **Oxygen.** When oxygen is in use, cigarette smoking is not allowed (and is generally not allowed in hospitals unless there is a designated smoking area) and 'Hazard' notices are prominently displayed in the patient's room or by the bedside. If spanners (wrenches) are needed for oxygen tanks, 'non-sparking' wrenches must be used.
- **Equipment.** All equipment must be carefully put away after use so that it does not present a hazard to patients who are ambulatory. It is essential that a clear pathway is maintained between the patient's bed and the toilet.
- **Bedrails.** If patients are confused or sedated, bedside rails are kept in the upright position when they are in bed, the bed is kept in the low position and the patients are closely observed. More patients probably suffer accidents trying to get out of bed when the bedrails have been raised than those who fall out of bed when there are no bedrails in place, so it is important to remain vigilant if the bedrails have been raised. This is especially so for those patients with diarrhoea or frequency and urgency associated with urination, who may suddenly need to get out of bed to use the toilet and who are reluctant to use the nurse-call system.
- **Fire.** In addition to the risk of fire associated with the use of medical gases such as oxygen, fires can occur from a variety of sources in all healthcare facilities. Nurses need to know, and have frequent drills in, how to respond appropriately to different types of fires, locate and activate fire alarms, appropriately use available fire-fighting equipment and safely and efficiently evacuate patients from an area where they are in danger from fire. During evacuations, it is important not to forget to evacuate patients in single rooms, especially those in negative pressure rooms into which smoke and fire will quickly be drawn because they have a lower atmospheric pressure than the outside corridor.
- **Noise.** Hospital activities are frequently noisy and patients need protection from this, as noise can cause irritation, difficulty in concentrating and thinking, discomfort, stress and lack of rest and sleep. Although noise may not directly cause accidents, it is detrimental to care and recovery and every effort must be made by nurses to identify potential sources of noise and develop strategies to decrease noise as an environmental pollutant.

- **Miscellaneous**. Floors need to be kept clean and dry and corridors need to be well lit and free of clutter. The nurse-call system should be checked to ensure that it is working properly and positioned within easy reach of the patient.

Evaluation

The patient will be assessed frequently and appropriately to ensure that objectives of care are being achieved, such as:

- patient factors that may predispose to accidents or infections and potential environmental safety hazards are identified and documented by a comprehensive nursing and environmental risk assessment and, where possible, rectified;
- good standards of infection prevention and control practices reduce the risk of patients acquiring healthcare-associated infections;
- consequently, the patient does not have an accident while in hospital and does not acquire a new infection.

The need for personal cleansing and dressing

Potential problems	Possible causes
Poor oral hygiene	Dehydration
	Malnutrition
	Infections
	Pain
	Oral or peri-oral lesions
	Inflammatory conditions of the oropharynx
Inadequate body hygiene	Dependence
	Immobility
	Lack of privacy
	Confusion
	Lethargy
	Incontinence
Loss of skin integrity	Infections
	Psoriasis, eczema, dermatitis
	Pressure ulcers
	Molluscum contagiosum
	Scabies
	Drug reactions

Objectives of care

- Maintain good oral hygiene.
- Preserve the integrity and cleanliness of the integumentary system (skin).

Assessment

- Assess the need for mouth care, identifying the current state of oral health, usual mouth care routine (tooth brushing, dental flossing), fluid and dietary intake, underlying physical and mental conditions that may interfere with maintaining good oral health, and medications that may affect the oral mucosa.
- Determine the level of independence/dependence being experienced by the patient and assess the need for personal care assistance to help the patient maintain body hygiene.

- Identify any underlying medical conditions that may disrupt the integrity of the skin.
- Assess the need for pain control.

Nursing interventions

Mouth care

Mobile patients should be encouraged to brush their teeth with a soft toothbrush after each meal (or at least twice daily) and taught how to use dental floss or dental tape to keep the teeth clean. Patients on bed rest or who are chair bound should be assisted with tooth brushing after each meal (or at least twice daily). Glycerine and lemon mouth care swabs may be used for those patients who are not able to brush their teeth, and mouthwash solutions may be useful for patients who have a dry mouth or halitosis (bad breath).

Patients who are *nil by mouth* or who have painful oral conditions, such as aphthous ulcers, that prevent brushing can clean and refresh the mouth using mouth care swabs and mouth rinses. Analgesia may be needed for patients with painful oral conditions.

Candida albicans is a common opportunistic infection that may cause thrush or other forms of stomatitis. Sometimes this is the result of therapy with broad-spectrum antibiotics, but in most patients with HIV disease it simply reflects their degree of immunosuppression. Treatment with antifungal preparations such as nystatin (Nystan®) or amphotericin (Fungilin®) lozenges or oral suspension, miconazole oral gel (Daktarin®) or systemic anti-fungal medication may be needed. If miconazole oral gel is used, nurses need to be aware that this is absorbed systemically and potential drug interactions need to be considered. Oral ketoconazole (Nizoral®) or oral or (less commonly) intravenous fluconazole (Diflucan®) or itraconazole (Sproanox®) is sometimes used. These drugs are discussed in more detail in Chapter 7, where Table 7.5 lists the common antifungal drugs currently in use and Table 7.6 describes the interactions between the 'azole' (imidazole) group of antifungal drugs (flu-conazole, ketoconazole, itraconazole) and some antiretroviral drugs. Candidal oesophagitis may occur, as may disseminated candidiasis, in some patients with late symptomatic HIV disease and both of these serious conditions require systemic antifungal therapy.

Body hygiene

Cleansing and grooming are both individual and personal. Although patients with fever or incontinence or seriously ill and/or weak patients may require specific interventions to maintain cleanliness, the regularity and timing of personal cleansing should be left to the discretion of each individual patient whenever possible. Those confined to bed should be offered a daily bed bath and the opportunity to wash their hair once or twice per week. If a patient declines, or asks to be helped later, this should be respected whenever possible. Patients must also be given the opportunity to wash their hands before eating and after toileting. Those with fever and/or night sweats may need assistance in washing and drying, and a change of nightclothes and bed linen will be needed after an episode of diaphoresis (sweating).

Patients should be encouraged or helped to keep the skin well moisturized, and the use of a simple moisturizer, such as aqueous cream, is ideal.

Those who are ambulatory should be encouraged to wear their ordinary, outdoor clothes during the day, and to be as mobile as their condition permits.

Preventing pressure ulcers

Regular assessment and preventative measures, as described previously, for preventing pressure ulcers are needed for all patients except those who are fully ambulatory.

Skin conditions

As people with HIV disease become progressively more immunocompromised, they frequently develop various skin conditions, such as seborrhoeic dermatitis, psoriasis and eczema, that are uncomfortable and distressing. Additionally, severely immunosuppressed patients are prone to a variety of infectious skin diseases, such as staphylococcal infection (impetigo), acneform folliculitis, and herpes simplex and varicella zoster viral infections. Fungal infections, such as tinea cruris (Jock itch), are also relatively common. Patients with these conditions can be helped by the provision of reassurance, comfort and advice and by prescribed medications and treatments. Itching and irritation can often be relieved by a cool bath (the water being just slightly lower than room temperature). Patients need to be encouraged not to scratch skin lesions because this delays healing and may cause secondary infection and scarring.

Some rashes and more serious skin conditions may occur as adverse effects of antiretroviral therapy and other drugs used for the prevention or treatment of opportunistic infections. **Stevens–Johnson syndrome** is a severe (and potentially life-threatening) form of erythema multiforme, an inflammatory eruption of large, fluid-filled blisters (bullae) on the oral mucosa, pharynx, anogenital region and conjunctiva. Patients with this serious condition are febrile and will have 'target-like' lesions on the skin. This condition can occur with the administration of several antibiotics, especially sulphonamides such as co-trimoxazole (Septrin®). In people with HIV disease, this syndrome may also occur as an adverse effect of treatment with some non-nucleoside reverse transcriptase inhibitors, such as nevirapine (Viramune®) and, less commonly, efavirenz (Sustiva®). The syndrome is also seen as an adverse effect of treatment with some antituberculosis drugs, especially with the use of thiacetazone in people co-infected with HIV. Thiacetazone is only used in some countries in the industrially developing world and is not used in the EU, North America or Australasia. The occurrence of this syndrome is a medical emergency, and the physician will discontinue any offending drugs and prescribe immediate intravenous or intramuscular corticosteroid therapy with drugs such as hydrocortisone or dexamethasone. Intravenous fluids are usually commenced and, when the patient can swallow, prednisolone gradually replaces parenterally administered steroids.

Shingles (herpes zoster) is caused by a reactivation of varicella-zoster virus (VZV) infection (the same virus that causes chickenpox), usually acquired during childhood. Shingles is frequently seen in people with both early and late symptomatic HIV disease, in whom it may cause severe illness because of the underlying immunosuppression. This condition is generally treated with high-dose aciclovir (Zovirax®) and analgesia is usually required.

Infection prevention

Patients with infectious skin conditions should be nursed in a single room with en suite toilet and bath/shower facilities and encouraged to shower rather then bathe. If they cannot use the shower, the addition of an antibacterial agent such as triclosan 2 per cent (Ster-Zac Bath Concentrate®) to their bath may be useful in preventing secondary infection.

Patients with unhealed zoster lesions (or chickenpox) are isolated in a single room and preferably one with negative-pressure ventilation. VZV is an airborne infection and can be transmitted from unhealed zoster lesions to other immunocompromised vulnerable individuals, in whom it may cause primary VZV infection, i.e. chickenpox, a potentially devastating condition in HIV-infection individuals. Nurses and other healthcare professionals without a previous history of chickenpox, or who are serologically negative for VZV antibodies, are excluded from caring for a patient with shingles (or chickenpox) until zoster lesions have healed. Visitors without a previous history of chickenpox, especially if they may be immunocompromised, need to be alerted to this risk.

Personal clothing from people with infectious skin conditions which becomes contaminated can safely be disinfected by washing in a washing machine with ordinary detergents, on the hot cycle. Patients should have their own toothbrush and razor; these should not be shared with anyone else.

Evaluation

The patient will be assessed frequently and appropriately to ensure that objectives of care are being achieved, such as:

- cleaning and grooming are carried out according to the patient's wishes;
- any impediments to good oral and body hygiene are identified and a plan of care implemented that ensures mouth care and assistance with body hygiene;
- the mouth and skin remain clean, intact and free of secondary infections;
- treatment and reassurance are given as appropriate where skin integrity is compromised;
- pain associated with oral or skin lesions is controlled.

The need for expression and communication

Potential problems	Possible causes
Impaired cognition	
Disorientation	HIV-related neurological conditions, medication, fever, pain, stress, dehydration, hypoxia, substance misuse, e.g. alcohol
Isolation and loneliness	Depression, fear of contagion by family, friends, healthcare workers
	Being nursed in a single room
	Excessive or inappropriate infection prevention precautions

Objectives of care

- Promote effective communications and supportive relationships with healthcare professionals.
- Minimize the effects of neurological dysfunction.
- Encourage the maintenance of social contacts with people important to the patient.
- Prevent the deleterious effects of social isolation.

Assessment

- Establish the patient's usual communication patterns and first language.
- Assess the patient's orientation to time, place and events.
- Confirm and document visitors the patient wishes to see (and any he or she does not wish to see).
- Document carefully and clearly who is aware of the patient's diagnosis (HIV status).

Nursing interventions

Reality orientation

All patients need to be orientated to the ward and the daily ward routine. Basic information needs to be given, such as where the toilets and shower/bathing facilities are, meal times, visitor regulations, fire precautions and evacuation procedures and, importantly, when the patient can expect to see their doctor. Patients who are confused need to be gently reminded of their environment, day and date and reassured that they are safe.

During the initial assessment, it is important to find out how the patient wishes to be addressed. It is generally useful if first names are used when speaking to the patient unless he or she has objected to this. There is nothing wrong in nurses using their own first names when talking to patients and this will generally help build a better relationship between nurse and patient. The patient should be introduced to other patients and healthcare professionals and to the nurse in charge and the nurse principally responsible for their care (the 'named nurse' or primary nurse). All healthcare staff should wear identification badges and/or badges that state their name and role.

Communication aids

The patient should have easy access to a telephone, stamps and stationery. If in a single room, it may be possible for the patient to have a television set. The patient should have a bedside radio (with earphones), newspapers and magazines. The nurse-call system must always be within easy reach of the patient. There should be a clock and a calendar in the patient's room.

If a patient has difficulty communicating in English, interpreters should be arranged and visitors should be encouraged to provide newspapers and magazines in the patient's first language.

The use of technical language and jargon should be kept to a minimum and, when used, carefully explained to the patient.

Time for talking/listening/touching

Nursing care plans must take into account the fact that patients need to talk to their nurses. Listening, holding a patient's hand and just quietly being with the patient are necessary aspects of nursing art. Complex social or psychological concerns may be appropriately referred to a counsellor or mental health nurse consultant.

Visitors

Caring for the patient's visitors is often a delicate task, especially if they do not know the patient's diagnosis, sexual orientation or usual lifestyle. **No information on any aspect of the patient's condition may be given to any visitors, no matter who they are, without the patient's express consent**. With the patient's permission, visitors should be encouraged. The partner of a homosexual patient often assumes the role of the patient's next of kin, which must be respected. As always, all visitors to the hospital must be treated with respect and consistent courtesy. An officious or abrupt manner displayed by healthcare workers to visitors can do immeasurable damage to their willingness to visit and is demoralizing to the patient. If possible, friends and family should be encouraged to visit throughout the day and early evening. If the patient is seriously ill, arrangements should be made for visitors to stay throughout the night.

Some patients may have been abandoned by both friends and family. With the patient's permission, it is possible to contact voluntary support groups who can arrange for members from their organization to visit the patient. The hospital's voluntary services may also be able to provide this service.

Infection prevention

Patients with HIV disease generally do not require any infection prevention precautions in addition to those for other patients, and the use of Standard Principles (Universal

Precautions) for preventing infections is sufficient to prevent nosocomial and healthcare-associated infections in hospital, community and primary care settings.[6,11] Excessive infection prevention precautions, such as inappropriate isolation or protective clothing, are barriers between the patient and other human beings and must be avoided. Patients who are fully ambulatory should be encouraged to use communal ward facilities, such as sitting rooms and television rooms, and to mix with other patients.

Evaluation

The patient will be assessed frequently and appropriately to ensure that objectives of care are being achieved, such as:

- care is planned to allow patients both space and time to communicate with their families, friends and healthcare workers and to remain orientated to their environment and condition,
- the disorientating and isolating effects of any neurological dysfunctions are minimized.
- feelings of loneliness, rejection and isolation are addressed.

The need for working and playing

Potential problems	Possible causes
Economic hardship	Loss of employment
Mental deterioration	Boredom, neurologic disease, loneliness

Objectives of care

- Provide access to appropriate financial resources.
- Minimize effects of boredom and loneliness.

Assessment

- Assess the effects of absence from usual employment and lifestyle. The nursing history should include information relating to any dependants the patient may have and how loss of earnings will affect the patient.
- Document the patient's past leisure time activities, hobbies and interests.
- Assess the patient's neurological status and the presence of any sensory deficits or physical disablement.
- Ascertain whether the patient expects visits from partner, friends and family.

Nursing interventions

Financial problems

It is probable that all patients with long-term illness, including HIV disease, will eventually need to claim various state benefits to which they are entitled. As the social security system is confusing and complex, the patient should be interviewed by a social worker as soon as possible following admission.

In the UK, individuals with HIV disease can obtain information about benefits and entitlements from specialist welfare advisers at a variety of non-governmental organizations, including the Terrence Higgins Trust (Telephone 020 7831 0330). In addition, advice is available from the Citizen's Advice Bureau (CAB), which has several centres in cities throughout England (London, Brighton, Birmingham, Carlisle) that specialize in providing HIV-related benefits advice. The prompt issue of medical and sickness certificates while the patient is in hospital is important and should not be left until the patient asks for them. Another real issue for some patients who are having financial difficulties is their ability to maintain rent or mortgage payments. The hospital social worker will be able to advise patients about their housing situation and may also be able to assist those who have been dismissed by their employers as a result of illness.

Leisure-time activities

It is important that patients have access to television viewing and a radio. The library services of the hospital should be explained and arrangements made for the patient to purchase newspapers and magazines. A comfortable area for sitting and socializing can provide patients with a change of scenery and promote social interaction. This room needs to be accessible at all times and patients need to be made aware of its location. An occupational therapy assessment may be indicated for some patients. Special interests and hobbies should be encouraged.

Visitors

Visiting times must be flexible and visitors encouraged. Where appropriate, visitors can be encouraged to take patients off the ward, as this can provide a very welcome break from the monotony of ward life. It is also necessary to respect the patients' privacy when partners are visiting and allow them the time and space to be with one another without interruption.

If the patient has no visitors, with his or her permission, the volunteer services or a voluntary organization may be able to arrange for someone to visit. The largest voluntary organization in the UK for patients with AIDS is the Terrence Higgins Trust. It is also important for patients to have visits from healthcare workers, especially if they are being nursed in single rooms. Time must be made available to visit and talk to the patient rather than only entering the room to 'do' something.

Evaluation

The patient will be assessed frequently and appropriately to ensure that objectives of care are being achieved, such as:

- all necessary assistance to deal with claiming benefit entitlements, planning leisure-time activities and arranging for visitors has been facilitated;

The need to maintain psychological equilibrium

Potential problems	Possible causes
Ineffective coping	Loss of control
Social isolation	Withdrawal of social supports Isolation in hospital
Loss of self-esteem	Guilt, altered body image, stigma of HIV infection, perception of self as contagious
Anxiety	Stress associated with progressive, chronic illness, fear of loss of confidentiality
Depression	Helplessness, grief associated with loss of: personal relationships, self-esteem, physical potency, control, sexuality, effective role in life

Objectives of care

- Allow the patient to express feelings and emotions.

- Participate in therapeutic strategies designed to alleviate predisposing factors to psychological dysfunction.
- Facilitate referrals to appropriate support personnel/agencies.

Assessment

- Assess for any indications of psychological distress, such as anxiety, depression, ineffective coping, feelings of isolation and low self-esteem.
- Ascertain the patient's level and source of emotional and social support.

Nursing interventions

Anxiety

Anxiety is neither inappropriate nor uncommon in people with serious chronic illness, including those with HIV disease, especially during periods of hospitalization. Manifestations of anxiety occur on several levels, ranging from mild tension to sympathetic nervous system overflow and panic (Table 16.10). Most patients will require assistance in coping with excessive anxiety.

TABLE 16.10 Levels of anxiety

Level 1 (Mild)

The patient is alert, enquiring, relatively relaxed and defence mechanisms are working well. In this level, patients are receptive to information.

Level 2 (Moderate)

Increased alertness and heightened emotional state. The patient is more receptive to sensory information than factual information and is able to learn relaxation techniques. In this level, patients are able to solve most problems on their own.

Level 3 (Severe)

Sympathetic nervous system overflow is present, with typical fight-or-flight responses. With severe anxiety, patients are no longer able to solve problems on their own, needing the advocate skills of the nurse. Physical signs and symptoms of anxiety are often present such as tachycardia, restlessness, irritability and a feeling of 'butterflies in the stomach'. The patient is frightened.

Level 4 (Panic)

The patient is overwhelmed by fear and is unable to concentrate, having more pronounced physical signs of sympathetic over-activity, such as insomnia, tachycardia, profuse perspiration (especially on the palms and forehead), frequency of micturition and defaecation, rapid breathing and vertigo.

Patients do not progress from level 1 through to level 4, but fluctuate from one level to another. Stressful events (Table 16.11) occurring during illness may precipitate progression to more severe levels of anxiety. Interventions designed to alleviate excessive anxiety include discussing patients' fears with them, rationally highlighting their identifiable strengths to cope with stressors, and encouraging socialization and leisure-time activities. Most hospitals have qualified counsellors and clinical psychologists on their staff who can offer more skilled assistance to the patient in alleviating anxiety and teaching relaxation techniques. Severe anxiety or panic generally requires anxiolytic medication (Table 16.12), which is more useful for the short-term management of acute anxiety than for long-term use.

Depression

Clinical depression is common in people with chronic illness and its early recognition allows prompt treatment. Patients may despair, complain of sleep disturbances (early morning

offer spiritual as well as physical support to patients by such simple activities as just listening and talking, especially at times of increased stress and worry, 'being there' for a patient when they need support and creating an environment in hospital in which the patient is facilitated to worship, pray and observe religious practices and rites.

Facilitating worship

Chaplains and other religious advisers must, at the patient's wish, have complete access. Patients should not be visited by religious advisers whom they have not requested to see. Often patients can be taken to the hospital chapel for religious services or to pray. It is essential that Christian patients have the opportunity of attending Confession and of receiving holy sacraments. The Sacrament of the Anointing of the Sick (Extreme Unction or Last Rites) is extremely important for many Christian patients, and the wish to be administered this sacrament should be documented in the patient's nursing notes. The Sacrament of Holy Communion is important to members of the Church of England and the Roman Catholic Church and of many other Christian religions. At the patient's request, chaplains can make available religious literature and a Bible. Religion is diverse and it is important to respect individual religious beliefs. Every effort should be made by healthcare professionals to recognize and encourage the practices involved within all of the diverse religious beliefs that patients may have. The opportunity to participate in religious worship is a tremendous comfort to many patients who are ill in hospital with HIV-related conditions.

Evaluation

The patient will be assessed frequently and appropriately to ensure that objectives of care are being achieved, such as:

- the patient has opportunities to worship and be comforted by his or her religious beliefs.

The need to express sexuality

Potential problems	Possible causes
Need to modify sexual behaviour	Infectious nature of HIV disease
Development of unsafe patterns of sexual behaviour	Lack of awareness of safer forms of sexual practices, denial, rebellion, anger
Loss of libido and/or erectile dysfunction	Progressive illness, guilt, anxiety, depression
Grief associated with perceived loss of sexuality	Infectiousness, changing body image, loss of sexual partner

Objectives of care

- Facilitate sexual health.
- Provide patients with information about safer sex.

Assessment

- Assess current sexual health status.
- Ascertain the patient's attitude to and knowledge of safer sexual practices.
- Identify any underlying physical or mental health problems that may be interfering with the patient's ability to express his or her sexuality.

Nursing interventions

Sexuality and sexual health

Sexuality is at the core of our personality and it is an essential element of our personhood.[27] It is 'a powerful and purposeful aspect of human nature and it is an important dimension of our humanness'[28] It is the way we individually and uniquely express and project our identity and inter-relate our physiological and psychosocial processes, which are inherent in the way we sexually develop and sexually respond, both to ourselves and to others.[27,28]

Sexuality is more than just overt sexual behaviour; it spans and underlies the complete range of human experience and contributes to our lives, and to the lives of our family, friends, neighbours, colleagues and clients in many ways.

In positively expressing our sexuality, we are able to build our unique identity, to communicate subtle, gentle or intense feelings, to realize sexual pleasure and physical release, to emotionally bond with others, to achieve a sense of self-worth and, for many, to link with the future through their children.[27] Being able to positively express our sexuality is one of the most joyful and enriching aspects of the human experience, which for many people in socially and economically deprived communities and countries helps compensate for many of the less positive aspects of living in our world today. It is an aspect of life to which all people are entitled and which, for many, makes waking up in the morning worthwhile, purposeful and exciting. Being able to positively express our individual sexuality is an essential component of experiencing a healthy sexual life (Table 16.14) and informs the whole of our lives.

TABLE 16.14 Positive sexuality

Experiencing a healthy sexual life includes:

- having access to sexual information and developing knowledge in relation to sexual and reproductive phenomena
- freedom from unwanted pregnancies and abusive sexual behaviour *and*
- being able to integrate the physical, emotional, intellectual and social aspects of sexual being, in ways that are positively enriching and that enhance personality, communication and love[29] *and*
- having an ability to create effective relationships with members of both sexes
- developing a self-awareness and appreciation of our feelings and attitudes towards sexuality and sexual behaviour
- having a positive self-image *and*
- developing a value system that can assist sexual decision-making
- having some degree of emotional comfort, interdependence and stability with respect to the sexual activities in which we participate[27] *and*
- a capacity to enjoy and control sexual and reproductive behaviour in accordance with a social and personal ethic
- freedom from fear, shame, guilt, false beliefs and other psychological factors inhibiting sexual response and impairing sexual relationships *and*
- freedom from organic disorders, diseases and deficiencies that interfere with sexual and reproductive functions[30]

Positive sexuality is associated with high self-esteem, respect for self and others, non-exploitive sexual satisfaction, rewarding human relationships and, for many, the joy of desired parenthood.

Sexuality is socially and culturally constructed, and concepts of sexuality have changed over time and remain dynamic today. There are significant individual, social and cultural variations in sexual values, accepted behaviour and sexual practices in different communities throughout the world, which will impact on the ability of an individual to positively express their sexuality.

However, most people would agree that the ability to positively express our sexuality is a major determinant of our sexual and reproductive health, which in turn is an important element of our physical and mental health. Everyone has an inalienable right to health, including sexual health (Table 16.15), and being able to positively express our sexuality is a natural aspiration for most people. HIV disease can have a significant impact on an individual's ability to achieve or sustain an adequate level of sexual health and may require adjustments to how an affected individual expresses his or her sexuality.

TABLE 16.15 Sexual health

Sexual health is an important part of physical and mental health. It is a key part of our identify as human beings, together with the fundamental human rights to privacy, a family life and living free from discrimination. Essential elements of good sexual health are equitable relationships and sexual fulfilment with access to information and services to avoid the risk of unintended pregnancy, illness or disease.

Department of Health (England) 2001.[31]

Patient education

Everyone, including those living with HIV disease, can benefit from being able to positively express their sexuality and participate in activities designed to promote and enhance their sexual health. Knowing how to protect one's self from sexually transmitted infections (STIs), including HIV infection, is an important feature of an overall strategy designed to maintain the best possible level of sexual health.

Because an HIV-infected person will have some degree of immunosuppression, newly acquired STIs may be more problematic than they would be in a non-HIV-infected person who is fully immunocompetent. Many STIs, including genital warts, herpes virus infections and various fungi and bacterial infections, may be more aggressive in HIV-infected people, more difficult to treat and more likely to result in more frequent recurrent disease. In addition, new STIs can stimulate HIV replication, increasing the viral load and accelerating HIV disease progression. The presence of either an ulcerative or inflammatory STI makes it more likely that HIV will be transmitted during unprotected sexual intercourse. For those HIV-infected people who have not previously been infected with herpes simplex viruses or cytomegalovirus, hepatitis B or hepatitis C viruses, becoming infected with these viruses can immensely complicate HIV disease and worsen clinical outcomes. Finally, having unprotected penetrative sex with another HIV-infected person may result in becoming re-infected with a more pathogenic or drug-resistant strain of HIV that may increase the rate of disease progression and significantly limit future treatment options.

Although it is everyone's responsibility to protect themselves from STIs, those HIV-infected people who know their infection status may be more acutely aware of the need to protect their sexual partners from infection. This concern may result in disclosure of one's HIV status and negotiation around the level of acceptable risk that each partner is comfortable with.

Nurses can offer factual advice on reducing the risk of sexual transmission of HIV and the prevention of STIs (Table 16.16) and can direct the patient to additional sources of reliable information (Table 16.17). The skills needed to engage in effective patient education encounters are discussed in detail in Chapter 19.

TABLE 16.16 General guidance for reducing the risk of acquiring or transmitting sexually transmitted infections (STIs)

■ Advise men to use a rubber latex or polyurethane male condom for each and every episode of insertive (penetrative) vaginal, anal or oral sex and for each and every episode of receptive anal or oral sex.

■ If men do not use a condom, women can be advised to consider using a polyurethane female condom (Femidom®) for vaginal sex and they should be advised to encourage men to use a rubber latex or polyurethane male condom for each episode of oral or anal sex.

■ The use of non-spermicidal lubricated condoms and additional water-based lubrication, such as KY Jelly® or other condom-compatible lubricants, should be encouraged. Patients are advised *not* to use oil-based lubricants, such as massage oil, Vaseline or baby oil, when using latex condoms, as they weaken rubber latex, resulting in a burst condom. Oil-based lubricants can be used with polyurethane condoms such as the Avanti® male condom and the Femidom® female condom.

■ If condoms are not used during sex, men should be advised not to ejaculate semen into their partner's vagina, rectum or mouth.

■ The use of spermicides (such as nonoxynol-9) should not be recommended, as they may cause irritation and ulcers in genital mucosa and increase, rather then decrease, the risk for STIs.

■ Patients should be advised that penetrative and oral vaginal sex should be avoided during the period in which a female partner is menstruating as, if she is infected with any blood-borne virus, the risk of transmitting the infection to her partner will be increased.

■ Patients should be cautioned that oral–anal sex should be avoided due to the potential for infection with enteric pathogens, such as hepatitis A or F viruses, *Shigella*, *Campylobacter*, *Salmonella*, *Giardia*.

■ All patients should be encouraged to seek prompt medical diagnosis and treatment for any suspected STI.

■ Reducing the number of sexual partners and/or using non-penetrative sexual activities, such as mutual masturbation, mouth to mouth contact, body rubbing, hugging and massage, can significantly reduce the risk for STIs.

TABLE 16.17 Some UK sources of reliable information on preventing sexually transmitted infections (including HIV infection)

■ *AIDS Reference Manual*, regularly published by the National AIDS Manual (NAM) Publications, 16a Clapham Common Southside, London SW4 7AB. Telephone: 020 7627 3200; e-mail: info@nam.org.uk; website: www.aidsmap.com

■ *Terrence Higgins Trust*, 52–54 Grays Inn Road, London WC1X 8JU. Telephone (THT Direct: 0845 1221 200); e-mail: info@tht.org.uk; website: www.tht.org.uk

■ *Gay Men Fighting AIDS* (GMFA), Unit 43, Eurolink Centre, 49 Effra Road, London SW2 1BZ. Telephone: 020 7738 6872; e-mail: gmfa@gmfa.demon.co.uk; website: http://www.metromate.org.uk/

■ *Public Health Laboratory Service* (PHLS) England. Website: http://www.phls.org.uk/advice/index.htm

■ *National HIV Prevention Information Services* (NHPIS), a free specialist information service on HIV health promotion, serving people with a professional interest in HIV prevention across England. Health Development Agency, Trevelyan House, 30 Great Peter Street, London SW1P 2HW. Telephone: 020 7413 2001; e-mail: nhpis@hda-online.org.uk; website: http://www.hda-online.org.uk/nhpis/

■ *The Body*, the most comprehensive HIV and AIDS information resource on the internet at: http://www.thebody.com/index.shtml

Patients need to be encouraged to seek prompt diagnosis and treatment if they suspect they may have been exposed to an infectious disease, as untreated STIs increase their risk of becoming infected with a new variant of HIV or transmitting HIV infection to others. Additionally, it is important that HIV-infected people receiving antiretroviral treatment realize that **a low or undetectable plasma HIV viral load does not mean that they are no longer infectious**. They may be less infectious,[32] but they are still potentially infectious, as the level of virus in plasma does not necessarily reflect the level of virus in semen or vaginal secretions, which may be higher due to poor penetration in these biological compartments by antiretroviral drugs. Consequently, all infected individuals need to take precautions to avoid infecting others, regardless of their plasma viral load measurement.

It is widely accepted that receptive unprotected anal intercourse is the highest risk sexual activity for HIV transmission, followed by unprotected vaginal intercourse. Unprotected means the male insertive partner not wearing a good-quality intact rubber latex or polyurethane condom, or the female partner not wearing a polyurethane vaginal condom for vaginal intercourse. Oral sex, especially receptive oral sex where semen is ejaculated into the mouth, is less risky then either anal or vaginal sex but can result in HIV infection. The only way to minimize the risk for infection in all three forms of penetrative sexual intercourse (vaginal, anal, oral) is by the use of a condom. For many people throughout the world, the greatest protection from the risk of STIs is afforded by establishing an exclusive monogamous sexual relationship with another uninfected person.

Loss of libido and erectile dysfunction

Patients who have lost their interest in sexual intercourse or male patients who have erectile difficulties will be fully investigated by the physician and referred appropriately if necessary. Medication may be prescribed for underlying chronic depression or anxiety (see Table 16.12) and sildenafil (Viagra®) may be prescribed for erectile dysfunction. The usual dose of Viagra® is 50 mg (up to 100 mg) taken orally 30–60 minutes prior to sexual intercourse. Nitrates, including inhaled amyl or isobutyl nitrate products ('poppers', 'aromas'), must not be used by patients taking Viagra®, as the two may interact and cause a sudden drop in blood pressure (hypotension). Additionally, some antiretroviral drugs, such as saquinavir (Fortovase®, Invirase®) and ritonavir (Norvir®), and some other drugs commonly used by people with HIV disease, such as ketoconazole (Nizoral®), itraconazole (Sproanox®) and erythromycin, are metabolized by the same enzyme system in the liver and the interaction between any of these drugs and Viagra® may result in high levels of Viagra® in the blood, which may increase the side effects from Viagra®. In this situation, patients will be advised to use a lower dose (25 mg) of Viagra® and not to use it more than once every 48 hours.

Referrals

Nurses may refer patients to health advisers, counsellors, psychologists or an appropriate community-based organization (Table 16.18) for further information and ongoing support in adopting a healthy sexual lifestyle.

Evaluation

The patient will be assessed frequently and appropriately to ensure that objectives of care are being achieved, such as:

- any underling physical or mental health problems that may be interfering with the patient's ability to express his or her sexuality are identified;
- the patients has an opportunity to discuss and explore issues surrounding the development of a healthy sexual lifestyle;
- appropriate referrals are made to the health adviser, counsellor, psychologist or relevant community-based organization;
- there are adequate support and health educative efforts to enable patients to adjust to their changing sexuality and modify future sexual behaviour to protect themselves and others.

TABLE 16.18 Community-based organizations in the UK that provide information and support for adopting a healthy sexual lifestyle

■ *Terrence Higgins Trust*, 52–54 Grays Inn Road, London WC1X 8JU.Telephone (THT Direct: 0845 1221 200); e-mail: info@tht.org.uk; website: www.tht.org.uk

■ *Gay Men Fighting AIDS (GMFA)*, Unit 43, Eurolink Centre, 49 Effra Road, London SW2 1BZ. Telephone: 020 7738 6872; e-mail: gmfa@gmfa.demon.co.uk; website: http://www.demon.co.uk/gmta

■ *London East AIDS Network* (LEAN), 35 Romford Road, Stratford, London E15 4LY. Telephone: 020 8519 9545; e-mail: info@lean.org.uk; website: www.lean.org.uk

■ *The Naz Project* (Support for Black and Asian HIV+ People), Palingswick House, 241 King Street, London W6 9LP. Telephone: 020 8741 1879

■ *Blackliners* (Support for Black and Afro-Caribbean HIV+ People), 46 Eurolink Centre, 49 Effra Road, London SW2 1BZ. Telephone: 020 7738 5274; e-mail (African Community Health Advisor): acha@blackliners.org; website: http://blackliners.mappibiz.com/home.htm

■ *Positively Women* (Support for HIV+ Women); 347–349 City Road, London EC1V 1LR. Telephone: 020 7713 0222; e-mail: poswomen@dircon.co.uk; website: http://www.csoft.co.uk/loving_and_living/pw.html

The needs associated with dying

Potential problems	Possible causes
Fear, anxiety and loneliness	Impending death, manner of death, loss of power and control
Physical problems associated with dying	Pathophysiology of end-stage HIV disease
Inability to adjust to impending death	Fear, regrets, unfinished business

Objectives of care

■ Negotiate and agree with the patient the plan and objectives of care.
■ Alleviate or control physical problems associated with the terminal stages of end-stage HIV disease.
■ Support, comfort and reassure the patient journeying towards death.

Assessment

■ Assess (and frequently re-assess) physical symptoms associated with the terminal stages of HIV disease.
■ Ascertain and anticipate the patient's existential, psychosocial, emotional and spiritual needs as they near the end of their life and identify opportunities for support.

Nursing interventions

Since the introduction of highly active antiretroviral therapy in the early to mid-1990s, the death rate from HIV disease has dramatically fallen in countries in the industrially developed world. However, no one knows yet how long end-stage disease can be postponed with the use of these complex and powerful therapies. If drug resistance is ultimately inevitable, and if unacceptable or severe side effects preclude life-long drug therapy, health will eventually fail and patients will then require nursing care and support as they near the end of their lives.

Death is part of life, and dying is simply 'living the end of life'. Everyone who has thought about their inevitable death shares a common wish to 'live the end of their life' well. Supporting patients during the final phase of their lives requires the best nursing skills and a heightened awareness of the unique needs of the person nearing death. These include the need to be safe and not to be hurt, to be given refuge or sanctuary and to be comforted, and the need to be accepted, to belong, and to give and receive love. Palliative and terminal nursing care is not then about death, but rather about supporting patients to 'live the end of their life' well.

Caring for patients living the end of their life is not just about physical care; it is also about nurses and other healthcare professionals meeting a variety of psychosocial, emotional, spiritual and existential needs patients may have. Nurses cannot do this alone, but they can co-ordinate the multidisciplinary and interdisciplinary support needed from members of the healthcare team.

A variety of physical and psychological problems that may impede patients from living the end of their lives well are typically manifested during the terminal stages of illness (Table 16.19). Almost all of them are generally amenable to skilled medical and nursing interventions and symptom management. In addition, several societal concerns and issues, including legal and ethical dilemmas, frequently need to be confronted and addressed, by both patients and their carers as the end of life draws near.

TABLE 16.19 Patient problems and concerns – end-stage HIV disease

Physical
Anorexia/weight loss
Fatigue/weakness
Pain
Incontinence
Dyspnoea
Cough
Pressure ulcers
Constipation
Nausea and vomiting
Dehydration
Bowel colic
Excessive respiratory secretions
Hiccup
Convulsions

Psychological
Restlessness and confusion
Depression
Stess/anxiety

Ethical and legal concerns
Euthanasia
'Living Wills'/Advanced Directives
Health Care Proxy

Agreeing the plan and objectives of care

Everyone approaches the end of their life differently, with unique needs and aspirations for this important and final stage of living. They need to make decisions about their treatment and care and, in discussion with their doctors, nurses and other members of the healthcare team, clarify and confirm their wishes. Some treatment and care issues that commonly need confronting are the discontinuation of many treatments, including antiretroviral therapy, treatment and/or chemoprophylaxis for various opportunistic infections, the use of corticosteroids and artificial nutrition and hydration, and cardiopulmonary resuscitation. A plan of care needs to be negotiated and agreed and the patient needs to be reassured that the objectives of care can be re-discussed at any time. Competent and effective symptom management is what most patients desire during this phase of their life.

Physical problems — symptom control

Nursing and medical interventions focused on the relief of most of the physical problems listed in Table 16.19 have been discussed previously in this chapter. However, the management of some of these problems within the context of palliative care deserves further elaboration. Although only briefly discussed in this chapter, nurses are encouraged to explore symptom management further in more comprehensive texts on palliative care recommended at the end of this chapter.

Pain   Pain, often severe, is a common patient problem and frequently persists, not because it is refractory to analgesia but because of various misconceptions patients, their friends and families and healthcare professionals have about pain and the drugs, especially opioids, that are used to alleviate it. **Analgesics are more effective in preventing pain than in relieving it.** Consequently, the initiation of an opioid analgesic should not be delayed by concern over tolerance or dependence, because these do not occur in the palliative care setting. The physician will order appropriate analgesia (Table 16.20) according to the type (neuropathic, visceral, somatic, bone), severity and intensity of the pain.

TABLE 16.20 Some analgesics commonly used in palliative care

Non-opioid analgesics	Opioid analgesics
Paracetamol	Codeine
Non-steroidal anti- inflammatory drugs (NSAIDs), e.g.	Dihydrocodeine tartrate
aspirin	Morphine
naproxen	Hydromorphone hydrochloride
flurbiprofen	Oxycodone
	Diamorphine hydrochloride
	Fentanyl (transdermal)
	Dextromoramide
	Dipipanone hydrochloride
	Methadone
	Dextropropoxyphene

Morphine is probably the most useful and commonly used analgesic and is best given orally as a solution or immediate-release tablet and, when the patient's 24-hour morphine requirement is established, as a modified-release preparation (12-hour or 24-hour preparations) either once or twice daily. Patients need daily pain assessment and dosage adjustment. If the patient cannot swallow, fentanyl transdermal patches (Durogesic®) can be used in place of morphine. Alternatively, morphine can be given parenterally by subcutaneous injection. However, in the UK diamorphine is preferred for subcutaneous injection (and for continuous subcutaneous infusion) because, being more soluble, a larger dose can be given in a smaller volume. However, diamorphine is only available in the UK; morphine is used in the rest of the world.

Frequently, morphine (or diamorphine) is administered by a **continuous subcutaneous infusion** via a portable **syringe driver**, which provides good control of pain with little discomfort or inconvenience to the patient.

The incorrect use of syringe drivers is a common cause of drug errors, and staff using these devices need to be adequately trained in their use. Additionally, it is important that the different rate settings on the device are clearly identified and differentiated. Finally, staff caring for patients for whom syringe drivers are being used need to be alert to the potential problems encountered with these devices (Table 16.21).

TABLE 16.21 Problems encountered with syringe drivers[9]

The following are problems that may be encountered with syringe drivers and the action that should be taken.

- If the subcutaneous infusion runs *too quickly*, check the rate setting and the calculation.
- If the subcutaneous infusion runs *too slowly*, check the start button, the battery, the syringe driver, the cannula, and make sure that the injection site is not inflamed.
- If there is an *injection site reaction*, make sure that the site does not need to be changed – firmness or swelling at the site of injection is not in itself an indication for change, but pain or obvious inflammation is.

N.B. Subcutaneous infusion solution should be monitored regularly, both to check for precipitation (and discolouration) and to ensure that the infusion is being administered at the correct rate.

Diazepam, prochlorperazine, chlorpromazine are not administered by continuous subcutaneous infusion via a syringe driver, as they tend to cause skin reactions at the injection site.

Other drugs, such as haloperidol, hyoscine hydrobromide, levomepromazine (methotrimeprazine) and midazolam, can also be given by continuous subcutaneous infusion via a syringe driver. The general principle that injections should be given into separate sites (and should not be mixed) does *not* apply to the use of syringe drivers in palliative care. As long as there is no known mixing incompatibility, many drugs used in terminal care may be combined with morphine or diamorphine in a syringe driver (Table 16.22).[9] Injections are usually dissolved in water for injection or sodium chloride 0.9 per cent (physiological saline

TABLE 16.22 Drugs that can be safely mixed with diamorphine in a syringe driver for continuous subcutaneous infusion[9]

- Cyclizine[a]
- Dexamethasone[b]
- Haloperidol[c]
- Hyoscine butylbromide
- Hyoscine hydrobromide
- Levomepromazine
- Metoclopramide[d]
- Midazolam

[a]Cyclizine may precipitate at concentrations above 10 mg/mL *or* in the presence of physiological saline *or* as the concentration of diamorphine relative to cyclizine increases; mixtures of diamorphine and cyclizine are also liable to precipitate after 24 hours.

[b]Special care is needed to avoid precipitation of dexamethasone when preparing. In many palliative care services, dexamethasone is frequently given by a separate infusion.

[c]Mixtures of haloperidol and diamorphine are liable to precipitate after 24 hours if haloperidol concentration is above 2 mg/mL.

[d]Under some conditions, metoclopramide may become discoloured; such solutions should be discarded.

solution). However, drugs dissolved in water for injection may cause pain at the injection site (perhaps not important if the drug being infused is an analgesic), and drugs dissolved in sodium chloride 0.9 per cent tend to precipitate more frequently than drugs dissolved in water for injection.

Neuropathic pain, caused by damage to the central or peripheral nervous system, can be severe and is often described by patients as a burning, scalding or stinging; it may be experienced as a shooting or sharp and cutting (lancinating) pain. If the pain originates from sympathetic nervous system damage, it is generally described as a burning pain and may be accompanied by other sympathetic nervous system symptoms, such as sweating.[9,33] Neuropathic pain is less responsive to non-opioid and opioid analgesics but may respond better when these analgesics are given with 'analgesic adjuvants', that is, analgesics enhanced with a tricyclic antidepressant (amitriptyline, nortriptyline) and/or gabapentin (Neurontin®), an anticonvulsant. Other types of adjuvant analgesia may be used under specialist supervision. Transcutaneous electrical nerve stimulation (TENS) and nerve blocks may also be helpful for some patients.[9,33]

Nurses need to consult the 'Prescribing in palliative care' section of the current issue of the BNF[9] for important information about the route of administration, typical doses and dosing regimens, side effects and drug interactions of these analgesics. Additionally, the Palliative Care Formulary[34] is an essential resource for nurses and other healthcare professionals and can be accessed online (see 'Internet resources' at the end of this chapter). As already mentioned, analgesics may be used in combination with anxiolytic and antidepressant drugs (see Table 16.12), or with corticosteroids, muscle relaxants and, occasionally, anticonvulsant drugs.

Cough   Intractable cough can often be relieved by the use of moist inhalations or oral morphine. For patients who cannot swallow, chronic intractable cough can be relieved by the use of morphine or diamorphine by continuous subcutaneous infusion via a syringe driver.

Dyspnoea   Regular doses of oral morphine every 4 hours may help the patient breathe more easily. Corticosteroids, such as dexamethasone, may also be helpful if there is bronchospasm or partial obstruction. Oxygen is often helpful and is administered most comfortably by nasal cannulae. Sedatives, such as diazepam, and diuretics may be prescribed and, if death is imminent, intravenous fluids or nasogastric tube feeds are discontinued because fluids worsen congestion and increase discomfort. The physician may prescribe anxiolytic medication, such as diazepam, to relieve anxiety associated with dyspnoea.

Excessive respiratory secretions and bowel colic   Excessive respiratory secretions cause respiratory 'rattling', a wet, bubbly sound that is distressing to conscious patients and to their visitors. Bowel colic frequently occurs and is uncomfortable and agitating to patients. Both of these conditions are often relieved by the use of hyoscine hydrobromide, which is generally given by continuous subcutaneous infusion via a syringe driver.

Restlessness and confusion   Patients nearing the end of their lives are often restless and confused. This can be caused by a variety of factors, including correctable causes such as anxiety and fear, unrelieved retention of urine and faecal impaction, and drug side effects (especially from opioid analgesics) and drug withdrawal symptoms following the extended use of drugs such as benzodiazepines, alcohol and nicotine. If restlessness and confusion continue despite alleviating any potential correctable causes, the administration of haloperidol, levomepromazine or midazolam by continuous subcutaneous infusion via a syringe driver may be helpful.

Nausea and vomiting   Haloperidol, levomepromazine, cyclizine or metoclopramide may be prescribed to be given orally, parenterally or by continuous subcutaneous infusion via a syringe driver. Cyclizine is particularly liable to precipitate if mixed with diamorphine or other drugs.

Convulsions   Anticonvulsants will be prescribed and midazolam may be ordered to be given by continuous subcutaneous infusion via a syringe driver.

Pressure ulcers   Regular relief of pressure as previously described in this chapter is important because patients in the end-stage of HIV disease are generally immobile and at risk of developing pressure ulcers.

Anorexia   Every opportunity to encourage patients in pre-terminal stages of HIV disease to eat should be taken and patients are often tempted (and appreciative of) special foods that they enjoy. Steroids (prednisolone or dexamethasone) may be prescribed for anorexia. However, in the terminal stages of illness, it should be noted that intravenous fluids, total parenteral nutrition (TPN) and nasogastric tube feedings do not prolong the lives of dying patients, and all are associated with increased discomfort and may decrease survival. Families and friends need to be comforted and told gently that the patient is dying and food will not help the patient's strength or substantially delay death. Dehydration and starvation typically occur in dying patients and are associated with an analgesic effect and an absence of any associated discomfort.

Constipation   Constipation is a common and distressing problem in end-stage HIV disease, often due to dehydration, anorexia and (especially) the use of opioid analgesics. It can be prevented by the regular use of a laxative that combines a faecal softener with a peristaltic stimulant, such as docusate sodium (Dioctyl®, Docusol®), or lactulose solution with a senna preparation. A small-volume enema containing docusate sodium with stool-softening agents (Fletchers' Enemmete®) may also be used.

Dry mouth   A dry mouth may be caused by mouth breathing, oxygen therapy, fungal infections and many of the drugs used for palliative care, such as opioid analgesics, hyoscine, some antidepressants and anti-emetics. Regular and appropriately frequent mouth care is essential and the patient's partner, family members or close friends can be taught how to do this. Measures such as the sucking of ice or pineapple chunks, or the use of artificial saliva, are often useful. Candidiasis should be treated appropriately with antifungal drugs.

Hiccup   Hiccups are often due to gastric distension and can be helped by the use of an antacid with an anti-flatulent. Metoclopramide or chlorpromazine may also be prescribed.

Psychological, emotional and social needs
Insight into impending death   It is important to ascertain the extent of the patient's knowledge about their own impending death. It is rare that a patient who is seriously ill with end-stage HIV disease is unaware that he or she is dying. However, if the assessment indicates that this is the case, this fact should be made known to the physician who has the primary

responsibility of discussing the patient's prognosis with him or her. If (or when) the patient's level of comfort permits, practical aspects of his or her death may be gently discussed. This may include referral to a legal adviser or social worker for patients who have not made a will. Nurses must never become involved in either helping a patient draw up a will or witnessing it.

It is extremely important that the nursing notes indicate who is to be informed when the patient dies. This information should come from the patient. It would be tragic simply to inform the family, when the most significant relationship may be the patient's partner. Because of the high incidence of cognitive impairment in the terminally ill, this discussion should take place at the earliest appropriate opportunity.

Coming to terms with dying   Dying is as important as being born, only this time, most people have an opportunity to contemplate the final weeks and days of their life. Although it is true that no two individuals react in the same way to impending death, there seem to be commonalities in their reactions. Dr Elisabeth Kübler-Ross has elegantly described these as the 'five stages of dying'[35] (Table 16.23), and this model helps healthcare professionals and the significant people in the patient's life to understand the various reactions many people experience as they attempt to come to terms with the end of their life. In reality, patients go back and forth, from one stage to another, not necessarily in consecutive order. In Stage 4, nurses can be helpful in reminding patients of the achievements of their lives and of the impact that all human beings have by living a life, however short. If the patient has not been abandoned, loved ones have time to express their love and respect, reassuring the patient that he or she will be remembered.

TABLE 16.23 Psychological stages of dying[35]

1. **Denial**: 'No, not me.' This is a typical reaction when a patient learns that he or she is terminally ill. Denial is important and necessary. It helps cushion the impact of the patient's awareness that death is inevitable.

2. **Rage and anger**: 'Why me?' The patient resents the fact that others will remain healthy and alive while he or she must die. God is a special target for anger since He is regarded as imposing, arbitrarily, the death sentence. To those who are shocked at her claim that such anger is not only permissible but inevitable, Dr Ross replies succinctly, 'God can take it'.

3. **Bargaining**: 'Yes me, but . . .' Patients accept the fact of death but strike bargains for more time. Mostly they bargain with God – even people who have never talked with God before. Sometimes they bargain with the physician. They promise to be good or to do something in exchange for another week or month or year of life. Notes Dr Ross: 'What they promise is totally irrelevant, because they don't keep their promises anyway'.

4. **Depression**: 'Yes me.' First, the person mourns past losses, things not done, wrongs committed. Then he or she enters a state of 'preparatory grief', getting ready for the arrival of death. The patient grows quiet, does not want visitors. 'When a dying patient doesn't want to see you any more,' says Dr Ross, 'this is a sign he has finished his unfinished business with you and it is a blessing. He can now let go peacefully'.

5. **Acceptance**: 'My time is very close now and it's all right.' Dr Ross describes this final stage as 'not a happy stage, but neither is it unhappy. It's devoid of feelings but it's not resignation, it's really a victory'.

Euthanasia and assisted suicide

Many analgesics and sedatives used in the terminal stages of HIV disease may accelerate death. These and other drugs and treatments must be used carefully and appropriately and in accord with good medical and nursing practice. In these circumstances, their use is permitted on the understanding that they are intended to relieve pain or other distressing symptoms, such as dyspnoea. They must never be used in such a manner that it could be construed that they were being administered to hasten death. Euthanasia has been defined by the UK House of Lords as 'a deliberate intervention undertaken with the express intention of ending a life so as to relieve intractable suffering'.[36] If requested by a dying patient (or with their consent), it is 'voluntary'; otherwise, it is 'non-voluntary'. If a patient requests information and equipment or drugs to end their own life, it is referred to as physician-assisted suicide.[33] Both of these acts are illegal in the UK and in most countries in the European Union, except in the Netherlands. Becoming involved in euthanasia or assisting with suicide, or colluding with anyone to hasten death, is a criminal act in the UK and may result in criminal charges of contributing to wrongful death or homicide.

Clearly, this needs to be carefully and sensitively explained to patients who request such help and, equally important, they need to be reassured that skilful palliative care will help them live the end of their life well. The patient's partner, family and close friends need to be involved in this discussion with the patient and other members of the multidisciplinary team, including spiritual adviser(s).

'Living Wills', advanced directives and healthcare proxies

Many patients in end-stage HIV disease will have made a 'Living Will', which is sometimes called an advanced directive. In the event that the patient is mentally incapable of making decisions about their treatment and care because they are unconscious or otherwise incapacitated, a 'Living Will' informs doctors about which treatments a patient does not want to artificially extend the end of their life, such as haemodialysis, endotracheal intubation and respiratory ventilation, nasogastric, enteral or parenteral nutrition and hydration and cardiopulmonary resuscitation. 'Living Wills' are legally enforceable in the UK under common law (that is, law decided by the Courts) if they meet certain criteria. The Department of Health (England) advises healthcare professionals that 'if an incompetent patient has clearly indicated in the past, while competent, that they would refuse treatment in certain circumstances (an "advance refusal"), and those circumstances arise, healthcare professionals must abide by that refusal'.[37] If patients enquire about making a 'Living Will', they can be referred to the Terrence Higgins Trust or the Voluntary Euthanasia Society (see 'Internet resources' at the end of this chapter) and can download forms and obtain comprehensive information free of charge. If a patient has made a 'Living Will', it is important that healthcare professionals are aware of it, that a copy of it is in the patient's records, and, ideally, that they have had an opportunity to discuss it with the patient before he or she loses the ability to make decisions about their care.

Sometimes patients appoint a 'Health Care Proxy', a relative, partner or friend empowered by them to make decisions about their treatment and care should they lose the ability to do this themselves. In the UK, these appointments are not legally binding on physicians but may usefully inform any decisions made with regard to continuing treatments at the end of a patient's life.

If the patient has a 'Living Will' and/or has appointed a Health Care Proxy, it is essential that they discuss this with their general practitioner and hospital healthcare staff so that everyone is clear about the patient's wishes, and distress and embarrassment are avoided at this sensitive and important time. Nurses can consult the current edition of the *AIDS Reference Manual*[38] for further information on these issues.

Last offices

The usual last offices are carried out. The patient is washed and the room tidied. Family, partners and close friends are allowed to see the body before any further procedures take place. The nurse must be accessible during this time to support those grieving for their loss. After the body has been viewed, it is placed in a shroud and then gently placed in a heavy-duty plastic body bag. It is both unnecessary and inappropriate to attach warning labels such as 'Infection risk' or 'BioHazard' to the body bag. Mortuary staff need to assume that all patients are potentially infected with blood-borne viruses and take appropriate precautions to prevent exposure to them. Nurses must wear disposable gloves and a plastic apron when carrying out last offices. Once the body has been placed in the body bag, no further infection prevention precautions are required.

Evaluation
The patient will be assessed frequently and appropriately to ensure that objectives of care are being achieved, such as:

- patient problems and symptoms associated with the end of life are controlled or alleviated;
- the patient is free of psychological distress and feels safe, comfortable and well supported by friendly and caring nurses as death approaches;
- grieving family, partner, relatives and friends are supported before and after the patient's death.

Summary

The individualized care of patients with HIV disease requires skill, competence and confidence. These attributes are based on a factual understanding of the pathophysiology of HIV infection and a comprehensive knowledge of relevant models of nursing care, designed to offer all patients, regardless of race, age, creed, gender, sexual orientation or disease, the highest quality of compassionate, non-judgemental nursing care.

REFERENCES

1. Henderson V. *Basic Principles of Nursing Care*. Geneva: International Council of Nurses, 1972.
2. Henderson V. The nature of nursing. *American Journal of Nursing* 1964; **64**:62–8.
3. Roper N, Logan WW, Tierney AJ. *The Elements of Nursing*, 4th edn. London: Churchill Livingstone, 1996.
4. Orem DE. *Nursing: Concepts of Practice*, 2nd edn. New York: McGraw Hill, 1980.
5. John C. *The Burford NDU Model; Caring in Practice*. Oxford: Blackwell Sciences, 1994.
6. Pratt RJ, Pellowe C, Loveday HP, Robinson N, Smith GW, and the **epic** Guideline Development Team. The **epic** Project: Developing National Evidence-based Guidelines for Preventing Healthcare Associated Infections. Phase 1: Guidelines for Preventing Hospital-acquired Infections. *Journal of Hospital Infection* 2001; **47**(Suppl.):S1–82. Available on: http://www.doh.gov.uk/hai/epic.htm
7. Pratt R, Pellowe C, Loveday HP, Harper P, Robinson N. The **epic** Project: Developing National Evidence-based Guidelines for Preventing Healthcare Associated Infections. Preventing infections associated with the use of central venous catheters. *Nursing Times* 2001; **97**:36–9.

8. Pellowe C, Loveday HP, Harper P, Robinson N, Pratt R. The **epic** Project: Developing National Evidence-based Guidelines for Preventing Healthcare Associated Infections. Preventing infections from short-term indwelling urethral catheters. *Nursing Times* 2001; **97**:34–5.

9. Mehta DK (Executive Editor). *British National Formulary (BNF)*, 42nd edn. London: British Medical Association and the Royal Pharmaceutical Society of Great Britain, March 2002. Updated and published every 6 months. Available from: BMJ Books, PO Box 295, London WC1H 9TE, UK, or from their website www.bmjbookshop.com. The BNF is also available online at: www.BNF.org

10. Alcorn K (ed.). *HIV & AIDS Treatments Directory*, 20th edn. London: National AIDS Manual (NAM) Publications, February 2002. Information also available online at: http://www.aidsmap.com

11. Loveday HP, Pellowe C, Harper P, Robinson N, Pratt R. The **epic** Project: Developing National Evidence-based Guidelines for Preventing Healthcare Associated Infections. Standard principles for preventing HAIs. *Nursing Times* 2001; **97**:36–7.

12. Norton D, McLaren R, Exton-Smith A. *An Investigation of Geriatric Nursing Problems in Hospital*. London: National Corporation for the Care of Old People, 1962 (re-issued 1975; Edinburgh: Churchill Livingstone).

13. Waterlow J. Prevention is cheaper than cure. *Nursing Times* 1988; **84**:69–70.

14. Waterlow J. A policy that protects. *Professional Nurse* 1991; **6**:258–64.

15. Clark M. Pressure ulcer prevention. In: Morrison M (ed.), *The Prevention and Treatment of Pressure Ulcers*. London: Harcourt Health Sciences, 2000, 75–98.

16. European Pressure Ulcer Advisory Panel (EPUAP). *Pressure Ulcer Prevention Guidelines*. London: EPUAP, 1998.

17. Torrance C. *Pressure Sores: Aetiology, Treatment and Prevention*. London: Croom Helm, 1983.

18. Meers PD, Ayliffe GA, Emmerson AM et al. Report on the national survey of infection in hospitals 1980. *Journal of Hospital Infection* (Supplementary) 1981; **2**:1–11.

19. Emmerson AM, Enstone JE, Griffin M, Kelsey MC, Smyth ETM. The second national prevalence survey of infection in hospitals – an overview of results. *Journal of Hospital Infection* 1996; **32**:175–90.

20. Teare EL, Cookson B, French G, Jenner EA, Scott G, Pallett A. UK Handwashing Initiative. *Journal of Hospital Infection* 1999; **43**:1–3.

21. Doweiko JP. Hematologic manifestations of HIV infection. In: Merigan TC, Bartlett JG, Bolognesi D (eds), *Textbook of AIDS Medicine*, 2nd edn. Baltimore: Williams & Wilkins, 1999, 611–27.

22. Wilson J. *Clinical Microbiology: An Introduction for Healthcare Professionals*, 8th edn. Edinburgh: Baillière Tindall, 2000.

23. Nauseef WM, Maki DG. A study of the value of simple protective isolation in patients with granulocytopenia. *New England Journal of Medicine* 1981; **304**:448–53.

24. Pizzo PA. The value of protective isolation in preventing nosocomial infections in high risk patients. *American Journal of Medicine* 1981; **70**:631–7.

25. Armstrong D. Protected environments are expensive and do not offer meaningful protection. *American Journal of Medicine* 1984; **76**:685–9.

26. Helminiak DA. *The Human Core of Spirituality: Mind as Psyche and Spirit*. Albany, NY: State University of New York Press, 1996, 307 pp.

27. Fogel CI. Human sexuality and health care. In: Fogel CI, Lauver D (eds), *Sexual Health Promotion*. Philadelphia: W.B. Saunders Company, 1990 Chapter 1.

28. Fonseca JD. Sexuality – a quality of being human. *Nursing Outlook* 1970; **18**:25.
29. Langfeldt T, Porter M. *Sexuality and Family Planning. Report of a Consultation and Research Findings*. Copenhagen: World Health Organization Sexuality and Family Planning Programme, 1986.
30. World Health Organization *Technical Report Series No 572*. Geneva: WHO, 1975.
31. Department of Health. *The National Strategy for Sexual Health and HIV*. London: Department of Health (England), 2001. Available from: www.doh.gov.uk/jointunit/jip.htm
32. Quinn TC, Wawer MJ, Sewankambo N et al. Viral load and heterosexual transmission of human immunodeficiency virus Type 1. *New England Journal of Medicine* 2000; **342**:921–9. Available online at: http://content.nejm.org/cgi/content/abstract/342/13/921
33. Woodruff R. *Palliative Medicine*, 3rd edn. Melbourne: Oxford University Press, 1999.
34. Twycross R, Wilcock A, Thorp S. *Palliative Care Formulary*. Oxford: Radcliffe Medical Press, 1998. Also available online at: http://www.palliativedrugs.com
35. Kübler-Ross E. *On Death and Dying*. London: Tavistock Publications, 1969.
36. House of Lords. *Report of the House of Lords' Select Committee on Medical Ethics*. Session 1993–94. Paper HL21-I. London: Her Majesty's Stationary Office (HSMO), 1994.
37. Department of Health (England). *12 Key Points on Consent: The Law in England*. London: HMSO, April 2001. Available online at: http://www.doh.gov.uk/consent
38. Fieldhouse R (ed.). *AIDS Reference Manual*, 24th edn. London: National AIDS Manual (NAM), October 2001.

FURTHER READING

Adler MW (ed.). *ABC of AIDS*, 5th edn. London: BMJ Publishing Group, 2001, ISBN 0-7279-1053-7.

Alexander MF, Fawcett JN, Runciman PJ. *Nursing Practice, Hospital & Home – The Adult*, 2nd edn. London: Churchill Livingstone, 2000, ISBN 0-443-06013-4.

Dickman A, Varga J. *The Syringe Driver – Continuous Subcutaneous Infusions in Palliative Care*. Oxford: Oxford University Press, 2002, ISBN 0-19-851550-2.

Fieldhouse R (ed.). *AIDS Reference Manual*, 24th edn. London: National AIDS Manual (NAM), October 2001, ISBN 1 898 397 08 2. A new edition is published by NAM each year and is available from: NAM, 16a Clapham Common Southside, London SW4 7AB. Telephone: 020 7627 3200; fax: 020 7627 3101; e-mail: info@nam.org.uk; website: www.aidsmap.com

George R, Farnham C, Schofield L. Palliative care and pain control in HIV and AIDS. In: Adler MW (ed.), *ABC of AIDS*, 5th edn. London: BMJ Publishing Group, 2001, 126 pp, ISBN 0-7279-1053-7.

Hinchliff S, Norman S, Schober J. *Nursing Practice & Health Care – a Foundation Text*, 3rd edn. London: Arnold (Hodder Headline Group), 1998, ISBN 0-340-69230-0.

Kübler-Ross E. *On Death and Dying*. London: Tavistock Publications, 1969, ISBN 0-422-75490-0.

Lugton J. *Communicating with Dying People and their Relatives*. Oxford: Radcliffe Medical Press, 2002, ISBN 1-85775-584-7.

Morrison M (ed.). *The Prevention and Treatment of Pressure Ulcers*. London: Harcourt Health Sciences, 2000, ISBN 0-7234-31582.

Neuberger J. *Dying Well: A Guide to Enabling A Good Death*, 3rd edn. Oxford: Radcliffe Medical Press, 2002, ISBN 1-8577-59400.

Neuberger J. *Caring for Dying People of Different Faiths*, 3rd edn. Oxford: Radcliffe Medical Press, 2002, ISBN 1-8577-59451.

Roper N, Logan WW, Tierney AJ. *The Elements of Nursing*, 4th edn. London: Churchill Livingstone, 1996, ISBN 0-443-05201-8.

Sherr L (ed.). *Grief and AIDS*. Chichester: John Wiley & Sons, 1995, ISBN 0-471-95346-6.

Sims R, Moss VA. *Palliative Care for People with AIDS*, 2nd edn. London: Edward Arnold, 1995, ISBN 0-340-61371-8.

Twycross R, Wilcock A, Charlesworth S, Dickman A. *Palliative Care Formulary*, 2nd edn. Oxford: Radcliffe Medical Press, 2002, ISBN 1-857-75511-1.

Weston A (ed.). *Sexually Transmitted Infections – a Guide to Care*. London: Nursing Times Books, 1999, ISBN 1-902499-09-3.

Woodruff R. *Palliative Medicine*, 3rd edn. Melbourne: Oxford University Press, 1999.

INTERNET RESOURCES

- *British National Formulary (BNF)*, published by the British Medical Association and the Royal Pharmaceutical Society of Great Britain, provides up-to-date information in relation to the drugs used in the UK to treat HIV infection and HIV-related diseases. Both the hard copy and the online version are updated every 6 months. The online version is available at:
  http://www.BNF.org/
- For a comprehensive guide to drugs used for the prophylaxis and treatment of opportunistic infections and other HIV-related illnesses, see the current edition of the *HIV & AIDS Treatments Directory*, published twice yearly by the National AIDS Manual (email: info@nam.org.uk), and the monthly *AIDS Treatment Update*, available online at:
  http://www.aidsmap.com

NAM also publishes the excellent and authoritative *AIDS Reference Manual*, which is updated each year.

- A website offering detailed information on drugs used for palliative care (including comprehensive information on using syringe drivers for the continuous subcutaneous infusion of drugs), based on the *Palliative Care Formulary* (see Twycross, Wilcock and Thorp above), can be found at:
  http://www.palliativedrugs.com
- *Living Wills, Advance Directives and Healthcare Proxies*: for detailed information and downloadable forms, direct patients to the London-based website of The Terrence Higgins Trust or the Voluntary Euthanasia Society. Patients and healthcare professionals can consult the Department of Health (England) website for guidance on consent and the requirement to abide by 'advance refusal' ('Living Wills'):
  http://www.aidsmap.com
  http://www.ves.org.uk
  http://www.doh.gov.uk/consent

CHAPTER 17

Nutrition and HIV disease

It was hoped that the advent of new treatments, particularly protease inhibitors, mixed with other agents to produce highly active antiretroviral therapy (HAART), would curtail weight loss and return persons with HIV to their earlier body composition. While HAART has undeniably lowered mortality, controlled opportunistic infections, and reduced hospitalization, it has not, unfortunately, had a major impact on weight loss and compromised nutritional status in persons with HIV. These nutritional issues continue virtually unabated.

Tracie Miller & Sherwood Gorbach[1]

Introduction

Malnutrition is a common feature of human immunodeficiency virus (HIV) disease and further compounds patient problems and immune system incompetence. Nurses and other healthcare professionals need to be able to assess the nutritional status of their patients and to participate effectively with other members of the care team in nutritional interventions.

Learning outcomes

After studying and reflecting on the material in this chapter, you will be able to:

- describe common mechanisms of malnutrition in human immunodeficiency virus (HIV) disease and identify associated risk factors;
- outline the elements of a nutritional assessment;
- discuss appropriate advice to give to patients for preventing gastrointestinal infections from food;

- describe the drugs used to prevent or alleviate malnutrition;
- discuss the care of patients with oral, enteral or intravenous nutritional supplementation.

BACKGROUND

Weight loss and thinness are common in all stages of HIV disease. In Africa, weight loss and emaciation, associated with diarrhoea ('slim disease'), are some of the most frequent manifestations of HIV disease.[2] In the Western world, weight loss is also common, and an HIV wasting syndrome has been an AIDS-defining indicator of disease since 1987.[3] A progressive, involuntary weight loss typically appears in the early stages of HIV disease and increases in severity as the disease progresses. In addition, metabolic changes and deficiencies of specific nutrients, vitamins and minerals are frequently associated with HIV disease, especially in late-stage illness.[4] HIV disease has a significant impact on the nutritional status of the individual, usually resulting in various types of malnutrition. In turn, malnutrition has an equally deleterious impact on immune function, morbidity and mortality in people with HIV disease. Iatrogenic factors (e.g. drugs used in the treatment of HIV disease) may also adversely influence nutritional status, and the efficacy of drug therapies currently used in HIV disease may be affected by the underlying nutritional status of the individual (Figure 17.1).

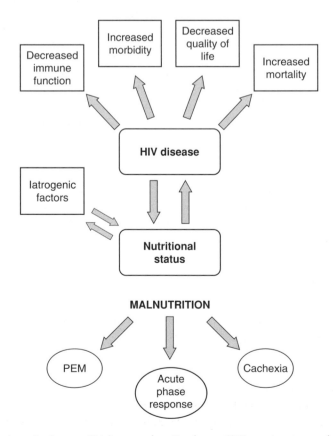

FIGURE 17.1 *The relationship between HIV disease and nutritional status. PEM, protein–energy malnutrition.*

Nutrition refers to the processes involved in taking in, assimilating and utilizing nutrients. Nutrients include both **macronutrients** (carbohydrates, proteins and fats) and **micronutrients** (vitamins, minerals and trace elements). Nutritional processes include ingestion, digestion, absorption, metabolism and effective utilization of nutrients. Nutrients are needed for tissue growth and repair and for maintenance of functional systems in the body. Each individual process may be impaired during HIV disease. A variety of external factors (economic, socio-cultural, behavioural etc.) may also influence nutritional status.

Malnutrition results from a change in any of the above processes or factors and may lead to either **over-nutrition** or **under-nutrition**. The primary causes of under-nutrition are well defined and are associated with deficiencies of one or more nutrients, due to inadequate ingestion, absorption or utilization and/or increased excretion or requirements.[5]

Different types of malnutrition in chronic disease are characterized in terms of both metabolic and nutritional changes (Table 17.1). All the following forms of malnutrition can be seen in HIV disease.

TABLE 17.1 Different types of malnutrition[4]

Type	Cause and characterization
Protein–energy malnutrition	Starvation – the body's needs for protein, energy fuels, or both, cannot be met by diet[8] Primary cause may be inadequate intake or secondary to malabsorption, decreased utilization or changes in metabolism, resulting in weight loss and wasting
Acute phase response	Metabolic changes, which occur as a result of tissue injury, infection, stress or inflammation and characterized by weight loss and changes (i.e. decreases) in the circulating levels of various plasma proteins, e.g. albumin[9]
Cachexia	A clinical syndrome involving a mixture of metabolic abnormalities that lead to a marked and sudden weight loss through accelerated wasting of host tissue mass, failure of adequate nutrient intake absorption and utilization[7] Cachexia is often a feature of late HIV disease

Protein–energy malnutrition

Protein–energy malnutrition (PEM) may be seen in patients in all stages of HIV disease, resulting in involuntary weight loss or wasting.[6] It is similar to starvation, and lean body mass is preserved relative to fat by adaptive mechanisms, e.g. decreased basal metabolic rate or resting energy expenditure.[1]

Acute phase response

This is a type of malnutrition seen in both acute and chronic illnesses, including HIV disease, in which patients experience weight loss and loss of lean body mass. It occurs during acute episodes of opportunistic infections or periods of stress.

Cachexia

This is frequently linked with end-stage HIV disease and is characterized by a profound and sudden depletion of lean body mass, especially muscle, and a variety of metabolic disorders. The changes associated with cachexia cannot usually be reversed by nutritional interventions.[7]

MECHANISMS OF MALNUTRITION IN HIV DISEASE

A variety of mechanisms of malnutrition in HIV disease have been defined,[4] including reduced food intake, drug–nutrient interactions, malabsorption and altered metabolism (Figure 17.2), and one or more of these components may be involved.

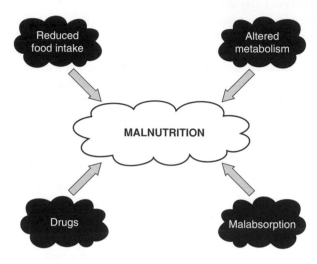

FIGURE 17.2 *Mechanisms of malnutrition.*

Reduced food intake

Several factors may lead to a reduced dietary intake during HIV disease. Anorexia (loss of appetite) may result from the disease process itself, mediated by a variety of cytokines (as discussed in Chapter 5), including tumour necrosis factor (TNF), interleukin-1 (IL-1) and interferons (IFNs). These cytokines are frequently elevated in patients with HIV disease[10] and have been associated with anorexia.[11] **Pain** and dysphagia (difficulty in swallowing) secondary to a number of opportunistic conditions or lesions, e.g. buccal candidiasis, various herpesvirus infections, Kaposi's sarcoma, aphthous ulcerations etc., may contribute to a reduced dietary intake. **Nausea** and **vomiting**, due to infections, tumours or drug treatment, are a frequent cause of reduced food intake, as is **diarrhoea**. Decreased neurological function, especially the AIDS–dementia complex, can affect food intake due to changes in both cognition and behaviour. Psychosocial causes, e.g. intentional weight loss, stress associated with bereavement, loss of employment etc., have also been identified as significant factors in weight loss due to a reduced food intake in some individuals with HIV disease.[12]

Drug–nutrient interactions

Many drugs used for treatment or prophylaxis in HIV disease potentially affect the processes of nutrition.[13,14] The side effects of these drugs may include **gastrointestinal symptoms**, e.g. amphotericin B, sulphadiazine and etoposide can cause **nausea**, **anorexia** and **vomiting**. Other drugs, e.g. trimethoprim-sulphamethoxazole and pentamidine, can cause a variety of **micronutrient imbalances**, such as glucose intolerance, folate deficiency etc., and are noxious to various organs (pancreas, liver, kidneys), which play a major role in digestion. Antiretroviral drugs such as zidovudine (AZT) are extremely toxic agents and can have a profound effect on nutritional status. In addition, zidovudine causes **myopathy** (muscle weakness), **anaemia** and **gastrointestinal symptoms**. Antibiotics may disrupt the normal flora of the gastrointestinal tract, increasing the risk of both diarrhoea and further gastrointestinal opportunistic infections.

Malabsorption

Malabsorption commonly occurs as a result of various gastrointestinal infections that cause **inflammation** and **diarrhoea**. Common gastrointestinal infections seen in patients with HIV disease include *Cryptosporidium* spp., *Isospora belli*, *Microsporidium*, *Salmonella* spp. and environmental mycobacteria, e.g. *Mycobacterium avium* complex (MAC). Opportunistic infections associated with diarrhoea are the most frequent cause of malabsorption and weight loss in patients with HIV disease.[12] Kaposi's sarcoma can also occur in the gastrointestinal tract, causing diarrhoea and subsequent malabsorption. Antacids, H2 antagonists, e.g. cimetidine, and other drugs that alter the pH and secretory function of the gastrointestinal tract may contribute to malabsorption.

Altered metabolism

Opportunistic infections result in **fever** and **hypermetabolic states** in which excessive calories are burned, leading to rapid wasting (acute phase response). Stress can also produce hypermetabolism. Various cytokines, e.g. TNF, IL-1 and IFNs, also influence metabolic processes. As these cytokines are often inappropriately produced during HIV disease, they may alter normal metabolic regulation, including fat (lipid) metabolism, leading to weight loss and cachexia.

THE EFFECTS OF MALNUTRITION ON HIV DISEASE

Malnutrition is either directly or indirectly the cause of significant patient problems frequently encountered in HIV disease. These problems are described in Table 17.2 and may result in a debilitated patient, unable to function optimally and at risk of losing his or her independence. Essential elements in patient care are the prevention of malnutrition and the restoration of nutritional adequacy to malnourished patients.

ASSESSMENT

Nutritional evaluation should be carried out early, soon after HIV disease is diagnosed. Elements of a comprehensive assessment include the items in Table 17.3. A multi-disciplinary approach to both assessment and intervention is needed. However, an early referral to a dietician is essential.

Ideal body weight can be estimated using the formulae in Table 17.4,[16] remembering that weight in pounds is converted to kilograms – 1 kilogram (kg) equals 2.2046 pounds (lb). Nutritional assessment data that indicate nutritional depletion might include the items shown in Table 17.5.

TABLE 17.2 Consequences of malnutrition in HIV disease

Malnutrition in HIV disease:

Further depresses an already compromised immune system, increasing both frequency and severity of opportunistic events[15]

Increases morbidity, which in turn:

  lessens effectiveness of drug treatments

  decreases ability to withstand opportunistic events

  prolongs periods of hospitalization

  increases cost of treatment

  decreases many indicators of quality of life:

    increases dependency on others and decreases self-care ability

    reduces muscle strength, energy and mobility

    alters body image

    increases despondency and decreases general enjoyment of life

Increases mortality:

  nutritional status is the most important determinant of both survival and mortality[16,17]

TABLE 17.3 Nutritional assessment evaluation

History

Normal weight; recent weight loss

Usual diet composition; current use of supplements

Average caloric intake

Anorexia, nausea, vomiting and/or diarrhoea

Systemic and local pain

Depression

Current chemotherapy

Economic status in relation to being able to buy food

Patient's ability to prepare food

Physical assessment – anthropometrics

Body weight and height

Estimated ideal body weight (see Table 17.4)

Per cent body weight change over time

Measurements of:

  triceps skinfold

  mid-arm muscle circumference

Body temperature and heart rate

Laboratory investigations (as ordered by physician)

24-hour nitrogen balance determination

Serum albumin (and pre-albumin) and transferrin levels

Total protein

Haemoglobin and haematocrit

White cell and total lymphocyte count

Risk factors

TABLE 17.4 Estimating ideal body weight

Men	106 lb (48.1 kg) for first 5 feet in height 6 lb (2.7 kg) for each inch over 5 feet
Women	100 lb (45.4 kg) for first 5 feet in height 5 lb (2.3 kg) for each inch over 5 feet
Example	The ideal weight for a man measuring 5 feet, 8 inches in height would be 106 lb + 48 lb (6 lb × 8 inches) = 154 lb (or 70 kg)

TABLE 17.5 Data indicative of nutritional depletion

Recent weight loss	>10%
Serum albumin	<35 g/L
Serum transferrin	< 2 g/L
Triceps skinfold thickness	
Males	<10 mm
Females	<13 mm
Upper arm circumference	
Males	<23 cm
Females	<22 cm
Lymphopenia	Present
Skin anergy	Present

RISK FACTORS

Important risk factors for malnutrition in HIV disease are **anorexia** (most frequent), **diarrhoea** and **fever** (most severe), although many patients have combined risk factors.[18] As opportunistic infections (especially those associated with diarrhoea) are a frequent cause of weight loss in patients with HIV disease, any unexplained weight loss should alert nurses to the possibility of covert infection.[12] Weight loss of 10 per cent or more can have a significant impact on the patient's functional status and survival prospects.[13,19]

Malnutrition can occur in patients with a seemingly adequate caloric intake who do not have significant weight loss; consequently, decisions to intervene nutritionally must be based upon the results of a valid assessment by a dietician.[20] The physician, in liaison with the dietician, may order a variety of laboratory investigations, especially serum albumin, an important tool used to monitor malnutrition.

NUTRITIONAL INTERVENTIONS

Early assessment allows for early intervention. Intervention areas include dietary counselling and patient education, drug therapy, oral supplements, enteral feeding and total parenteral nutrition.

Dietary counselling and patient education

Patients need to have a good understanding of the nutritional implications of HIV disease and the importance of maintaining body weight by eating a balanced diet, especially high-protein, calorifically dense foods. They need to have the opportunity to consult a dietician periodically. This will allow an opportunity for ongoing monitoring and space to discuss alternative diets patients may be contemplating. Patient education might also focus on sensible measures that may promote a healthier lifestyle, e.g. stress management and the need for regular exercise, and practical aspects of nutrition, especially food safety. Food safety is particularly important in HIV-infected individuals who, as a result of a progressive decrease in the effectiveness of their immune system, are more prone to food-borne illnesses as a consequence of eating contaminated food. These illnesses often present with nausea and vomiting, fever, diarrhoea, abdominal pain (cramping) and headache. They are often difficult to treat and can be extremely serious (even fatal) in an individual who is immunocompromised. Patient education can help patients to 'eat defensively', avoiding the potential for food poisoning. The following recommendations can be made.

- **Shopping**. Buy perishable foods (those that require refrigeration or freezing) last and check that the 'sell by date' of all foods is current. Ensure that safety seals on tins and jars are intact and that tins are not dented or otherwise damaged.
- **Fridges and freezers**. Ensure that refrigerators are kept between 0 and 5 °C and that freezers are kept at 0 to −18 °C. Refrigerator and freezer thermometers are inexpensive and should be used.
- **Food storage**. Store cooked and uncooked (raw) foods separately in the refrigerator. All raw meats should be stored in plastic bags and kept in the lower part of the refrigerator to prevent possible contamination of other foods by drippings.
- **Frozen foods**. Some frozen foods, e.g. vegetables, fish fingers etc., can be cooked from frozen. Foods that need defrosting should be thawed out in the refrigerator (or microwave oven on the defrost setting), not at room temperature.
- **Handwashing**. Wash hands thoroughly in warm, soapy water and rinse well prior to and after handling all food, especially raw meats! Cover any cuts or lesions with a waterproof bandage or wear a disposable plastic glove (available from supermarkets for catering use). Use paper towels or cloth towels once only!
- **Chopping (cutting) boards**. Use a separate chopping board for raw meats. Chopping boards made from hard plastic or marble are easier to clean and disinfect than those made from wood. Disinfect chopping boards daily with a weak solution of bleach (or put in a dishwasher, if appropriate).
- **Meats, poultry, fish, eggs**. Ensure that these are all well cooked and are consumed soon after cooking and not left at room temperature.
- **Raw foods**. Do not eat raw eggs or soft-boiled eggs or omelettes (unless they are well cooked). Do not eat homemade mayonnaise. Avoid pâtés, raw or partially cooked poultry, meats (e.g. steak tartare), fish (e.g. sushi, partially cooked or steamed clams, oysters, prawns etc.).
- **Leftovers**. These are safe if they are kept in the refrigerator for no longer than 3 days. Heat thoroughly (75 °C) before eating and do not reheat more than once. It is often better to put leftovers in a plastic bag and put them in a freezer.
- **Milk, cheese and yoghurt**. Eat only those products that have been **pasteurized**. Avoid eating blue vein cheeses, e.g. Stilton.
- **Vegetables and fruits**. Wash all fruit and vegetables thoroughly before use. It is a good idea to wash them in cooled, boiled water or a disinfecting solution, e.g. 1 gallon of water and 20 drops of 2 per cent iodine (available at any pharmacy). Let produce stand in the solution for about 10–15 minutes and rinse well.

- **Drinking water**. Do not use tap water or even **bottled water**. Tap water should be used after it has been boiled, cooled and then stored in the refrigerator. It should be prepared daily.
- **Eating out**. Be careful! Avoid eating salads (choose hot soups instead) and avoid drinking water.

Both dieticians and nurses will be able to suggest ways to manage nutritionally related symptoms or side effects such as lack of appetite, mouth soreness, difficulty in swallowing (dysphagia), nausea and diarrhoea. Practical advice is available in the form of patient education booklets, both in the UK[21] and the USA,[22] and copies can be easily obtained for patient distribution.

Drug therapy

Drugs that control nausea, vomiting and diarrhoea or that act as appetite stimulants are commonly used to help improve the patient's nutritional status.

Anti-diarrhoea drugs

Patients should be encouraged not to use anti-diarrhoea drugs that are available over the counter without first consulting their medical practitioner. These drugs are often contraindicated for treating the diarrhoea caused by enteric pathogens until the infection has been treated. The most common anti-diarrhoea drugs used are anti-motility agents, such as **co-phenotrope** (Lomotil®), **loperamide hydrochloride** (Imodium®, Arret®, Diocalm Ultra®) and **codeine phosphate**. Absorbents and bulk-forming drugs, e.g. kaolin, are not useful for acute diarrhoea. **Octreotide** (Sandostatin®) is sometimes used for severe diarrhoea, especially cryptosporidium-induced secretory diarrhoea.[23] For the prevention and treatment of fluid and electrolyte imbalance in patients with acute diarrhoea, especially those who are frail and undernourished, **oral rehydration therapy (ORT)** may be helpful. Nurses can teach patients how to make up a sugar and salt ORT solution, or advise them on using proprietary preparations, e.g. Dioralyte®, Rehidrat® etc.

Anti-emetic drugs

Several drugs are available that are useful in managing nausea and vomiting. Some of the more commonly used agents include **metoclopramide** (Maxolon®), **domperidone** (Motilium®), and **prochlorperazine** (Stemetil®). Some of these drugs are also available in an injectable form and as suppositories or in buccal preparations. Side effects include extrapyramidal reactions (especially in children and young adults), which are manifested by Parkinson-like dystonic muscular spasms. This is an important and distressing side effect, which can be successfully terminated by the administration of an antimuscarinic drug, e.g. **benzhexol hydrochloride** (Artane®) or **procyclidine hydrochloride** (Kemadrin®), once recognized.

Many patients use **cannabis** (marijuana) to control nausea. However, it is an illegal substance in the UK and cannot be prescribed, although its use is widespread and it probably has no significant side effects, other than being mildly hallucinogenic in some individuals. A desire to increase the dose and withdrawal symptoms are unusual.[24]

Appetite stimulants

The appetite may be stimulated by small doses of **alcohol**, e.g. sherry or wine, by **cannabis** and by a variety of 'tonics', which probably owe their alleged efficacy to the power of suggestion rather than any inherent property of the preparation. **Megestrol acetate** (Megace®) is used for the treatment of anorexia, weight loss and cachexia in patients with HIV disease. It is supplied as an oral suspension (40 mg/mL) and the usual prescribed dose is 400–800 mg/10–20 mL per day. Side effects are generally mild but varied. However, occasional, more serious side effects include venous thrombosis and impotence. Nurses should consult the product insert for detailed information on side effects. Megace® is not given to pregnant women.

Oral supplements

Oral supplements are often used at an early stage for patients with HIV disease to help maintain weight, reverse nutritional deficiencies and promote anabolism (growth and repair of body tissue).

Supplements of micronutrients

Malnourished patients with HIV disease develop a variety of micronutrient deficiencies, which further depress their immune system and adversely affect both their ability to recover from opportunistic events and their response to chemotherapy.[23] Possible deficiencies include minerals, vitamins (A, C, E and B groups) and trace elements (iron, copper, zinc, iodine, selenium, magnesium etc.). In addition, any infection, including HIV infection, speeds up the production of **oxidants**, which are **free radical molecules** produced by various cellular–enzymatic reactions in the body. Free radicals both damage and reduce the ability of tissues to resist infection and tumours. Increased free radical activity may also trigger programmed cell death (apoptosis), as discussed in Chapter 5, causing a further depletion of CD4+ T-lymphocytes.

Consequently, oral supplementation of micronutrients may be useful, especially in ensuring adequate intake of **beta-carotene** (precursor to vitamin A), **zinc** and various **anti-oxidants** such as vitamins C and E. Trace elements thought to be important in effective immune system function include **zinc** and **selenium**. Finally, increasing the levels of **essential polyunsaturated fatty acids (EFAs)**, e.g. **omega-6** (linoleic acid, derived from vegetable oils such as corn, safflower, sunflower and soybean oils) and **omega-3**, which is present in coldwater fish oils and includes eicosapentaenoic acid (EPA) and **docosahexaenoic acid (DHA)**, may improve immune function.

It would seem sensible for most patients to take a comprehensive over-the-counter **multiple vitamin and mineral preparation** and ensure an adequate supply of **anti-oxidants** and an adequate intake of essential polyunsaturated fats by taking a **fish oil** and **linoleic acid** (e.g. **soya lecithin**) capsule each day.

Enteral feeding

A regular diet may be supplemented with calorie-counted high-energy and protein-rich foods eaten as snacks between meals. However, supplementation is generally better accomplished by using commercial products and, as a wide variety of nutritionally complete foods is available, a dietician's advice is essential.

Enteral supplementation or total nutrition

These formulae may be given via a soft, small-calibre nasogastric or nasoduodenal tube or through an endoscopically or surgically placed gastrostomy or jejunostomy tube. They may be given as additions to a regular diet or as total nutrition.

The choice of oral or enteral supplements, or products used for enteral nutrition, will be based on what the patient is able to tolerate. Different types of formulae include the following.

- **Milk-based polymeric formula**. Polymeric formulae provide protein and other nutrients intact or in a partially hydrolysed form. They require normal gut function for maximum digestion and absorption. If patients can tolerate lactose, milk-based products are less expensive, easily available and often more palatable than lactose-free polymeric formulae.
- **Lactose-free polymeric formula**. When lactose causes diarrhoea, lactose-free polymeric formulae are given and milk drinks avoided. Calcium supplementation may be required in lactose-free diets.
- **Elemental formula**. Unlike polymeric formulae, the protein in elemental formulae is provided in the form of peptides or free amino acids (peptide-based formulae are sometimes referred to as semi-elemental). These formulae require less effective gut functioning before absorption and are commonly used for patients with malabsorption and diarrhoea.

Each commercially prepared enteral formula varies in relation to the composition of carbohydrates and fats, the caloric and protein content and its osmolality. The specific content of each formula is listed in the *Monthly Index of Medical Specialities (MIMS)* (UK), the *British National Formulary (BNF)* and the *Physicians' Desk Reference (PDR)* (USA), but the following general comments can be made.

- **Carbohydrates**. Carbohydrates may include lactose (if tolerated) or, in lactose-free diets, they are supplied in the form of maltodextrin, modified starch, sucrose, corn syrup and/or hydrolysed cornstarch.
- **Fats**. Two types of fats are included in enteral formulae: **long-chain triglycerides (LCTs)** and **medium-chain triglycerides (MCTs)**. Fat is an excellent source of calories; however, LCTs are not well tolerated by patients with impaired gut function and cause mucosal irritation, further compromising nutrient absorption. MCTs are better tolerated and, consequently, are more commonly used in enteral formulae. In addition, the **total fat content** is important. High fat content (i.e. >15 per cent) can promote immunosuppression, and fat intolerance is common in patients with small bowel involvement.[15] Consequently, low-fat enteral formulae (i.e. fat content < 5 per cent) are usually used. As MCTs do not contain linoleic acid, supplements of EFAs, especially omega-6, should be given.
- **Caloric/protein content**. Most enteral formulae are designed to deliver 1.0–1.5 kcal (and 0.02–0.04 g of protein) per mL. Special enteral formulae usually deliver 1.5–2.0 kcal (and 0.06–0.08 g of protein) per mL.[23]
- **Osmolality**. The concentration of osmotically active particles in solution determines its infusion rate. **Isosmolar** formulae are routinely given to patients with relatively intact gut function and are infused at full strength at an initial rate of approximately 40 mL/hour. **Hyperosmolar** formulae are given to patients with gut dysfunction and are initially infused at quarter strength. As tolerance develops, the strength of hyperosmolar diets may be advanced to half to quarter strength, and eventually to full strength. Both types of formulae are infused at an initial rate of 40 mL/hour, the eventual infusion rate being (up to 100–125 mL/hour) dependent upon the patient's tolerance and calculated total caloric and protein requirements.[23]

Caring for patients with feeding tubes

Following insertion of a nasogastric or nasoduodenal tube, an abdominal X-ray is ordered to ensure that the tube has been properly positioned. Continuous feeding is achieved by use of a volumetric pump, and the formula, strength and rate of infusion will be prescribed by the physician. The head of the bed is elevated 30° or more while the infusion is being administered. The tube should be aspirated and the amount of content (residuals) noted every 2 hours. If more than 150 mL, the infusion should be discontinued for 2 hours. After this time, residuals should be re-checked and if <150 mL, the infusion is re-started, otherwise the physician must be consulted. The tube is flushed every 4 hours with 20 mL of sterile water. Intake and output records are maintained and the patient's weight is recorded (in kilograms) weekly on the vital signs chart. The patient's urine should be tested for sugar and acetone each shift and if the urinary sugar is 4+, a serum glucose test should be done immediately. A normal laboratory value for (fasting) serum glucose is 3.9–5.6 mmol/L (or 70–110 mg/dL). If the serum glucose level is >6 mmol/L (or >160 mg/dL), the physician must be notified for treatment orders. The patient must be observed for an increase in temperature, increasing abdominal distension, nausea, vomiting or diarrhoea. Extra supplements of minerals (e.g. zinc, calcium, phosphate, magnesium) may be ordered and vitamin supplements may also be prescribed. Regular blood tests, e.g. full blood count and biochemical assays, are used to monitor the patient.

Parenteral nutrition

Intravenous nutrition may be given as **supplemental parenteral nutrition** or, where it is the sole source of nutrition, as **total parenteral nutrition (TPN)**. Parenteral nutrition requires the intravenous infusion of solutions containing glucose, fat, amino acids, electrolytes, trace elements and vitamins. Because of the high concentration of glucose (10–50 per cent) and protein in these solutions, which cause venous thrombosis, they are normally administered via a central venous catheter. The objectives of TPN in severely malnourished patients with HIV disease include slow, continued gains in weight, lean body mass and quality of life. TPN is initiated in hospital and can be continued in an out-patient or community setting.[16,25]

Central venous catheter

In England, national evidence-based guidelines for preventing bloodstream infections from the insertion and maintenance of central venous catheters[26] are available online from: www.doh.gov.uk/HAI.

Catheter insertion requires full aseptic conditions and is never appropriately done as an emergency procedure. The catheter is not inserted on the wards, but either in the operating theatre (operating room) or in a specialized area, e.g. angiography department, where maximum barrier precautions can be observed. Various catheters are available, e.g. Teflon, silicone and polyurethane, some of which (e.g. Hickman Catheter®) incorporate a Dacron cuff for siting at the distal exit of the skin tunnel, where it provokes a sterile inflammatory process, causing the surrounding tissues to adhere to and anchor the cuff into position.

Central venous access

The catheter is placed in the superior or inferior vena cava or right atrium, or in a large vein leading to these vessels. The catheter may also be inserted via the internal jugular vein, femoral vein or the cephalic vein. However, both neck and antecubital fossa insertion sites are uncomfortable and difficult to manage. Inserting a catheter in the groin (femoral vein) increases the risk of infection. Consequently, most physicians choose to insert the catheter **infraclavicularly** into the **subclavian vein**, positioning the tip of the catheter in the mid-portion of the **superior vena cava**. Triple-lumen catheters are associated with increased risk of infection and are not generally used in patients requiring long-term parenteral nutrition.

A single-lumen catheter (e.g. Hickman®, Silastic Broviac® etc.) is burrowed through the subcutaneous tissue in the anterior chest wall and exits away from the site of subclavian vein puncture. Some silicone catheters (Port-a-Cath®, Mediport®) have a portal that is placed under the skin and sutured to the chest wall. Access to the portal is via a special Huber point needle, which may remain in place for up to 1 week. If the brachial vein in the antecubital fossa or the femoral vein is used, a special 'long line' will be required.

The catheter is inserted under local anaesthesia, with the patient sedated and in the head-down position (unless contraindicated) as a precaution against the risk of air embolism during the negative-pressure phase of respiration[27] and to permit dilatation of the neck and shoulder vessels. During the procedure, the nurse instructs the patient to turn his or her face away from the insertion area to prevent possible contamination of the insertion site. The patient will need to be supported during the procedure to permit hyperextension of the shoulder. This can be facilitated by placing a rolled sheet or towel vertically along the spinal column. The insertion site should be shaved, if necessary, and an appropriate skin disinfectant used, e.g. chlorhexidine 0.5 per cent in 70 per cent spirit. During the insertion, the physician may instruct the patient to bear down with his or her mouth closed (**Valsalva's manoeuvre**) to increase intrathoracic pressure and distend the neck veins. The nurse must help the patient to remain still during the procedure. Following insertion (and after re-positioning of the catheter), a chest X-ray is taken to confirm correct catheter placement before TPN commences. In-line filters are not used, as the particles to be infused are too large to go through a filter. A special occlusive dressing covers the insertion site.

Caring for a patient receiving TPN via a central venous catheter

Following commencement of TPN, the appropriate ongoing assessment, nursing interventions and evaluation are as shown in Table 17.6. Hospital and home-care units should have current protocols for caring for patients having TPN and these should be reviewed on a regular basis. TPN solutions are prepared either commercially or in a pharmacy under a laminar flow hood and are normally supplied in a 3-litre bag, sufficient for one 24-hour period. Pharmacy departments normally supply the infusion with the administration set attached. The nurse must prime the tubing and connect it to the TPN catheter. The inside and outside of the hub of the catheter and the end of the administration set are sprayed with an appropriate disinfectant, e.g. chlorhexidine gluconate, and allowed to dry before the connection is made.

Standard composition of TPN

A standard TPN solution contains protein, carbohydrates, electrolytes and micronutrients (vitamins, minerals and trace elements).

- **Protein.** Protein is utilized by the body in the form of **nitrogen** and is needed for tissue (especially muscle) growth and repair. Protein is the only source of nitrogen and each 6.25 g of whole protein contains 1 g of nitrogen$_2$ (10 g nitrogen$_2$ = 62.5 g protein). Most adult patients with HIV disease require 2.0–2.5 g/kg of protein daily,[23] which is given as mixtures of essential and non-essential synthetic L-amino acids.

TABLE 17.6 Nursing protocols: total parenteral nutrition (TPN)

1. Infuse TPN solution and 20% fat emulsion as per physician's orders, using an alarmed volumetric pump, and check infusion rate every hour. Standard infusion rates are:

TPN solution

Day 1	40 mL/hour	
Day 2	80 mL/hour	by volumetric pump
Day 3	80–125 mL/hour	

Fat emulsion solution

Infuse 500 mL of 20% fat emulsion over 6–8 hours at least three times per week by volumetric pump.

Do not make any rapid changes to infusion rate; adjustments to rate must not exceed 10% of the original rate.

2. Monitor vital signs 4 hourly and notify the physician if the oral temperature is >38 °C.

3. Record fluid intake and output.

4. Weigh daily (at the same time) and record weight in kilograms on patient's observation flow sheet; when stable, weigh twice weekly.

5. Initiate 24-hour urine collections for estimation of urea nitrogen and electrolyte excretion twice weekly, e.g. commencing at 6:00 a.m. every Monday and Thursday.

6. Test blood glucose concentration four times a day, using test strips (e.g. BM-Test 1-44®, Dextrostix® etc.) and a meter. If these are not available, test urine for sugar and acetone four times daily and record on patient's observation flow sheet. If urine sugar is 4+, request a STAT serum glucose test. If the serum glucose is >6 mmol/L (or >160 mg/dL), contact the physician for further instructions.

7. The insertion site is covered with a sterile, semi-occlusive transparent dressing, e.g. Opsite IV3000® or sterile gauze, according to the TPN protocol. Inspect site daily for signs of inflammation and lack of integrity of dressing.

8. When necessary, change dressing according to TPN protocol, using full aseptic technique. Standard protocols include cleaning the entry site with an aqueous solution of chlorhexidine and then dressing it with Opsite IV3000®. Send a swab from the site to the microbiology department for culture and sensitivity.

9. Ensure a pair of atraumatic clamps are kept at the bedside for emergency use.

10. No medications or blood products are given via the TPN catheter. The TPN catheter is not used for central venous pressure (CVP) measurements or withdrawing blood samples. The only time a blood sample from the catheter may be required is if catheter infection is suspected.

11. Change the administration set every 24 (or 48–72) hours as per TPN protocol, only using administration sets with a Luer Lock fitting.

12. If TPN is temporarily stopped, the catheter should be flushed with 5–10 mL of normal saline when the feed is discontinued, and again prior to recommencing TPN.

13. A single bag of TPN solution must not be infused over a period longer than 24 hours. If any feed remains after this time, it is discarded.

14. Ensure standard TPN laboratory examinations are drawn weekly according to TPN protocols for comprehensive biochemical monitoring.

Test for:[23,28]

Daily	Glucose, electrolytes and blood urea nitrogen (when patient is stable, change from daily monitoring to twice weekly)
Baseline then twice weekly	Serum albumin, transferrin, liver function studies, serum creatinine, haemoglobin, haemocrit, white blood cell count, calcium, phosphate and magnesium levels
Baseline then weekly	Prothrombin time, micronutrient tests, e.g. copper, zinc, transferrin, triglyceride, pre-albumin, retinol binding protein

- **Carbohydrate.** This is given for energy and heat production and is measured in kilocalories (kcal). A sufficient amount of non-protein carbohydrate calories (protein sparing) must be given to ensure that the amino acids are used for tissue growth and repair and not energy. Glucose (dextrose) is the preferred source of carbohydrate and is used in various strengths, from 10 to 50 per cent. The usual energy requirement for adults with HIV disease[23] is 35–40 kcal/kg, i.e. approximately 2500–3000 kcal daily.

■ **Fat.** Fat is also given for protein-sparing energy and has the advantages of a high energy to fluid volume ratio, neutral pH, iso-osmolarity with plasma and provides essential fatty acids. Patients undergoing standard TPN therapy should receive 3–5 per cent of their daily caloric intake in the form of fat. This may be achieved by routinely administering 500 mL of a 20 per cent fat emulsion (usually derived from soya bean oil) containing 2 kcal/mL over 6–8 hours at least three times a week.[23] Several days of adaptation may be needed to attain maximal utilization of fat emulsions. Reactions to a 20 per cent fat emulsion include episodes of pyrexia and, rarely, anaphylactic responses.[24] Additives are never mixed with fat emulsions unless their compatibility has been approved by a pharmacist.

■ **Micronutrients.** Micronutrients (e.g. vitamins, minerals and trace elements) and **electrolytes** (e.g. sodium, chloride, potassium etc.) are added by pharmacy to the daily infusion as prescribed.

Complications of central TPN therapy

A variety of complications are associated with central TPN administration. Complications can be technical, infectious or metabolic.

Technical complications

Important technical complications include catheter misplacement, pneumothorax, thrombosis, catheter embolism and, importantly, **air embolism**.

Air embolism can be fatal and may occur when the patient is in the upright or semi-upright position and the integrity of the subclavian venous catheter infusion system is disrupted (disconnected).[23] This event is characterized by the sudden onset in the patient of severe respiratory distress, associated with both cardiac and neurologic deficits. Treatment involves the immediate positioning of the patient in the Durant position (lying on the left side with the head down and the feet elevated) and prompt syringe aspiration of blood and air from the subclavian catheter. Prevention relies on ensuring the integrity of the catheter system, i.e. secure fixation of all catheter connections and using only Luer Lock (never 'male–female') catheter connections.

Infectious complications

Infectious complications include insertion-site infection, primary catheter infection and secondary infections.

Localized **insertion-site infection** is easily detected, as the surrounding skin becomes erythematous and tender and the catheter tract may exude purulent drainage. **Primary catheter infection** is more difficult to detect. However, the key diagnostic triad of catheter infection (in order of occurrence) is:[23]

1. a 'plateau' temperature pattern (38.0–38.5 °C) for 12–24 hours;
2. unexplained hyperglycaemia (>6 mmol/L or 160 mg/dL);
3. an increased number of leucocytes (white blood cells) – leucocytosis (<11.0 × 10^9/L).

Both insertion-site and primary catheter infections, when diagnosed, require that the TPN catheter be removed (and the tip sent to the microbiology department for culture and sensitivity). A new central TPN catheter must be inserted at a new site. The physician will prescribe appropriate antibiotic therapy for the infection.

Metabolic complications

A range of metabolic complications are associated with TPN therapy, including high and low serum levels of glucose, sodium, potassium, phosphates, chloride, calcium etc.

Hyperglycaemia is the most frequent metabolic complication of TPN therapy, even in non-diabetic patients. Insulin may be prescribed to be given concurrently with the TPN solution and it is usually given separately by a syringe pump. The blood glucose level should be maintained at ≥6 mmol/L (160 mg/dL). Insulin may be added to the TPN solution, but no more than 40 units of insulin should be added to 1 litre of solution. If insulin is added to the TPN solution, it is added as 10-unit increments (i.e. 10 units in each litre of TPN solution) and the blood glucose level is maintained by giving additional insulin intravenously until control is achieved by the insulin in the TPN solution.

Hypoglycaemia (blood glucose level <3.9 mmol/L or <70 mg/dL) often occurs when the TPN solution is suddenly discontinued. Hypoglycaemia is usually prevented by 'tapering off' TPN therapy, ensuring that oral carbohydrate intake is sufficient before discontinuing TPN. If hypoglycaemia occurs, it is generally treated by infusions of 10 per cent dextrose in normal saline.

During TPN therapy, patients should be as ambulatory as possible and, if being discharged, intensive patient education programmes can prepare them to take a large share of the responsibility for successful home treatment.

Peripheral parenteral nutrition

Short-term (not more than 5–7 days) peripheral parenteral nutrition (PPN) may be given through an 18-gauge intravenous cannula inserted into a peripheral vein, but the parenteral nutrition solution has a lower concentration of glucose. A standard litre of PPN solution contains 500 mL 20 per cent dextrose in water and 500 mL 10 per cent amino acids, plus vitamins, minerals and trace elements. In addition, a daily infusion of 500 mL of 20 per cent fat emulsion is given. The cannula is re-sited every 48–72 hours and the insertion site is routinely dressed with a transparent polyurethane film dressing, e.g. Op-Site®.

REFERENCES

1. Miller T, Gorbach S (eds.). *Nutritional Aspects of HIV Infection*. London: Arnold (Hodder Headline Group), 1999, 216 pp.
2. Colebunders R, Mann JM, Francis H et al. Evaluation of a clinical case definition of acquired immunodeficiency syndrome in Africa. *Lancet* 1987; I:492–4.
3. Centers for Disease Control. Revision of the CDC surveillance case definition for acquired immunodeficiency syndrome: a report by the Council of State and Territorial Epidemiologists, AIDS Program. *Morbidity and Mortality Weekly Report (MMWR)* 14 August 1987; **36**(Suppl. 1):1–15S.
4. Raiten DJ. *Nutrition and HIV Infection: a Review and Evaluation of the Extant Knowledge of the Relationship between Nutrition and HIV Infection*. Bethesda, MD: LSRO, Federation of American Societies for Experimental Biology, 1990.
5. Herbert V. The five possible causes of all nutrient deficiency: illustrated by deficiencies of vitamin B12 and folic acid. *American Journal of Clinical Nutrition* 1973; **26**:77–88.
6. Kotler DP. Malnutrition in HIV infection and AIDS. *AIDS* 1989; **3**(Suppl. 1):S175–80.

7. Kern KA, Norton JA. Cancer cachexis. *Journal of Parenteral and Enteral Nutrition* 1988; **12**:286–98.

8. Torun B, Viteri FE. Protein–energy malnutrition. In: Shils ME, Young VR (eds), *Modern Nutrition in Health and Disease*, 7th edn. Philadelphia: Lea & Febiger, 1988, 746–73.

9. Fleck A. Acute phase response: implications for nutrition and recovery. *Nutrition* 1988; **4**:109–17.

10. Lahdevirta J, Maury CPJ, Teppo AM et al. Elevated levels of circulating cachectin/tumor necrosis factor in patients with acquired immunodeficiency syndrome. *American Journal of Medicine* 1988; **85**:289–91.

11. Grunfeld C, Palladino MA Jr. Tumor necrosis factor; immunologic, antitumor, metabolic and cardiovascular activities. *Advances in Internal Medicine* 1990; **35**:45–71.

12. Summerbell DC, Perett JP, Gazzard BC. Causes of weight loss in human immunodeficiency virus infection. *International Journal of STD & AIDS* 1993; **4**:234–6.

13. Fields Newman C, Horn B. Drug–nutrient interactions. In: *AIDS Guidebook*. Freemont, CA: The Cutting Edge Consulting, 1988.

14. Ghiron L, Dwyer J, Stollman LB. Nutrition support of the HIV-positive, ARC and AIDS patient. *Clinical Nutrition* 1989; **8**:103–13.

15. Andrassy RJ. Nutrition and immunocompromise: an overview. *AIDS Patient Care* 1990; **4**(Suppl. D):S9–12.

16. Ellis W, Basinger G, Paul J et al. The use of home total parenteral nutrition in a patient with AIDS. *AIDS Patient Care* 1994; **8**:6–10.

17. O'Sullivan P, Linke RA, Dalton S. Evaluation of body weight and nutritional status among AIDS patients. *Journal of the American Dietetic Association* 1985; **85**:1483–4.

18. Schwenk A, Burger B, Wessel D et al. Clinical risk factors for malnutrition in HIV-1 infected patients. *AIDS* 1993; **7**:1213–19.

19. Mascioli E. Nutrition and HIV infection. *AIDS Clinical Care* 1993; **5**:85–7.

20. McQuiggan M. Enteral nutrition for the hospitalized HIV patient. *AIDS Patient Care* 1990; **4**(Suppl. D):S13–16.

21. Ross H. *Nutrition & HIV Infection*. The AIDS Education and Research Trust (AVERT), UK, 1993.

22. Physicians' Association for AIDS Care. *HIV Disease: Nutrition Guidelines: Practical Steps for a Healthier Life*. Stadlanders Pharmacy, USA, 1993.

23. Hickey MS. *Handbook of Enteral, Parenteral and ARC/AIDS Nutritional Therapy*. St Louis, MO: Mosby Year Book, 1992.

24. British Medical Association and the Royal Pharmaceutical Society of Great Britain. *British National Formulary*, March 1994, No. 27.

25. Mughal M, Irving M. Home parenteral nutrition in the United Kingdom and Ireland. *Lancet* 1986; **ii**:383–7.

26. Pratt RJ, Pellowe C, Loveday HP, Robinson N, Smith GW and the **epic** Guideline Development Team. The **epic** Project: Developing National Evidence-based Guidelines for Preventing Healthcare associated Infections. Phase 1: Guidelines for Preventing Hospital-acquired Infections. *Journal of Hospital Infection* 2001; **47**(Suppl.):S1–S82. Available online at: www.doh.gov.uk/HAI

27. Taylor M. Total parenteral nutrition (Parts 1 & 2). *Nursing Standard* 1994; **8**(23):25–8 and **8**(24):37–9.

28. Howard LJ. Parenteral and enteral nutrition and therapy. In: Wilson JD, Braunwald E, Isselbacher KJ et al. (eds), *Harrison 's Principles of Internal Medicine*, Vol. 1, 12th (International) edn, Part 4(75). London: McGraw-Hill, 1991, 427–34.

FURTHER READING

Miller T, Gorbach S (eds). *Nutritional Aspects of HIV Infection*. London: Arnold (Hodder Headline Group), 1999, 216 pp.

CHAPTER 18

Discharge planning and community care

Introduction

Many patients with late symptomatic disease (AIDS) will require community nursing services at some point in their illness. Successful community nursing care is in part dependent upon good discharge planning procedures when patients are in hospital. This chapter discusses the discharge planning that is in use in the UK; however, the principles of how to discharge patients safely to their homes that are dealt with here apply in most countries.

Learning outcomes

After studying and reflecting on the material in this chapter, you will be able to:

- discuss a policy for the safe discharge of patients from hospital to the community;
- identify nursing practice issues in caring for patients in the community.

DISCHARGE PLANNING

Effective discharge planning requires strategic planning by hospitals and health authorities and, just as there is often an admissions policy, there must be a discharge policy. Table 18.1 can serve as a model for this policy.[1]

On admission, the nursing assessment must include the relevant social history of the patient. This should include an assessment of the requisites for health described in Chapter 16, which can then be reassessed and documented upon discharge. A standard format can be

TABLE 18.1 Discharge policy

Aims

1. The safe discharge of all adults to situations where:
    (a) their treatment and recovery will be continuous with that given in hospital
    (b) their immediate needs for warmth, food and relief from pain are met
    (c) they have shelter and are safe from molestation
2. The implementation of procedures for safe discharges for adults, and the monitoring of practices and progress
3. Close co-operation with local authority (municipal) services
4. Co-ordination of effort between hospital and community-based healthcare professionals
5. Establishing effective lines of communication with all parties involved

Objectives commensurate with these aims are to ensure that:

1. Each individual patient receives the care and attention necessary without having to compete with others
2. Where a patient is found to need nursing care, he or she will not be discharged unless there is suitable provision
3. All vulnerable patients (and those living alone) have someone to see them into their home
4. Planning for discharge starts as soon as possible (preferably before admission)
5. The handover of the care of the patient from hospital to the community should provide for continuous cover for the patient

Planning process

1. Weekly planning meetings are held by the ward team to co-ordinate and take responsibility for the recovery and safe discharge of all patients; it is essential that relevant community nursing staff attend these meetings
2. The planning meeting will assess the ability of the patient to manage the situation that will be encountered on discharge and advise the responsible physician accordingly
3. The planning meeting will decide which pre-discharge preparations are required and the ward sister (head nurse) is responsible for seeing that these preparations are put into effect and for setting a target date for the patient's discharge
4. The responsibility for successful discharge shall fall to the nurse in charge of the ward at the time of the patient's discharge; this nurse will have the authority to cancel the discharge if the arrangements agreed by the planning meeting are not yet completed
5. The discharge is not effective until the persons/agencies in the community have taken over any of the caring duties deemed necessary and, until that time, responsibility for the patient's continuing care shall remain with the hospital
6. Responsibility for medical cover must be transferred to the patient's general practitioner (family doctor) in advance of the patient's discharge
7. It is the responsibility of the nurse in charge to see that all parties concerned have been informed of the patient's discharge by the end of the discharge day

used to detail the social history aspects of the nursing assessment if it is carefully designed so that it can be individualized for each patient. The Social History Form in Figure 18.1 outlines some of the essential information that will be needed and this form can also serve as a permanent record of the patient's discharge plans.

Procedures for safe discharge should be established and should include guidance for hospital nursing personnel, community nursing personnel and local authority staff. Table 18.1 is a suggested model for effecting the safe discharge of patients with HIV disease.

Preparing for discharge from hospital

A Social History Form can be initiated in the out-patients department or the accident and emergency department by the nurse effecting the admission. It remains the responsibility of the nurse admitting the patient to the ward to complete the form as far as possible during the

SOCIAL HISTORY

Name _____ _____ Age _____

Hospital identification number _____ Ward _____

Date of admission/nursing assessment _____

Address _____ _____

_____

_____ _____ (Telephone number) _____

Next of kin and address _____

_____

_____ _____ (Telephone number) _____

General practitioner and address _____

_____

_____ (Telephone number) _____

Admitting consultant _____

Next of kin informed of admission: YES/NO

Comment _____

_____

GP informed of admission: YES/NO

Comment _____

_____

Reason for admission _____

_____

FIGURE 18.1 *Social History Form.*   contd ▶

Accommodation

Own   Rented   Private   Council   Sheltered

House   Flat   Room   Which floor? _____

Stairs _____

Toilet (which floor?) _____

Heating _____ Central heating

Cooking facilities _____

Coin Metres for   Heating   YES/NO   Electricity   YES/NO

Accommodation shared with _____

_____

Pets _____

Pets being looked after by _____

Keys to accommodation with _____

Is accommodation now secure?   YES/NO

If no, what action being taken? _____

Employer and address _____

_____

_____ (Telephone number) _____

Does employer need to be informed of admission?   YES/NO

If yes, who is informing employer? _____

Date employer notified _____

Name/position of individual notified _____

_____

contd ▶

COMMUNITY SERVICES

Service	On admission			On discharge	
	Known	Frequency	Informed of admission	Needed	Arrangement
District Nurse					
Health Visitor					
Home Help					
Community Physiotherapist					
Community Occupational Therapist					
Social Worker					
Meals on Wheels					
Volunteer					
Other (Specify)					
Comments:					

contd ▶

SOCIAL HISTORY/DISCHARGE PLANS

Medications	
Medication being taken on admission	Medication to be taken home on discharge

Medications (patient education)

Date/Time/Name and position of individual instructing patient on discharge medications

Date _____ Time _____ Health professional _____

Assessment of patient education:

Does patient understand how to self-administer medications?	YES/NO
Is patient aware of common side-effects of medication and how to detect signs/symptoms of side-effects and reactions?	YES/NO
Has patient been given *written* instructions on how to self-administer medications, their side-effects and how and when to obtain new supply?	YES/NO
If patient on zidovudine (Retrovir – AZT), has he/she been issued with a timed medication device and instructed on how to use it?	YES/NO
Have all medications/instructions been listed on discharge summary to community nursing services?	YES/NO

Transportation: Indicate below arrangements made for patient's transportation home

Ordered by _____ Date _____

If patient lives alone, who will accompany patient home and see him/her safely in their home?

contd ▶

Requisites for health: State discharge status for the following self-care requisites

The need for adequate respiration:

The need for adequate hydration:

The need for adequate nutrition:

The need for urinary and faecal elimination:

The need to control body temperature:

The need for movement and mobilization:

The need for a safe environment:

The need for personal cleansing and dressing:

The need for expression and communication:

The need for working and playing:

The need for adequate rest and sleep:

The need to maintain psychological equilibrium:

The need to worship according to his/her own faith:

The need to express sexuality:

Has patient education on safer sex been implemented?   YES/NO

Needs associated with dying:

contd ▶

DISCHARGE PLANNING MEETINGS

Notes of Discharge Planning Meetings. Enter summary of Discharge Planning arrangements agreed (date and sign each entry)

Original social history assessment completed by:

_____ Date _____

(Nurse to *print* name)

Signature _____

Final Social History/Discharge Plans completed by:

_____ Date _____

(Nurse responsible for safe discharge of
patient – to *print* name)

Signature _____

NB   A copy of this form is to be sent to Community Nursing Service on
     day of discharge and original filed in patient's case notes.

initial nursing assessment. The nurse in charge of the ward is responsible for ensuring that the Social History Form has been initiated by the end of the first day of admission.

As soon as it becomes clear that either local authority or community nursing services are currently being provided on a regular basis, these agencies are notified of the admission. This should occur within 24 hours of admission or, if at the weekend, as soon as the offices open. The Hospital Admissions Office must send notification of the patient's admission to their general practitioner (GP) or health centre as soon as possible, on the day after admission.

For patients living alone at the time of admission, the nurse in charge should ensure that: a set of house keys has been located and kept either with the patient or in a safe place; arrangements are made through friends/neighbours/relatives to look after the accommodation; any pets will be cared for and, if not, that the social services are notified immediately; any documents or valuables are itemized and kept with the patient or in the hospital's security department.

Any information about a patient that is received from a relative/friend/neighbour should be recorded by nursing staff. All relevant information about the social circumstances of the patient should be collected, and sought if not offered, from relevant agencies by the time of the first planning meeting after admission.

At the planning meeting, a provisional plan is made for:

- any likely treatment,
- anticipated length of hospital stay,
- the direction of discharge (e.g. own home, convalescence, extended care facility),
- the patient's need for care at point of discharge,
- any agencies that might offer care.

The plan is reviewed at each planning meeting subsequently and, as the patient returns to fitness, action is delegated to alert and involve relatives/friends of the patient and agencies as appropriate.

The patient's consent is required before his or her medical details are given to any outside agencies. It should be explained to any patient who is unwilling to give this consent that without it the necessary community services cannot be adequately arranged. Representatives of all community agencies involved should be invited to planning meetings.

The decision about an appropriate avenue for discharge is made by the planning team in consultation with the patient and his or her family and friends. All action necessary to prepare the patient and the home environment is instigated at the planning meeting. If the community agencies/family and friends are not able to attend the meetings themselves, their views should be given by the social work member of the team or, if this is not possible, by others who have met them. It is the responsibility of the social worker to see that these views are represented in some way at the planning meetings.

For patients being discharged to convalescence or extended care facilities, the date is set by the receiving facility. It must be clear that the hospital will re-admit the patient if convalescence breaks down prior to his or her return home date.

If the patient is to return directly home and needs support, referrals to the relevant agency should be made at least 2 weeks in advance of any likely discharge date. These referrals should be conducted in terms of a request for assessment of the patient whilst in hospital, i.e. before the next planning meeting. At the planning meeting, a date is fixed, depending on service provisions, and all relevant agencies are notified of the decision on the same day.

The date of the discharge, if it involves community services, should be fixed at least 1 week in advance and, if possible, at the penultimate planning meeting, so that the final planning meeting confirms all arrangements. As soon as the date of the discharge is set, all relevant parties are notified, including transportation services, if required. The decision as to who notifies whom is made at the planning meeting.

During the last week in hospital, the patient should be visited by representatives of any agencies providing community care, and preferably by the individual carer. Prior to discharge, each patient should receive written confirmation, on one document, of the dates and times of relevant visits to them by community services. Before the patient leaves the ward, it is the responsibility of the nurse in charge on that day to ensure that:

- the patient has all necessary drugs and dressings and has been instructed (preferably by a pharmacist) how to use them;
- all valuables and effects held by the hospital are given to the patient or his or her escort;
- the patient has access to his or her home accommodation;
- there is someone to see the patient inside safely (other than transportation personnel);
- the patient is equipped with a written document of agencies who will be visiting him or her, with dates and times;
- where relevant, a letter for the receiving nursing adviser accompanies the patient;
- the patient has adequate supplies of food to last until the next visit by someone providing a shopping service, where needed;
- power, heating and water supplies in the accommodation are fully operational;
- the patient has enough money for essential needs to last until the next day when banks/post offices are open;
- all relevant agencies have been fully informed;*
- all equipment and adaptations have been provided.

Responsibility for the care of the patient is transferred to the escort and then to the person settling the patient into the home. Before leaving the patient, that person must ensure that all the checks described above (except*) have been completed and are satisfactory. The escort or the receiver of the patient should take responsibility for notifying the discharging ward immediately of any deficiencies in the provision.

The patient can be said to have been safely discharged only when comfortably settled, with immediate needs for food, warmth and relief from pain met, and there is a comprehensive plan for the continuing care of that individual within the community that is understood by all parties.

Discharge against medical advice

Attempts should be made to dissuade patients from discharging themselves against medical advice. The patient may agree to see a counsellor or psychiatrist prior to leaving and, if so, this should be facilitated. In every case, the patient is told (and this is documented in writing) that the hospital will accept no responsibility for the consequences of patients discharging themselves and that community services cannot be guaranteed.

COMMUNITY SERVICES

Where a known patient is admitted to the hospital, the district nurse should notify the ward of the service being provided, including treatment given prior to admission. Where possible, this should be done by a visit to the ward. If the patient is known to live alone, social services should be notified as soon as possible if arrangements are needed to protect the patient's home. Any action taken in this way must also be notified to the ward.

When a known patient is to be discharged to the care of a district nurse, the district nurse should visit the hospital during the week preceding discharge in order to discuss the continuing care needs of the patient with both the ward nursing staff and the patient. All home assessments should be carried out within 24 hours of the discharge. The district nurse should notify the ward of the first day the visit can be made to the patient being discharged.

Local authority staff (community municipal services)

For a patient who is receiving any social or municipal services, e.g. home help, home meals, day centre attendance, and is known to have entered hospital, notice of the involvement should be sent to the ward immediately. If the patient lives alone, the agent of social services should ensure that arrangements have been made to protect the property. Any other personal details can only be disclosed with the consent of the patient. The agent should telephone the ward to arrange a time to visit and to attend the next planning meeting. The agent should also notify the hospital social worker. Agents may decide it is appropriate for a hospital social worker to convey their views at the planning meeting and can negotiate with the hospital social work department for this to be done.

The agent should visit the patient in hospital as soon as possible and negotiate the release of information to the ward staff. This information is then given to the nurse in charge.

During the patient's stay in hospital, any information or developments that occur in the home, including the care of any children, should be notified to the ward immediately.

All improvements to the home that are essential to the patient's safe return should be initiated as soon as they are identified, and completed prior to the safe discharge of the patient. Adaptations in the home may be initiated by the hospital occupational therapy department and paid for by the local authority.

As soon as a discharge date is foreseeable, the hospital will contact the relevant community agencies. If the patient has not received a service within the last 3 months (including time in hospital), the agencies will make an assessment of the level of need within 1 week of a request. Ideally, this will entail a visit to the patient in hospital and a report within no more than a week on the level of service that will be offered.

One week after the initial request for an assessment has been made, a discharge date may be arranged depending on the findings and the views of the community agencies involved. Any objections or other pertinent information should be communicated to the ward before or at the discharge planning meeting. For extremely dependent/handicapped patients, this may involve a separate conference at the hospital, which all agencies should endeavour to attend.

If a patient goes to a convalescent facility without being visited in hospital, the community agencies should have 2 weeks' notice of the return home date, and should carry out an assessment on the first working day after return with a view to starting the service as soon as possible.

Community nursing services

Clearly, there should be enough community nurses in a Primary Care Trust to be able to offer a nursing visit at any time of the day or night and at weekends. Many patients with end-stage

HIV disease can only be cared for safely in the community if they have access to round-the-clock nursing care. A central contact point that can identify and locate any community nurse in the area, 24 hours a day, is required. This involves clerical support and a paging system.

Nursing care in the community

All members of the primary healthcare team may be involved in the care of people with HIV-related illnesses, e.g. GP, health visitor, community nurse, family planning nurse, school nurse, practice nurse and community psychiatric nurse. Clearly, their involvement in the discharge planning process is essential if continuity of care is to be realized. Patients should be encouraged to give permission for their GP to be fully informed of their condition so that meaningful community nursing care can be assessed and planned with the support of their medical adviser. On occasion, patients refuse to give permission for their GP to be informed of their diagnosis and, although the patients' wishes must be absolutely respected, this situation is fraught with real difficulties and the patient should be explicitly made aware that there are potential problems involved. In these circumstances, district nurses will have to liaise with hospital medical staff in caring for these individuals. However, most GPs establish trusting relationships with their patients and it is becoming more unusual for patients to refuse permission for their GP to be informed of their medical condition.

People with HIV disease can live safely with healthy members of the family in the community without any fear of HIV transmission from them to family and friends. In advising HIV-infected patients, community nursing staff should take the following points into consideration.

Personal hygiene

Good general personal hygiene practices should be adopted. Razors, toothbrushes or other implements that could become contaminated with blood should not be shared. Sanitary towels must be disposed of in heavy-duty plastic bags, which can be discreetly collected and sent for incineration along with other contaminated wastes. Tampons may be flushed down the toilet. Individuals with HIV infection should wear gloves when cleaning fish bowls or bird cages, gardening and dealing with cat litter trays because of the risk of contamination with potential parasitic pathogens, e.g. *Toxoplasma gondii, Cryptococcus neoformans*.

General hygiene

Individuals with HIV infection can safely prepare, cook and serve food for others, observing the usual standards of good hygiene (i.e. hands washed prior to food preparation and after handling any uncooked foods). Special crockery and cutlery are not necessary, and all crockery and cutlery should be washed after use in hand-hot water with a detergent (a disinfectant is not needed) and left to drip dry.

Linen visibly contaminated with blood, body fluids, excretions or secretions can be safely washed in a washing machine on the hot cycle. The hot cycle on standard washing machines exceeds the Department of Health recommendations of 71 °C (160 °F) for not less than 3 minutes plus mixing time. This temperature and the addition of a detergent will inactivate any HIV, and added disinfectants are not necessary. If the patient is too ill to do his or her own laundry, it can be done by a home help, friends or, if necessary, arrangements can be made by the district nurse to have it processed at a local authority laundry. In this case, it is ideally first placed in a water-soluble plastic bag, which is put in an appropriately colour-coded nylon (or heavy-duty plastic) bag. In general, community nurses make arrangements with the environmental health department in their local authority to collect the laundry. This must be done discreetly; colour-coded bags of contaminated laundry or rubbish must not be left outside the patient's home, visible to neighbours, and collection personnel must be well educated so that they do not arrive wearing bizarre protective clothing (which, of course, is not necessary). If this point is not attended to, inadvertent breaches of confidentiality might result, with disastrous consequences for the patient.

Individuals with HIV infection can use the same toilet and bath or shower as anyone else in the household; normal domestic cleaning is adequate after use (disinfectants are not necessary).

Clearly, individuals with HIV infection may use, for example, the library, pub, restaurant, cinema, as any other member of the community might. There is no possibility of HIV transmission in public swimming baths.[2]

In general, individuals with HIV infection should be encouraged to continue their usual employment and they may have to be discreet about informing their employer and fellow workmates of their medical condition.

Patient education

Health education designed to promote the primary prevention of others and secondary prevention for the patient should be implemented. Community nurses may need to discuss 'safer sex' practices with patients, and leaflets are available from a variety of sources, for example the Terrence Higgins Trust in London. Individuals with HIV infection should be advised not to donate blood, tissues, organs or semen or to carry donor cards. They should not breast-feed infants (see Chapter 12). Patient education is discussed in more detail in Chapter 19.

Dental treatment

Ideally, people who are infected with HIV should inform their dentist of this fact when presenting for treatment. However, this has often resulted in a refusal by a dentist to treat an infected individual. All dentists have been advised by the Department of Health in the UK, and the Centers for Disease Control and Prevention (CDC) in the USA, to observe universal precautions with all patients, all the time, regardless of what they know or do not know about their serological status for HIV infection.[3,4]

Planning for home care

The following points should be considered when assessing and planning care for patients in the community. It is essential that community nurses caring for patients with HIV infection are themselves free of any infectious illness (e.g. colds, herpes labialis) so as not to transmit any infections to the patient. Good hand-washing technique prior to nursing the patient and on completion of nursing care is required. Community nursing staff (and their managers) must know and understand the local operational policies and procedures for the community nursing care of patients with HIV-related illness. If no operational policies and procedures exist, they should be urgently prepared.

Sharps and injections

Community nurse managers should ensure that all equipment needed for caring safely for patients is readily available to community nurses.

Extreme caution must be taken when dealing with or disposing of needles and other sharp instruments. A suitable sharps container can be left in the patient's home until it is two-thirds full, when it is sealed and arrangements are made for it to be collected for incineration. Small portable sharps containers are available, which can be safely carried by community nurses.

Needles must never be re-capped or re-inserted into their original sheaths, and the needle is not disengaged from the syringe prior to disposal, but is disposed of as a single unit into the sharps container. The only exception is after the collection of blood, when the needle is carefully disengaged from the syringe (preferably with a needle holder) to avoid a microscopic aerosol contamination when the blood is injected into the specimen container. Vacuum collection devices (e.g. Vacutainers) are preferable to a syringe and needle for venesection.

Preventing and managing occupational exposure to blood-borne pathogens

It is important that nurses and others involved in caring for patients at home take appropriate precautions to prevent exposure to blood-borne pathogens. These precautions are comprehensively described in Chapters 14 and 15. Should mucous membranes (e.g. eyes, nose, mouth) be accidentally splashed with blood or other potentially infectious body fluids, or should a needle-stick injury occur, the procedures outlined in Chapter 15 should be followed.

Cuts

Any cuts or open lesions on the arms or hands of nursing personnel must be covered with a waterproof, occlusive bandage. Nurses with eczema on their hands should not deliver direct personal care to any patient, including those with known HIV infection.

Infection control precautions

No protective clothing or infection control precautions are required to enter the patient's home, for introductions (shaking his or her hand) or for talking to the patient. Community nurses must observe the infection control precautions discussed in Chapters 14 and 15. The patient should be encouraged to maintain social relationships and not to become isolated. Family and friends frequently require reassurance regarding the infectious nature of the patient's condition.

Toilets

If the patient has restricted mobility and cannot use the toilet, a bedside commode or 'chemical toilet' may be useful. Bedpans and urinals should be carefully emptied into the toilet (avoiding splashing), rinsed and stored dry (i.e. they must not be left soaking in a disinfectant). Community nurses should wear disposable gloves when handling bedpans and urinals and when dealing with incontinent patients. After flushing, it is not necessary to pour disinfectants into the toilet.

Spillages

Spillages of blood or other bloody body fluids from any patient, including those known to be infected with HIV, should be carefully covered with a suitable disinfectant, left for 5–10 minutes and then carefully wiped up with disposable paper towels, which are disposed of into a plastic bag. Nurses should wear gloves and a plastic apron when dealing with spillages. If spillages occur on carpets, they should be carefully mopped up with paper towels; chlorine-based disinfectants should not be used. After wiping up the spillage, the area of carpet can be cleaned with a detergent and hot soapy water.

Palliative and terminal care

Many patients with end-stage HIV disease will require palliative and terminal care at home, which are much the same as they are for any other patient. Attention to symptom control is paramount, and this will require a twilight or night community nursing service.

Death at home

The usual last offices are carried out, observing the same infection control precautions as those in operation when the patient was alive. Disposable gloves and aprons should be worn by those performing last offices. Undertakers will bring a plastic cadaver bag and will put the body into it. Once the body is in the cadaver bag, transport personnel do not require any protective clothing to handle it.

Summary

Operational policies must exist that allow community nurses the time to complete a home-care nursing assessment prior to the patient's discharge from hospital. The actual delivery of nursing care to patients with HIV disease in the home is exactly the same as that required for the nursing care of any other patient. Because of the various opportunistic infections patients with HIV disease may present with, additional infection control precautions beyond the Standard Principles of infection prevention may be needed. Community nurses have an immense role to play in this epidemic – perhaps the most critical role of all. Every opportunity for health education must be embraced and, with careful discharge planning, community nurses will be able to coordinate all the services patients require. These nurses are strategically placed to make a real impact on the quality of care delivered, and evidence to date indicates they are responding to this challenge with their usual brand of improvisation, courage and compassion.

REFERENCES

1. Crowther P, Donnelly D, Hill P et al. (1987). *Discharge from hospital.* A discussion document with reference to the Riverside (West) Health Authority, 2 February 1987. London: Riverside Health Authority.
2. Royal Society of Medicine. Public swimming pools and AIDS. *The AIDS Letter* 1987; **1**:8.
3. DHSS (1986). Guidance for surgeons, anaesthetists, dentists and their teams in dealing with patients infected with HTLV-III. Acquired immune Deficiency Syndrome AIDS, Booklet 3 (April), CMO (86)7, 6.
4. Centers for Disease Control. Recommendations for prevention of HIV transmission in health-care settings. *Morbidity and Mortality Weekly Report (MMWR)* 21 August 1987; **36**(2S):S7–8.

The nurse as a health educator

Introduction

The concept of the nurse as a 'health educator' is emphasized in most descriptions of the role of the professional nurse. In the UK, university educational programmes that prepare students to become registered professional nurses stress the importance of ensuring that they acquire skills in relation to the identification of the health-related learning needs of patients, their families and friends and to participation in health promotion. Today, the skilled participation of nurses in primary, secondary and tertiary prevention is essential. This chapter is designed to illustrate effective patient/client education techniques that nurses can use as 'educators for health' (Figure 19.1).

Learning outcomes

After studying and reflecting on the material in this chapter, you will be able to:

[Short-term goal]	**understand** the underlying principles and practice of patient education and **have an opportunity** to demonstrate the technical skills needed to effectively participate in primary, secondary and tertiary health promotion activities;
[Long-term goal]	**practise** the skills of health education and fulfil the educative role of the professional nurse;
[Objectives]	**describe** a systematic model of health education appropriate for use in a clinical setting;
	identify the critical elements of:
	(a) assessing learning needs,
	(b) planning an educational response,
	(c) implementing patient education encounters,
	(d) evaluating learning;

demonstrate practice techniques related to effective patient education;
discuss obstacles to patient learning;
outline a strategy for patient education activities in your own practice setting.

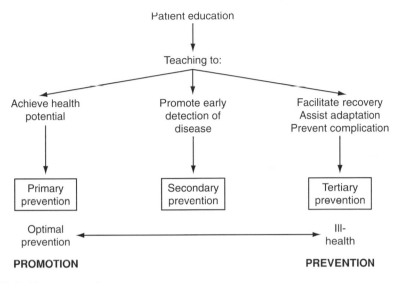

FIGURE 19.1 *Health education and prevention.*

BACKGROUND

There are various models of health education available, all having relevance and uses for different individuals, cultures and situations. Although no single model of health education is always ideal in the variety of situations found in clinical practice, probably the most useful for nurses is an eclectic 'educational model' (Table 19.1). This is based on the belief that health behaviour is a product of prior learning and that this behaviour can be changed by educational processes. In this model, the nurse acts as a teacher and the patient accepts the role of the learner. This approach has been labelled 'teaching for health' and has been extensively described by Coutts and Hardy.[1] Their model sets out the following activities designed to identify and solve health-related problems:

- informing (giving information);
- advising;

TABLE 19.1 Educational model

Assess learning needs/potential learning opportunities
Plan education programmes
Implement appropriate teaching
Evaluate effectiveness of encounter

- helping with the acquisition of skills;
- assisting with the process of clarifying beliefs, feelings and values;
- enabling the adaptation of lifestyle;
- promoting change in the structures and organizations that influence health status;
- providing a model of values and behaviour related to health.

Inherent in an educational model is the ability of the nurse to **assess** the learning needs of patients and relatives and the potential learning opportunities available, **plan** patient education programmes, **implement** appropriate teaching methods and techniques that promote health, and **evaluate** the effectiveness of the patient/client educational encounters.

ASSESSING LEARNING NEEDS

In order to assess the learning needs of patients and relatives, the nurse must first identity:

- prior knowledge and use of language;
- what the patient needs/wants to know;
- the optimum teaching and learning; and
- any barriers to learning.

Different individuals will have different learning needs, often based on their intelligence, education, social and cultural background. The patients' perception of what they need to know is often different from that of the nurse. The best way to establish what a patient needs to know is just to ask him or her, for example, 'What is your understanding of high-risk sexual behaviour?' or 'Can you explain to me how your discharge medications are to be taken?'. This allows the nurse an opportunity to ascertain prior knowledge and to assess the language (i.e. the words) the patient uses to communicate and to describe behaviour. This will assist in determining what learning deficits exist and inform as to how much the patient wants, needs and is able to learn.

It is essential to provide privacy and time to define learning needs adequately and to give the patient permission and opportunity to ask questions. It is axiomatic that the nurse must know the patient and his or her individual circumstances, have clinical confidence and competence to engage in an educational encounter in relation to the specific issue being discussed, and is comfortable in using language familiar to the patient.

During this phase it is important to assess the optimum circumstances in which effective patient education encounters can be initiated. Learning can only occur when the individual is ready to learn. Barriers to learning include:

- differences between teacher and patient in cultural, social and educational background and differences in primary language;
- differences between teacher and patient in values, sex, sexual orientation, religion and beliefs;
- distractions due to confusion, pain, depression, fatigue or anxiety;
- contradictory messages received from other sources;
- faults in the teaching plan/technique: lack of privacy, time, competence and/or confidence of teacher;
- differences in language: nurse's language not understood by patient or patient's language not understood by nurse.

PLANNING AN EDUCATIONAL RESPONSE

Planning a patient education activity takes into account the educational technique to be used, the timing of the activity and the end product (i.e. the goals) (Table 19.2). **Goals** are sometimes referred to as 'aims' and are defined as **broad, general statements of goal direction, which contain reference to the worthwhileness of achieving it**.[2] Just as the assessment phase involves the patient, so too must the planning stage (to the extent his or her clinical condition permits). The goals/aims of the activity must be negotiated with the patient. This involves asking patients what they want to know, what they think they should know or offering possible learning options. In addressing learning needs, the patient and the nurse should negotiate both short-term and long-term goals, i.e. what the patient will be able to do or accomplish as a result (both in the short term and in the longer term) of the educational encounter. For example, a short-term goal that might be negotiated with a patient in reference to safer sexual behaviour might be that at the end of the session the patient would understand the sexual means of HIV transmission. The long-term goal might be that the patient would be enabled to adopt safer ways of expressing his or her sexuality in order to prevent secondary infectious disease acquisition and transmission of HIV to another individual.

TABLE 19.2 Planning an educational response – the goals

Negotiate:	goals (aims), i.e.	broad general statements of goal direction, which contain references to the worthwhileness of achieving it
	short-term goal(s) & **long-term goal(s)**, i.e.	what the patient **will be able to do** as a result of the teaching/ learning encounter
	e.g. teaching session	safer sexual behaviour
	short-term goal	'At the end of this session, the patient will *understand* the sexual means of HIV transmission'
	long-term goal	'At the end of this session(s), the patient will be *enabled* to adopt a safer means of expressing his/her sexuality in order to prevent secondary infectious disease acquisition and transmission of HIV to others'

Once the goals have been negotiated, the intended learning outcomes (i.e. objectives) of the session are derived and can be specified. **Objectives are carefully constructed statements that indicate with precision what the patient will be able to do at the end of a teaching/learning session.** Objectives are written for and directed at the patient and are action verb statements, i.e. they describe what behaviour the patient will be able to achieve at the end of the session. For example, a specific objective might be 'At the end of this session, the patient will be able to describe high-risk sexual behaviours', or 'with the use of an anatomical model, demonstrate the correct use of a condom' (Table 19.3). Each action verb used in objective statements describes a specific behaviour that is observable, measurable, logical, feasible, unequivocal and relevant (Figure 19.2). The 'goals' and 'objectives' at the beginning of this chapter offer another example of setting the intended learning outcomes of a planned educational initiative. Objectives are usually constructed to describe **cognitive** (i.e. thinking) and **psychomotor skills** that will result from the teaching/learning process and, as such, have a built-in evaluation facility. Objectives can also be directed at different cognitive levels, for example knowledge, comprehension, application, analysis, synthesis and evaluation. More difficult to evaluate, but also useful, are objectives that can be directed towards **affective** (i.e. valuing, feeling and attitude formation) domains (Table 19.4).

TABLE 19.3 Teaching session: safer sexual behaviour – short-term goal

Short-term goal	At the end of this session, the patient will understand the sexual means of HIV transmission
Objectives	At the end of this session, the patient will:
	1. *List* the body fluids that may transmit HIV
	2. *Describe* the types of sexual behaviour that will facilitate HIV transmission
	3. *Discuss* ways in which he/she can adopt a safer form of sexual expression
	4. *Identify* potential problems with partner(s) in changing to a safer sexual lifestyle
	5. *Demonstrate* (on an anatomical model) the correct use of a rubber condom

Objectives have a built-in evaluation facility.

Goals and specific objectives are much like a brick wall. The wall itself is the goal (or aim) and each individual brick is an objective. Initially, the short-term and long-term goals, along with the specific objectives, should be written down by the nurse in order to have a checklist to evaluate the degree of learning that has taken place after the encounter(s). Once the goals and objectives have been negotiated and specified, the nurse can select the appropriate teaching method. In patient education encounters, the most common methods are **one-to-one discussions** in which the current knowledge, attitudes and behaviour of the patient are assessed, clarifying or giving additional information or facilitating the development of skills (e.g. decision-making, psychomotor, assertion skills etc.). **Demonstrations** are also a method

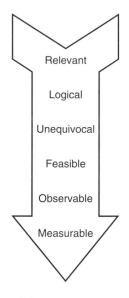

Relevant

Logical

Unequivocal

Feasible

Observable

Measurable

FIGURE 19.2 *Qualities of a specific educational objective.*

TABLE 19.4 Types and levels of learning

Cognitive	Process of thinking, of acquiring information and working with it
Affective	Incorporates values, attitudes, beliefs and feelings that create idiosyncratic reactions Has important motivation influences
Psychomotor	Acquisition of a motor skill perfected through practice

commonly used in patient education encounters (e.g. the use of camouflage make-up, using a condom). In the planning stage, any teaching equipment/aids, written guidelines or literature may also be considered. A simple and brief teaching plan should be constructed, which includes the goals and objectives of the session, the step-by-step implementation of the session and a brief evaluation of what learning took place. This teaching plan should form part of the documentation of care given in the nursing care plan.

PREPARING A TEACHING PLAN

This plan should first consider the teaching method or techniques that seem best suited to achieve the goals negotiated with the patient. The first consideration is that the method or technique chosen allows for maximum involvement of the patient. This is facilitated by using effective non-verbal communication skills, building into the plan opportunities for frequent question and answer periods and by being involved in the verbal summary of the session. If the goal is directed towards enabling the acquisition of a psychomotor skill (e.g. preparing intravenous medication for administration through a Hickman catheter), the teaching plan should include an opportunity for immediate supervised practice following the demonstration.

The teaching plan should include a short introduction, the main body of the teaching material, a summary and a question and answer period (Table 19.5).

TABLE 19.5 Planning an educational response – the teaching plan

Prepare:	Teaching plan	
	Introduction	Establish significance of session and clarify goals and objectives
	Main body	Work from:
		■ known to the unknown
		■ familiar to the unfamiliar
		■ knowledge to concepts
		■ basic to advanced
		■ questions to answers
		■ problems to solutions
	Summary	Review goals and objectives
		Repeat important points
	Questions and answers	Clarify information

The introduction should include the goals (both short term and long term) and objectives of the session and should establish the importance of the session.

The material in the main body of the session should follow a logical sequence. As the nurse will have established how much the patient knows during the assessment period, the teaching session should be directed at working from the known to the unknown, from familiar to unfamiliar knowledge and concepts, from basic to advanced material, from questions to answers and from identified problems to solutions.

The summary should include a review of the original goals and objectives of the session and repeat the important points made during the main body of the talk.

Finally, questions and answers will help clarify information for the patient and allow for the first evaluation of the achievement (or non-achievement) of the short-term goal(s).

IMPLEMENTING PATIENT EDUCATION

Effective teaching requires effective communication skills, both verbal and non-verbal. Non-verbal communications (i.e. body language) are critical and include the following.

- **Proximity, i.e. how close you are to the patient**. Individuals with HIV infection and AIDS often feel isolated and stigmatized, and effective teaching means being close to the patient, without invading his or her personal space. Teaching sessions should not be conducted from the foot of the bed or with the nurse standing over a patient lying in bed. Either both the nurse and the patient should be sitting in chairs relatively close to each other or, if the patient is in bed, the nurse should sit near the patient's head.
- **Body contact, i.e. touching**. Although in formal teaching practice body contact is not generally useful, in patient education, especially with an individual who has HIV-related conditions, touching can convey many effective messages, such as 'I care and I'm here for you' and 'I'm not afraid to be close to you'. Touching has to be done sensitively and is often over-done, resulting in counter-productive reactions.
- **Facial expressions**. These convey a wealth of information, and a 'deadpan', non-reactive facial expression is not useful. Nurses who practise good listening skills, as described by Ewles and Simnett,[3] and who are enthusiastic and responsive to the patient and the issues being discussed, convey a real sense of sincerity.
- **Eye contact**. This should be scanning in nature, not staring, which would make the patient feel uncomfortable. Good, intermittent eye contact is needed from speaker to listener during educational encounters. Generally, the listener (be it the nurse or the patient) will look directly (straight in the eyes) at the speaker. If this does not happen, it is an indication that, for one reason or another, the listener is not paying attention to the speaker. There may be many reasons for inattention (e.g. the issues being discussed are uncomfortable to the listener, the language used is not being understood, the patient is in pain, etc.) and this is an important clue for the speaker.
- **Posture**. This sends messages to both the health educator and the patient. Sitting with arms crossed and fists clenched may signal significant anxiety, which precludes learning until the underlying cause is addressed.

Many other aspects of body language, e.g. hand and head movements, orientation (i.e. the layout of the room), physical appearance (e.g. uniform versus casual/professional clothes) and movements, are important in teaching and learning, especially in semi-formal and formal teaching environments.

Maintaining good listening skills is an essential ingredient at all stages of the teaching process. It is an active process, which helps the patient talk, ask questions and participate in the learning process. Effective listening assists in clarifying the patient's attitudes, beliefs and values. These skills include the following.

- **Expressive concentration** on what the speaker is saying. This involves the non-verbal body language skills discussed previously, e.g. good eye contact, reactive facial expressions, posture and head movements (e.g. nodding in understanding) etc.
- **Inviting the patient to talk**, e.g. 'How do you feel about what I've just said?' or 'How can you use the information we've discussed this morning?'.
- **Being attentive**, e.g. maintaining steady eye contact, making neutral noises such as 'I see...' or 'yes...', etc.

- **Paraphrasing** involves re-stating the essential aspects of what the patient is saying, e.g. 'So, you're worried your partner will be put off having sex if you wear a rubber condom'.
- **Reflecting feelings verbally** mirrors back to the patient the feelings you perceive he or she is communicating, e.g. 'You are clearly worried about how your parents will react to the news that you are gay'.
- **Reflecting meanings** adds content to feelings, e.g. 'You are frightened because you are scheduled for a bronchoscopy this afternoon'.
- **Summarizing** is useful in clarifying the information the patient is giving you and should be used throughout active listening, not just at the end of the teaching session. Summarizing involves making brief statements that reflect the salient points the patient has made, e.g. 'So far, it seems that what you are saying is . . .'.

In implementing the main body of the teaching session, the following principles are useful to consider.

- **Time.** Negotiate with the patient when the session will start and ensure that you are there on time. Keep the session brief. It is far better to have several brief sessions that the patient can concentrate on, rather than a long, tiring session. People who are ill or worried or who have some degree of subclinical cognitive dysfunction as a result of HIV infection often find it difficult to concentrate for more than 15 or 20 minutes at a time.
- **State the most important things first.** Patients will often remember the first things said, and objectives should be prioritized so that critical points are discussed first.
- **Repeat and stress critical points.** Without being tedious, it is important to repeat and re-emphasize critical points, e.g. 'The most important aspect in adopting safer sexual behaviour is to avoid penetrative sex without using a rubber condom'.
- **Give clear, precise and specific advice**, for example 'You will be taking foscarnet through your Hickman catheter every day, except Saturday and Sunday. It is important that you adjust your administration set so it takes 2 hours to run the foscarnet in, rather than 'Take your foscarnet 5 days a week and run it in slowly'.
- **Avoid using jargon and long words and sentences.** It may be appropriate to use medical terminology in order to help the patient communicate easily with other healthcare professionals, but if medical terminology is used, it must be carefully explained to the patient and, during the evaluation stage, any terminology used must be re-checked to ensure the patient actually understands it.
- **Give written information** to the patient and go through the information with him or her. It is sometimes possible to ask the patient to write down the important points covered and, as this actively involves the patient in the learning process, it can be useful. Obviously, asking the patient to take dictation is not useful.

If the learning goals include teaching a psychomotor skill, the following essential principles must be included in the teaching plan.

- Demonstrate skill, using a skill analysis approach.
- Ensure demonstration is clearly visible to patient.
- Maintain a non-threatening atmosphere.
- Allow immediate supervised practice.
- Provide written information.

In demonstrating the skill, it is important that all the equipment (if any) used is prepared and at hand and that the demonstration is easily visible to the patient. Part of the demonstration should include a skills analysis, i.e. the components of the skill are broken down into stages, starting with component 1, then component 2 and so on, until the totality of the components equals the skill being taught. For example, if the patient is being taught to administer his or her own aerosolized pentamidine, the skills analysis might be as follows.

1. Attach a needle to 10 mL syringe.
2. Wipe off the rubber top of the vial of bacteriostatic water with an alcohol swab and let it dry.
3. Uncap the needle guard from the needle.
4. Insert the needle into the rubber top of the vial of water.
5. Pull back on the plunger of the syringe and draw up 6 mL of water.
6. Carefully withdraw the needle and syringe from the vial of water.
7. Put the needle guard back on the needle.
8. Wipe off the rubber top of the lyophilized pentamidine with an alcohol swab and let it dry.
9. Take the needle guard back off the needle.
10. Insert the needle into the rubber top of the pentamidine vial and inject the 6 mL of water.
11. Withdraw the needle and syringe and cover the needle again with the needle guard.
12. Shake the vial of pentamidine and water until the pentamidine is fully dissolved.
13. Etc.

Full, simple, written instructions as per the skills analysis should be left with the patient.

During the learning session, the teacher needs to ensure that the atmosphere is friendly and relaxed (i.e. non-threatening) and should remain enthusiastic in order to keep the patient motivated.

Following the demonstration, it is essential that an opportunity is built into the learning session for immediate supervised practice by the patient so that the skills can be consolidated and reinforced. This is also part of the evaluation stage of the teaching/learning process.

If one of the learning goals is directed towards teaching the patient both affective (feeling) and cognitive (thinking) skills, e.g. decision-making skills, the following points are important.

■ Help the patient to define the problem, e.g. 'I can't find a way to tell my wife I'm infected with HIV'.
■ Clarify the patient's goals, e.g. 'I don't want to infect my wife'.
■ Help the patient to define alternative methods of achieving the goal, e.g. 'Maybe the doctor should tell her', or 'I won't tell her, but I'll only have safer sex with her in the future'.
■ Help the patient to identify the advantages and disadvantages of each method, e.g. 'If I don't tell her myself, she won't trust or respect me in the future'.
■ Let the patient decide which is the best course of action, based on the above, and discuss with the patient his or her perception of the likely results of that decision.

Finally, in implementing planned teaching, barriers to effective communication should be identified and addressed, as discussed previously.

EVALUATING THE TEACHING SESSION

After summarizing the main points of the session and answering the patient's questions, the short-term goals and specific learning objectives are reviewed with the patient and an evaluation assessment is made, i.e. the patient did or did not achieve the learning objectives and the short-term goal. The long-term goals are evaluated at future teaching/learning sessions. The nurse should revisit the patient the next day, if possible, to re-check the evaluation assessment and to answer any further questions that may have arisen. On-going assessment will identify further learning needs, and the process described in this chapter is repeated.

DOCUMENTATION OF TEACHING

The teaching plan is entered into the patient's notes and the teaching/learning session is documented in the Nursing Care Plan.

REFERENCES

1. Coutts LC, Hardy LK. *Teaching For Health; The Nurse as Health Educator*. London: Churchill Livingstone, 1995.
2. Quinn FM. *The Principles and Practice of Nurse Education*, 4th edn. London: Croom Helm, 2000.
3. Ewles L, Simnett I. *Promoting Health: A Practical Guide to Health Education*. Chichester: John Wiley & Sons, 1985.

FURTHER READING

Coutts LC, Hardy LK. *Teaching For Health; The Nurse as Health Educator*. London: Churchill Livingstone, 1995.
Ewles L, Simnett I. *Promoting Health: A Practical Guide to Health Education*, 5th edn. London: Baillière Tindall, 2003.
Quinn FM. *The Principles and Practice of Nurse Education*, 4th edn. London: Croom Helm, 2000.

Understanding antiretroviral therapy

Introduction

In 1987, the first drug that could target the human immunodeficiency virus (HIV) and inhibit its replication cycle was introduced into clinical practice. Known then as AZT but now referred to as zidovudine (ZDV), monotherapy with this drug produced remarkable, if unsustainable, clinical improvements in many patients desperately ill and nearing the end of their lives. This was a significant turning point in HIV management, which heralded the dawn of a new era in which an impressive and expanding range of specific antiretroviral drugs would become available to effectively treat HIV-infected people, at least in the wealthier nations of the world. These drugs have revolutionized the treatment of people with HIV disease and have had a truly remarkable impact on reducing HIV-related morbidity and mortality.[1]

Today, treatment protocols, regimens and associated laboratory assays for monitoring treatment efficacy have become more sophisticated. So too has our awareness of the emergence of viral resistance to antiretroviral drugs and our understanding of the importance of the need for almost total adherence to prescribed therapy.

In this chapter, we will review the principles of treatment and the different types of antiretroviral agents that are now available for the management of people with HIV disease. We will then examine the nursing care and adherence issues associated with treatment regimens and explore the factors associated with the emergence of drug resistance. Because chemotherapy for HIV disease is a fast-moving and ever-changing field, we will identify how nurses and other healthcare professionals (and their clients) can access continuously updated treatment information.

Learning outcomes

After studying and reflecting on the material in this chapter, you will be able to:

- discuss the principles of treatment for HIV disease and explain the pharmacological activity of the different classes of antiretroviral drugs;
- describe the laboratory methods used to monitor treatment efficacy;
- discuss the side effects and drug interactions associated with antiretroviral therapy;
- outline factors associated with the emergence of drug-resistant viral variants and describe the clinical impact of resistance; and
- identify how you can access current treatment information.

BACKGROUND

During the early years of the global pandemic, great strides were made in quickly identifying HIV as the viral cause of AIDS and then understanding the pathogenesis of HIV disease (Chapters 3 and 6). It was clear that the adverse clinical outcomes of HIV infection were a consequence of progressive and unrelenting viral replication. Knowing this, it was then possible to plot the predictable stages and events associated with a changing inverse relationship between a rising viral load and a falling CD4+ T-lymphocyte cell count (see Figure 7.1). The higher the viral load, the greater the fall in CD4+ cells and the more likely the emergence of opportunistic infections and other adverse events and the worsening of the patient's health. Laboratory techniques for monitoring CD4+ cell counts and plasma viral load (HIV RNA) were developed and are now routinely used to monitor treatment efficacy.

With the advent of different types of antiretroviral agents, physicians saw that they could use these drugs in combinations to slow or halt this destructive viral replication. By the mid-1990s, complex regimens of antiretroviral drugs, known as highly active antiretroviral therapy (**HAART**), were in widespread use in industrially developed countries. However, it was not long before the phenomenon of drug resistance was experienced, and assays to detect and monitor resistance to antiretroviral drugs were quickly developed and introduced into routine clinical practice.

Patients on long-term therapy also frequently experienced serious late side effects, which, in addition to the development of drug resistance, often curtailed their ability to benefit from therapy.

PRINCIPLES OF ANTIRETROVIRAL TREATMENT

Antiretroviral treatment is aimed at reducing the plasma HIV RNA level (viral load) to the lowest possible level, preferably below the level of detection, as quickly as possible for as long as possible. An increasing variety of different types of antiretroviral agents is currently either licensed in the UK for the treatment of HIV disease or available through expanded access schemes (Table 20.1).

Currently available drugs target two specific viral enzymes necessary for HIV replication: reverse transcriptase (RT) and protease (Figure 20.1). New types of drugs, such as integrase inhibitors, attachment and fusion inhibitors, antisense drugs and immune system stimulators, are either in various stages of development or have advanced to clinical trials.

Reverse transcriptase inhibitors

As previously discussed in Chapter 6, when HIV enters a cell, it takes along with its ribonucleic acid (RNA) genome several viral enzymes which are essential for viral

TABLE 20.1 Antiretroviral drugs used in the UK (2003)

Generic name	Proprietary name	Other names	Manufacturer
Nucleoside reverse transcriptase inhibitors (NRTIs)			
Zidovudine	Retrovir®	ZDV/AZT	GlaxoSmithKline (GSK)
Lamivudine	Epivir®	3TC	GSK
	Zeffix®		GSK
Zalcitabine	HIVID®	ddC	Roche Products Ltd
Didanosine	Videx®	ddI	Bristol-Myers Squibb
Stavudine	Zerit®	d4T	Bristol-Myers Squibb
Abacavir	Ziagen®	ABC	GSK
(Lamivudine with zidovudine)	Combivir®		GSK
(Abacavir with lamivudine & zidovudine)	Trizivir®		GSK
Nucleotide reverse transcriptase inhibitors			
Tenofovir	Viread®	PMPA	Gilead Sciences
Non-nucleoside reverse transcriptase inhibitors (NNRTIs)			
Nevirapine	Viramune®	NVP	Boehringer Ingelheim
Efavirenz	Sustiva®	EFV	Du Pont Pharmaceuticals
Delavirdine°	Rescriptor®	DLV	Pharmacia Ltd
Protease inhibitors (PIs)			
Amprenavir	Agenerase®		GSK
Saquinavir		SQV	Roche Products Ltd
(hard gel caps)	Invirase®		
(soft gel caps)	Fortovase®		
Ritonavir	Norvir®	RTV	Abbott Laboratories
Indinavir	Crixivan®	IDV	Merck Sharp & Dohme
Nelfinavir	Viracept®	NFV	Roche Products Ltd
Lopinavir/ritonavir	Kaletra®		Abbott Laboratories
Atazanavir°	Reyataz®	ATV	Bristol-Myers Squibb

°Not currently licensed in the UK but available through an expanded access programme or trials.

replication. The viral enzyme RT is needed almost immediately after the virus gains entry into the cell in order for HIV to transcribe (copy) its genetic code from RNA to proviral DNA (deoxyribonucleic acid). If prevented from effectively 'reverse transcribing' itself, HIV would be unable to infect the cell, as viral RNA cannot be integrated into the host cell nucleus (which is composed of DNA). By 2003, an expanding repertoire of nucleoside, nucleotide and non-nucleoside reverse transcriptase inhibitors had been developed and had become an essential component of modern antiretroviral drug regimens.

Nucleoside RT inhibitors

Nucleoside RT inhibitors (NRTIs) are also known as nucleoside analogues, or by the term used by many patients – 'nukes'. Nucleosides are derivatives of nucleotides, which are the four base molecules (adenine, thymine, cytosine, guanine) that form the rungs of the sugar–phosphate twisted ladder (double helix) that makes up DNA. In the host cell, nucleotides are split into nucleosides by the action of a cellular enzyme (nucleotidase) and are known as natural or endogenous nucleosides.

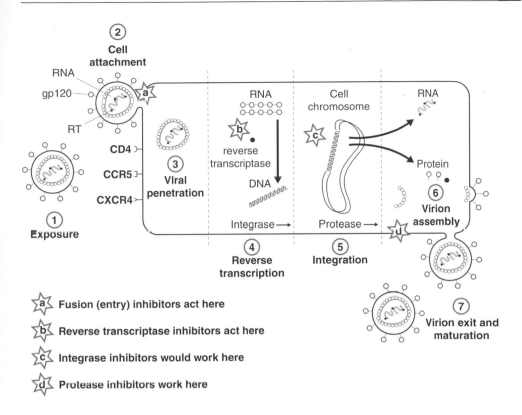

FIGURE 20.1 *Life cycle of HIV showing opportunities for drug intervention.*

Scientists have chemically developed nucleoside analogues, which are similar (analogous) to but slightly different from the natural endogenous nucleosides. When administered as an antiretroviral drug, they enter cells and undergo a chemical transformation (phosphorylation) that changes them into active triphosphate metabolites, which are 'fake' nucleosides. They then successfully compete with natural endogenous nucleosides during reverse transcription. When selected as one of the building blocks for the new proviral DNA that is being constructed, nucleoside analogues inhibit DNA synthesis by a process known as chain termination. This causes the formation of an abnormal DNA transcript, which cannot be integrated into the host cell DNA. As a result, HIV replication is halted.

In general, NRTIs are not as potent as other classes of antiretroviral drugs and they also interfere with other cellular enzymes in the body that have a similar action to that of RT.

Nucleotide RT inhibitors

These RT inhibitors have the same mode of action as nucleoside analogues, but they are already monophosphorylated and require fewer metabolic steps to achieve their active form.

Non-nucleoside RT inhibitors

Non-nucleoside RT inhibitors (NNRTIs – sometimes referred to by patients as 'non-nukes') also inhibit reverse transcription but do so by a different method. When these drugs enter a cell, they bind directly to RT, causing conformational changes to this enzyme, which inhibits its activity. They are extremely effective at slowing down viral replication.

Protease inhibitors

Protease inhibitors (PIs) work entirely differently from the RT inhibitors. After HIV has infected the host cell nucleus, it will, on stimulation, reactivate and go into 'forward transcription', changing the DNA back into HIV RNA. In addition, during replication, HIV will manufacture new structural and core proteins along with the necessary viral enzymes. These proteins, which have been initially produced during forward transcription in long chains, will need to be sliced (cleaved) into smaller pieces before all of these new components can be assembled into a mature, competent virion. This cleaving (or cutting up) is done by a viral digestive enzyme known as protease. PIs prevent the 'protease scissors' from carrying out this essential function and, consequently, prevent mature virions from being formed. These are extremely effective antiretroviral agents and their introduction into clinical practice has revolutionized therapeutic outcomes.

HIGHLY ACTIVE ANTIRETROVIRAL THERAPY – HAART

Today, patients are treated with a combination of three (or more) different types of anti-retroviral drugs (see Table 20.1), usually two nucleoside reverse transcriptase inhibitors with *either* a non-nucleoside reverse transcriptase inhibitor *or* one or two protease inhibitors.[2-4]

Although immensely effective, these powerful drugs are associated with a wide range of both short-term and long-term toxicities and drug interactions. Table 20.2 describes typical dosing regimens and some of the more important side effects, drug interactions and other information that nurses and their patients need to be aware of. As drug information is continually evolving, healthcare professionals and patients need to ensure that they have access to the most current information, especially from high-quality reputable online resources (see 'Internet resources' at the end of this chapter).

TABLE 20.2 Antiretroviral drugs: side effects and drug interactions[3,5,6]

Drug and usual dose[a] in adults and adolescents	Side effects[b] (not an all-inclusive list)	Some important nursing information[a]
NRTIs Nucleoside reverse transcriptase inhibitors		
Zidovudine *Retrovir®* ZDV/AZT **One 300 mg tablet twice a day** Oral solution available as well	Low red blood cell count (anaemia), headache, nausea, muscle soreness and inflammation (myopathy), weakness, lactic acidosis, possible elevated liver enzymes or more severe problems (hepatomegaly with steatosis), fingernail, skin and oral mucosa discolouration, diarrhoea, fever, seizures, anorexia and neuropathy	Monitor haemoglobin for anaemia Take with meals or within an hour following meals **Contraindications**: low neutrophil counts or haemoglobin values; monitor liver function enzymes **Drug interactions**: *Warning: do not use with*: ganciclovir, stavudine **Increased risk of toxicity if used with**: methadone (increases ZDV plasma levels), NSAIDs, valproate, fluconazole, probenecid, phenytoin

Drug and usual dose[a] in adults and adolescents	Side effects[b] (not an all-inclusive list)	Some important nursing information[a]
Lamivudine *Epivir®, Zeffix®* 3TC **One 150 mg tablet twice a day** Oral solution available as well	Side effects overall rare Headache, fatigue, nausea, diarrhoea, insomnia, low white blood cell count (neutropenia), low red blood cell count (anaemia)	May 'reverse' resistance of HIV to ZDV when used together Monitor triglycerides for pancreatitis, especially in children Can be taken with or without food Also active against hepatitis B virus (HBV) **Contraindications:** breastfeeding **Drug interactions:** *Warning: do not use with:* trimethoprim and co-trimoxazole at high doses, and do not use with intravenous ganciclovir or foscarnet
Zalcitabine *HIVID®* ddC **One 0.75 mg (750 micrograms) tablet three times a day**	Peripheral neuropathy (nerve damage): tingling, numbness or pain in the hands or feet; pancreatitis, mouth and oesophageal ulcers (canker sores), lactic acidosis, possible elevated liver enzymes or more severe problems (hepatomegaly with steatosis)	Women should avoid pregnancy while taking this drug because of a potential risk of birth defects Can be taken with or without food but absorption improved when taken on an empty stomach **Contraindications:** peripheral neuropathy **Drug interactions:** *Warning: do not take with:* magnesium/ aluminium-containing antacids Should not be used with didanosine or other antiretroviral drugs that may cause peripheral neuropathy The following drugs may increase plasma levels of zalcitabine: trimethoprim and co-trimoxazole, cimetidine, probenecid
Didanosine *Videx®* ddI **Adult (dosage based on body weight)** **>60 kg: 250 mg daily as one dose or two divided doses** **<60 kg: 250 mg daily as one dose or two divided doses; or one 400 mg enteric-coated (EC) capsule once daily** Oral solution available as well	Peripheral neuropathy (nerve damage): tingling, numbness or pain in the hands or feet; pancreatitis (nausea, abdominal pain), GI upset, diarrhoea, headache, vomiting, rash, dry skin, lactic acidosis, possible elevated liver enzymes or more severe liver problems (hepatomegaly with steatosis)	Tablets must be taken at least 30–45 minutes prior to eating New EC capsules need to be taken 1 hour before or 1 hour after food Use cold (non-carbonated) water or cold apple juice to swallow tablets Take at least 1 hour apart from indinavir Alcohol may increase risk of pancreatitis; increased risk of pancreatitis with concurrent use of stavudine or hydroxyurea Monitor liver function enzymes **Contraindications:** breastfeeding **Drug interactions:** *Warning: do not take with:* magnesium/ aluminium-containing antacids Plasma didanosine concentration possibly increased by ganciclovir and is increased by tenofovir

TABLE 20.2 – continued

Drug and usual dose° in adults and adolescents	Side effects[b] (not an all-inclusive list)	Some important nursing information°
Stavudine *Zerit®* d4T **One 40 mg capsule twice a day (30 mg capsule for people weighing <60 kg)** Oral solution available as well	Peripheral neuropathy (nerve damage): tingling, numbness or pain in the hands or feet; pancreatitis, insomnia, headache, nausea, diarrhoea, lactic acidosis, possible elevated liver enzymes or more severe problems (hepatomegaly with steatosis), dyspnoea, influenza-like syndrome, vertigo, chest pain	Take 1 hour before food **Contraindications**: breastfeeding **Drug interactions**: *Warning: do not take with*: zidovudine Doxorubicin may inhibit the effect of stavudine
Abacavir *Ziagen®* ABC **300 mg every 12 hours**	Hypersensitivity reaction, headache, nausea, vomiting, shortness of breath, abdominal pain, lactic acidosis, possible liver problems (severe hepatomegaly with steatosis)	Hypersensitivity (serious allergic reaction) reported in 3–5% of people People who experience increasing nausea, abdominal pain, fever, fatigue, shortness of breath and/or skin rash within 6 weeks after starting abacavir may be experiencing a hypersensitivity reaction and the patient's physician must be contacted immediately Once a patient has stopped taking abacavir, he/she should not restart the drug, as this may result in a life-threatening reaction Can be taken with or without food **Contraindications**: pregnancy, breastfeeding **Drug interactions**: plasma concentration of methadone may be decreased by abacavir
Lamivudine 150 mg *with* **zidovudine 300 mg** *Combivir®* CBV (*Combivir®* is a combination of two drugs in one tablet) **One tablet is taken twice a day**	As for zidovudine and lamivudine	Monitor haemoglobin for anaemia Can be taken with or without food but preferentially take with food to minimize stomach discomfort **Contraindications and drug interactions**: as for each of the drug components
Abacavir 300 mg *with* **lamivudine 150 mg** *and* **zidovudine 300 mg** *Trizivir®* TZV (*Trizivir®* is a combination of three drugs in one tablet) **One tablet twice a day**	As for zidovudine, lamivudine and abacavir	This medication contains abacavir, which can cause a serious allergic reaction in some people (read the warning above for abacavir) Contact physician immediately if any sign of allergy occurs (fever, nausea, dizziness, vomiting, abdominal pain, fatigue, shortness of breath and/or skin rash within 6 weeks after starting) Once a patient has stopped taking *Trizivir®* for this reason, he/she should not restart the drug without a doctor's permission, as this may result in a life-threatening reaction Can be taken with or without food but preferentially take with food to minimize stomach discomfort **Contraindications and drug interactions**: as for each of the drug components

Drug and usual dose[e] in adults and adolescents	Side effects[b] (not an all-inclusive list)	Some important nursing information[a]

NNRTIs (Non-nucleoside reverse transcriptase inhibitors)

Nevirapine Viramune® NVP **Initially, one 200 mg tablet daily for first 14 days and then, if no rash present, 200 mg tablet twice a day** Oral solution available as well	Rash (including Stevens–Johnson syndrome and, rarely, toxic epidermal necrolysis), abdominal pain, nausea and vomiting, diarrhoea, fever, drowsiness, fatigue, headache, low white blood cell count (neutropenia), increased liver enzymes, hepatitis (rare)	Lowers blood levels of protease inhibitors Notify physician if rash develops Can be taken with or without food Liver enzymes should be monitored, especially when used in pregnancy **Contraindications**: breastfeeding, severe hepatitis impairment **Drug interactions**: *Warning: do not use with*: rifampicin, St John's wort, ketoconazole May reduce or increase plasma levels of some other antiretroviral drugs Nevirapine reduces plasma concentration of methadone and may reduce efficacy of oral contraceptives
Efavirenz Sustiva® EFV **600 mg once daily** Bedtime dosing is recommended due to side effects	Central nervous system (CNS)-related symptoms: dizziness, somnolence, insomnia, vivid dreams, impaired concentration, light headedness; rash (including Stevens–Johnson syndrome), nausea, diarrhoea, depression, hepatitis, pancreatitis, raised serum cholesterol levels and elevated liver enzymes (especially if sero-positive for hepatitis B or hepatitis C)	Women should avoid pregnancy because of potential drug-related fetal injury High-fat meals may increase side effects Can be taken with or without food Grapefruit juice may affect plasma-efavirenz levels **Contraindications**: breastfeeding **Drugs interactions**: *Warning: do not use with*: terfenadine, midazolam, St John's wort, ergot derivatives (e.g. ergotamine tartrate) May reduce or increase plasma levels of some other antiretroviral drugs Rifampicin and clarithromycin reduce plasma levels of efavirenz, and rifabutin plasma levels are decreased by efavirenz therapy Efavirenz reduces plasma concentration of methadone and may reduce efficacy of oral contraceptives
Delavirdine Rescriptor® DLV **400 mg taken three times daily**	Rash, headache, fatigue, nausea, elevated liver enzymes	Should be taken at least 1 hour before and after didanosine and antacids Raises blood levels of some protease inhibitors Notify doctor if rash develops Can be taken with or without food **Drugs interactions**: *Warning: do not use with*: simvastatin, lovastatin, rifampicin, rifabutin, terfenadine, midazolam, H2 blockers, proton pump inhibitors, ergot derivatives (e.g. ergotamine tartrate) Levels of clarithromycin, dapsone, quinidine and warfarin are increased when taking delavirdine May reduce or increase plasma levels of some other antiretroviral drugs

TABLE 20.2 – continued

Drug and usual dose[a] in adults and adolescents	Side effects[b] (not an all-inclusive list)	Some important nursing information[a]
Nucleotide RT inhibitors		
Tenofovir *Viread®* **One 245 mg tablet once daily**	Nausea, vomiting, flatulence, diarrhoea, headache, lactic acidosis, possible liver problems (severe hepatomegaly with steatosis), hypophosphataemia	Can increase the blood levels of didanosine when co-administered Take with food, preferably a meal containing some fat Also active against hepatitis B virus (HBV) **Contraindications**: severe renal impairment, breastfeeding **Drug interactions**: may reduce or increase plasma levels of some other antiretroviral drugs
Protease inhibitors (PIs)		
Amprenavir *Agenerase®* **1.2 g every 12 hours** Oral solution available (N.B. bioavailability of *Agenerase®* solution is lower than that of capsules; the two formulations are not interchangeable on a milligram for milligram basis May be combined with other protease inhibitors at a lower dose	Nausea, diarrhoea, headache, stomach pains/gas, rash (including, rarely, Stevens–Johnson syndrome), and numbing sensations (on the skin, usually around the mouth – perioral paraesthesia), tremor, depression	Avoid during pregnancy Can be taken with or without food but do not take within 1 hour of a high-fat meal **Contraindications**: breastfeeding Oral solution contains propylene glycol – avoid in hepatic impairment and severe renal impairment **Drug interactions**: *Warning: do not use with*: simvastatin, atorvastatin, fluvastatin, pravastatin lovastatin, terfenadine, midazolam, ergot derivatives (e.g. ergotamine tartrate), rifampicin, St John's wort, pimozide and vitamin E Amprenavir may increase plasma concentrations of sildenafil, cimetidine, erythromycin, rifabutin, dapsone, carbamazepine, itraconazole, clozapine, thioridazine, some calcium channel blockers Risk of prolonged sedation and respiratory depression when used with alprazolam, clorazepate, diazepam, flurazepam, midazolam May reduce or increase plasma levels of some other antiretroviral drugs
Saquinavir SQV (soft gel caps) *Fortovase®* **1.2 g every 8 hours** May be combined with other protease inhibitors at a lower dose	Nausea, diarrhoea, gas, rash, abdominal pain, headache, mouth ulcerations, peripheral neuropathy, mood changes, fever, kidney stones (nephrolithiasis)	Take with food or within 2 hours of eating Saquinavir taken without food may be less potent *Fortovase®* replaces older, less potent hard gel saquinavir formulation (*Invirase®*) **Contraindications**: breastfeeding, severe hepatic impairment **Drug interactions**: *Warning: do not use with*: simvastatin, lovastatin, terfenadine, midazolam, ergot derivatives (e.g. ergotamine tartrate), rifamycins, St John's wort, tolterodine, pimozide

Drug and usual dose[a] in adults and adolescents	Side effects[b] (not an all-inclusive list)	Some important nursing information[a]
		Saquinavir increases the plasma concentrations of thioridazine, sildenafil Ranitidine, ketoconazole, and possibly other imidazoles and triazoles, increase the plasma concentration of saquinavir; whereas carbamazepine, phenobarbital, phenytoin, dexamethasone may reduce the plasma concentration of saquinavir May reduce or increase plasma levels of some other antiretroviral drugs
Ritonavir *Norvir®* · RTV **600 mg every 12 hours** Oral solution available as well May be combined with other protease inhibitors at a lower dose.	Nausea, diarrhoea, abdominal pain, weakness, numbness around mouth, throat irritation, change of taste, syncope (fainting), hypotension, seizures, cough, anxiety, fever, decreased thyroxine, sweating, pancreatitis	Dose may be gradually increased over the first week to reduce side effects Separate **didanosine** dosing by at least 2 hours Should be taken with a full meal **Contraindications**: breastfeeding, severe hepatic impairment **Drug interactions:**[a] *Warning: do not use with*: simvastatin, lovastatin, terfenadine, ergot derivatives (e.g. ergotamine tartrate), rifabutin, St John's wort, pimozide, clozapine, tolterodine, dextropropoxyphene, pethidine, piroxicam, bupropion, eletripan, sildenafil, amiodarone, flecainide, propafenone, quinidine Risk of prolonged sedation and respiratory depression when used with alprazolam, clorazepate, diazepam, flurazepam, midazolam, zolpidem – avoid concomitant use Ritonavir may increase plasma concentrations of: SSRIs and tricyclic antidepressants, warfarin and other anticoagulants, tolbutamide, disopyramide, mexiletine, opioid analgesics (but not methadone), NSAIDs, sildenafil, antifungal drugs such as ketoconazole and possibly other imidazoles and triazoles, cimetidine, erythromycin, clarithromycin, cyclosporin, carbamazepine, clozapine, thioridazine, some calcium channel blockers Contraceptive effect of combined oral contraceptives reduced May reduce or increase plasma levels of some other antiretroviral drugs Extensive drug interactions; check current issue of *BNF*[3]

TABLE 20.2 – continued

Drug and usual dose° in adults and adolescents	Side effects[b] (not an all-inclusive list)	Some important nursing information°
Indinavir *Crixivan®* IDV **800 mg every 8 hours** May be combined with other protease inhibitors at a lower dose	Kidney stones (may have back/flank pain), elevated bilirubin level (bile pigment), rash, nausea, diarrhoea, dry skin, hyperpigmentation, alopecia (hair loss)	Drink at least six glasses (1.5 litres) of water daily to avoid kidney stones Preferentially, take on empty stomach with water 1 hour before or 2 hours after eating However, if stomach problems arise, indinavir may be taken with a light low-fat snack **Contraindications**: breastfeeding **Drug interactions**: *Warning: do not use with*: simvastatin, atorvastin, lovastatin, terfenadine, alprazolam, midazolam, ergot derivatives (e.g. ergotamine tartrate), rifampicin, St John's wort, tolterodine, pimozide, eletripan Indinavir may increase plasma concentrations of: rifabutin, thioridazine and sildenafil Plasma concentrations of indinavir may be decreased by St John's wort, carbamazepine, phenobarbital, phenytoin, dexamethasone May reduce or increase plasma levels of some other antiretroviral drugs
Nelfinavir *Viracept®* NFV **750 mg three times a day or 1.25 g twice daily** Oral powder available May be combined with other protease inhibitors at a lower dose	Diarrhoea, nausea, rash, headache, stomach cramps, fever	Tablets are coated to prevent dissolving while swallowing Take with a meal or light snack **Contraindications**: breastfeeding **Drug interactions**: *Warning: do not use with*: amiodarone, quinidine, simvastatin, atorvastin, lovastatin, terfenadine, midazolam, ergot derivatives (e.g. ergotamine tartrate), rifampicin, St John's wort, tolterodine, pimozide, eletripan Nelfinavir may increase plasma concentrations of: rifabutin, thioridazine, sildenafil, carbamazepine, phenytoin Phenobarbital reduces plasma concentration of nelfinavir May reduce or increase plasma levels of some other antiretroviral drugs Nelfinavir may reduce efficacy of oral contraceptives
Lopinavir (133.3 mg) combined with **ritonavir** (33.3 mg) *Kaletra®* **Three capsules twice daily** Oral solution available as lopinavir 400 mg with ritonavir 100 mg per 5 mL	Loose stools, diarrhoea, nausea, headache, influenza-like syndrome, appetite changes, hypertension, palpitations, chest pain, dyspnoea, agitation, anxiety, ataxia, confusion, depression, peripheral neuritis, sexual dysfunction, dry skin, sweating	**May interact with many other drugs** Preferentially, take with food Oral solution contains 42.4% alcohol **Contraindications**: breastfeeding **Drug interactions**: *Warning: do not use with*: (as for ritonavir) plus: rifampicin Efavirenz, nevirapine and tenofovir reduce plasma lopinavir concentrations and lopinavir increases plasma tenofovir concentration

Drug and usual dose[a] in adults and adolescents	Side effects[b] (not an all-inclusive list)	Some important nursing information[a]
		Dexamethasone, carbamazepine, phenytoin and phenobarbital all reduce plasma concentration of lopinavir
Atazanavir *Reyataz®* In early 2003, this drug was still in clinical trials but the dose is likely to be 400 mg once daily	Diarrhoea; reportedly fewer side effects than other PIs Further information when clinical trials are completed	Taken with food No significant drug interactions reported to date

[a]Check all dosages and potential drug interactions with the current online edition of the *British National Formulary*: www.bnf.org.
[b]Check online sources for further information on side effects at: www.aidsmap.com or www.netdoctor.co.uk/medicines and www.bnf.org.
NSAIDs, non-steroidal anti-inflammatory drugs; SSRIs, selective serotonin re-uptake inhibitors.

Starting HAART

Decisions about when to initiate treatment need to be individualized and carefully arrived at, by both patient and physician. Once committed to HAART, the commitment is for life.

In general, HAART is commenced in all symptomatic patients and in those people in whom there is a high rate of viral replication and before there is irreversible damage to the immune system, e.g. before the CD4+ T-lymphocyte cell count falls below 200 CD4+ cells per cubic millimetre (mm³) of peripheral blood. Patients who are asymptomatic and who have a CD4+ cell count between 200 and 350 mm³ are closely monitored for their rate of CD4+, cell loss and their plasma HIV RNA viral load. Those with a rapidly falling CD4+ count and a high viral load will generally be advised to commence antiretroviral therapy.[2–4]

HAART is not generally prescribed for asymptomatic patients who have a CD4+ cell count of <350 per mm³.[2–4] Various issues need to be factored into the decision to commence treatment. These include the preference of the patient and his or her perceived ability to adhere to therapy. The benefits of treatment in improving health and immune function and delaying end-stage disease must also be weighed against the risks of both early and late toxicities associated with HAART. The long-term adverse effects of HAART are serious in some patients and may limit their future treatment opportunities. Additionally, there may be significant psychological implications for patients in committing themselves to fairly complicated life-long drug regimens.

Monitoring treatment

There are three essential laboratory tests used to monitor the patient's immune status, disease progression, treatment efficacy and drug resistance:

- CD4+ T-lymphocyte cell counts,
- plasma HIV RNA level (viral load),
- genotypic and phenotypic viral resistance assays.

Healthy adults who are not immunosuppressed will, on average, have a CD4+ T-lymphocyte cell count of between 600 and 1200 cells/mm³ of peripheral blood, or generally around 1000 CD4+ cells/mm³. As HIV infects these cells and uses them for replication, there is an increase in the number of new viruses being produced, which are able to infect yet more

CD4⁺ cells. The budding out of new viruses from infected CD4⁺ cells will ultimately destroy those cells. This leads to a progressive decline in the number of CD4⁺ cells over time. This, as discussed in Chapters 6 and 7, is the principal cellular pathology in HIV disease. The lower the CD4⁺ cell count, and the higher the plasma HIV viral load, the nearer the patient is to developing the opportunistic infections and neoplasms that define end-stage disease, i.e. AIDS (see Figure 7.1).

Two essential assays are used to monitor both the rate of disease progression and the efficacy of antiretroviral treatment: CD4⁺ T-lymphocyte cell counts and plasma HIV RNA levels (viral load).

Plasma HIV RNA levels (viral load) indicate the magnitude of HIV replication and its associated rate of CD4⁺ T-lymphocyte destruction. To illustrate the relationship between these two measurements, an analogy of a train travelling towards the edge of a cliff (tumbling over the cliff representing AIDS) has been described (Figure 20.2).[7] The CD4⁺ T-cell count is the distance to the edge of the cliff, i.e. the point where a patient is at that moment in time on a continuum from infection to end-stage disease (AIDS) and death. The lower the CD4⁺ T-cell count, the closer the train is to disaster. The viral load is the speed of the train, i.e. how fast a patient is progressing towards AIDS. The higher the plasma HIV RNA viral load, the faster the train is moving towards the edge of the cliff. Antiretroviral therapy aims to slow down or halt the train by depressing viral replication. This often gives the immune system some respite, allowing it to partially recover, and this is reflected in an increasing CD4⁺ cell count.

These two measurements need to be obtained on a periodic basis to determine both the risks for disease progression and when to initiate or modify antiretroviral treatment regimens.

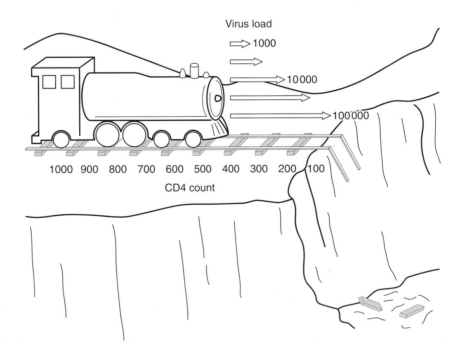

FIGURE 20.2 *Train analogy relating HIV progression to viral load and CD4 count. (Coffin JM. HIV viral dynamics. Reprinted from AIDS 1996; **10**(Suppl. 3):S75–84. Used by permission of Lippincott, Williams & Wilkins.)*

DRUG RESISTANCE

As previously discussed in Chapter 6, HIV makes billions of copies of itself each day, which means that 99 per cent of the virus present in an infected person at any one moment in time has been produced by infected cells within the previous 2 weeks. HIV, like all retroviruses, makes frequent errors in transcription, i.e. it produces imperfect copies of itself – viral variants which are called mutants. This tendency for inaccuracy in transcription, coupled with such a rapid rate of viral replication, ensures that there is always a varied pool of mutants in any infected person. Some of these mutants may be resistant to some types of antiretroviral drugs. Drug-resistant mutations happen randomly and, with billions of viruses being produced every day, it is likely that at least one or two of the new viruses will be resistant to an antiretroviral drug.

For example, if by chance a few of the newly produced mutant viruses are resistant to one type of antiretroviral drug, say ritonavir, then their replication cycle will not be suppressed by this drug. However, ritonavir will continue to inhibit the viral enzyme protease in all of the other more numerous viruses that make up the viral pool in that person and suppress viral replication – but not in those few ritonavir-resistant mutants. These mutants will go on to replicate, eventually making hundreds of millions of new copies of themselves every day, almost all of which will be ritonavir resistant. Ultimately, they will become the dominant virus in the pool, and the infected person's viral load will climb back up to pre-treatment levels, with a corresponding drop in CD4+ T-cells. Clearly, this is a perilous situation for any patient.

An obvious way to prevent the emergence of drug-resistant viral variants is to suppress the volume of HIV replication. If, instead of allowing HIV to replicate at full speed and produce 9–11 billion new copies daily, some of which are bound to be mutants, its ability to replicate was suppressed by effectively using HAART, there would be dramatically less virus produced and fewer potentially drug-resistant mutants emerging.

A number of factors influence the speed and extent of viral resistance, including: the patient's prior treatment history and disease stage, his or her ability to adhere fully to HAART, the potency of the treatment regimen, individual variation in drug metabolism and pharmacodynamics, and the kinetics of viral replication. There are significant consequences of an expanding population of drug-resistant, and multiple drug-resistant, HIV-infected individuals. Not only are their treatment options severely limited (or non-existent), but also they are able to transmit drug-resistant HIV to others.[8]

Using potent combinations of antiretroviral drugs to initially and then consistently suppress HIV replication below the level of detection (>50 copies/mL) offers the best chance of preventing, or at least postponing, viral resistance.

Genotyping or phenotyping assays are now in widespread use in clinical practice to monitor drug resistance (Table 20.3).

HAART-RELATED ADVERSE CLINICAL EVENTS

There is a range of (sometimes serious) adverse clinical events associated with the use of HAART, some of the more important of which are listed in Table 20.4.[4,10] Avoiding and managing these side effects have been described in the continuously updated UK **HIV i-Base** publication,[8] which is available online from http://www.i-Base.org.uk/.

TABLE 20.3 Assays for monitoring drug resistance[4,9]

Assay	Method	Some advantages and disadvantages
Genotypic	Detects drug-resistant mutations that are present in the relevant viral genes, i.e. reverse transcriptase and protease	*Advantages* Can be performed rapidly, results available within 1–2 weeks of sample collection May detect presence of resistant mutants before they have resulted in phenotypic resistance Less expensive then phenotypic assays *Disadvantages* Requires a viral load >1000 copies/mL Detects resistance only in dominant species (>20%) Technician experience influences results Interpretation requires knowledge of mutational changes, e.g. expertise
Phenotypic	Measures the ability of a virus to grow in different concentrations of antiretroviral drugs	*Advantages* Interpretation more analogous to resistance testing of bacteria. Assesses the total effect, including mutations, mutational interactions Reproducibility is good Advantage over genotype when there are multiple mutations *Disadvantages* Requires a viral load >500–1000 copies/mL Longer delay in reporting (2–3 weeks) Thresholds to define susceptibility are arbitrary, non-standardized, and do not always reflect achievable drug concentrations Detects resistance only in dominant species (>20%)

ADHERENCE TO HAART

The effective treatment of any condition requires patients to adhere to prescribed therapy. In many chronic illnesses, e.g. hypertension, it is recognized that less than perfect adherence may be adequate in controlling the disease and preventing unfavourable outcomes, a phenomenon sometimes known as 'pharmacological forgiveness'. HIV disease, on the other hand, is unforgiving; it requires total life-long adherence to continually suppress viral replication, delay disease progression and prevent the emergence of drug-resistant variants. There are many barriers to achieving this standard of adherence, and general practitioners and practice nurses need to be fully aware of these and develop strategies to support patients in adhering to HAART regimens.[11] The issues associated with adherence to therapy are discussed in detail in Chapters 13 and 21.

Summary

More and more patients with HIV disease are living good-quality lives for a previously inconceivable longer period of time, thanks to the breathtaking advancements in antiretroviral treatment. Techniques to monitor treatment efficacy are improving rapidly, e.g. ultra-sensitive plasma HIV RNA viral level assays and new assays to identify drug resistance. Everything, however, hinges on the ability of patients to fully adhere to treatment regimens,

TABLE 20.4 HAART-associated adverse clinical events[4,10]

Clinical event	Associated antiretroviral drugs
Lactic acidosis and hepatic steatosis	Nucleoside analogues
Pancreatitis	Nucleoside analogues
Fatty liver	Nucleoside analogues
Liver toxicity	Most HIV drugs can damage the liver, but ritonavir, nevirapine and efavirenz frequently cause liver damage
Nephrolithiasis (kidney stones)	Indinavir
Lipodystrophy – fat maldistribution (fat gain, fat loss and high plasma levels of triglycerides and cholesterol, along with insulin resistance)	Unsure – both protease inhibitors and nucleoside analogues have been suggested to be associated with this syndrome
Hyperglycaemia	Protease inhibitors
Hypersensitivity reactions (rash, fever, diarrhoea and abdominal pain, fatigue, nausea and vomiting, headache, flu-like symptoms, cough, dyspnoea and sore throat)	Abacavir, Trizivir® (which contains abacavir) Potentially fatal; consult physician immediately
Skin rash	Abacavir, nevirapine, efavirenz, delavirdine, amprenavir
Peripheral neuropathy	Zalcitabine, stavudine, didanosine, lamivudine
Central nervous system side effects	Efavirenz
Insomnia	Efavirenz
Sexual problems	Unsure – perhaps protease inhibitors involved, but many other factors play a part in the development of sexual problems
Dry skin and chapped lips	Indinavir, epivir (and hydroxyurea)
Capsulitis (frozen shoulder)	Indinavir
Alopecia (hair loss)	Indinavir, epivir (and hydroxyurea)
Paronychia (fingernail and toenail inflammation/infections)	Indinavir, epivir (and hydroxyurea)
Nausea and vomiting	Most antiretroviral drugs
Fatigue	Most antiretroviral drugs
Diarrhoea	Most antiretroviral drugs, but frequently associated with: nelfinavir, saquinavir, amprenavir, ritonavir, abacavir and didanosine

and general practice staff can play a decisive role in supporting patients to maintain the challenging level of drug adherence necessary to prevent drug resistance and progression to end-stage HIV disease.

REFERENCES

1. Palella FJ, Delaney KM, Moorman AC et al. Declining morbidity and mortality among patients with advanced human immunodeficiency virus infection. *New England Journal of Medicine* 1998; **338**:853–60.
2. British HIV Association (BHIVA). *Guidelines for the Treatment of HIV-infected Adults with Antiretroviral Therapy*, 2001. Available online at: http://www.bhiva.org/guidelines.html

3. Mehta DK (Executive Editor). *British National Formulary (BNF)*, 44th edn. London: British Medical Association and the Royal Pharmaceutical Society of Great Britain, September 2002. Available from: BMJ Books, PO Box 295, London WC1H 9TE, UK, or from their website: www.bmjbookshop.com. The BNF is also available online at: www.BNF.org

4. Centers for Disease Control and Prevention. Guidelines for using antiretroviral agents among HIV-infected adults and adolescents: Recommendations of the Panel on Clinical Practices for Treatment of HIV. *Morbidity and Mortality Weekly Report (MMWR)* 17 May 2002; **51**(RR-7):1–64. Available online at: http://www.cdc.gov/mmwr/PDF/rr/rr5107.pdf

5. National AIDS Manual (NAM). *HIV & AIDS Treatment Directory*, 22nd edn. London: NAM Publications, December 2002, 698 pp. Updated and published every 6 months. Details from: NAM, 16a Clapham Common Southside, London SW4 7AB. Telephone +44 (0)20 7627 3200; fax. +44 (0)20 7627 3101; e-mail: info@nam.org.uk; website: www.aidsmap.com

6. AIDS Project – Los Angeles. Medications used in the treatment of HIV. *Positive Living* March 2002. Online publication (cited 5 January 2003), available at: http://www.thebody.com/apla/apr02/hiv_medications.html

7. Coffin JM. HIV viral dynamics. *AIDS* 1996; **10**(Suppl. 3):S75–84.

8. Cohen OJ, Fauci AS. Transmission of multidrug-resistant human immunodeficiency virus – the wake-up call. *New England Journal of Medicine* 1998; **339**:341–3.

9. Bartlett JG. *The 2002 Abbreviated Guide to Medical Management of HIV Infection*. Baltimore, MD: Johns Hopkins University (Division of Infectious Diseases), 2002, 154 pp. Available from the Johns Hopkins AIDS Services online at: http://hopkins-aids.edu

10. i-Base. *Avoiding and Managing Side Effects*. London: HIV i-Base Publications, August 2002. Available online from: http://www.i-Base.org.uk/

11. Leake H, Horne R. Optimising adherence to combination therapy. *Journal of HIV Therapy* 1998; **3**:67–71.

INTERNET RESOURCES

- The *British National Formulary (BNF)*, published by the **British Medical Association** and the **Royal Pharmaceutical Society of Great Britain**, provides up-to-date information in relation to the drugs used in the UK to treat HIV infection and HIV-related illnesses. The online version is updated every 6 months. Available from: BMJ Books, PO Box 295, London WC1H 9TE, UK, or from their website www.bmjbookshop.com: http://www.BNF.org/

- Online continuously updated guidelines on using antiretroviral drugs in children are available as a **Living Document** from the US Department of Health and Human Services. *Guidelines for the Use of Antiretroviral Agents in Pediatric HIV Infection*: Working Group on Antiretroviral Therapy and Medical Management of HIV-infected Children convened by the National Institutes of Health, National Pediatric and Family HIV Resource Center, and the Health Resources and Services Administration. December 14, 2001: http://www.aidsinfo.nih.gov/guidelines

- Information from The UK National AIDS Manual (NAM), the International HIV/AIDS Alliance and the British HIV Association (BHIVA) covers the entire spectrum of the

prevention, care and treatment of adults and children and is available on the premiere UK HIV website. Publications include the *HIV & AIDS Treatment Directory*, which is updated and published every 6 months. Details from: NAM, 16a Clapham Common Southside, London SW4 7AB; Tel. +44 (0)20 7627 3200; fax +44 (0)20 7627 3101; e-mail: info@nam.org.uk; or their website:
http://www.aidsmap.com

- In the UK, a range of current, continuously updated and free treatment information is available from **i-Base**, either in hard copy or downloadable from their excellent website. Included in their information database is an introduction to antiretroviral therapy, information on avoiding and managing side effects from antiretroviral treatment and on 'salvage' therapy following the development of drug resistance. To contact i-Base, telephone +44 (0)20 7407 8488 or fax +44 (0)20 7407 8489 or, better still, e-mail them at: admin@i.Base.org.uk or visit their website:
http://www.i-Base.org.uk/

- 'NetDoctor' is a UK independent health website that provides easy access to clear and reliable information, including information on all antiretroviral drugs used in Europe and North America:
http://www.netdoctor.co.uk/medicines/

Adherence to antiretroviral therapy

Heather Loveday

> To write prescriptions is easy, but to come to an understanding with people is hard.
>
> A Country Doctor, *Franz Kafka*

Introduction

The advent of highly active antiretroviral therapy (HAART) in the latter half of the 1990s transformed both the clinical care and the health outlook for people living with HIV infection. Although HAART regimens have produced dramatic reductions in HIV-related mortality in countries where they are available, there is also considerable evidence that strict adherence is a crucial factor in maximizing the benefits of therapy. In the developed world, the challenge for both healthcare practitioners and people living with HIV infection is how to sustain a life-long commitment to near-total adherence to potent, toxic and often complex regimens of antiretroviral therapy.

In this chapter we will identify what is meant by the term adherence; discuss its importance in HAART; explore the factors that facilitate and hinder a person's ability to adhere to therapy; and discuss interventions that can be used by nurses and patients to support and sustain adherence to therapy and maintain an acceptable quality of life.

Learning outcomes

After studying and reflecting on the material in this chapter, you will be able to:

- discuss with patients and their carers the importance of adhering to HAART;
- identify factors in patients' everyday lives that may create barriers to successful adherence;
- assist patients in planning strategies to support and sustain medication adherence.

COMPLIANCE, ADHERENCE AND CONCORDANCE

Compliance has been defined as 'the extent to which a person's behaviour (in terms of taking medications, following diets or executing lifestyle changes) coincides with medical or health advice'.[1] This definition provides a traditional and predominantly paternalistic view of the therapeutic relationship between the doctor and patient and implies that the patient is subservient to the clinician. In this model, the role of the patient is to follow instructions, and failure to do so is often construed as obstructive or recalcitrant behaviour. The problems that arise from non-compliance are laid firmly at the door of the patient.[1,2-4] From the perspective of the patient, the terminology used to describe people's efforts to follow prescribed therapy is important, and 'compliance' suggests disempowerment and the relinquishment of decision-making to an authority figure.[5] In contrast, the term **adherence** has been adopted to indicate greater collaborative involvement of patients in planning and implementing regimens.

A move away from the traditional model of compliance towards a model of adherence that places greater emphasis on the patient's role in achieving the optimum therapeutic outcome is now generally advocated.[6] In the UK, The Royal Pharmaceutical Society suggests that this process is best achieved through a therapeutic partnership termed **concordance**.[7] This is felt to promote a better understanding of both the patient's and the professional's health beliefs in order to assist the patient in making an informed choice.

Adherence to therapy in chronic illness

Difficulty in adhering to treatment regimens is more prevalent when illness is chronic and the treatment recommendations are largely prophylactic. Experiences with other chronic illnesses, such as diabetes, renal failure, hypertension and rheumatoid arthritis, indicate that patient adherence has a direct effect on clinical outcome. In these illnesses, adherence to treatment is estimated at between 20 and 80 per cent, and authors have identified a number of factors that are consistently associated with poor adherence.[8-10] These include: anxiety associated with taking medication; the impact of side effects; health beliefs; complexity of regimens; and poor clinician–patient relationships. Other authors suggest that at times patients choose not to adhere to treatment in order to maintain some control over their lives or coping with their illness.[11,12]

Adherence to HAART

The therapeutic success of HAART is dependent upon the continual suppression of HIV RNA viral load to levels that cannot be detected by current assays. This requires the maintenance of optimum therapeutic drug levels to ensure effectiveness. The pharmacodynamics of antiretroviral medications and the relative inflexibility of regimens mean that patients must achieve near-perfect adherence to give themselves the best chance of achieving sustained viral suppression.

The development of drug resistance has been covered in detail in Chapter 20. In summary, the failure of HAART to bring about a sustained reduction in HIV RNA viral load may be related to a number of factors, including: individual patient characteristics that affect the activity of the drug, such as poor absorption and increased drug clearance; the choice of sub-optimal combinations or dose prescribing; pre-existing resistance to one or more of the drugs in the HAART regimen; and, finally, the patient being unable to adhere to the medication regimen. Once developed, drug resistance limits future treatment options due to cross-resistance to drugs in the same group.

Measuring adherence

The degree to which patients adhere to therapy is difficult to measure accurately. Methods used to determine adherence include: self-reporting by the patient; clinician estimates; pill counts and determining prescription refills; and medication event monitoring through electronic devices that track the date and time of opening and closing of medication containers. Each of these approaches is problematic, as they assume that reports or estimates are accurate, or that the patient has taken the medication that has been removed from the container. Adherence may also be measured through laboratory measurements such as blood or urine levels, and although they may indicate that medication has been taken in the recent past, they may also be misleading, as patients may be more adherent immediately prior to clinic appointments than at other times.

Adherence to HAART, as with other medications, is difficult to measure, primarily because there is no agreed level at which patients can be considered to be adherent. In studies associated with other chronic diseases, patients who take 80 per cent or more of their prescribed medication are considered to be adherent. Although many early studies of HIV adherence used 80 per cent as a crude marker, it has become clear that this is insufficient to achieve the desired outcomes of treatment. Research shows that even occasional missed doses of HAART adversely affect clinical outcomes. Table 21.1 shows that the 80 per cent level of adherence, seen as optimum in many chronic illnesses, will result in some level of treatment failure for 50 per cent of the patients taking HAART.[13]

TABLE 21.1 Level of adherence needed to effectively reduce viral load

Adherence rate (%)	Percentage of people with undetectable plasma HIV RNA
>95	81
90–95	64
80–90	50
70–80	25
<70	6

Several studies have shown that a large percentage of patients who are not being supported in clinical trials have difficulty in consistently adhering to antiretroviral therapy regimens exactly as prescribed.[14–17] This is, perhaps, understandable considering the various side effects, drug interactions, complicated dosing regimens and dietary restrictions associated with therapy and the need to take these drugs for life. However, low levels of treatment adherence have serious clinical consequences.

Treatment failure or breakthrough occurs most often when people miss sufficient doses to result in the development of drug resistance. However, there is little indication from research of how many doses may be missed or the influence of the pattern of missed doses on virological failure. It is likely that this will vary among patients and be related to factors such as stage of disease, previous medication history and resistance profiles.

What are the facilitators and barriers to adherence?

Much of the early research into HIV adherence concentrated on attempting to find factors that might predict non-adherence. However, the results of these studies and those in other chronic diseases fail to identify any socio-demographic, clinical or lifestyle predictors of non-adherence. The only consistent factor across studies seems to be depressed mood.[18] For most people, patterns of adherence vary with the circumstances of their lives. Few people claim to be 100 per cent adherent; most people are adherent for 70–99 per cent of the time, and about 30 per cent of patients are poor adherers, taking less than 60 per cent of prescribed doses.[19] Adherence or lack of it is therefore dynamic, changing and varying within individuals according to circumstances at given points in time.

Although not predictive of adherence levels, there are a number of factors that need to be considered by patients and clinicians in order to promote adherence and give patients their 'best shot' at sustained viral suppression.

The regimen

Adherence literature has shown consistent associations between problems of adherence and the complexity of regimens, the number of pills being taken and, perhaps most importantly, the impact of regimens on people's everyday lives.[20] However, complexity does not simply refer to the number of different medications or pills, but also encompasses the dosing schedule, the duration of therapy and dietary or lifestyle restrictions. HAART regimens contain all these elements and as such present a major barrier to sustained adherence. Most current treatment regimens involve at least three medications, and some, particularly salvage therapies, continue to involve numerous pills, capsules or tablets with restrictions related to mealtimes and food selections.

There is an assumption that reducing the medication burden in terms of pill count or dose events will resolve adherence problems. Indeed, since the advent of HAART, there have been considerable advances in terms of combining medications such as zidovudine and lamivudine (Combivir®) and zidovudine combined with lamivudine and abacavir (Trizivir®) in order to make the regimen more 'forgiving'. However, studies suggest that this is not necessarily the case, and that **it is the ease with which regimens can be accommodated within an individual's daily routine that is crucial.**[21–24] This is reinforced by more recent work which suggests that regimens with two or fewer dose events without food restrictions are more likely to be adhered to.[25]

The side effects associated with HAART have been shown to influence adherence. In patients with asymptomatic disease, side effects can be perceived as worse than the disease and consequently may lead to missed doses. Most HAART regimens produce side effects, particularly during the early stages of therapy. The specific side effects associated with individual medications are discussed in Chapter 20. Common problems include: nausea, vomiting, diarrhoea, headache, rash, paraesthesia in the hands and feet (leading to peripheral neuropathy), and general fatigue. Long-term side effects include liver toxicity, neutropenia and anaemia and hyperlipidaemia. Additionally, body fat changes (lipodystrophy), including fat accumulation, especially around the neck and upper back and abdomen, and fat wasting (known as lipoatrophy), especially from the face and buttocks, commonly occur.

Patient characteristics

Perhaps the single most important factor in adherence to HAART is the patient's health beliefs and experiences in relation to medication and HIV disease. There is good-quality research that demonstrates that many HIV-infected people understand the seriousness of their illness, recognize the importance of adherence and are aware of the virological consequences of poor adherence.[17,26] In these studies, 97 per cent of those taking HAART felt that HIV was still a serious illness, and 94 per cent were aware of the danger of developing drug resistance. A positive outlook can be influential, and studies suggest that people who perceive that they have more control over their health and are optimistic about the future are more likely to adhere to therapy.[27] There is also evidence that those people who perceive the benefits of HAART may be more adherent than those with reservations about the effectiveness of therapy.[28,29] However, this is far from conclusive, and there is contradictory evidence that healthy scepticism may result in greater personal responsibility and therefore greater adherence.[30]

The only consistent predictor of poor adherence in the research literature, across many chronic conditions, is depressed mood and mental health problems. The prevalence of depression in people with HIV disease has been estimated as between 20 and 52 per cent,[31–36] compared with those in the general community amongst whom the prevalence of major depression is 3–10 per cent.[37] The symptoms of depression include lack of motivation, poor organization and difficulty in concentrating and remembering. Clearly, having to maintain adherence to complex treatment regimens that require a positive approach to all of the above may prove problematic.

Social support

The presence of stable relationships and having access to social and emotional support are also an important factor in maintaining adherence.[17] People who live alone and have poor social networks are more likely to have problems with adherence than those who do not.[38] In addition, fear of stigma and being noticed when taking medication by those outside one's immediate social networks present a barrier to normalizing adherence behaviour.

Levels of knowledge and understanding

The patient's ability to make decisions and participate in discussions related to treatment is central to achieving good patterns of adherence. There is a widely held belief that patients who are well informed are more likely to be adherent because they understand the reasoning behind treatment and appreciate the consequences of poor adherence. Patients need clear and understandable information before they can make the decisions needed to commence HAART. There is some evidence that those people who feel well informed about their therapy are more likely to feel in control of their illness and are more likely to be adherent.[27] However, even the most knowledgeable and well-informed person may forget to take a particular dose or make an informed decision to miss a particular dose.

Lifestyle factors

There is little consistent evidence that substance or alcohol misuse are predictors of non-adherence. However, both of these factors may be significant in people's ability to cope with complex regimens that require a high degree of organization. A recent study suggests that these difficulties are associated with the chaotic lifestyle of people who misuse drugs and alcohol rather than having a direct relationship with substance misuse.[39] There is evidence that those who are drug or alcohol dependent are no more likely to be non-adherent than those who are not.[40]

Healthcare provider factors

The qualities of the healthcare provider (HCP) are an important factor in helping patients to adhere to HAART.[41–43] Much of the early adherence literature focused entirely on the role of the patient in maintaining adherence and failed to recognize that the HCP has clear responsibilities in facilitating adherence. The collaborative nature of treatment decisions in HIV care, as in other chronic illnesses, is central to current trends in managing adherence and requires a degree of 'engagement' between patient and HCP. In order to achieve engagement with the patient, the HCP needs to use a range of interpersonal and clinical skills, including: listening; being sensitive to the needs and limitations of the patient; developing an understanding of the patient's situation; good communication skills, in particular the ability to translate complex information into a format that is both detailed and understandable; and the ability to recognize the patient as a partner in clinical decisions. In order for this type of engagement to develop, the patient needs to have continuity of care so that expectations are consistent and experiences can be shared.[44,45] Finally, evidence suggests that those patients who perceive that the HCP/patient relationship is one of mutual respect and trust are more likely to be adherent[27] and to feel that they are able to be open and honest about problems associated with adherence to HAART.

The nursing role in supporting adherence to HAART

Strategies to support adherence to HAART need to be implemented from an early stage in the patient's treatment journey. In the same way that adherence behaviour is multi-factorial and dynamic, approaches to supporting adherence need to be multi-focused and flexible in order meet the changing needs of individuals.

A major problem facing clinicians is the amount of time needed to help patient's to come to decisions about their treatment options and to provide appropriate advice and support once those decisions have been taken. The nurse is ideally placed to support patients through many of the difficulties associated with HAART. These include: the decision-making process associated with starting or changing therapy; identifying with patients how best to integrate medication taking into daily routines; providing advice and adjuvant therapy during the initial stages of HAART; and providing long-term adherence support. Nurses can also provide advice on accessing additional sources of information, including Internet resources. However, while clinicians or nurses initiate and co-ordinate interventions, other members of the multidisciplinary team, such as health advisers, pharmacists, dieticians and clinical psychologists, play a key role in supporting adherence.

Skills development for supporting adherence

The major obstacle facing most nurses is the lack of time to consult with patients on a regular and meaningful basis. In a busy outpatient clinic, a 10-minute consultation may be the best that a patient can expect with a doctor or nurse. In a recent survey conducted by the Adherence Strategy Panel, although 97 per cent of clinicians identified that they were personally involved in discussing adherence, they only spent a fifth of the available consultation time doing so, and a staggering 75 per cent identified that they had had no formal preparation for dealing with adherence issues.[46] Figures are not available for nursing involvement, but one might expect similar findings.

The development of competency frameworks and in-service education such as that developed by nurse specialists at the Chelsea and Westminster Hospital in London help nurses to develop the necessary knowledge and skills to support patients taking HAART.[47] While most patients consider their clinician to be their key HCP, many consider nurses and pharmacists to be central to their care. The development of clinics led by nurses and pharmacists to support patients in adhering to HAART regimens means that valuable skills and knowledge can be used for the patient's benefit.[48,49] Such clinics also ensure that patients have continuity of care and are able to access HCPs more easily if they encounter problems between clinic appointments.

Assessment of patient's readiness to start therapy

'Individualize the drugs to fit the patient and not the patient to fit the drug'[50] is an important principle for the nurse to apply with patients when discussing the initiation of therapy. In order to tailor therapy to meet individual requirements, the nurse needs to have a detailed knowledge of the patient's clinical history, psychological state, lifestyle, health beliefs and support mechanisms. This information needs to be collected systematically and recorded accurately so that potential barriers to adherence can be identified. Nursing assessment tools can be used to explore adherence issues with patients and highlight potential problems so that options can be reviewed or interventions employed. It is worth acknowledging that empowering patients to decide not to embark on therapy or to delay starting it may be in their best interests if commencing therapy is jeopardized by major barriers to adherence.

Following assessment, the patient and clinician discuss the treatment options that take account of the various factors identified during assessment. This enables barriers to adherence to be considered and the patient to be a partner in the decision-making process.

Promoting knowledge and understanding

Patient knowledge and understanding are the foundation of all strategies to support adherence to HAART.[42] Information enables patients to participate in the decision-making process and to take responsibility for their choices. Information can be provided in a range of formats and media in order to facilitate understanding and involvement. Many pharmaceutical companies and community-based organizations such as (in the UK) the National AIDS Manual, the Terrence Higgins Trust, and Positively Women, provide written information in readable and clearly illustrated booklets which are available free of charge to patients. There is also a wide range of resources available on the Internet that provide answers to questions frequently asked about HAART. A computer-based program known as 'The Wheel' is available on the Internet (see 'Internet resources' at the end of this chapter), which helps people to explore the impact of various treatment options on their everyday lives and highlights where potential clashes between daily routines and the demands of therapy may occur.[51] This approach involves patients in the selection of medications that they think can be accommodated within their daily lives and may help to establish positive adherence behaviours in the early stages of therapy. Providing information in a variety of formats will help to reinforce messages and can be useful in pro-viding material for discussion and for assessing the patient's readiness to embark on therapy.

INITIATING THERAPY

Once an assessment has been made and the patient has taken the decision to commence HAART, he or she may benefit from participating in a trial run, substituting dummy medication for the real thing. While this will not produce the possible side effects patients may experience when starting or changing therapies, it does enable them to check out how the selected regimen fits in with their everyday routines.

In the early stages of therapy, patients need to be closely monitored and supported. Regular clinic appointments and/or telephone follow-up provide nurses with the opportunity to check how strategies are working. In addition, asking patients to describe the medications they take and when and how they should be taken can reinforce knowledge and understanding. Confusion about how many pills to take and the appearance of different pills and lack of understanding of the instructions associated with medication taking are more frequently reported by patients who are considered to be non-adherent than by those who are adherent.[50]

DEVELOPING CUES FOR MEDICATION ADHERENCE

Many patients state that they simply forget to take medications at certain times. This tendency can be reduced by a process of identifying 'cues' that help to remind patients about taking their medications at the correct time and to overcome unintentional non-adherence. Cues involve linking the taking of medication to everyday objects or routine behaviours, such as making the first cup of tea in the morning, going to the bathroom, watching particular television programmes, or letting the dog out last thing at night. The aim of cueing is to remind the patient to take the medication before carrying out the associated routine.

ORGANIZING MEDICATION

One of the practical problems faced by patients involves making multiple medications easily accessible at the correct time of day. Strategies to help with the organization of medications include the provision of daily or weekly dosset boxes, which allow medications to be taken at the appropriate time without having to deal with two or three different medication containers. Developing routines associated with organizing medications, such as filling dosset boxes each night or at the beginning of each week, can help some patients. For others, such routines may be too intrusive into the normal rhythm of their lives.

The use of watch alarms or bleeps can act as a reminder to take medications, and some medication containers have built-in alarms. This strategy can be particularly useful for the difficult to remember or inconvenient doses such as at lunchtime or late at night. Using medication reminder charts or diaries may help patients to keep track of their medication-taking behaviour and record when doses are taken or missed. The latter is important, as it may help to determine patterns of missed doses that will help patients and clinicians to develop strategies for overcoming problems. Nurses can also advise on planning ahead for disruptions to daily routines such as holidays abroad, return to employment or the development of new relationships.

ADHERENCE PROGRAMMES

Structured programmes of adherence support at strategic points in therapy may provide crucial assistance in establishing and maintaining adherence. The literature describes many nurse-led programmes that provide support in formal clinic settings, either in groups or as individuals, or as consultations by telephone or email.[52] These programmes offer patients the opportunity to discuss difficulties with regimens and nurses the chance to monitor adherence. In addition, there is a current trend to develop community-led programmes, outside the clinical setting, for groups of patients in order to assist them in decision-making and to support them in the initial stages of HAART. The aim of such programmes is to maintain quality of life and help patients 'live well' while taking therapy. The content of these programmes may vary according to patient groups, but most involve aspects of patient education already discussed as well as opportunities for patients to discuss therapy with people already taking medication. Programmes may also include self-management skills and opportunities to access social support. Although healthcare practitioners may deliver some of the content of the programme, most chronic disease self-management courses are led by lay facilitators who are experiencing chronic illness, and also involve considerable input from group members themselves and from voluntary organizations.[53–55] The 'Expert Patient' programmes in the UK, such as 'Living Well', are examples of second-generation chronic disease self-management courses.[56]

Social support

In addition to formal clinics or structured programmes, it is important to make use of patients' existing social support networks. Encouraging patients to involve partners, family members and friends in providing practical and informational support can improve adherence to therapy. Practical support may involve providing reminders or checking that medications have been organized correctly. Informational support may involve being available on the telephone to give advice. If patients lack established social networks, the use of 'buddy' systems may help to support them through the initial stages of therapy, while structured group programmes may provide the opportunity to construct more supportive networks for themselves.

Ongoing monitoring and support

Establishing adherence in the early stages of therapy is often accompanied by high levels of motivation on behalf of patients to do well. Goals such as bringing RNA viral load to levels that are undetectable give patients a target for achievement. As therapy progresses, the long-term nature of medication taking and the effort required to sustain therapy can have negative effects on patients and result in lapses in adherence. The temptation to 'take a holiday' may be compelling if side effects become intolerable or the impact of the regimen on everyday life is overly restrictive. The role of the nurse in providing ongoing monitoring and support is central to the durability of medication regimens.

The side effects of medications have been discussed in detail in Chapter 20, and assessment and prompt management of side effects are essential if adherence is to be sustained. Nurses need to be aware of the patient's levels of tolerability in relation to individual experience and use clinical and supportive interventions to help patients cope with distressing short-term effects such as nausea and diarrhoea. It is also imperative that nurses be critically aware of the mood of their patients so that early signs of depression, such as mood swings, sleeplessness and loss of attention, are recognized and treated, as depression provides a major threat to medication adherence.

The use of screening tools at every clinic visit to assess levels of adherence, tolerability of side effects and psychological state may help to give structure to monitoring and provide the prompts for nurses and clinicians to explore particular problems in more detail. It is important that these tools are validated and provide accurate assessments of adherence and quality-of-life factors.

Providing feedback to patients about their plasma RNA viral load and $CD4^+$ T-lymphocyte cell count levels will help to reinforce the relationship between adherence and the durability of treatment. Where patients report that sustaining the regimen is becoming impossible, nurses need to highlight this to clinicians so that strategies such as structured treatment interruptions might be considered.

Summary

Adherence to HAART is essential if treatment is to be durable. Although a number of factors contribute to poor adherence, the only factor that is consistently predictive of non-adherence is depression. A patient's first treatment regimen is often the most effective in lowering the RNA viral load to undetectable levels, and therefore the decision to initiate therapy must be carefully considered by the clinician and the patient. The patient's readiness and ability to maintain near-perfect adherence need to be assessed, and the nursing role is central to providing patients with the information and support they need to make informed decisions. Nurses need to make an accurate assessment of the barriers and supports to adherence with individual patients and develop treatment plans that will sustain motivation and maintain quality of life. Interventions such as integrating treatment into daily activities, making medications accessible in the correct dose and at the right time, and providing ongoing peer or healthcare provider support will assist in the establishment and sustainability of adherence behaviours. Nurses also need to create a climate of trust and collaboration with patients, so that reasons for non-adherence can be monitored and clinical management can be modified, where possible, when adhering to regimens has a negative impact on quality of life. These approaches will help to build a partnership approach to medication adherence that moves away from the out-dated concepts of compliance.

REFERENCES

1. Haynes RB. Introduction. In: RB Haynes, DW Taylor, DC Sackett (eds), *Compliance in Health Care*. Baltimore: Johns Hopkins University Press, 1979.
2. Varni JW, Wallander JL. Adherence to health-related regimes in paediatric chronic disorders. *Clinical Psychology Review* 1984; **4**:585–96.
3. Donovan JCL, Blake DR. Patient non-compliance: deviance or reasoned decision-making. *Social Science and Medicine* 1992; **34**:507–13.
4. Stimson G. Obeying doctors' orders: a view from the other side. *Social Science and Medicine* 1975; **8**:97–104.
5. Grahame-Smith H. Compliance: the patient's perspective. *Journal of HIV Therapy* 1998; **3**:72–5.
6. Sumartojo E. When tuberculosis treatment fails. A social behavioural account of patient adherence. *American Review of Respiratory Disease* 1993; **147**:1311–20.
7. Royal Pharmaceutical Society. *From Compliance to Concordance: Achieving Goals in Medicine Taking*. London: Royal Pharmaceutical Society, 1996.
8. Eraker SA, Kirscht JP, Becker MH. Understanding and improving adherence. *Annals of Internal Medicine* 1984; **100**:258–68.

9. Meichenbaum D, Turk DC. Treatment and adherence: terminology, incidence and conceptualisation. In: *Facilitating Treatment Adherence*. New York: Plenum Press, 1987, 19–39.
10. DiMatteo MR, Friedman HS. Patient co-operation with treatment. In: *Social Psychology and Medicine*. Cambridge, MA: Oelgeschlager, Gunn and Hain, 1982, 35–58.
11. Conrad P. The meaning of medications: another look at adherence. *Social Science Medicine* 1985; **20**:29–37.
12. Samet JH, Libman H, Steger KA, Rajeev K. Adherence with zidovudine therapy in patients infected with human immunodeficiency virus, type 1: a cross-sectional study in a municipal hospital clinic. *American Journal of Medicine* 1992; **92**:495–502.
13. Paterson DL, Swindells S, Mohr J et al. Adherence to protease inhibitor therapy and outcomes in patients with HIV infection. *Annals of Internal Medicine* 2000; **133**:21–30.
14. Altice FL, Friedland GH. The era of adherence to HIV therapy. *Annals of Internal Medicine* 1998; **129**:503–5.
15. Hecht F, Colfax G, Swanson M, Chesney MA. Adherence and effectiveness of protease inhibitors in clinical practice. Paper presented at the Fifth Conference on Retroviruses and Opportunistic Infections, February 2–6 1998, Chicago, Illinois.
16. Gray L, Edmondson E, Lemke AL. *HIV Treatment Adherence: A Guide for Program Development*. HIV/AIDS Project Development and Evaluation: http://www.hapdeu.org/adherence
17. Anderson W, Weatherburn P. *Taking Heart? The Impact of Combination Therapy on the Lives of People with HIV*. London: SIGMA Research, 1999.
18. Dunbar Jacob J, Burke LE, Puczynski S. Clinical assessment and management of adherence to medical regimens. In: PM Nicassio, TW Smith (eds), *Managing Chronic Illness*. Washington, DC: American Psychological Society, 1998, 313–49.
19. Flexner C. Practical treatment issues and adherence: challenges from the clinic. Presented at the ICAAC 1997 Satellite Symposium: Evolving HIV Treatments: Advances and the Challenge of Adherence: www.healthcg.com/hiv/treatment/icaac97/adherence/flexner.html
20. Dunbar Jacob J, Erlen JA, Schlenk EA, Ryan CM, Sereika SM, Doswell WM. Adherence in chronic disease. *Annual Review of Nursing Research* 2000; **18**:48–90.
21. Samet JH, Libman H, Steger KA, Rajeev K. Adherence with zidovudine therapy in patients infected with human immunodeficiency virus, type 1: a cross-sectional study in a municipal hospital clinic. *American Journal of Medicine* 1992; **92**:495–502.
22. Singh N, Squier C, Sivek C, Wagener M. Determinants of adherence with antiretroviral therapy in patients with human immunodeficiency virus: prospective assessment with implications for enhancing adherence. *AIDS Care* 1996; **8**:261–9.
23. Wenger N. Patient characteristics and attitudes associated with antiretroviral adherence. *6th Conference on Retroviruses and Opportunistic Infections*, Abstract No. 98, Chicago, Illinois, February 1999.
24. Myers ED, Branthwaite A. Outpatient compliance with antidepressant medication. *British Journal of Psychiatry* 1992; **160**:83–6.
25. Stone VE, Hogan JW, Schuman P et al. Antiretroviral regimen complexity, self-reported adherence, and HIV patients' understanding of their regimens: survey of women in the HER study. *Journal of Acquired Immune Deficiency Syndromes* 2001; **28**:124–31.
26. Anderson W, Weatherburn P. *The Impact of Combination Therapy on the Lives of People with HIV*. London: SIGMA Research, 1998.

27. Loveday HP, Pratt RJ, Robinson N, Pellowe CM, Franks PJ, Loveday C. Patient active coping, optimism and physician support are all vital to adherence to medication. Programme and Abstracts of the *12th International AIDS Conference*, Abstract No. 24378, Geneva, June 28–July 3, 1998.

28. Agnoletto V, Hollander L, Calvi G et al. Compliance in HIV. Programme and Abstracts of the *12th International AIDS Conference*, Abstract No. 32386, Geneva, June 28–July 3, 1998.

29. Jones AM, Thaker H, Foley B et al. A qualitative study on retroviral therapy: drug compliance in IVDU patients. Programme and Abstracts of the *12th International AIDS Conference*, Abstract No. 32361, Geneva, June 28–July 3, 1998.

30. Weiss JJ, Antoni MH, Mulder CL, Garssen B. Attitudes and age are related to adherence to combination therapy in HIV-positive gay men. Programme and Abstracts of the *12th International AIDS Conference*, Abstract No. 32331, Geneva, June 28–July 3, 1998.

31. Belkin GS, Fleishman JA, Piette J. Physical symptoms and depressive symptoms in individuals with HIV infection. *Psychosomatics* 1992; **33**:416–27.

32. Burack JH, Barrett DC, Stall RD, Chesney MA, Ekstrand ML, Coates TJ. Depressive symptoms and CD4 lymphocyte decline among HIV infected men. *Journal of the American Medical Association* 1993; **270**:2568–73.

33. Hoover DR, Saah AF, Bacellar H et al. Signs and symptoms of 'asymptomatic' HIV-1 infection in homosexual men. Multi-center AIDS Cohort Study. *Journal of Acquired Immune Deficiency Syndromes* 1993; **6**:66–71.

34. Lyketsos CG, McHugh PR, Hanson A. Screening for psychiatric morbidity in a medical outpatient clinic for HIV infection: the need for a psychiatric presence. *International Journal of Psychiatry in Medicine* 1993; **24**:103–13.

35. Katz MH, Douglas JM, Bolan GA et al. Depression and use of mental health services among HIV-infected men. *AIDS Care* 1996; **8**:433–42.

36. Low-Beer S, Chan K, Yip B et al. Depressive symptoms decline among persons on protease inhibitors. *Journal of Acquired Immune Deficiency Syndromes* 2000; **23**:295–301.

37. Elliot A. Depression and HIV. Project Inform's depression and HIV. HIV/AIDS Treatment Information: http://wwwprojinf.org/fs/depression.html, 1997.

38. Pratt RJ, Robinson N, Loveday HP et al. Improvement in sexual drive and a falling viral load are associated with adherence to anti-retroviral therapy. Programme and Abstracts of the *12th International AIDS Conference*, Abstract No. 32343, Geneva, June 28–July 3, 1998.

39. Chesney MA, Ickovics J, Hecht GS, Rabkin J. Adherence a necessity for successful HIV combination therapy. *AIDS* 1999; **13**(Suppl. A):S271–8.

40. Turner JG, Nokes KM, Corless IB et al. History of drug use and adherence in HIV+ persons. Programme and Abstracts of the *12th International AIDS Conference*, Abstract No. 32366, Geneva, June 28–July 3, 1998.

41. Treisman GA. A behavioural approach for the promotion of adherence in complicated patient populations. Presented at the *ICAAC 1997 Satellite Symposium: Evolving HIV Treatments: Advances and the Challenge of Adherence*: www.healthcg.com/hiv/treatment/icaac97/adherence/treisman.html

42. Williams A, Freidland G. Adherence, compliance, and HAART. *AIDS Clinical Care* 1997; **9**:51–5.

43. Ickovics JR, Meisler AW. Adherence in AIDS clinical trials: a framework for clinical research and clinical care. *Journal of Clinical Epidemiology* 1997; **50**:385–91.

44. Pattullo ALS. Heterogeneity of care for HIV-infected individuals decreases with the physician knowledge. *International Journal of STD and AIDS* 1998; **7**:435–8.
45. Holzemer WL, Corless I, Noakes K, Predictors of self-reported adherence in persons living with HIV disease. *AIDS Patient Care and STDs* 1999; **3**:185–97.
46. Walsh JC, Sherr L, and The Adherence Strategy Group. An assessment of current HIV treatment adherence services in the UK. *AIDS Care* 2002; **14**:329–34.
47. Allom J. Empowering nurses to provide adherence support. *HIV Nursing* 2001; **1**:4–5.
48. Horne R, Leake H. Optimising adherence to combination therapy. *Journal of HIV Therapy* 1998; **3**:67–71.
49. Loughlin E, Jensen H. Patient adherence to medication for HIV. *Professional Nurse* 2000; **16**:897–901.
50. Chesney MA. Factors affecting adherence to antiretroviral therapy. *Clinical Infectious Diseases* 2000; **30**(Suppl. 6):171–6.
51. Graeme-Smith H. *The Wheel.* Available on: http://www.aidsmap.com/wheel/starthere.htm
52. *HIV Treatment Adherence Development Guide.* Available at: http://www.hapdeu.org
53. Gifford AL, Laurent DD, Gonz´alez VM, Chesney MA, Lorig KR. Pilot randomized trial of education to improve self-management skills of men with symptomatic HIV/AIDS. *Journal of Acquired Immune Deficiency Syndrome and Human Retrovirology* 1998; **18**:136–44.
54. The Stanford Patient Education Research Center – Chronic Disease Self-Management Courses. See: http://www.stanford.edu/group/perc/programs.html
55. Long Term Medical Conditions Alliance (UK) and the Living with Long Term Illness Project (Lill). See: http://www.lmca.demon.co.uk
56. Department of Health (England). *The Expert Patient: A New Approach to Chronic Disease Management for the 21st Century.* London: Department of Health, August 2001. Available on: http://www.doh.gov.uk/healthinequalities

INTERNET RESOURCES

- 'Medicines **partnership**' is a 2-year initiative, supported by the Department of Health (England), aimed at putting the principles of concordance into practice: http://www.medicines-partnership.org
- 'The Wheel' is a confidential, interactive program that shows you how well any combination of drugs would fit into your everyday life (available in English, French, Spanish, Italian, Portuguese): http://www.aidsmap.com/wheel/starthere.htm
- 'AIDSmap' is the premiere UK website for comprehensive information on all aspects of antiretroviral treatment: http://aidsmap.com
- 'Project Inform' is a major USA website dedicated to providing information and support for people taking antiretroviral therapy: http://www.projinf.org/fs/adherence.html
- The 'Treatment Adherence Project' (TAP) is another USA website which offers an online and downloadable guide for the development of HIV antiretroviral treatment adherence programmes and a wide range of fact sheets: http://www.hapdeu.org/adherence

- The 'San Francisco AIDS Foundation' website provides comprehensive information on adherence to treatment:
http://www.sfaf.org
- Patients and healthcare providers need to agree on the health outcomes that the patient desires and on the strategy for achieving them. This has become known as 'concordance', and further information on how this relates to adherence can be accessed from the concordance website:
www.concordance.org

22 CHAPTER

Complementary and alternative approaches to care

Nicola Robinson and Robert Pratt

> Health is dependent upon a state of equilibrium among the various internal factors which govern the operations of the body and the mind: this equilibrium in turn is reached only when man lives in harmony with his external environment.
>
> *Hippocrates (c.460–377 BC)*

Introduction

In the early years of our experience with HIV disease, conventional (orthodox) medical treatments focused on preventing and managing predictable opportunistic infections and cancers resulting from a progressive decline in immune system function due to the effects of unrelenting HIV replication. Then, within just a few short years of the advent of national epidemics of HIV infection and AIDS, a variety of antiretroviral drugs aimed at halting, or at least slowing, viral replication were developed and rapidly introduced into clinical practice in the industrially developed world. For most people, these new drugs allowed the damaged immune system a chance to partially recover and protect against further opportunistic events. However, these drugs were also associated with an impressive range of serious toxicities and were intolerable to some.

Because of this, and other reasons, many people with HIV disease choose various complementary and alternative approaches to therapy as either a substitute for or an addition to conventional medical treatment. Many others explore these seemingly more natural therapies simply as an adjuvant to better health and an improved sense of well-being, hoping to maximize their immune responses.

Complementary and alternative medicine (CAM) is the term now most commonly used to refer to this range of health-related therapies usually considered to lie outside of Western orthodox medical care. These therapies encompass a range of disciplines and are commonly used by people with HIV disease and other chronic medical conditions in many countries. Although the practices used in CAM are all quite diverse, most emphasize the holistic and individualized nature of treatment and tend to focus on the 'whole' person: body, mind and spirit, rather than just HIV infection itself.

This chapter provides an introduction to the range of CAM therapies frequently accessed by people with HIV disease and discusses the underlying evidence for their effectiveness, anticipated benefits, contraindications and potential adverse outcomes.

Learning outcomes

After studying and reflecting on the material in this chapter, you will be able to:

- respond to patient enquiries regarding commonly used CAM therapies;
- discuss with patients any contraindications or potential adverse consequences of CAM practices within the context of their current medical condition and treatment regimens;
- refer patients to further reliable sources of information and advice.

COMPLEMENTARY AND ALTERNATIVE MEDICINE

The use of CAM is growing in the UK, North America and Australia.[1-3] In a recent UK survey, one in five Britons had used a CAM therapy in the previous year – twice as many compared to a similar survey conducted 6 years previously.[1] Although a wide range of CAM is available (Table 22.1), in this survey herbal medicine (the most popular), aromatherapy, homeopathy and acupuncture were the most commonly used CAM therapies in the UK.

Similarly, a survey in England showed that more than one in four adults will use one or more of the six most well-established and popular CAM therapies (Table 22.2) during their lifetime (increasing to one in three if aromatherapy and reflexology are included) and that, in any year, 11 per cent of the adult population will access one of the most popular CAM therapies.[4]

Use of CAM by people with HIV disease

Since the beginning of the HIV/AIDS pandemic, people affected by HIV disease have often looked beyond traditional systems of healthcare for other therapies that they could use to complement conventional treatment regimens or as an alternative to antiretroviral treatment. The main reasons people with HIV disease use CAM therapies are to reduce stress and improve psychological health, provide pain relief, alleviate the side effects of antiretroviral therapy, improve immune responses, slow or delay HIV disease progression, and because they perceive that 'natural is best'.[5] Additionally, CAM therapies are often used to prevent or manage the symptoms or adverse effects of a range of other health problems that frequently occur as HIV disease progresses, such as fatigue, weakness and lack of energy, weight loss and decreases in lean muscle mass, skin problems, declining libido or sexual dysfunction, nausea and vomiting, anorexia, diarrhoea, insomnia and thrush.

TABLE 22.1 Commonly available CAM therapies in the UK

Group 1	
Herbal medicine	Acupuncture
Osteopathy	Homeopathy
Chiropractic	
Group 2	
Bodywork therapies	Aromatherapy
(includes massage)	Reflexology
Shiatsu	Alexander technique
Hypnotherapy	Meditation
Bach flower remedies	Nutrition medicine
Counselling stress therapy	Yoga
Maharishi ayurvedic medicine	Spiritual healing, also known as therapeutic touch
Group 3a	
Ayurvedic medicine	Chinese herbal medicine
Anthroposophical medicine	Eastern medicine (Tib)
Traditional Chinese medicine	Naturopathy
Group 3b	
Crystal therapy	Dowsing
Iridology	Radionics
Others	
Therapeutic touch	Autogenic therapy/training
Biofeedback	Music as therapy
Humour and laughter therapy	T'ai Chi and Qi Gong
Relaxation and visualization	Chelation therapy
Craniosacral therapy	Applied kinesiology

The evidence for effectiveness and safety

Western orthodox medical treatments, for example antiretroviral drugs, are only introduced into clinical practice following rigorous scientific research. In general, this usually involves testing interventions by using a double-blinded, randomized, controlled clinical trial (RCT) to demonstrate the limits of safety of the treatment, establish the correct dose of a medication, and to prove conclusively that the treatment will result in the promised effect. A well-designed RCT is the only way to establish the effectiveness and safety of treatment interventions. A detailed description of clinical trial methods within the context of HIV prophylaxis and treatment has been published by the National AIDS Manual in the UK[6] (see also recommendations for 'Further reading' at the end of this chapter).

Some CAM therapies involving the use of substances, such as herbal medicine, homoeopathy and ayurvedic medicine, can and have been assessed by clinical trials.[7] However, it is difficult to test most CAM therapies using an RCT approach because they are

TABLE 22.2 Most popular complementary and alternative therapies in the UK[1,4]

Acupuncture	*also*
Chiropractic	Aromatherapy
Herbal medicine	Reflexology
Homeopathy	*plus*
Hypnotherapy	Autogenic training
Osteopathy	Bach flower remedies

holistic in nature, that is, they are designed to treat the whole person, not just a disease or infection. Additionally, CAM therapies are rarely standardized, for example different brands of herbs and various nutritional supplements can have different amounts of the active ingredient. Evaluation is also complex due to the holistic nature of CAM practices that are individualized and based on the needs of each client. Two patients with back pain, for instance, may require slightly different osteopathic manipulations, making it difficult to test effectiveness. Because CAM practices commonly incorporate multiple interventions, it is difficult to assess which particular intervention produced the desired outcome, especially if some interventions enhance others (synergy).

Most CAM therapists lack research training and as a result there has been a poor research infrastructure and inadequate research funding within the CAM field.

Many CAM practitioners believe that conventional research methods are inappropriate to investigate CAM. Consequently, there is a paucity of good-quality clinical trial research to show that most CAM therapies are either safe or effective. This does not mean that they are not; it simply means that there is little reliable evidence to show that they are. It is worth remembering that qualitative research methods can also be used to provide reliable information about the benefits of an intervention.

In the UK, a parliamentary committee (House of Lords Select Committee on Science and Technology) held an extensive enquiry into the use of CAM and published its Report in November 2000.[8] The committee classified CAM therapies according to the evidence available for their effectiveness (see Table 22.1). Group 1 therapies included the most professionally organized CAM disciplines that incorporated their own diagnostic approaches, where there was some scientific evidence of effectiveness and where a recognized system of training for practitioners was in place. CAM therapies in this group included acupuncture, chiropractic, herbal medicine, homeopathy and osteopathy. CAM therapies that lack a firm scientific basis and are not regulated to protect the public but that did give help and comfort to many people, such as massage, reflexology and healing, were assigned to Group 2. Other CAM therapies that have no established evidence base to support their claims for safety and efficacy were assigned to Group 3. Within this group, long-established and traditional disciplines with very specific philosophies, such as Traditional Chinese Medicine (TCM), Chinese herbal medicine and ayurvedic medicine, were placed in Group 3a, and other alternative disciplines, such as crystal therapy, dowsing, iridology and radionics, were classified as Group 3b. This classification has been criticized by some practitioners, notably the categorization of TCM, which includes acupuncture and herbal preparations in its approach, and the different classification for Maharishi ayurvedic medicine and ayurvedic medicine.

CAM THERAPIES AND HIV DISEASE

Some of the CAM therapies most frequently accessed by people with HIV disease are described below. However, more comprehensive information on all CAM practices can be found in recent authoritative and highly recommended UK guides to using CAM[5,9,10] (see also recommendations for 'Further reading' at the end of this chapter). Most of the evidence for efficacy cited in this section is taken from a recent definitive UK review of CAM therapies.[9] This brief discussion focuses principally on the most commonly used CAM therapies in the UK (see Table 22.2). It is important for nurses to encourage patients to keep their general healthcare provider informed of their CAM therapies, as many of these are used by some practitioners as a complete medical system and this may increase the risk of delaying more appropriate conventional diagnosis or treatment in some situations. It is important to remember that some substances used in some CAM therapies can interact with antiretroviral and other drugs used by patients with HIV disease, for example the herbs St John's wort and garlic. Both the patient's primary conventional medical adviser (usually their hospital doctor or general practitioner) and CAM therapist(s) need to be aware of each regimen in order to ensure that harmful interactions are avoided.

COMMONLY USED CAM THERAPIES

Acupuncture

Acupuncture originates from China and usually involves the insertion of small needles into specific points located around the body on 'energy channels' called meridians. Traditional Chinese acupuncture is based on the idea that the body's vital energy (called Qi) flows through these channels and, when someone is ill, the balance of this energy is blocked.

Acupuncture has been used for at least 5000 years as a method of rebalancing the body's energy and encouraging the vital life force to circulate freely around the body through various channels. The state of health or energy balance of an individual is assessed by taking a detailed history and examining the tongue and pulse for diagnostic information. There are different types of acupuncture, including Chinese whole body acupuncture, electro-acupuncture and Japanese acupuncture. **Acupressure** does not employ needles, but practitioners use finger pressure on acupuncture points, and laser acupuncture uses low-dose laser light to stimulate acupuncture points. All of these and more techniques are described in the current *Directory of Complementary Therapies*, published by the UK National AIDS Manual[5] (see also recommendations for 'Further reading' at the end of this chapter).

Acupuncture is used frequently by people with HIV disease for its reputed ability to improve well-being, relieve symptoms, boost immunity and reduce stress levels. One of the symptoms commonly reported by many people with HIV disease is pain as a result of peripheral neuropathy (PN; see Chapters 7 and 9) and many people with this condition seek relief from acupuncture.

Effectiveness

Although there is good-quality evidence to show that acupuncture is effective in reducing dental pain[11] and chemotherapy-induced and postoperative nausea and vomiting,[12,13] there is limited information on the efficacy of acupuncture in relieving pain from HIV-related PN. One relatively recent and frequently cited large multi-centre RCT found no evidence that acupuncture was effective in relieving pain from HIV-related PN.[14] There is, however, anecdotal evidence which suggests that some people with PN may experience pain relief, and others report having increased physical strength and better mobility and in general feeling better following acupuncture.

Safety

Acupuncture is relatively safe when administered by properly trained practitioners.[15] However, the use of needles presents the potential risk of transmitting blood-borne infections, and at least one person has acquired HIV infection from acupuncture treatment.[16]

Strict asepsis and sterile, disposable needles should be used to prevent cross-infections, and acupuncture should not be used for people who have bleeding disorders, such as HIV-related thrombocytopenia (see Chapter 7).

Aromatherapy

Aromatherapy involves the controlled use of essential oils (plant essences) for therapeutic purposes. The oils are inhaled, used for massage or added to baths and compresses. Essential oils are sometimes used for wound care and as mouth rinses for the relief of mouth ulcers following chemotherapy. Each oil is thought to have a different healing effect on the mind or body and can be used to alleviate specific symptoms or as a relaxant.

Aromatherapy tends principally to be used as a way of treating stress, promoting relaxation and helping muscle fatigue. Each essential oil is believed to have its own energetic properties and specific therapeutic indications. Nurses have traditionally used the essential oils of eucalyptus or benzoin (Friar's Balsam) for respiratory inhalations.[17] Other frequently used essential oils include lavender to treat insomnia and tea tree oil for wound care.[18]

Effectiveness

There is some evidence that aromatherapy massage can reduce anxiety and stress.[17] There is weak evidence that topical applications of tea tree oil may be helpful in acne and fungal infections, although a systematic review concluded that the evidence for this was 'promising but not compelling'.[18] There is scant good-quality evidence for any other therapeutic benefits associated with the use of plant essences, but its popularity must mean that many people do feel benefits from using this therapy.

Safety

Aromatherapy is considered generally safe, but some adverse reactions can occur, such as phototoxicity, nausea, headaches and various allergic reactions. Although suitable for use with most therapies, aromatherapy should not be used in conjunction with homeopathy. The use of many essential oils is contraindicated in pregnancy and many others are toxic to infants and young children. Essential oils should be kept away from the eyes and mucous membranes. As many essential oils are very potent, such as thyme, sage and hyssop, their source, use and safety should be discussed with an experienced practitioner.

Autogenic training

Autogenic training involves a set of mental exercises designed to reduce stress and provide deep relaxation of both the body and the mind, an important component of healing.

The biofeedback techniques used in autogenic training aim to balance the sympathetic nervous system (which is responsible for 'flight or fight' responses such as stress, anxiety, anger) and the parasympathetic nervous system (responsible for relaxation and recuperation). Autogenic training exercises are intended to give users feedback and control over the mental, physical and emotional aspects of their lives and address the buried issues that may be contributing to their symptoms. Exercises include training on how to deal with emotions such as fear, anger, depression and anxiety. These exercises are often more effective when carried out in a group situation, which also provides friendship and support.

Autogenic training is often used for anxiety, hypertension, asthma, eczema, glaucoma and intestinal diseases. People with HIV disease may use it to help relieve breathing problems, night sweats, diarrhoea and weight loss and for reviving energy and assisting sleep. This therapy appears to work best when individual self-motivation is high and there is a commitment to self-healing. This is due to the time needed to carry out the exercises, preferably two 20-minute sessions a day. The technique is versatile and can be tailored to individual needs.

Effectiveness

Systematic reviews of controlled trials showed that although autogenic training was helpful in treating hypertension, stress and anxiety, the quality of the evidence showing efficacy was weak.[19,20]

Safety

Autogenic training should not be used for those with serious mental health problems, insulin-dependent diabetes, epilepsy and alcoholism.

Bach flower remedies

Bach flower remedies are based on the theory that flowers contain the life force of the plant and this in turn is imprinted into water through sun infusion to yield the flower remedy. The preparations are usually ingested and used to help balance physical and emotional conditions.

Bach flower remedies were discovered in the 1930s by Dr Edward Bach, who identified the need for natural remedies based on the individual emotional condition of the patient. He developed a method of preparing remedies from 37 wild flowering plants and one remedy from a natural spring attributed with healing properties.[10] The best known remedy is the Rescue Remedy (a combination of five single remedies), which is used in dealing with shock, distress and anxiety. These remedies are readily available from chemists and health food shops.

Effectiveness

Although many people believe in Bach flower remedies and there are many anecdotal reports of their effectiveness, clinical trials have shown that any efficacy is probably due to a placebo effect.[21,22]

Safety

Bach flower remedies are extremely safe and have just one contraindication. Because these remedies contain small amounts of alcohol, they must not be used by patients receiving disulfiram (Antabuse®) treatment for alcohol dependence, as the interaction of even the minute amounts of alcohol and disulfiram will result in a severe reaction.

Chiropractic

Chiropractic diagnoses and treats mechanical disorders of the joints, muscles and ligaments of the body by manual adjustment. This therapy is based on the premise that dysfunction of the spine, pelvis and extremity articulations may disturb associated nerve function. This in turn may lead to specific types of pain syndromes, and in some cases, ill health, and chiropractic treatment consists mainly of specific manipulation adjustments.[23]

These mechanical disorders may also be treated by the other principal manipulative therapies, osteopathy and massage.

Chiropractic is principally used to treat acute low back pain (LBP) and neck pain, although practitioners will also treat a wide variety of other patient problems, including asthma, cardiovascular problems, migraine, headache and irritable bowel syndrome. Diagnosis is established from history, examination and, if appropriate, radiographic examinations (X-rays) of the spine. Treatment consists mainly of different types of spinal manipulations.

Effectiveness

Many systematic reviews over the last decade have analysed clinical trial evidence in relation to the effectiveness of chiropractic therapy and have arrived at mixed conclusions. One of the most recent and rigorous reviews, which synthesized the best available evidence, concluded that there was moderately good evidence to show that chiropractic therapy was effective in LBP but inconclusive evidence that it was helpful in mixed acute and chronic LBP and for sciatica.[24] There is some weaker evidence to show that chiropractic may also be effective in treating non-migrainous headache.[25] There is, however, no good-quality evidence to prove that chiropractic therapy is effective in any other conditions, although, as for most CAM therapies, it must be remembered that patients frequently feel their conditions have been improved as a result of these highly individualized therapeutic interventions.

Safety

Chiropractic therapy is generally safe but is contraindicated in patients with advanced osteoporosis, bleeding abnormalities, malignant or inflammatory spinal disease and for those receiving anticoagulants.[9]

Herbalism (Western)

Medicinal herbs and plants have been used for centuries to alleviate symptoms and treat illness. Different ways of using medicinal herbs have evolved in various countries, for example Chinese herbalism, Indian ayurveda, Japanese kampo and European herbalism. Today, modern Western herbalism (sometimes referred to as phytomedicine) has been incorporated into conventional medicine in many Western European countries.

Each patient is assessed by a practitioner (traditional herbalist) and prescribed treatment appropriate to their general health status, current health problems and lifestyle. A variety of different and often very potent herbs is used (Table 22.3), either as single agents or in combination with other herbs.

Effectiveness

In the first dozen years of the HIV/AIDS pandemic, a variety of herbs and other substances that allegedly had antiretroviral activity were promoted as either treatment or a 'cure' for AIDS. Some, like compound Q (trichosantin), an extract of the Chinese cucumber (*Trichosanthes kirlowii*), and hypercin, the active ingredient in St John's wort (*Hypericum triquethrifolium*), were shown to have *in vitro* (laboratory experiments) antiviral activity. However, there is no evidence that in clinical use they have any effect on HIV disease, and many, like compound Q, have serious toxicities. Chinese herbs have also been widely used for the symptomatic treatment of patients with HIV disease. In one well-designed placebo-controlled clinical trial, a mixture of 31 Chinese herbs was effective in decreasing the

TABLE 22.3 Some herbs commonly used in Western herbalism[9]

Herb	Most common indication	Side effects	Drug interactions
Aloe vera *Aloe barbadensis*	Topical gel: various skin conditions, e.g. sunburn, rash, genital herpes, psoriasis	None reported for topical gel; many side effects follow oral use and should not be taken by injection!	None for topical gel
Artichoke *Cynara scolymus*	Dyspepsia, hyperlipidaemia	Flatulence, allergic reactions; not given if gallbladder disease present	None known
Asian ginseng *Panax ginseng*	Increased vitality, immune function, sexual function	Insomnia, diarrhoea, vaginal bleeding, mastalgia, swollen tender breasts, mania, possible cause of Stevens–Johnson syndrome; not used if hypertension present	Monoamine oxidase inhibitors, such as phenelzine; increases effect of hypoglycaemic drugs
Cannabis *Cannabis sativa*	Pain, anxiety, insomnia, anorexia	Occasionally chronic use can impair co-ordination, cause nausea and vomiting, and anxiety and paranoia; memory loss and shortened attention span may occur with long-term use	None known
Cranberry *Vaccinium marcocarpon*	Preventing recurrent urinary tract infections	None	None known
Echinacea *Echinacea* spp.	Prevention and treatment of common infections, e.g. the common cold	Uncommon; diarrhoea sometimes reported; patients with HIV infection should not use echinacea for prolonged periods of time	May interact with immunosuppressants such as corticosteroids, and also with cyclosporin
Garlic *Allium sativum*	High serum cholesterol (hyperlipidaemia), hypertension, prevention of arteriosclerosis	Breath and body odour, allergic reactions, nausea, heartburn, flatulence; should not be taken by people with bleeding disorders or before major surgery	Potentiates effect of anticoagulants, may enhance hypoglycaemic effects of antidiabetic medication
Ginger *Zingiber officinale*	Prevention of motion sickness, dyspepsia, loss of appetite; postoperative nausea and vomiting	Occasionally heartburn	Increases effects of anticoagulants; may interfere with cardiac and antidiabetic therapy; not given for 'morning sickness' in pregnancy
Ginkgo *Ginkgo biloba*	Intermittent claudication, dementia, memory impairment, tinnitus	Occasionally gastrointestinal complaints, diarrhoea, vomiting, allergic reactions, pruritus, headache, dizziness, nose bleeding	Potentiates anticoagulants
Horse chestnut *Aesculus hippocastanum*	Symptoms (pain, fatigue, pruritus, oedema) or trophic changes associated with chronic venous insufficiency; haematoma	Occasionally pruritus, nausea, stomach complaints, bleeding, nephropathy, allergic reactions	Potentiates anticoagulants and anticoagulant effect of aspirin
Kava Kava *Piper methysticum*	Anxiety, insomnia	Occasionally stomach complaints, restlessness, mydriasis, allergic skin reactions, dermatomyositis, hepatitis; may cause serious (and potentially fatal) liver disease; in 2002, Kava Kava was withdrawn from sale in the UK	Potentiation of drugs acting on the central nervous system, e.g. alcohol, benzodiazepines and barbiturates; may reduce the effects of levodopa

TABLE 22.3 – continued

Herb	Most common indication	Side effects	Drug interactions
Milk thistle *Silybum marianum*	Liver disease, in particular hepatitis and (alcoholic) cirrhosis	Occasionally diarrhoea	None reported
Phyllanthus *Phyllanthus amarus, niruri, urinaria*	Hepatitis B infection		
Saw palmetto *Serenoa repens*	Benign prostatic hyperplasia	Occasionally gastrointestinal complaints, constipation, diarrhoea, dysuria, decreased libido	May limit iron absorption
Siberian ginseng *Eleutherococcus senticosus*	Increased vitality, exercise performance, immune function, sexual function	Diarrhoea, dizziness, hypertension, pericardial pain, tachycardia, extrasystole, insomnia, headache	Anxiolytic or sedative agents, anticoagulants, hypoglycaemic agents; hypotensive and hypertensive drugs; may increase serum digoxin levels
St John's wort *Hypericum triquethrifolium (perforatum)*	Mild to moderate depression	Occasionally photosensitization, gastrointestinal symptoms, allergic reactions, fatigue, anxiety	HIV protease inhibitors, warfarin, digoxin, anticonvulsants, antidepressants, iron
Valerian *Valeriana officinalis*	Insomnia, anxiety, nervous tension	Occasionally headache, gastrointestinal symptoms, morning hang-over	May potentiate the effects of other sedatives and hypnotics
Yohimbe *Pausinystalia yohimbe*	Erectile dysfunction	Occasionally insomnia, anxiety, hypertension, tachycardia, bronchospasm, nausea, vomiting	Potentiates some antidepressants, central nervous system stimulants, phenothiazines; reduces effects of antihypertensive drugs; may interact with sildenafil

number and severity of HIV-related symptoms and in increasing 'life satisfaction' but did not change more objective end-point outcomes, such as CD4+ T-cell counts and weight.[26]

Clinical research in patients has shown that no herbal treatment to date has: any significant *in vivo* antiretroviral activity; delayed progression from primary HIV infection to AIDS; any restorative effect on a damaged immune system; any significant therapeutic effectiveness for HIV-related opportunistic events; or any decrease in infectiousness or increased protection against HIV infection on exposure.

However, herbs do play an important role in people's self-care strategies in and practitioner-directed healthcare regimens, especially in alleviating many of the health problems associated with symptomatic HIV disease. The herbs in Table 22.3, with the exception of some forms of ginseng, all have some RCT evidence indicating their effectiveness in the conditions listed.[9]

Safety

The manufacture of herbal medicines is not well regulated, and the quality and amount of the active ingredient in different brands of commercially available herbs may vary considerably. A recent NAM report warns that 'Contamination, adulteration and misidentification of herbs may all be responsible for causing side-effects and, in severe cases, poisoning'.[5]

Herbal medicines are not free of toxicity, and they frequently interact with conventional medications. Some, like St John's wort, can significantly reduce the plasma level of the antiretroviral drug indinavir.[27] Garlic can increase the potential gastrointestinal side effects of ritonavir and may affect the plasma levels of saquinavir, both of which are important antiretroviral drugs.[28] There are several excellent accounts in the literature of herb–drug interactions,[29,30] and nurses should refer patients contemplating or using medicinal herbs to reliable guidance and information on potential herb–drug interactions and side effects.[5,9]

Other herbs are also toxic. One particular herb, *Aristolochia*, used in some Chinese herbal medicines as an anti-inflammatory agent for gout, arthritis, rheumatism and chronic inflammatory skin diseases, can cause serious and often fatal kidney damage.[31] The use of this herb is currently prohibited in the UK and in most other countries within the European Union (EU).[32,33] Finally, the UK government is advising consumers to avoid taking the herb Kava Kava, which has been implicated in causing serious liver disease in some countries in the EU.[32]

Homeopathy

Homeopathy became popular in Europe in the middle of the nineteenth century and continues today as an important therapeutic option for many people in the UK and the EU. This CAM approach is based on the theory of treating like with like, i.e. using a substance to cure a disease that produces symptoms similar to those the person is experiencing. Homeopathic remedies are derived from a variety of substances that are highly diluted and used to treat people with matching symptoms. For example, a substance that causes a rash if administered to a healthy person is used to treat a person complaining of a rash. In assessing the patient, homeopaths take into account a range of physical, emotional and lifestyle factors, which contribute to the diagnosis.

Homeopathic remedies are made from plant, animal and mineral sources by a process of dilution and shaking in the presence of light. Each dilution increases the potency of the remedy. Highly individualized remedies are prescribed, as homeopaths take into account the smallest variations occurring in reported symptoms, such as whether the symptoms are worse at any particular time of day, with specific climatic changes and emotional changes.

Homeopaths do not usually classify patients according to conventional diseases, but rather match symptoms with homeopathic remedies. These remedies are used to treat a wide range of acute and chronic physical and emotional symptoms, although they are most effective in treating conditions with an allergic component.[9]

Patients with HIV disease often seek homeopathic treatment for a variety of HIV-related symptoms, including night sweats, fatigue, nausea and weight loss. Interestingly, in a recent (but small) RCT, individualized homeopathic remedies had positive effects on CD4+ T-cell counts in a randomized trial of 100 people with HIV disease.[34]

Effectiveness

The evidence of effectiveness is, like much of the evidence for many other CAM therapies, inconclusive. One meta-analysis of all homeopathic, placebo-controlled RCTs concluded that clinical improvement was almost two and a half times more likely in those receiving homeopathic treatment than in those receiving a placebo.[35] Other analyses of a specific remedy[36] or condition[37] failed to demonstrate evidence of efficacy.

Safety

Although treatment may worsen the presenting symptoms (which is considered a positive sign by homeopathic practitioners), there seem to be no adverse effects associated with the administration of homeopathic remedies other than the occasional allergic response. Similarly, there are no known interactions between homeopathic remedies and conventional drugs, although many homeopaths believe that some medicines, such as antibiotics and corticosteroids, may block the action of homeopathic remedies.[9]

Hypnotherapy

Hypnotherapy induces a trance-like state during which the person becomes deeply relaxed and the unconscious becomes accessible to therapeutic suggestions. It can be used to reduce or eliminate symptoms or to assist the unconscious mind to help individuals change addictive behaviours that are harming health, such as cigarette smoking and alcohol abuse.

Hypnotherapy is principally used to treat stress and anxiety, pain, various phobias, addictions, and psychosomatic conditions such as asthma and irritable bowel syndrome.[9,23]

Effectiveness

The evidence for hypnotherapy has recently been reviewed.[9] Many meta-analyses and other reviews of RCTs tend to be inconclusive in showing whether hypnotherapy is effective for a wide range of conditions in which it is used. However, one often-cited meta-analysis of 18 controlled trials concluded that hypnotherapy was effective for various conditions, including anxiety, insomnia, pain, hypertension and obesity.[38] Additional evidence is available supporting the effectiveness of hypnotherapy for treating pain,[39] and for asthma, irritable bowel syndrome, dermatological conditions, and nausea and vomiting in oncology patients.[40]

Massage

Massage involves manipulating the soft tissues and muscles of the body, using pressure and traction.

Different massage techniques are used, including aromatherapy massage, shiatsu, holistic massage, Swedish massage, biodynamic massage and therapeutic massage. Swedish massage is the most commonly used technique in the UK and involves a variety of manual techniques which aim to relax, strengthen and stimulate the muscles.[5]

Shiatsu is a system of massage originating from Japan which uses finger pressure (acupressure) on acupuncture points. It relies on affecting the body's energy, or Qi, as referred to in Traditional Chinese Medicine. Shiatsu is reputed to be effective in 'tonifying' the body by increasing the flow of blood and energy and dispersing blockages, and in treating specific conditions such as asthma, migraine, rheumatic and arthritic complaints, digestive disorders and, in particular, stress and anxiety.

The benefits of massage reported by clients include a great sense of relaxation, which allows deep breathing, stimulation of the oxygen supply and the restoration of strength and mobility. The importance of touch in reassurance and support cannot be overestimated, particularly for those feeling lonely, stigmatized and isolated. Massage is frequently used in conjunction with other CAM therapies.

Effectiveness

The evidence for the effectiveness of massage therapy has been reviewed,[9] and various studies cited describe positive evidence for the use of massage to alleviate stress, anxiety, depression, LBP and fibromyalgia, and to improve quality of life. Anecdotally, it is almost universal for clients to report feeling better following competent massage therapy.

Safety

Massage therapy given by a skilled therapist is very safe. However, it is generally contraindicated for people with phlebitis, deep vein thrombosis, burns, advanced osteoporosis, open wounds and some infectious skin conditions.[9] It is important that massage is given by a person who has been appropriately trained. There are no reported interactions between massage therapy and other CAM practices or conventional treatment.

Osteopathy

Osteopathy is a system of diagnosis and treatment that uses techniques to manipulate the musculo-skeletal system (principally the spine) to correct the underlying cause of various symptoms such as pain, anxiety and stress.

Patients have osteopathic treatments for musculo-skeletal problems such as low back and neck pain, shoulder, elbow, knee and hip pain. Osteopathy acts to balance mechanical dysfunctions that are impairing healing abilities. Treatment can improve the functioning of the nervous system, blood circulation and lymphatic drainage. Osteopathy is a holistic therapy and also recognizes the role played by other factors such as diet, psychological causes, the environment and genetics.

Cranial osteopathy is a gentler therapy in which manipulation of the skull enhances the body's vitality. It can be used for stress-related conditions, including depression, anxiety and insomnia. Recurrent chest pains, neck pains, breathing and bowel function may be improved with osteopathic intervention. Circulation and nerve function may also be improved, and night sweats may be alleviated by restoring the balance between the sympathetic and para-sympathetic nervous systems.

Effectiveness

There is RCT evidence which shows that osteopathy does help to alleviate LBP (particularly acute and sub-acute).[41,42] However, there is little good-quality evidence to show that this form of therapy is effective in any other conditions.

Safety

Osteopathy is relatively safe when administered by trained practitioners. Spinal trauma is a potential risk, and osteopathy is contraindicated for patients with osteoporosis or bleeding disorders.

Reflexology

Reflexology is a system of massage of the feet based on the belief that there are zones running vertically through the body and that each organ has a corresponding location in the foot.

Reflexology practitioners believe that any disease or damage in the body can be identified on the foot and may be influenced by careful massage and pressure on the relevant zone. Treatment is gentle and relaxing and is often accompanied by a sense of well-being. The 'hands-on' element and calming effect of reflexology are useful to many clients for alleviating stress. Anecdotally, success has been reported with neck stiffness and backache, respiratory, circulatory and digestive problems and insomnia. Reflexologists also work on zones associated with the lymphatic and endocrine systems, which they feel may strengthen immune function.

Effectiveness

A review has shown that most evidence for effectiveness comes from poor-quality RCTs and, consequently, is weak.[9]

Safety

Although generally a safe therapy, reflexology is sometimes contraindicated for patients with gout or venous ulceration of the feet.

Diet and micronutrient supplements

The role of diet and health is emphasized by most CAM therapies. Dietary adjustments include: macrobiotic diets, anti-*Candida* diets, organic, whole food and raw food diets, exclusion diets, micronutrients, vitamins and minerals.

Nutrition undoubtedly has an effect on immunity, and has been suggested to have been an important factor in the reduction of infectious disease in the twentieth century. CAM therapists have a range of views on the effect of diet on health.

Macrobiotic diets, based on Chinese and Japanese beliefs about food, advocate that a diet which balances *yin* and *yang* energies is the key to good health. Many people with HIV disease have reported that such diets have helped them. Yin foods tend to be fruit, vegetables, pulses and sugary foods. Yang foods are meat, grains, fish and some seasonings. However, there are real concerns that this type of diet may lack the calories necessary to maintain stable weight as well as essential micronutrients such as some important B-complex vitiamins.

Candida albicans causes thrush, which is a common health problem for people with HIV disease. Increasingly, CAM practitioners have felt that this organism is responsible for a great deal of illnesses. Avoidance of sugar and simple carbohydrates in processed food, such as white bread, white flour, white pasta, white rice and alcohol, is encouraged. This diet is a restrictive, cleansing diet based on fresh vegetables, lightly cooked whole grains and easily digested proteins such as white meat and fish. Yoghurt is allowed but no other dairy products or tofu. The effectiveness of this diet in people with HIV has not been studied, but anecdotal reports suggest that it is helpful in preventing recurrences of thrush. This diet may, however, present problems for those who are losing weight and rely on the energy provided by carbohydrates.

Organic, raw and whole food diets are advocated, particularly by naturopaths (see below), but may take more time for preparation and result in too much loss of weight. Many raw foods may represent risks to people who are immunocompromised, and nurses must ensure patients are aware of the essentials of food safety (see Table 7.16 in Chapter 7).

People with diarrhoea may benefit from general food hygiene principles: wash food thoroughly, do not reheat food, avoid take-away foods. Reducing the intake of fat and insoluble fibre (such as bran and brown bread), while increasing the intake of soluble fibre (such as apples, bananas, potatoes, pulses) and ensuring an adequate fluid intake may help.

Late HIV disease is usually associated with malnutrition and a wasting condition known as cachexia, which in turn further impairs immune function. Various nutritional supplements are suggested as being helpful, including glutamine and carnitine.

Effectiveness

There is some evidence that glutamine-antioxidant supplementation may prevent further weight loss or facilitate weight gain,[43] and that carnitine supplementation may have a beneficial effect on zidovudine-related myopathies and improve immune function.[44]

Safety

Raw food may cause serious gastrointestinal (and systemic) infections in immuno-compromised individuals. Food supplements may be toxic in large amounts, for example fat-soluble vitamins such as vitamins A and D, and some diets may restrict the intake of essential fatty acids and other micronutrients, leading to nutritional deficiencies and malnutrition. The conventional nutritional support of people with HIV disease is discussed in Chapter 17.

Exercise and movement

Exercise and movement can improve mood, help self-image, enhance immunity and maintain and build muscle mass.

Treatments which provide regular exercise can improve muscle tone, which helps where there is weight loss and wasting in HIV disease. Lung function can be improved by techniques such as T'ai Chi and Qi Gong, which help in directing the Qi. Similarly, yoga acts to relax the mind and body, increases suppleness and improves breathing control and posture. The Alexander technique, a taught technique, acts to correct problems with posture, the theory being that health problems are related to posture. The technique encourages people to optimize their health by teaching them to stand, sit and move according to the body's natural design and function.

Effectiveness

There is good clinical trial evidence to suggest that exercise and movement, especially techniques such as T'ai Chi, can help people maintain balance (and prevent falls) and strength,[45] improve cardiorespiratory function,[46] and have a beneficial effect in depression, anger and fatigue.[47]

Healing

This is a system of spiritual healing, sometimes based on prayer and religious beliefs, that attempts to treat illness through non-physical means, usually by directing thoughts towards an individual. It often involves 'the laying on of hands'.

Healing can be used for any condition and it is not necessary for the client to have any religious beliefs for it to be effective. Some people may experience a major health improvement, be more able to cope, feel calmer and have an improved quality of life after healing. Some healers apply direct touch and some work with the 'aura' or energy field around the client and sense the imbalances in their flow or energy. Healing may be combined with the use of crystals or coloured lights.

Effectiveness

There is ample evidence that spiritual healing can be effective. One systematic review, which included 23 placebo-controlled RCTs and almost 3000 people, showed that half of those involved experienced a positive result following healing.[48] Another similar review found much the same.[49]

Safety

There are no adverse effects of healing, but it is probably contraindicated for people with significant mental health disorders.

Naturopathy

This is an eclectic healing system based on the principle that the body is able to heal itself.

The history of 'nature care' goes back to Ancient Greece but was more formalized during the nineteenth century. Naturopaths believe that the natural equilibrium and harmony of the body is needed to nurture the 'vital force'. The body's equilibrium can be disrupted by toxin build up, which results in disease when the body tries to eliminate the toxins. Presenting symptoms and the underlying causes of illness are addressed by naturopathic treatment which involves using various CAM practices such as lifestyle and dietary adjustments, fasting, sweating, herbal medicine, hydrotherapy, spa therapy, exercise, osteopathy and stress management. Naturopathic practice also involves the integration of appropriate conventional medicine into individualized treatment programmes.

Effectiveness and safety

The effectiveness, safety and contraindications of many of the individual CAM practices used in naturopathic therapy have been discussed previously. Because an individualized holistic treatment regimen is developed for each patient, it is difficult to assess the effectiveness and safety of this eclectic combination of CAM practices by RCT methods.

Relaxation therapy (stress management)

The stress often associated with living with chronic illness can impair immune function and further worsen the clinical course of HIV disease. Using a variety of techniques to manage stress effectively can be beneficial for most people.

Stress is typically manifested by sympathetic nervous system responses, including sweating and tachycardia, and those affected frequently complain of headache, musculoskeletal pain, an inability to concentrate, anxiety and panic.

Stress management and relaxation therapy strategies use a variety of CAM approaches, including hypnotherapy, autogenic training, meditation, biofeedback, refocusing, breathing control, and progressive muscle relaxation.

Effectiveness

A recent overview[9] of research has described relatively good systematic review evidence for the effectiveness of many of the techniques used in stress management to control symptoms such as such as anxiety and panic that are sometimes associated with serious illnesses. This overview also highlighted some evidence of effectiveness, showing a beneficial result from using relaxation techniques for depression, insomnia and menopausal symptoms, but results were less conclusive for their use in managing both acute and chronic pain. There is additional evidence to show the effectiveness of guided imagery as a means to improve quality of life in people living with HIV disease.[50]

Safety

Relaxation and stress management techniques are generally safe and without any adverse effects. However, these techniques may be contraindicated for people with severe mental health disorders.[9]

Visualization and imagery

Visualization uses mental imagery to fight illness. This technique may take the form of conjuring mental images of HIV-infected cells being eliminated from the body or imagining the whole body as healthy and active once more.

Effectiveness

A RCT comparing guided imagery or progressive muscle relaxation with no intervention observed no beneficial effects in terms of quality of life.[50] Perceived health was, however, best in the group treated with guided imagery.

Safety

There are no untoward side effects from using this technique, but perhaps patients with serious mental health problems should avoid it.

Summary

Most CAM therapies seem relevant to the treatment, palliative and supportive care of people living with HIV disease. However, there are few reliable and rigorous data from clinical trials on the use of CAM in the treatment of people with HIV disease, and it is unclear whether CAM treatments offer any scientifically measurable benefit over and above conventional approaches in this group. However, it often seems that most people who use CAM feel that they have benefited from these therapies and find relief with CAM that eludes them when using more orthodox treatments. The popularity and frequently reported positive health outcomes of CAM may result from the relationship clients have with their practitioners and the power of the placebo effect.[51] In some CAM practices, human touch may also be beneficial and contribute to clients developing a sense of well-being.

The nursing history must detail any CAM treatments patients are receiving, and nurses need to be alert in identifying potential interactions between CAM therapies and conventional medical regimens. Patients considering the use of CAM can be referred to reliable sources of information (see listings at the end of this chapter) and nurses can help patients explore the evidence that a particular CAM approach actually works and is safe within the context of their own circumstances and current medical treatments.

Patients also need to be aware that training and education for CAM practices are mainly unregulated in the UK and in many other countries in the EU and vary widely in content, depth and duration.[8,52] They should be encouraged to discuss with practitioners their training, qualifications and experience and to check out their registration or membership with the relevant professional organization (see 'Contact organizations' and 'Internet resources' at the end of this chapter). Finally, patients also need to be encouraged to seek early medical advice from their conventional healthcare providers for their illnesses or any other healthcare problem irrespective of whether or not they are receiving CAM therapy.

ETHICAL ISSUES FOR NURSES

The new *Code of Professional Conduct*, published by the UK Nursing and Midwifery Council, sets out the ethical principles for using CAM therapies in professional practice.[53] The code says quite clearly that nurses and midwives must ensure that the use of CAM therapies is safe and in the interests of patients and clients. These issues must be discussed with the healthcare team as part of the therapeutic process, and the patient or client must consent to their use.

REFERENCES

1. Ernst E, White A. The BBC survey of complementary medicine use in the UK. *Complementary Therapies in Medicine* 2000; **8**:32–6.
2. Eisenberg D, David RB, Ettner SL et al. Trends in alternative medicine use in the United States, 1990–1997. *Journal of the American Medical Association* 1998; **280**:1569–75.
3. McLennan AH, Wilson DH, Taylor AW. Prevalence and cost of alternative medicine in Australia. *Lancet* 1996; **347**:569–73.
4. Thomas KJ, Nicholl JP, Coleman P. Use and expenditure on complementary medicine in England: a population based survey. *Journal of Complementary Therapies in Medicine* 2001; **9**:2–11.
5. Poppa A (ed.). *Directory of Complementary Therapies in HIV & AIDS*, 2nd edn. London: National AIDS Manual (NAM) Publications, March 2002, 39 pp. Available from: NAM, 16a Clapham Common Southside, London SW4 7AB, UK. Tel. +44 (0)20 7627 3200, fax: +44 (0)20 7627 3101, e-mail: info@nam.org.uk; website: http://www.aidsmap.com
6. Alcorn K. *Clinical Trials*, 3rd edn. London: National AIDS Manual (NAM) Publications, 2002. Available from: NAM, 16a Clapham Common Southside, London SW4 7AB, UK. Tel. +44 (0)20 7627 3200, fax: +44 (0)20 7627 3101. e-mail: info@nam.org.uk; website: http://www.aidsmap.com
7. Ozsoy M, Ernst E. How effective are complementary therapies for HIV and AIDS? A systematic review. *International Journal of STD & AIDS* 1999; **10**:629–35.
8. House of Lords Select Committee on Science and Technology. *Complementary and Alternative Medicine*, Sixth Report. London: Stationery Office, 21 November 2000, 140 pp. Available online from: http://www.parliament.the-stationery-office.co.uk/pa/ld199900/ldselect/ldsctech/123/12301.htm
9. Ernst E. *The Desktop Guide to Complementary and Alternative Medicine: an Evidence-based Approach*. Edinburgh: Mosby (Harcourt Publishers Ltd), 2001, 444 pp.
10. Rankin-Box D. *The Nurse's Handbook of Complementary Therapies*, 2nd edn. Edinburgh: Baillière Tindall (in association with the Royal College of Nursing), 2001, 289 pp.
11. Melchart D, Linde K, Fischer P et al. Acupuncture for recurrent headaches: a systematic review of randomized controlled trials. *Cephalagia* 1999; **19**:779–86.
12. Vickers A. Can acupuncture have specific effects on health? A systematic review of acupuncture antiemesis trials. *Journal of the Royal Society Medicine* 1996; **89**:303–11.
13. Lee A, Done ML. The use of nonpharmacologic techniques to prevent postoperative nausea and vomiting: a meta-analysis. *Anesthesia and Analgesia* 1999; **88**:1362–9.

14. Shlay CJ, Chaloner K, Max MB et al. Acupuncture and amitriptyline for pain due to HIV-related peripheral neuropathy. A randomized controlled trial. *Journal of the American Medical Association* 1998; **280**:1590–5.

15. MacPherson H, Thomas K, Walters S, Fitter M. The York Acupuncture Safety Study: prospective survey of 34 000 treatments by traditional acupuncturists. *British Medical Journal* 2001; **323**:486–7.

16. Vittecoq D, Mettetal JF, Rouzioux C, Bach JF, Bouchon JP. Acute HIV infection after acupuncture treatments [Letter]. *New England Journal of Medicine*, 1989; **320**:250–1.

17. Cooke B, Ernst E. Aromatherapy: a systematic review. *British Journal of General Practice* 2000; **50**:493–6.

18. Ernst E, Huntley A. Tea tree oil: a systematic review of randomized clinical trials. *Forsch Komplementärmed Klass Naturheilkd* 2000; **7**:17–20.

19. Kanji N, White AR, Ernst E. Anti-hypertensive effects of autogenic training: a systematic review: *Perfusion* 1999; **12**:279–82.

20. Kanji N, Ernst E. Autogenic training for stress and anxiety: a systematic review. *Complementary Therapies in Medicine* 2000; **8**:106–10.

21. Armstrong NC, Ernst E. A randomized, double-blind, placebo-controlled trial of Bach Flower Remedy. *Perfusion* 1999; **11**:440–6.

22. Walach H, Rilling C, Engelke U. Bach flower remedies are ineffective for test anxiety: results of a blinded, placebo-controlled randomized trial. *Forsch Komplementärmed Klass Naturheilkd* 2000; **7**:55.

23. Department of Health (England) with the Foundation for Integrated Medicine, the NHS Alliance and the National Association of Primary Care. *Complementary Medicine – Information Pack for Primary Care Groups.* June 2000. Available from: http://www.fimed.org

24. Bronfort G. Spinal manipulation, current state of research and its indications. *Neurology Clinics of North America* 1999; **17**:91–111.

25. Vernon H, McDermain CS, Hagino C. Systematic review of randomized clinical trials of complementary/alternative therapies in the treatment of tension-type and cervicogenic headache. *Complementary Therapies in Medicine* 1999; **7**:142–55.

26. Burack JH, Cohen MR, Hahn JA et al. Pilot randomized controlled trial of Chinese herbal treatment for HIV-associated symptoms. *Journal of the Acquired Immune Deficiency Syndrome and Human Retrovirology* 1996; **12**:386–93.

27. Piscitelli SC, Burstein AH, Chaitt D et al. Indinavir concentrations and St John's wort. *Lancet* 2000; **355**:547–8.

28. Piscitelli SC, Gallicano KD. Interactions among drugs for HIV and opportunistic infections. *New England Journal of Medicine* 2001; **344**:984–6.

29. Fugh-Berman A, Ernst E. Herb–drug interaction: review and assessment of report reliability. *British Journal of Clinical Pharmacology* 2001; **52**:587–95.

30. Miller LG. Herbal medicinals: selected clinical considerations focusing on known or potential drug–herb interactions. *Archives of Internal Medicine* 1998; **158**:2200–11.

31. Lord G, Tagore R, Cook T, Gower P, Pusey C. Nephropathy caused by Chinese herbs in the UK. *Lancet* 1999; **354**:481–2.

32. Medicines Control Agency (MCA). *Licensing of Medicines: Policy on Herbal Medicines (Aristolochia and Kava Kava).* [serial online] 2001, cited 14 April 2002. Available from: Herbal Medicines Policy Unit, 16-1, MCA, Market Towers, 1 Nine Elms Lane, London SW8 5NQ; telephone +44 (0)20-7273 0404; fax +44 (0)20-7273 0387; e-mail info@mca.gov.uk or from MCA website at:

http://www.mca.gov.uk/ourwork/licensingmeds/herbalmeds/herbalmeds.htm

33. Working Party on Herbal Medicinal Products (European Agency for the Evaluation of Medicinal Products – EMEA). Position Paper on the Risks Associated with the Use of Herbal Products Containing Aristolochia species. EMEA/HMPWP/23/00. [serial online] October 2000, cited 14 April 2002. Available from: http://www.emea.eu.int/pdfs/human/hmpwp/002300en.pdf

34. Rastogi DP, Singh VP, Singh V, Dey SK, Rao K. Homeopathy in HIV infection: a trial report of double-blind placebo controlled study. *British Homeopathy Journal* 1999; **88**:49–57.

35. Linde K, Clausius N, Ramirez G et al. Are the clinical effects of homeopathy placebo effects? A meta-analysis of placebo-controlled trials. *Lancet* 1997; **350**:834–43.

36. Ernst E, Pittler MH. Efficacy of homeopathic arnica. A systematic review of placebo-controlled clinical trials. *Archives of Surgery* 1998; **133M**:1187–90.

37. Ernst E, Barnes J. Are homeopathic remedies effective for delayed-onset muscle soreness. A systematic review of placebo-controlled trials. *Perfusion* 1998; **11**:4–8.

38. Kirsch I, Montgomery G, Sapirstein G. Hypnosis as an adjunct to cognitive-behavioural psychotherapy: a meta-analysis. *Journal of Consultations in Clinical Psychology* 1995; **63**:214–20.

39. Montgomery GH, Du Hamel KN, Redd WH. A meta-analysis of hypnotically induced analgesia: how effective is hypnosis? *International Journal of Clinical and Experimental Hypnosis* 2000; **48**:138–53.

40. Pinnell CM, Covino NA. Empirical findings on the use of hypnosis in medicine: a critical review. *International Journal of Clinical and Experimental Hypnosis* 2000; **48**:170–94.

41. Lesho EP. An overview of osteopathic medicine. *Archives of Family Medicine* 1999; **8**:477–83.

42. Andersson GB, Lucente T, Davis AM, Kappler RE, Lipton JA, Leurgans SA. Comparison of osteopathic spinal manipulation with standard care for patients with low back pain. *New England Journal of Medicine* 1999; **341**:1426–31.

43. Wilmore DW. Glutamine-antioxidant supplementation increases body cell mass in AIDS patients with weight loss: a randomized double-blind controlled trial. *Nutrition* 1999; **15**:860–4.

44. Mintz M. Carnitine in human immunodeficiency virus type 1 infection/acquired immune deficiency syndrome. *Journal of Child Neurology* 1995; **10**(Suppl. 2):S40–4.

45. Wolf SL, Barnhart HX, Dutner NG et al. Balance and strength in older adults: intervention gains and tai chi maintenance. *Journal of the American Geriatric Society* 1996; **44**:489–97.

46. Lai JS, Lan C, Wong MK, Teng SH. Two-year trends in cardiorespiratory function among tai chi chuan practitioners and sedentary subjects. *Journal of the American Geriatric Society* 1995; **43**:1222–7.

47. Putai J. Changes in heart rate, noradrenaline, cortisol and mood during tai chi. *Journal of Psychosomatic Respiration* 1989; **33**:197–206.

48. Astin J, Harkness E, Ernst E. The efficacy of spiritual healing: a systematic review of randomised trials. *Annals of Internal Medicine* 2000; **132**:903–10.

49. Abbot NC. Healing as a therapy for human disease. *Journal of Alternative and Complementary Medicine* 2000; **6**:159–69.

50. Eller LS. Effects of cognitive–behavioural interventions on quality of life in persons with HIV. *International Journal of Nursing Studies* 1999; **36**:223–33.

51. Peters D. *Understanding the Placebo Effect in Complementary Medicine: Theory, Practice and Research*. Edinburgh: Churchill Livingstone, 2001, 235 pp.

52. Robinson N. Education and training in complementary medicine. *Holistic Health* 2001/2002; **71**:10–13.

53. NMC. *Code of Professional Conduct*. London: Nursing & Midwifery Council, April 2002, 12 pp. Available from: NMC, 23 Portland Place, London W1B 1PZ, UK; telephone 020 7637 7181; fax 020 7436 2924; e-mail: publications@nmc-uk.org; website: www.nmc-uk.org

FURTHER READING

Books

Alcorn K. *Clinical Trials*, 3rd edn. London: National AIDS Manual (NAM) Publications, 2002. Available from: NAM, 16a Clapham Common Southside, London SW4 7AB, UK; telephone +44 (0)20 7627 3200; fax +44 (0)20 7627 3101; e-mail: info@nam.org.uk; available from: http://www.aidsmap.com

Ernst E. *The Desktop Guide to Complementary and Alternative Medicine: an Evidence-based Approach*. Edinburgh: Mosby (Harcourt Publishers Ltd), 2001, 444 pp (plus CD-ROM), ISBN 0-7234-3207-4.

Ernst E, White A. *Acupuncture, a Scientific Appraisal*. Oxford: Butterworth Heinemann, 1999, 168 pp, ISBN 0-750641630.

Lewith G, Jonas WB, Walach H. *Clinical Research in Complementary Therapies – Principles, Problems and Solutions*. Edinburgh: Churchill Livingstone, 2002, 376 pp, ISBN 0-443-06367-2.

Peters D. *Understanding the Placebo Effect in Complementary Medicine: Theory, Practice and Research*. Edinburgh: Churchill Livingstone, 2001, 235 pp, ISBN 0-443-06031-2.

Poppa A (ed.). *Directory of Complementary Therapies in HIV & AIDS*, 2nd edn. London: National AIDS Manual (NAM) Publications, March 2002, 39 pp, ISBN 1-898397-92-9. Available from: NAM, 16a Clapham Common Southside, London SW4 7AB, UK; telephone +44 (0)20 7627 3200; fax +44 (0)20 7627 3101. e-mail: info@nam.org.uk; website: http://www.aidsmap.com

Rankin-Box D. *The Nurse's Handbook of Complementary Therapies*, 2nd edn. Edinburgh: Baillière Tindall (in association with the Royal College of Nursing), 2001, 289 pp, ISBN 0-7020-2651-4.

Standish LJ, Calabrese C, Galantino ML. *AIDS and Complementary & Alternative Medicine – Current Science and Practice*. New York: Churchill Livingstone, 2002, 360 pp, ISBN 0-443-05831-8.

Journals

Complementary Therapies in Nursing & Midwifery and *Complementary Therapies in Medicine*. Both journals available from: Harcourt Publishers Ltd, Harcourt Place, 32 Jamestown Rd, London NW1 7BY, UK; e-mail: journals@Harcourt.com; telephone (UK) +44 (0)20 8308 5700 (in the USA call Toll free: 1-877-839-7126).

Reports

Department of Health (England) with the Foundation for Integrated Medicine, the NHS Alliance and the National Association of Primary Care, have produced an authoritative, easy to understand report entitled *Complementary Medicine – Information Pack for Primary Care Groups* (June 2000). This report can be downloaded from http://www.fimed.org

House of Lords Select Committee on Science and Technology. *Complementary and Alternative Medicine*, Sixth Report. London: Stationery Office, 21 November 2000, 140 pp. Available from: http://www.parliament.the-stationery-office.co.uk/pa/ld199900/ldselect/ldsctech/123/12301.htm

INTERNET RESOURCES AND CONTACT ORGANIZATIONS (UK)[5,10,23]

- **British Acupuncture Council**, 63 Jeddo Road, London W12 9HQ; telephone: +44 (0)20 8735 0400:
  http://www.acupuncture.org.uk
- **International Federation of Professional Aromatherapists**, 82 Ashby Road, Hinckley, Leicestershire LE10 1SN; telephone: +44(0)1455 637987:
  http://www.ifparoma.org
- **General Chiropractic Council**, 344–354 Gray's Inn Road, London WC1X 8BP; telephone: +44 (0)845 601 1796; e-mail: enquiries@gcc-uk.org:
  http:www.gcc-uk.org
- **Faculty of Homeopathy**, 15 Clerkenwell Close, London EC1R 0AA; telephone: +44 (0)20 7566 7810:
  http://www.trusthomeopathy.org
- **The Society of Homeopaths**, 4a Artizan Road, Northampton NN1 4HU, UK; telephone: +44 (0)1604 621 400:
  http:www.homeopathy-soh.org
- **British Massage Therapy Council**, 17 Rymers Lane, Oxford OX4 3JU, UK; telephone: +44 (0)1865 774123:
  http://www.bmtc.co.uk
- **National Institute of Medical Herbalists**, 56 Longbrook Street, Exeter EX4 6AH, UK; telephone: +44 (0)1392 426 022:
  http://www.nimh.org.uk
- **Medicines Control Agency (MCA) Herbal Medicines Policy Unit**, 16-1, MCA, Market Towers, 1 Nine Elms Lane, London SW8 5NQ; telephone +44 (0)20-7273 0404; fax +44 (0)20-7273 0387; e-mail: info@mca.gov.uk:
  http://www.mca.gov.uk
- **The British Naturopathic Association**, Goswell Road, Street, Somerset BA16 0JG, UK; telephone: +44 (0)1458 840072:
  http://www.naturopaths.org.uk
- **British College of Osteopathic Medicine**, Lief House, 3 Sumpter Close, 120–122 Finchley Road, London NW3 5HR; telephone: +44 (0)20 7435 6464:
  http://www.bcom.ac.uk
- **The Association of Reflexologists**, 27 Old Gloucester St, London WC1N 3XX; telephone: +44 (0)870 5673320:
  http://www.aor.org.uk
- **British Reflexology Association**, Administration Office, Monks Orchard, Whitbourne, Worcester WR6 5RB, UK; telephone: +44 (0)1886 821207:
  http://www.britreflex.co.uk

- **The Prince of Wales Foundation for Integrated Medicine** promotes the development and integrated delivery of safe, effective and efficient forms of healthcare, including conventional and complementary medicine, to patients and their families through encouraging greater collaboration between all forms of healthcare. Their website has a wealth of information on CAM:
  http://www.fimed.org

CHAPTER 23

HIV disease in the industrially developing world

Carol Pellowe

AIDS cannot be controlled anywhere until it is controlled everywhere.
Jonathan Mann, London Lighthouse, 1996

Introduction

The United Nations Joint Programme on AIDS (UNAIDS) report on the global HIV/AIDS epidemic of 2002[1] acknowledges that the epidemic is at an early stage of development and the long-term outcome unclear. What is known is that the majority of people infected and affected by HIV disease live in the developing world and have little or no access to the antiretroviral treatments described in previous chapters. The impact of this pandemic is an economic and social crisis of unparalleled proportions, affecting those countries that are least equipped to cope. Contributing to this are several interlinked issues: prevalence of HIV infection, poverty, politics and the power and status of women. In combination, these factors create specific problems for each resource-poor country, presenting different challenges and demanding individual solutions. Although lessons can be learned from other areas, each country needs to create its own plan of action that is multi-faceted and takes account of the forces driving its own national epidemic. In this chapter, we explore the underlying political, economic and gender issues that impact on the prevalence and treatment of HIV infection in the industrially developing world.

Learning outcomes

After studying and reflecting on the material in this chapter, you will be able to:

- discuss the social, cultural and political issues affecting the growth of national epidemics of HIV disease in resource-poor countries;
- describe opportunities and challenges for the prevention and treatment of HIV disease in these regions;
- identify the critical role of nurses and the potential impact of professional nursing on affected communities.

THE GROWTH OF NATIONAL EPIDEMICS IN RESOURCE-POOR COUNTRIES

The UNAIDS report[1] is a stark reminder of the crisis to date. An estimated 5 million people became infected in 2001, 800 000 of whom were children. Mother-to-child transmission (MTCT) is the major cause of infection in children, and with 60 per cent of new infections occurring in women, predominantly aged 15–24 years, this remains a key issue.[1] Sub-Saharan Africa has been the worst affected area, where 28.5 million are currently living with HIV/AIDS. In four countries – Botswana, Lesotho, Swaziland and Zimbabwe – HIV prevalence exceeds 30 per cent in the adult population.[2] Although there have been encouraging signs of the situation being brought under control in Uganda and Senegal, other countries such as Botswana and Zimbabwe are facing an exponential rise, and a negative population growth is predicted by 2010.[1] In South Africa, where the epidemic is the most severe in the world, life expectancy has been reduced by 18 years and AIDS-related deaths in young people are not expected to peak until between 2010 and 2015.[1]

In other parts of the world, new epidemics are flourishing. Most countries in Asia appear to have low prevalence rates, but 1 per cent prevalence in a populous nation like India means it has 3.86 million people living with HIV disease.[3] The World Bank has already warned that India alone could have 37 million people infected with HIV by the year 2005, which is roughly the total number of HIV infections in the world today.[4] Low prevalence rates also conceal serious localized epidemics, for example HIV infections in injecting drug users in China has increased by 70 per cent.[1] In addition, the failure to ensure a safe blood supply for transfusions further exacerbates the situation. Henan Province in China has recently witnessed a serious epidemic in donors, caused by blood-collecting centres not following basic safety procedures,[5] and in Sindh, Pakistan, only 20 per cent of blood donations are currently screened for HIV infection.[6]

The effect of an increasing prevalence of HIV disease in a populous nation has a significant impact on that country's economy. With average life expectancy in sub-Saharan Africa down to 47 years, as opposed to 67 years without AIDS,[1] the loss of such a critical workforce not only disrupts the family unit but also threatens the nation's economic stability. Those who are dying are the breadwinners and taxpayers, and their death has a major impact on family income and the national economy. In Zambia, the death of a father reduces the disposable family income by 80 per cent[1] and, as household income falls, the demand for services and products reduces. Absenteeism due to sickness or caring for the sick is a critical problem for businesses, affecting costs, productivity and profit. Many African governments cannot cope with the persistent drain on their resources. Their health budgets are crippled by the demands of increasing numbers of men, women and children dying from AIDS and there are no resources to care for the increasing number of orphans, a problem which by 2010 is predicted to affect 21 per cent of all children, 89 per cent of whom will be orphaned due to AIDS.[1]

POVERTY AND POLITICS

Professor Stefano Vella, President of the International AIDS Society (IAS), has described the cost of HIV/AID epidemics in the developing world as 'the most challenging imperative of this century', and suggested that the cost should be borne by the wealthy countries.[7] In December 2001, a report from the World Health Organization (WHO)[8] clearly demonstrated that poverty causes disease and that disease causes poverty, a cycle that cripples economic growth in developing countries. It boldly suggested that if the richer nations were to allocate just 0.1 per cent of their collective general domestic product (GDP) in grants, so offering approximately £25 per head in the developing world, 8 million lives would be saved. Such ideas sound simple, but success will depend upon the richer nations making significant contributions totalling millions of pounds each year. In June 2001, the United Nations General Assembly held a special assembly session (UNGASS) on HIV/AIDS at which 180 countries agreed to launch a global fund to fight HIV/AIDS, malaria and tuberculosis (TGF) and agreed to increase annual expenditure on preventing and treating these diseases to $10 billion (£7 billion) a year by 2005.[3] Although there was some initial reluctance of richer nations to contribute the amounts needed in the first years following the launch of TGF,[9] it is anticipated that funding will continue to increase to the levels needed to achieve the objectives agreed at the UNGASS meeting.

The benefit of UNGASS was that it forced a response from each government and meant that AIDS could no longer be marginalized. The subsequent *Declaration of Commitment on HIV/AIDS*[10] describes a broad agenda for action, including measurable targets to be met by 2003 and 2005. It includes action on human resources and care of orphans, and predicts that if $4.8 billion can be raised, 29 million lives could be saved over the next 10 years.[11] The XIV International AIDS Conference in Barcelona in 2002 was the first opportunity to examine progress to date. Richard Feachem of the Global Fund announced that from the first proposals received, $16.6 million had been committed to 40 countries. HIV/AIDS projects will receive 76 per cent of the money, to be divided equally between prevention and treatment. Although the second round of bids was underway, he warned that unless the promised money was received soon, the sustainability of new projects would be uncertain.[11] The Global Fund represents a bold new approach, it would be a tragedy if it failed simply because of funding.

International aid is critical, but equally important is the political will within a country to address national epidemics of HIV/AIDS. Peter Piot, Executive Director of UNAIDS, described the XIII International AIDS Conference in Durban as 'the wake-up call',[12] yet at its opening session, President Thabo Mbeki of South Africa failed to acknowledge the link between HIV and AIDS. In October 2001, a report by the government-funded Medical Research Council in South Africa was suppressed, as its 'shocking' findings suggested that 40 per cent of deaths between the ages of 15 and 49 were AIDS-related and it predicted that, by the end of the decade, AIDS will cause in excess of 700 000 deaths a year in South Africa.[13] The South African Health Minister, Manto Tshabalala-Msimang, derided the report as a 'massive propaganda tool'.[14] As the UNAIDS report for 2002 notes, 'effective responses are possible only when they are politically backed and full-scale'.[1]

Where resources are scarce, the most disenfranchised and marginalized groups are least likely to be helped. One wonders if we really care about drug users. In many industrially developing countries, such as Vietnam, Thailand and India, injecting drug use has been a problem for years, and recent escalations in the prevalence of HIV infection are increasing due to needle sharing, yet these areas failed to respond with appropriate primary prevention initiatives. In Indonesia, HIV infection prevalence in the injecting drug user population was not even considered worth measuring until 1999/2000, and among those in treatment, prevalence rates were over 40 per cent by the end of 2001.[15] Without political commitment and action from governments, supported by governments in the industrially developed world that recognize that investment in the prevention of HIV infection among drug users is worthwhile, these epidemics will undermine any other public health initiative. It is to be hoped that the necessary action will follow the words of UNGASS.

UNEQUAL POWER AND GENDER INEQUALITY

Another important aspect driving the growth of national epidemics in the industrially developing world is women's position in society. The oppression of women by men has a major impact on a woman's ability to protect herself against infection or access treatment. While issues of 'gender and inequality' have frequently featured in conference programmes, the lack of a feminist perspective has reduced the context of discussions to interpersonal relations and self-esteem rather than consideration of the broader cultural systems of meaning that rank men over women. An international study of gender relations and sexual negotiation suggests that women are constrained in their sexual behaviour and choices by two major factors: economic dependence on men and gender stereotypes that inform expectations of male and female sexual behaviour and create barriers for sexual communication.[16]

The vulnerability of women to HIV infection is discussed in detail in Chapter 11, but in the industrially developing world women face additional dangers. The frequent use of injections and blood transfusions for women who give birth or develop anaemia poses a hazard where clean medical supplies cannot be assured. An association between HIV infection and contaminated medical supplies was established as early as 1986, yet in many areas insufficient attention has been paid to the easy and cost-effective remedy.[6,17]

Women affected and infected by HIV have been described as 'invisible',[18] for the impact on them is very different from that on other groups at increased risk of exposure and infection, such as men in urban environments in the industrially developed world who have sex with men. 'Isolation and invisibility "unite" women living with HIV … When they meet other women with HIV they may have nothing in common but the virus.'[18] For them, there are decisions to be made not only about themselves, but also often about their children and, in many cases, their unborn children. Prostitution is common among women whose husbands have been lost to war, genocide or AIDS, but this adds its own dangers of infection. Yet being a prostitute appears to be less of a stigma than being infected with HIV, and the main concern is for many prostitutes is who will care for their family after they have died.[19] With the average life expectancy of a Kenyan prostitute being 7 years, and most dying before their thirtieth birthday, time to make arrangements for the future care of their children is truly short.[20]

The gender power relations in a society also affect children and young people. One means of surviving poverty is for families to involve their children in prostitution, both girls and boys. This not only deprives them of their childhood, but also subjects them to abusive sexual relations. The unequal power relations between these children and their parents, pimps and clients means that they have no control over their own bodies or lives. The ensuing damage, sometimes including mutilation and castration, results in a complex matrix of psychological and physical problems. As one woman recalled: 'When I was 13 years old I was sold to an

Indian brothel. Thirteen is an age to go to school, to enjoy with friends, but I was in a dark room all the day and night, weeping'.[21]

PRIMARY PREVENTION IN RESOURCE-POOR SETTINGS

A key aspect in controlling the epidemic is prevention, and it is encouraging to note that UNGASS gave prevention equal status to care and treatment.[10] The traditional social safety net in many countries is the extended family, and where this is threatened by an overwhelming number of deaths, the whole fabric of society is threatened. Prevention of infection is the only measure currently available, and there have been some fine examples of innovative and effective campaigns.[22] However, first and foremost there must be a supportive policy context, for without political support, all efforts will be thwarted.[1]

Approaches to prevention

Having attained the political will, the following elements are key factors in any national effort.[23]

- General awareness-raising activities to provide information and counter negative reactions to HIV-infected people.
- Focus on persuasive action to meet the needs of specially vulnerable groups and communities, with steadily expanding coverage.
- Multi-sectoral and multi-level partnerships to deliver programmes and services across a range of contexts.
- Community involvement in programme and intervention development, and building upon the will of groups and individuals to contribute to national HIV prevention efforts.
- Greater integration between prevention and care to reduce costs and to reduce levels of discrimination and stigmatization.
- Action to build societal resistance to HIV transmission and reduce the systematic vulnerability of particular groups and sections of society.

Whether working at a community or group level, certain factors need to be taken into account if the prevention activities are to be effective, such as working through existing organizations and structures, building partnerships, and including people living with HIV and AIDS to enhance their visibility and benefit from their experience.[22] Several of the cited examples of good practice have relevance for nurses, in particular the International Planned Parenthood Federation's project in Jamaica, Honduras and Brazil to integrate HIV/AIDS prevention into the family planning service. Instead of 'adding' an HIV/AIDS component to the existing service, the project aimed to improve the overall quality of service by changing the manner in which it was provided and effecting changes in the interaction between clients and service providers. Considerable staff preparation and education was required, but the service now provides a holistic sexual health service covering risk behaviours, sexual relationships and even previously taboo areas such as anal and oral sex and sexual abuse.

Preventing sexual transmission

The theme of the World AIDS Campaign 2001 was 'I care ... do you?'. The aim was to involve men more fully in the effort to fight AIDS and to highlight the masculine behaviours and attitudes that contribute to the spread of HIV. In the early years of the epidemic, male condoms were promoted as the choice of protection but this ignored the fact that their use was male controlled and often inconsistent. Consequently, current programmes target men and their responsibilities and highlight the advantages to themselves, such as reduced risk of sexually transmitted infections (STIs). Persuading people to use condoms is only part of the solution. It is equally important to ensure an increased supply of affordable, good-quality condoms.[1] One innovative initiative recently reported from Livingstone, Zambia, involved taxi drivers distributing condoms and safer sex advice to their customers.[24]

An alternative to the male condom for some is the female condom. Its introduction was hailed as a major innovation providing protection against pregnancy and STIs. A study of its effect on sexual communication and negotiation showed that the female condom was most likely to be successfully utilized by sex workers who have experience of negotiation, or where it is a preferable alternative to unpopular male condoms.[16] Its introduction into a community without the accompaniment of context-appropriate education and promotion is unlikely to be successful. Brazil was the first country to allow government distribution of female condoms but, due to their costs compared with male condoms, the campaign tended to target female sex workers, women living with HIV/AIDS and drug users.[25]

Another long-awaited alternative to the male condom is a vaginal microbicide preparation (ointment, cream, pessary) that women could self-administer and control to protect themselves from HIV and other STIs. This would have distinct advantages over the female condom in that women could theoretically use it without discussion with their sexual partners. Several different types of microbicide preparations are now undergoing clinical trials.[26] Microbicides may also prove to be useful in preventing HIV and other STIs for other populations who do not use condoms, including men who have sex with men.

Preventing mother-to-child HIV transmission

Much of the prevention work to date has been focused on women and preventing MCT. Nurses and midwives have played a pivotal role in this respect, as they are key workers when women approach services seeking information about contraception and pregnancy. Providing mobile drop-in clinics for young people to discuss concerns and obtain contraceptives is just one example of their role in improving services to remote and marginalized women. Another example of nurses engaging in prevention initiatives is the STI–HIV intervention project in Kolkata, Tamil Nadu, which targeted women sex workers based in brothels to encourage them to seek treatment for sexually transmitted diseases and increase their use of condoms.[27] The policy of preventing MCT transmission depends upon midwives engaging in discussions with women about the advantages of HIV antenatal testing. With 20 million births per year in India and 1–4 per cent HIV prevalence among pregnant women, midwives there are playing a critical role in identifying those infected and offering appropriate interventions.[26] Currently, the favoured treatment is to administer one dose of the antiretroviral drug nevirapine to the woman during labour and give a dose to the baby within 72 hours of birth.[28] This treatment is relatively inexpensive and the manufacturer of nevirapine has agreed to provide it at no cost in some countries. Despite this, and mandates from the WHO and UNAIDS that the prevention of MCT transmission be included as a minimum standard of care, some governments in resource-poor countries have been slow in responding effectively.[29] While this represents an important step in managing the epidemic, it ignores two fundamental problems: the means for women to prevent infection in the first place, and the issue of child care. Unless these two issues are addressed within the broader context of women's lives, the full potential of initiatives focused on reducing MCT transmission of HIV will not be fully realized.

Preventing transmission through injecting drug use

The illicit drug trade is a global phenomenon and it is estimated that up to 10 million people worldwide inject illicit drugs.[1] Drug users are frequently marginalized in society and, although most governments officially support harm reduction programmes, inadequate resources and infrastructure often constrain successful implementation.[30] Drug users are often forced to pay for expensive rehabilitation treatments, such as methadone, and are wary of accessing needle exchange centres for fear of arrest.[30] A WHO study recommended that a quality comprehensive service should include offering syringes, needles and condoms free of charge.[30] In addition, healthcare workers need to feel safe from prosecution when working in needle exchange schemes. Where such services have been implemented, for example in Brazil, the incidence of HIV infection has fallen dramatically.[25]

Vaccine development

Given the urgent problem of prevention, it is not surprising that the development of a vaccine is regarded as a critical component of an effective primary prevention strategy for countries in the industrially developing world. Both parenteral and oral vaccines are now in clinical trials throughout the world. Oral vaccines may be more effective in establishing mucosal defences and also have the advantage of not being reliant on the use of syringes and needles for vaccination.[31]

When an effective vaccine is available, the deployment of a successful vaccine programme is dependent on finding answers to three questions:

- How long will it take?
- Who will pay for it?
- Who will have access to it?

Clinical testing of a vaccine takes a minimum of 6 years and more usually 9–10, so even if the current trials prove efficacious, we still have some way to go, and many more lives will be lost before its preventive value is felt. The companies involved in the production of vaccines are commercial organizations with an interest in a return on their investment. Vaccine development alone is estimated to cost $50–100 million, and without some form of tier pricing, whereby richer nations pay an excess for a small supply, allowing poorer nations to receive the bulk at minimal or low cost, this too will be elusive.[7]

Antiretroviral therapy

The treatment of people living with HIV disease involves two key issues – access to antiretroviral therapy (ART) and the treatment of opportunistic infection – and it is important that the latter is not overshadowed by debates about the former.

Antiretroviral therapy improves the health of those infected, and there is evidence that a reduction in viral load reduces the risk of additional transmission.[32] However, these drugs are expensive, and unaffordable in the poorer regions of the world. One of the key questions to breaking the cycle of poverty is how to access life-prolonging therapy. Most people in the world who are infected with HIV do not have access to ART because they live in economically deprived countries where these drugs cannot be provided. The debate over access continues among the drug companies, international organizations, pressure groups and others concerned with equality, equity and human rights.

International agreements on trade-related intellectual property rights (TRIPS) give pharmaceutical companies the right to determine the production, distribution, pricing and therefore availability of new medicines. Under this agreement, pharmaceutical companies have 20 years' exclusive rights to a drug, which is invariably put on the market at a high price to recoup the development costs. Oxfam and other noted charities have been concerned that TRIPS make the cost of some patent-protected drugs unaffordable to all but a privileged few. In Oxfam's report *Dare to Lead* (2001), it argues that GlaxoSmithKline has a moral duty to forego intellectual property privileges in developing countries if these are likely to result in an increase in prices.[33] Previously, India operated a process patent law, which enabled it to 'copy' new drugs, but it eventually signed TRIPS and it will remain to be seen if access to medicines for opportunistic diseases or ART will be adversely affected. By 2006, TRIPS will become legally binding on all World Trade Organization members, effectively preventing them from manufacturing cheap generic copies of new drugs. Even if antiretroviral drugs could be manufactured generically, or made available at 'no profit', the cost would still be beyond the means of many countries in the poorer regions of the world.[7] However, some countries have been successful in making ART available. In 1996, Brazil introduced universal and free distribution of a wide range of antiretroviral drugs through the national public health network for all those who require them.[25]

Where ART is made available, there are additional associated costs that also have to be met. Infrastructures need to be established to ensure that everyone on ART has reliable and continuing laboratory monitoring, such as CD4+ T-cell counts, measurements of plasma RNA viral load and drug resistance testing. These too are unaffordable in many resource-poor countries, and the companies marketing these tests will need to match the generosity of the pharmaceutical companies if the risk of worldwide blood-resistant virus is to be averted.

Opportunistic diseases

For the time being, treatment of HIV-related opportunistic conditions remains the mainstay of care. The same clinical manifestations seen in industrialized countries (as discussed in Chapter 7) occur in the developing countries. These are often the first indication that someone has HIV infection, and late presentation to a medical facility affects life expectancy.

Wasting

The background of poverty and lack of resources compounds the problems of progressive ill-health and immunosuppression, as rates of respiratory infections, tuberculosis and diarrhoeal disease are already high.[34] The condition was first described in Africa as 'slim disease' because of its association with weight loss and diarrhoea.[35] Wasting remains a key problem and, although the contributing factors are multi-factorial, lack of adequate nutrition compounds this progressive debilitation.

Skin disorders

Skin disorders are also frequently seen as early manifestations of HIV infection, particularly varicella zoster and fungal infections.[34]

Tuberculosis

Without doubt, tuberculosis remains the most important HIV-related opportunistic disease in most regions of the world. It appears early in the course of HIV disease and causes a rapid decline in immune system competence and health. UNAIDS aptly described HIV and tuberculosis as 'a deadly partnership'.[36] HIV increases a person's susceptibility to active disease following exposure and infection with *Mycobacterium tuberculosis*.[37] Additionally, active tuberculosis accelerates HIV replication, leading to further immune system damage. In the early phase of HIV disease, pulmonary tuberculosis is common, whereas later it tends to be disseminated.[39] (For more details on tuberculosis, see Chapter 8.)

Malaria

There is also a link between HIV infection and some tropical diseases. Malaria, one of the major causes of morbidity and mortality worldwide, causes anaemia in children, which is commonly treated with a blood transfusion, which poses a further risk if blood is not screened. Pregnant women (who also frequently receive unscreened blood during childbirth) infected with HIV also experience greater frequency and severity of malaria parasitaemia.[38] A study of co-infection of HIV and malaria in the Amazon region of Guyana suggests that, like co-infection with HIV and tuberculosis, malaria increases the rate of illness and death.[39]

From the conditions highlighted above, it is clear that people living with HIV disease require good-quality nursing care. As wasting is a common clinical outcome of HIV infection, nurses have a pivotal role in assessing their patients' nutrition and fluid intake, mouth care, skin integrity and diarrhoea, and in planning appropriate interventions. While the debate over access to ART continues, it is important to remember that managing many of the opportunistic infections is relatively inexpensive and greatly improves quality of life.

THE NURSING RESPONSE

The HIV/AIDS pandemic is the most serious threat to health of our time, and nurses have a major part to play in both prevention and care. The International Council of Nurses (ICN) revised its Code of Ethics for Nurses in 2000, which defines four universal, fundamental responsibilities for nurses: to promote health; to prevent illness; to restore health; and to alleviate suffering. This code identifies how nurses, educationalists and national organizations can work together to meet these responsibilities.[40]

A hierarchy of different care levels for resource-poor countries has been described and at each level nurses have a pivotal role.[34] For nurses working in countries in the industrially developing world, the most difficult problem is to provide sensitive care that respects human rights in an under funded, over burdened healthcare system. The arrival of large numbers of people presenting with symptomatic HIV disease opened the door to a situation in which ignorance, stigma and neglect prevailed and even basic care was lacking.[41] To help address this situation, a tripartite research collaboration was established involving Thames Valley University in the UK, the British Council in India and the Leelabai Thackersey College of Nursing at Shreemati Nathibai Domador Thackersey (SNDT) Women's University in Mumbai, India. It became known as the *Kaleidoscope* Project and was later extended to the Arabian Gulf and Nigeria.[42]

Following a training needs analysis, which highlighted a fear of contagion and deficits in knowledge, a 2-week, highly interactive educational programme was held for senior nurses and midwives. In the latter part of the programme, the participants were introduced to action research and change theory, which they used to construct an action plan for returning to their clinical areas. The groups devised their plans based on one of nine action fields: infection control; health education; mutual support; community action; pre-qualifying nurse education; post-qualifying in-service nurse education; nursing practice and research; policy development; and counselling support.

A second workshop was held 12 months later to report on progress and identify the factors that either helped or hindered achieving the objectives of their plans. This was also an opportunity to update the participants and encourage them to continue to develop their plans as part of their professional development.

The results from six cohorts in India clearly demonstrated significant success in achieving their plans and the importance of support from doctors and other nurses as well as their own status and confidence.[42] Conversely, lack of personal authority and resistance from managers were highly predictive of lack of achievement. Infection control was a key feature in many fields, and achievements ranged from increasing basic supplies of soap to the production of education materials. Considering the lack of status afforded nurses in India and the strong cultural barriers that prevent discussion of explicit sexual behaviour, these cohorts were powerful examples of what can be achieved by nurses, allowing them to make a defining contribution to the quality of care for patients with HIV disease. As the majority workforce in most healthcare systems, nurses must become increasingly involved in the politics of healthcare if they are to establish the systems best suited to addressing this crisis. They must continue to be assisted to provide competent and compassionate care not only to meet the ICN's code, but also because, for most people with HIV disease, nursing care is all the care they will ever receive.

Summary

The problems of HIV infection and AIDS in the industrially developing world are complex and will not be resolved by quick single solutions. These problems require a long-term commitment and multi-lateral thinking to provide sustainable and realistic results. Condom distribution and use may slow national epidemics, but can never halt an epidemic that is fuelled by poverty. Two keys to tackling the problem are resources and leadership, for without resources one cannot do anything, and without both political and cultural leadership one cannot mobilize resources. The issues are many and intricate, but by tackling the macroeconomics of debt relief and world trade, some of the more one-to-one interventions may stand a chance of success. This requires the world to unite and believe that all life has equal value now and not wait until it is too late.

> No nation can wall itself off from the rest of the world. Global issues are not 'over there' and 'later'. They are 'here' and they are 'now'.
>
> Senator Tim Wirth of Colorado, President of the United Nations Foundation[43]

REFERENCES

1. UNAIDS. *Report on the Global HIV/AIDS Epidemic*. Geneva: UNAIDS/WHO, 2002.
2. Monitoring the AIDS Pandemic (MAP). *The Status and Trends of the HIV/AIDS Epidemics in the World*. Washington, DC: MAP, 2002. Available from: http://www.mapnetwork.org
3. Boseley S. AIDS threatens to explode in east Europe. *The Guardian* 29 November 2001.

4. World Bank. *Project Appraisal Document on a Proposed Credit in the Amount of SDR 140.82 million to India for a Second National HIV/AIDS Control Project.* Washington, DC: World Bank, 1999.

5. UNAIDS. *AIDS Epidemic Update: December 2001.* Geneva: UNAIDS/WHO, 2001. Available from: http://www.unaids.org

6. IRIN-Asia. *Pakistan. Focus on HIV/AIDS Prevention.* [Serial online] 2002 [cited 16 April 2002]. Available from: http://www.healthdev.net./sea-aids

7. Vella S. Footing the bill for HIV/AIDS. Sixth ICAAP Conference, Melbourne, Australia, 5–10 October 2001. [Serial online] 2001 [cited 15 October 2001]. Available from: http://www.hdnet.org

8. World Health Organization. *Macroeconomics and Health: Investing in Health for Economic Development – Report of the Commission on Macroeconomics and Health.* Geneva: WHO, 2001.

9. Leader. A time for optimism: the world can solve its greatest problems. *The Guardian* 24 December 2001.

10. United Nations. *Declaration of Commitment on HIV/AIDS.* Geneva: United Nations & UNAIDS, 2001. Available from: http://www.unaids.org

11. Feachem R. *Update and Vision for the Global Fund,* TuOrG185. XIV International AIDS Conference, Barcelona, 7–12 July 2002. Available from: http://www.aids2002.com

12. Piot P. Are we accountable against our promises? *AIDS 2002 Today* (conference newspaper) 8 July 2002. XIV International AIDS Conference, Barcelona, 7–12 July 2002. Available from: http://www.aids2002.com

13. Medical Research Council. *Impact of HIV/AIDS on Adult Mortality in South Africa.* October 2001. Available from: http://www.mrc.ac.za/home.html

14. McGreal C. AIDS will kill 700,000 South Africans a year. *The Guardian* 17 October 2001.

15. Asian Harm Reduction Network. Who cares about the Asian epidemic? [Serial online] 2001 [cited 2 December 2001]. Available from: http://www.archives.healthdev.net/sea-aids

16. Aggleton P, Rivers K, Scott S. Use of the female condom: gender relations and sexual negotiation. In *Sex and Youth: Contextual Factors Affecting Risk for HIV/AIDS.* Geneva: UNAIDS, 1999.

17. Mann JM, Francis H, Davachi F et al. Risk factors for human immunodeficiency virus serpositivity among children 1–24 months old in Kinshasa, Zaire. *Lancet* 1986; **2**:654–7.

18. Gorna R. *Vamps, Virgins and Victims: How can Women Fight AIDS?* London. Cassell, 1996.

19. McGreal C. Struggle to save children of outcast women. *The Guardian* 29 December 2001.

20. Toolis K. Killer on the road. *The Guardian* 28 December 2001.

21. AIDS 2002 Today. Girls trafficked to Indian brothels. *AIDS 2002 Today* (conference newspaper) 11 July 2002. XIV International AIDS Conference, Barcelona, 7–12 July 2002.

22. UNAIDS. *Innovative Approaches to HIV Prevention: Selected Case Studies.* Geneva: Joint United Programme on HIV/AIDS and the World Health Organization, 2001.

23. Piot P, Aggleton P. The global epidemic. *AIDS Care* 1998; **10**(Suppl. 12):S200–8.

24. Meldrum A. Taxis carry condoms and hope in Zambia's war on AIDS. *The Guardian* 3 July 2002.

25. Ministry of Health. Response: *The Experience of the Brazilian AIDS Programme*. Brazil: Ministry of Health of Brazil, 2002.

26. Ramakant B. Microbicides: communities ready and trials moving forward. Third International Conference on AIDS in India, 2–5 December 2001, Chennai, India. [Serial online] 2002 [cited 11 February 2002]. Available from: http//archives.healthdev.net/sea-aids

27. Ramasundaram S. Can India avoid being devastated by HIV? *British Medical Journal* 2002; **324**:182–3.

28. Guay LA, Musoke P, Fleming T, Bagenda D, Allen M, Nakabiito C. Intrapartum and neonatal single dose nevirapine compared with zidovudine for prevention of mother-to-child transmission of HIV-1 in Kampala, Uganda: HIVNET 012 randomised trial. *Lancet* 1999; **354**:795–802.

29. Saloojee H, Violari A. A regular review: HIV infection in children. *British Medical Journal* 2001; **323**:670–4.

30. Perlis T, Des Jarlais D, Poznyak V et al. Cross-national research methods for adapting interventions for injecting drug users (IDUs), MoOrD1065. XIV International AIDS Conference, Barcelona, 7–12 July 2002. Available from: http://www.aids2002.com

31. Immunitor. *Press release: Immunitor Company Announces Publication of V-1 Immunitor Clinical Results*. [Serial online] 2002 [cited 7 February 2002]. Available from: http://www.thomasland.com

32. Dayton J, Merson M. The value of early detection of HIV in developing countries. *IAS Newsletter* 2001; **19**:8–10.

33. Oxfam. *Dare to Lead: Public Health and Company Wealth*. Oxfam Briefing Paper on GlaxoSmithKline. Oxford: Oxfam, 2001.

34. Gilks CF. HIV care in non-industrialised countries. In: Weiss RA, Adler MW, Rowland-Jones SL (eds), *The Changing Face of HIV and AIDS*. Oxford: Oxford University Press, 2001, 171–86.

35. Serwadda D, Mugerwa RD, Sewankanmbo NK et al. Slim disease: a new disease in Uganda and its association with HTLV III infection. *Lancet* 1985: **2**:849–52.

36. UNAIDS. *A Deadly Partnership: Tuberculosis in the Era of HIV*. Geneva: UNAIDS, 1996.

37. Harries AD, Maher D. *TB/HIV, A Clinical Manual*. Geneva: WHO, 1996.

38. Grant AD, De Cock KM. HIV infection and AIDS in the developing world. In: Adler MW (ed.), *ABC of AIDS*, 5th edn. London: BMJ Books, 2001, 59–64.

39. Palmer CJ, Validum L, Loeffke B et al. HIV prevalence in a gold mining camp in the Amazon region, Guyana. *Emerging Infectious Diseases*. Centers for Disease Control. [Serial online] 2002 [cited 12 March 2002]; **8**. Available from: http://www.cdc.gov/ncidod/EID

40. International Council for Nurses. *The ICN Code of Ethics for Nurses*. Switzerland: ICN, 2000. Available from http://www.icn.ch/ethics.htm

41. UNAIDS/WHO. *AIDS Epidemic Update: December 1999*. Geneva: Joint United Programme on HIV/AIDS and the World Health Organization, 1999. Available from: http:// www.unaids.org

42. Pratt RJ, Pellowe CM, Juvekar SK et al. Kaleidoscope: a 5-year action research project to develop nursing confidence in caring for patients with HIV disease in west India. *International Nursing Review* 2001; **48,:**164–73. Available from: www.blackwell-science.com/inr

43. Leader. Packed planet: So many people, so little time. *Star Tribune* 22 November 2001.

INTERNET RESOURCES

- Official UNAIDS website, contains latest global reports on HIV/AIDS statistics and the Global Fund, fact sheets, conference reports and details of next international conference:
  http://www.unaids.org
- A global campaign against poverty, it contains a specific section on HIV/AIDS with very useful reports on current issues and campaigns:
  http://www.actionaid.org
- An international non-governmental organization providing specialist financial support to other charities to increase their resources. It has an archive of reports relating to HIV/AIDS:
  http://www.cafonline.org

Glossary

Acquired immunodeficiency syndrome (AIDS) A late symptomatic stage of disease caused by infection with the human immunodeficiency virus (HIV), characterized by a high viral load, a profoundly depressed level of CD4⁺ T-lymphocytes, severe opportunistic infections and cancers.

Acute HIV infection The phase of rapid viral replication immediately following primary infection with HIV.

Adenopathy Enlargement of glandular tissue, e.g. lymph nodes (**lymphadenopathy**).

Adherence Usually refers to the extent to which people take their medication exactly as prescribed. Also called **compliance**.

Aetiology The study or theory of the factors that cause disease.

AFB Acid-fast bacilli, e.g. *Mycobacterium tuberculosis* complex. *See also* **mycobacteria**.

AIDS Acronym for **acquired immunodeficiency syndrome**. *See also* **SIDA**.

AIDS dementia complex (ADC) Now less frequently used term for (*see also*) **HIV-1-associated dementia (HAD)** in adults and **HIV encephalopathy** in children.

AIDS-related complex (ARC) Term used in the 1980s to describe symptomatic HIV disease, e.g. weight loss, night sweats, fatigue that had not yet progressed to AIDS-defining opportunistic infections, neoplasms and other end-stage pathology.

AIDS wasting syndrome Progressive involuntary weight loss of 10 per cent or more of baseline body weight plus a 30-day history of either chronic diarrhoea or chronic weakness and either intermittent or constant fever in the absence of any other illness or condition other than HIV infection that would account for this syndrome. This condition is commonly known as **slim disease** in tropical countries, e.g. Africa.

Alkaline phosphatase An enzyme found in the membranes of liver, bone, kidney and intestinal cells. Serum levels of alkaline phosphates are elevated in liver disease.

Amoebiasis (amebiasis) A parasitic infestation of the gastrointestinal tract with *Entamoeba histolytica*, which causes ulceration of the gastrointestinal mucosa and a profuse bloody diarrhoea (amoebic dysentery). Systemic spread to the liver and other internal organs sometimes occurs, leading to abscess formation.

Anaemia A deficiency in either quantity or quality of oxygen-carrying red blood corpuscles (erythrocytes) in the blood. Anaemia, commonly seen in HIV disease, is characterized by dyspnoea (breathlessness) on exertion, pallor and palpitations.

Anergy (anergic) From a Greek word meaning 'lack of energy'. In acquired (adaptive) immunity, anergy is used to describe a diminished immune response to antigens that a person has previously been exposed to (recall antigens), e.g. no immune response on purified protein derivative (PPD) skin testing in a person with HIV disease who has previously been infected with tubercle bacilli. Anergic is the opposite of allergic.

Anorexia Loss of appetite for food.

Antenatal Occurring before birth, e.g. antenatal screening for HIV infection.

Antibody Glycoprotein molecules in the blood produced from B-lymphocyte-derived plasma cells (**secreted antibody**) or found on the surface of B-lymphocytes (**membrane antibody**) that combine with antigens (forming **immune complexes**). Membrane antibodies act as B-lymphocyte receptors (**BCRs**) for antigens. There are five different types, or **classes**, of antibody, each named by the abbreviation for immunoglobulin (Ig) and a letter of the Greek alphabet, i.e. IgM, IgG, IgA, IgD, IgE. The terms **immunoglobulin** and **antibody** are used interchangeably.

Antigens A material or substance that has some surface feature detectable as foreign to the host which stimulates an adaptive immune response (*see also* **epitope**). Typically, antigens are foreign (i.e. non-self), either particulate (cells, microorganisms) or large protein or polysaccharide molecules.

Antigen-presenting cells (APCs) A broad spectrum of cells that present antigens to lymphocytes, e.g. interdigitating dendritic cells (IDCs), macrophages, monocytes. APCs that express major histocompatibility complex (MHC) class I complexes are known as **target cells** and present endogenous antigens (e.g. cells infected with viruses); APCs that express both MHC class I and II complexes can present both endogenous and exogenous antigens to lymphocytes, and are sometimes referred to as **professional APCs**.

APCs *See* **antigen-presenting cells**.

Aphthous ulcers (aphthae) Small, painful oral or oesophageal ulcers consisting of white circular lesions surrounded by erythematous margins with a central area of necrotic epithelial cells and debris (which, when wiped off, reveal a red base); common in HIV disease.

Apoptosis Programmed cell death (suicide), the mechanism by which natural killer (NK) cells and cytotoxic T-lymphocytes (CTLs) destroy virus-infected and tumour cells.

ART Antiretroviral therapy. *See also* **HAART**.

Aspergillosis A fungal infection of the lungs that can spread throughout the body; caused by species of *Aspergillus*.

Asymptomatic Without symptoms, e.g. asymptomatic HIV disease.

Ataxia Failure of muscular co-ordination; irregularity of muscular action.

B-lymphocytes One of two types of lymphocytes (the other being T-lymphocytes). Derived from bone marrow and spleen, they are involved in **humoral** immune responses.

Bactericidal A property of many cellular mechanisms or external agents (e.g. antibiotics, disinfectants) capable of killing bacteria, e.g. ampicillin has a broad spectrum of bactericidal activity.

Bacteriostatic A property of many cellular mechanisms or external agents (e.g. antibiotics, disinfectants) capable of inhibiting bacterial growth, e.g. tetracycline is a bacteriostatic antibiotic.

BCG (Bacillus Calmette Guérin) Vaccine used for preventing tuberculosis, developed by the French bacteriologists Albert Léon Calmette and Camille Guérin in 1921; an attenuated (weakened) form of *Mycobacterium bovis*, the TB bacilli usually found in cattle. The BCG vaccine remains in widespread use today and is recommended by the World Health Organization for use in infants at the time of birth. Not generally used in North America.

Beta-2 microglobulin (abbreviated to **β2M** or **β₂-microglobulin**) Naturally occurring major histocompatibility complex (MHC) class I molecules. These small proteins are released by many activated immune system cells (e.g. lymphocytes) and, in HIV disease, elevated plasma β2M levels above 5 micrograms (μg) may indicate a higher risk of disease progression. *See also* **neopterin**.

Billion The cardinal number equal to a thousand millions (1 000 000 000 in the USA and France, and to a million millions in the UK. In this text, the USA definition is used as it is the standard definition used by international scientific organizations, e.g. six billion = 6 000 000 000. *See also* **million**.

Bi-sexuality Refers to either men or women who are emotionally attracted to and may have physical sexual relations with individuals of the opposite and of the same gender.

Body fat redistribution *See* **lipodystrophy syndrome**.

Cachexia A profound state of ill-health, malnutrition and wasting.

Candidiasis Infection, usually of the oropharynx, oesophagus, trachea, bronchi, lungs or vagina, with yeast-like fungi of the *Candida* family, usually *Candida albicans*.

CCR5 *See* **chemokine receptors**.

CDC Centers for Disease Control and Prevention, Atlanta, Georgia, USA. Internet address on the worldwide web http://www.cdc.gov

CD4 Cell surface receptor molecules (part of the immunoglobulin G superfamily) expressed on some T-lymphocytes and other immune system cells, e.g. monocytes, tissue macrophages, dendritic cells, microglial cells, Langerhans cells. They participate in normal class II major histocompatibility complex (MHC) recognition in association with T-cell responsiveness to foreign antigens. They are the principal cell surface receptors for HIV. *See also* **CD8**.

CD4⁺ T-lymphocyte cell counts Laboratory estimates of the number of CD4⁺ T-lymphocytes in peripheral blood are generally reported as the number of cells per cubic millimetre (**cells/mm³**); less frequently, they are reported as the number of cells per microlitre (cells/μL) or per 10⁶/L. Estimates of the number of CD4⁺ T-lymphocytes in peripheral blood and their trends to decrease or increase over time comprise one of the most important laboratory assessments predicting disease progression and response to antiretroviral therapy.

CD4⁺ T-lymphocyte cell percentage The proportion of all T-lymphocytes that are CD4⁺ cells; in health, this is approximately 40 per cent, but progressively declines in HIV-infected people.

CD4⁺:CD8⁺ ratio Ratio of the number of CD4⁺ to CD8⁺ cells (normally approximately equal to 2:1). Alterations are not specific to HIV infection, and many other viral diseases (e.g. influenza, hepatitis B, CMV infection) may produce transient reductions in this ratio.

CD8 Cell surface receptor molecules expressed on some T-lymphocytes, e.g. cytotoxic and inducer/suppressor T-lymphocytes. *See also* **CD4**.

Chancroid Highly contagious sexually transmitted disease caused by the *Haemophilus ducreyi* bacterium. It presents as a genital ulcer accompanied by inflammation and suppuration of local lymph glands.

Chemokines A subgroup of **cytokines** (*see also*) that are principally responsible for the process of chemotaxis, i.e. chemical signals used to attract cells (chiefly leucocytes) to an area of infection. Also known as chemotactic cytokines or chemoattractant molecules. The two major groups of chemokines are referred to as **CXC (alpha chemokines)** and **CC (beta chemokines)**.

Chemokine receptors Seven transmembrane, G-protein-coupled cell surface receptors for chemokines. Important chemokine receptors associated with HIV infection include **CXCR4** (previously referred to as fusin or lester) and **CCR5**. *See also* **chemokines**.

Chemoprophylaxis The use of drugs or chemicals to prevent infection or disease

Chemotaxis A process by which phagocytic cells (e.g. neutrophils, monocytes) are attracted to sites of tissue damage or inflammation.

Chemotherapy The use of drugs to treat disease; usually refers to anti-cancer drug regimens. *See also* **cytotoxic**.

Circumoral paraesthesia An abnormal sensation, such as burning or prickling, around the mouth, sometimes caused by some antiretroviral drugs and other medications.

Clades Viral variants (*see* **variants**) of HIV-1 that occur as a result of geographical diversity in different regions of the world. Also called HIV-1 **subtypes** but not **quasispecies** (*see also*).

Cleavage, cleave To divide, split or sever by cutting, e.g. the viral enzyme protease cleaves large strands of viral protein in the maturing HIV virion, splitting it into the smaller core proteins.

Clinical latency Period following infection before the onset of symptoms, i.e. asymptomatic infection.

CMV *See* **cytomegalovirus**.

Coccidioidomycosis An infectious fungal disease caused by inhalation of spores of *Coccidioides immitis*. Also called desert fever, San Joaquin Valley fever, or valley fever. Seen mainly in the south-western regions of the USA and Central and South America. An opportunistic infection seen in patients with HIV disease.

Cognitive impairment Difficulty in thinking; specifically, a progress decline in the ability to process, learn and remember information.

Commensals Microorganisms that live in symbiosis on or within other organisms without harming them, e.g. the normal flora of the gastrointestinal tract is composed of harmless bacteria (commensals).

Condyloma acuminatum (genital warts) Warts in the genital or peri-anal area caused by the **human papilloma virus (HPV)**. The infection is principally sexually transmitted and infected patients can transmit the virus from one person to another and from one part of their own body to another part (auto-inoculable).

CSWs Acronym for **commercial sex workers**: individuals (male, female or transsexual/transgender individuals) who sell sex, i.e. prostitutes.

CTLs (cytotoxic T-lymphocytes) *See* **killer cells**.

Creatinine A breakdown product of creatine, an important constituent of muscle. The levels of creatinine in blood and urine are often measured to evaluate renal function. A **creatinine clearance test** measures the amount of creatinine in a 24-hour collection of urine (normal values: 10–20 mmol/24 hours).

Cryptococcosis Infectious disease caused by *Cryptococcus neoformans*, a fungus found in soil contaminated by bird faeces. It sometimes causes **cryptococcal meningitis** in immuno-compromised individuals, which is a serious, often life-threatening inflammatory disease of the central nervous system.

Cryptosporidiosis A serious diarrhoeal disease of immunocompromised people caused by the protozoon *Cryptosporidium parvum*, which infects the gastrointestinal tract. This parasite is naturally found in the intestines of animals and may be transmitted to humans by direct contact with an infected animal, by eating contaminated food, or by drinking contaminated water.

Cunnilingus Sucking, licking and/or kissing a woman's genitals to provide sexual stimulation. *See also* **fellatio**.

Cytokines Soluble protein molecules secreted by immune system cells that act as cell-to-cell messengers to stimulate or inhibit the growth of immune system cells and amplify or depress immune responses. *See also* **chemokines**.

Cytomegalovirus (CMV) A common human herpesvirus that causes a variety of multi-system opportunistic diseases in immunocompromised patients, e.g. retinitis, encephalitis and pneumonitis.

Cytotoxic A drug or process that is toxic or destructive to cells, e.g. cytotoxic drugs are used to treat many types of cancer.

Cytotoxic T-lymphocytes (CTLs) *See* **killer cells**.

CXCR4 *See* **chemokine receptors**.

Dendritic cells Antigen-presenting cells (APCs) originating in the bone marrow that have many long and branched (tree-like) flapping membrane extensions. They are found in both lymphoid and non-lymphoid tissues, and in the blood and lymph. Different types of dendritic cells include: **interdigitating dendritic cells (IDCs)** in the thymus, **follicular dendritic cells (FDCs)** in germinal centres of peripheral lymphoid tissues, **Langerhans cells** in the skin, **veiled cells** in lymph, and dendritic cells circulating in the blood (**blood dendritic cells**). They capture and bind to antigens (including high levels of HIV) and bring them to the lymphoid organ, where an immune response is initiated.

Diaphoresis Sweating; profuse perspiration.

Diplopia Double vision.

DNA Deoxyribonucleic acid; *see* **nucleic acids**.

DNA polymerase An enzyme that facilitates DNA to act as a template for making additional identical copies of itself. It works by adding nucleotides (the structural units of nucleic acids) and synthesizing new DNA. *See also* **polymerase chain reaction (PCR) tests**; **nucleotide**.

Dyspnoea Difficult or laboured breathing.

ELISA Acronym for enzyme-linked immunosorbent assay; a test used to detect and/or quantify the presence of an antibody or antigen using a ligand (e.g. anti-immunoglobulin) conjugated to an enzyme that changes the colour of a substrate. ELISA techniques are widely used to detect antibodies to HIV (and to many other pathogens) and are the principal diagnostic test for HIV infection.

Endemic A disease (or condition) present or habitually prevalent in a specified population or geographical region all of the time. *See also* **epidemic**; **pandemic**.

Endogenous Relating to or produced by the body, e.g. endogenous depression caused by factors within the body. *See also* **exogenous**.

Endothelium Refers to the layer of epithelial cells that lines the cavities of the heart, blood and lymph vessels, and the serous cavities of the body. *See also* **epithelium**.

Entry inhibitors Drugs designed to prevent HIV attaching to receptor sites on the surface of host cells that HIV targets for infection (e.g. CD4$^+$ T-lymphocytes) and entering cells. Also called **fusion inhibitors**. An example of this class of antiretroviral drugs is enfuvirtide, also called T-20 and Fuzeon™, which binds to the viral gp41 glycoprotein and prevents HIV from binding with the surface of host cells, thus preventing entry and infection.

Epidemic A sudden and significant increase (outbreak) in the incidence of a disease that is normally endemic in a population or of a new disease within a specified population during a specified period of time. *See also* **endemic**; **pandemic**.

Epidermis The outer and non-vascular layer of the skin.

Epithelium The covering of internal and external surfaces of the body composed of cells joined to each other by small amounts of cementing substances. Epithelium is classified into types on the basis of the number of layers deep and the shape of the superficial cells, e.g. simple squamous, simple columnar, transitional.

Epitope A unique shape or marker carried on an antigen's surface that the immune system recognizes and which triggers a corresponding antibody response. *See also* **antigen**.

Epstein–Barr virus (EBV) A human herpesvirus that can cause infectious mononucleosis (glandular fever) in adolescents in the industrially developed world, Burkitt's lymphoma in children in Africa and nasopharyngeal carcinoma in South East Asia and China. Also causes **oral hairy leucoplakia** and various types of **lymphomas** in HIV-infected people.

Erythema Redness of the skin as a result of injury, infection and/or inflammation.

Erythrocytes Red blood corpuscles whose major function is to carry oxygen to the cells.

Erythropoietin A naturally occurring hormone produced in the kidneys that stimulates the production of red blood corpuscles by the bone marrow. Recombinant human erythropoietin (**epoetin**) is frequently used to treat anaemia associated with HIV disease and with some antiretroviral drugs. *See also* **anaemia**.

Exanthem An infectious disease characterized by a skin eruption or rash.

Exogenous Developing or originating outside the body, i.e. external. *See also* **endogenous**.

Fat redistribution *See* **lipodystrophy syndrome**.

Fc receptors Receptors for the Fc portion (region, fragment) of antibodies (immuno-globulins) found on some phagocytic cells, allowing these cells to bind to antibody-coated targets and kill them by a process known as **antibody-dependent cell-mediated cytotoxicity (ADCC)**.

Fellatio Sucking or licking a man's penis to provide sexual stimulation. *See also* **cunnilingus**.

Floaters Drifting dark spots within the field of vision, often caused by CMV retinitis in HIV-infected people.

Fomites Inanimate objects, such as clothes or bedding, capable of harbouring and transmitting infectious microorganisms, e.g. MRSA, SARS virus.

Fusion inhibitors *See* **entry inhibitors**.

Gay *See* **homosexuality**; **MSM**.

Genes Short segments of DNA which are interpreted by the body as templates for building specific proteins. They are the smallest biological units of heredity. The information from all the genes, taken together, comprises the blueprint for the human body and its function.

Genotype The genetic composition of any organism.

Genus (plural **genera**) A group of closely related species.

Ghon focus Initial lesion in the lungs in tuberculosis, consisting of infected macrophages, provoking the formation of a **granuloma** (*see also*).

Gonorrhoea A sexually transmitted infection caused by *Neisseria gonorrhoeae*. It can also be transmitted from an infected mother to her newborn infant during the birth process.

Gram's stain A differential stain developed by the Danish bacteriologist Hans Christian Gram in 1884 that classifies bacteria into two large groups: Gram-positive and Gram-negative.

Gram-negative bacteria Bacteria that lose the crystal violet colour after decolourizing by alcohol; they stain pink after treatment with safranin (a basic red dye).

Gram-positive bacteria Bacteria that retain the crystal violet colour after decolourizing by alcohol; they stain dark purple.

Granulocyte A type of white blood cell (leucocyte) with characteristic granules in its cytoplasm which facilitate the digestion of microorganisms. There are three types of granulocytes (also known as **polymorphonuclear leucocytes**): **neutrophils**, **basophils** and **eosinophils**.

Granulocytopenia A marked reduction in the number of granulocytes in the blood, especially in the number of neutrophils (**neutropenia**).

Granuloma An organized collection of epithelioid cells which are modified plump macrophages (histiocytes), surrounded by lymphocytes and capillaries, usually having a central area made of caseum (consistency of soft cheese), an extracellular acidic environment with a low oxygen tension that inhibits both macrophage function and bacillary growth. Surrounding the caseum are activated and non-activated macrophages. Granulomas are characteristic of chronic infection (e.g. tuberculosis) and form to wall off and limit the infection.

HAART (highly active antiretroviral therapy) A treatment regimen that incorporates a combination of different antiretroviral drugs, sometimes referred to as **ART**, i.e. antiretroviral therapy.

Haematocrit A laboratory measurement of the volume of packed red blood corpuscles in the blood, usually expressed as a percentage of the total blood volume. Also called **packed cell volume (PCV)**. Normal values are: (men) 40–54 per cent of the blood (0.40–0.54) and (women) 37–47 per cent of the blood (0.37–0.47).

Haemoglobin The component of red blood corpuscles that carries oxygen. Normal range of laboratory measurements: (men) 130–180 g/L and (women) 115–165 g/L.

Haemophilia Hereditary bleeding disorders affecting mainly males and caused by clotting factor deficiencies of factor VIII, IX or XI.

Health Protection Agency (HPA) A new national organization for England and Wales, established on 1 April 2003. It is dedicated to protecting people's health and reducing the impact of infectious diseases, chemical hazards, poisons and radiation hazards. It brings together the expertise of health and scientific professionals working in public health, communicable disease, emergency planning, infection control, laboratories, poisons, chemical and radiation hazards. Further information is available from their website at: http://www.hpa.org.uk

Hepatitis Inflammatory disease of the liver, generally (but not exclusively) caused by the hepatotropic viruses, i.e. hepatitis A, B, C, D and E viruses. **HIV–hepatitis C virus co-infection** is frequently associated with a more rapid progression of chronic hepatitis C to cirrhosis and liver failure.

Herpesviruses A family of at least eight human viruses that establish life-long latent infection from which the virus can be re-activated, causing a recurrence of clinical disease. Includes herpes simplex viruses types 1 and 2, varicella-zoster virus, human herpesvirus 8 (Kaposi's sarcoma-related herpesvirus), cytomegalovirus, Epstein–Barr virus and human herpesviruses 6 and 7.

Heterodimer A **dimer** is a compound (a substance that consists of a union of two or more elements, or subunits) of two identical simpler molecules; a **heterodimer** (e.g. the HIV viral enzyme reverse transcriptase) is composed of two different types of subunits (p66 and p51).

Heterosexuality Refers to men and women who are emotionally and physically attracted to and have sexual relations with individuals of the opposite gender.

Histoplasmosis A fungal infection, usually of the lungs, caused by the fungus *Histoplasma capsulatum*. The major endemic areas for histoplasmosis are the Mississippi and Ohio River valleys of the eastern USA. A similar fungus (or variant of *H. capsulatum*), *H. duboisii*, is found in Africa.

HIV-associated dementia (HAD) A progressive degenerative neurological condition seen in adults in late symptomatic HIV disease which occurs as a direct result of HIV infection of central nervous system cells and structures in the brain. HAD is characterized by various neurological dysfunctions, including loss of coordination, mood swings, loss of inhibitions, and widespread cognitive dysfunction and personality changes. Also known (less frequently) as the AIDS dementia complex (ADC) and **HIV encephalopathy** in children.

HIV disease The entire spectrum of cellular and clinical pathology from initial infection to end-stage disease and death.

HIV encephalopathy Childhood form of **HIV-associated dementia (HAD)**, characterized by a loss of previously acquired cognitive and motor milestones and spastic paraparesis (or quadriparesis).

Homosexuality Refers to people who are physically and emotionally attracted to and have sexual relations with others of the same gender, e.g. man and man, woman and woman. In the Western world, male homosexuals are commonly referred to as **gay** men, and female homosexuals are commonly known as **lesbians**.

Human immunodeficiency viruses (HIV) – types 1 (HIV-1) and 2 (HIV-2) The viruses which cause AIDS in humans. In the early years of the pandemic, they were referred to as HTLV-III (USA), LAV (France) and ARV (USA).

Human papilloma virus (HPV) A sexually transmitted virus which causes genital warts, cervical dysplasia and cervical cancer.

Human T-cell lymphotropic virus type 1 (HTLV-1) A retrovirus that causes adult T-cell leukaemia/lymphoma (ATL) or myelopathy/tropical spastic paraparesis (HAM/TSP) in some infected people.

Human T-cell lymphotropic virus type 2 (HTLV-2) A retrovirus closely related to HTLV-1 which may cause neurological disease similar to HAM/TSP in some infected people.

Hyperlipidaemia Increase in the plasma concentrations of cholesterol (**hypercholesteraemia**) or triglycerides (**hypertriglyceridaemia**), or both. In patients with HIV disease, this is a frequent long-term side effect of antiretroviral therapy, especially associated with the use of protease inhibitors. Hyperlipidaemia is associated with an increased risk of cardiovascular disease and pancreatitis.

Hypogammaglobulinaemia A deficiency of plasma gamma globulin, an important immunoglobulin which protects against infection.

Hypoxia An insufficient supply of oxygen to the tissues.

Iatrogenesis Problems or any adverse condition occurring in patients as a result of treatment or care by healthcare providers.

Idiopathic Without a known cause, e.g. idiopathic diarrhoea.

IDU (injecting drug use/user) This term is preferentially used as it accurately describes the behaviour without using imprecise or judgemental words, e.g. addict, abuser, intravenous.

Immune complexes Clusters formed when antibodies and antigens bind together.

Immunoglobulin *See* **antibody**.

Incidence The rate at which a certain event occurs in a defined population during a specific period of time, e.g. the number of new AIDS cases which occurred in the UK during 2002. *See also* **prevalence**.

Infectious A property of human hosts that refers to their level of infectiousness. *See also* **infective, infectivity**.

Infective, Infectivity A property of an HIV (or any other) virus that refers to its ability to breach host defences and infect host cells. *See also* **infectious**.

Integrase (IN) A viral enzyme in HIV (also referred to as p32). Following reverse transcription, integrase acts as a 'tailor', cutting and joining the new HIV DNA viral genome and integrating it into the host cell chromosomes.

Integrase inhibitors An experimental class of antiretroviral drugs that prevent the viral enzyme integrase from inserting HIV DNA into the host cell chromosomes.

Interferons A group of naturally occurring antiviral proteins (cytokines) produced by activated T-lymphocytes in response to viral infections which modulate the immune response. Interferons prevent uninfected cells from becoming infected and hasten recovery following viral disease.

Interferon alpha (IFNα) Synthetic IFNα is used in the treatment of chronic hepatitis B and hepatitis C and is being investigated for use in the treatment of HIV disease, especially in the treatment of Kaposi's sarcoma, and in other forms of cancer. Long-acting **peginterferon alfa-2b** is used for the treatment of hepatitis C (usually in combination with the antiviral drug **ribarvirin**). IFNα is administered by subcutaneous, intramuscular or intravenous injection.

Interferon beta (IFNβ) Synthetic IFNβ is used in the treatment of multiple sclerosis. It is administered by subcutaneous injection.

Interleukin-2 (aldesleukin) Naturally occurring interleukin-2 is a cytokine produced by activated T-lymphocytes to stimulate the activation of cytotoxic killer cells in response to viral infections. Recombinant interleukin-2, also known as aldesleukin, is used in the treatment of metastatic renal cell carcinoma and is being investigated for its use as an immune system stimulant in people with HIV disease. It is no longer administered by intravenous infusion and is only given by subcutaneous injection.

Intrapartum Time during labour and delivery.

In vitro (Latin *vitreus* – glassy) The occurrence of a phenomenon in laboratory experiments (literally, 'within a glass', e.g. a test tube) and not necessarily reflecting what happens within the human body. For example, a drug may exhibit certain characteristics *in vitro* that may or may not occur inside the body. *See also* **in vivo**.

In vivo (Latin *vivere* – live) Occurrence of a phenomenon or effect within the living human body, as opposed to **in vitro**.

Jaundice A yellow discolouring of the skin, mucous membranes and whites of the eyes, caused by excessive amounts of bilirubin in the blood. Jaundice is caused by liver or gall-bladder disease or by excessive haemolysis (breakdown) of red blood corpuscles.

JC virus (JCV) A polyomavirus (a type of papovavirus) that causes **progressive multifocal leucoencephalopathy (PML)** in immunocompromised people, especially patients with late symptomatic HIV disease (AIDS).

Kaposi's sarcoma A type of cancer probably caused by infection with human herpesvirus 8 (Kaposi's sarcoma-related herpesvirus). A malignant neoplastic vascular proliferation characterized by the development of bluish-red cutaneous nodules, usually on the lower extremities (most often on the toes or feet), and slowly increasing in size and number and spreading to more proximal sites, especially on the face and nose. *See also* **sarcoma**; **herpesvirus**.

Killer cells Many different immune system cells that kill other cells, usually those infected with viruses or undergoing neoplastic change. Killer cells (also called **cytotoxic cells**) include **natural killer cells (NK cells)** and **cytotoxic T-lymphocytes (CTLs)**. Different cells kill by a variety of mechanisms, e.g. **apoptosis** (*see also*), antibody-dependent cell-mediated cytoxicity (ADCC) or killer cell (K cell) activity.

Kilodalton A dalton is an arbitrary (dimensionless) unit of mass, i.e. molecular weight (also called atomic mass unit); the term kilo (symbol k) is used in units of measurements to indicate a quantity one thousand (10^3) times the unit designated by the root (e.g. Dalton) with which it is combined. Kilodalton is the term used to describe the relative molecular mass (that is, molecular weight) of various components of the human immunodeficiency viruses, e.g. p17 is a core protein having a relative molecular mass of 17 kilodaltons.

Langerhans cells Epidermal dendritic antigen-presenting cells; frequently the first cells to encounter and latch onto HIV in the mucous membranes and transport it to the T-lymphocytes in lymphoid tissue (not to be confused with pancreatic insulin-secreting cells called *islets of Langerhans*) *See also* **dendritic cells**.

LAS (lymphadenopathy syndrome) *See* **PGL**.

Lentivirus A type of retrovirus characterized by a long interval between infection and the onset of symptoms; often referred to as a 'slow' virus. HIV is a lentivirus.

Leucocyte/leukocyte White blood cell.

Leucocytosis An abnormally high level of leucocytes in the blood, usually in response to infection.

Leucopenia Decreased number of leucocytes, principally granulocytes, in the blood.

Leucoplakia A pre-cancerous lesion that develops on the tongue or the inside of the cheek, usually as a response to chronic irritation. *See also* **oral hairy leucoplakia**.

Ligand (Latin *ligare* – to bind) A small molecule that binds specifically to a larger molecule (a receptor), e.g. an antigen (being a small molecule) binding to an antibody (a larger molecule) is the ligand for that antibody; a specific chemokine (a small molecule) binding to a specific chemokine cell surface receptor (a larger molecule) is the ligand for that receptor.

Lipid Groups of fats and fat-like compounds, including sterols, fatty acids and many other substances.

Lipoatrophy *See* **lipodystrophy**.

Lipodystrophy Abnormal fat changes in the body which may be associated with the long-term side effects of antiretroviral therapy. Lipodystrophy refers to several problems linked to this disorder of fat metabolism, including: (1) an accumulation of fat around the abdomen (crix belly, protease paunch), on the back of the neck and shoulders (buffalo hump); (2) loss of fat in the legs, arms, buttocks and face (**lipoatrophy**); (3) high levels of fat (triglycerides, cholesterol) in the blood; (4) high levels of sugar (and sometimes insulin) in the blood.

Litre (l, L) Metric unit of measurement of volume; 1 litre consists of 1000 millilitres (mL).

Lymphocytes White blood cells that play a major role in mounting a specific immune response to antigens. *See also* **B-lymphocytes**; **T-lymphocytes**; **natural killer cells**.

Lymphoid interstitial pneumonitis (LIP) A type of pneumonia common in HIV-infected children. It is an AIDS-defining condition in children.

Lymphoma Cancer of lymphoid tissues, including non-Hodgkin's lymphomas (also called B-cell lymphomas), which are frequently seen in HIV-infected people.

Lymphopenia Decrease in the proportion of lymphocytes in the blood, similar to **lymphocytopenia** – a reduced number of lymphocytes in the blood – both of which suggest immune system injury.

MAC *See **Mycobacterium avium** complex.*

Macrophage A phagocytic cell that is derived from a **monocyte** (a type of white blood cell, or leucocyte, that circulates in the blood) that has migrated into an organ or tissue. Macrophages and monocytes are collectively known as **mononuclear phagocytes**.

Magnetic resonance imaging (MRI) A non-invasive, non-X-ray diagnostic scan that provides computer-generated images of the body's internal tissues and organs.

MAI *See **Mycobacterium avium** complex.*

Major histocompatibility complex (MHC) Host molecules that associate intracellularly with antigen (peptide) fragments to form an antigen–MHC complex on the surface of the host cell, which allows T-lymphocyte receptors to recognize antigens.

Meninges Membranes surrounding the brain or spinal cord.

Meningitis Inflammation of the meninges, usually caused by pathogenic microorganisms.

Metastasis Spread of a disease, such as cancer, from its original site to other sites in the body.

MHC *See **major histocompatibility complex**.*

Microbicide Any agent that destroys microorganisms. Rectal and vaginal microbicides are being investigated for their use in preventing sexually transmitted infections.

Microgram (symbol **μg** or abbreviated **mcg**) Metric unit of mass (weight), being one-millionth of a gram (10^{-6} g) or one one-thousandth of a milligram (10^{-3} mg).

Micrometre (symbol **μm**) Unit of measurement: one-millionth (10^{-6}) of a metre or one-thousandth (10^{-3}) of a millimetre; formerly called a **micron** (symbol **μ**). It can also be expressed as one 25-thousandth of an inch.

Micron (symbol **μ**) *See **micrometre**.*

Microsporidiosis An intestinal infection caused by different protozoal parasites known as **microsporidia**. Infection results in (sometimes torrential) diarrhoea in severely immunocompromised people.

Milligram (abbreviated **mg**) Unit of measurement: one-thousandth of a gram.

Millilitre (abbreviated **ml, mL**) Metric unit of volume measurement, being one-thousandth of a litre (or one cubic centimetre).

Millimetre (abbreviated **mm**) Unit of measurement: one-thousandth of a metre. The level of CD4⁺ T-lymphocytes in peripheral blood is commonly reported as the number of cells per cubic millimetre, i.e. cells/mm³.

Million The cardinal number equal to a thousand thousands, i.e. 1000 000, e.g. ten million = 10 000 000. *See also* **billion**.

MSM (men who have sex with men) A more accurate description of this group, as many men who have sex with men may not self-identify as homosexual, bisexual or (in the Western world) **gay**.

M-tropic HIV-1 variants Those variants of HIV-1 that preferentially seek out, infect and replicate in macrophages and monocytes in addition to CD4⁺ T-lymphocytes. These variants do not generally form syncytia (*see also* **syncytia**), i.e. are non-syncytium-inducing (NSI), and use the CCR5 chemokine receptor to bind to and infect cells. *See also* **R5 viruses**; **T-tropic variants**.

Myalgia Muscle pain.

Mycobacteria Bacilli that are small (less than 0.5 μm in diameter), non-sporing, Gram-positive, oxygen-loving (aerophilic) bacilli; slender, curved (often beaded) rods, enveloped by acid-fast and alcohol-fast surface lipids, which reproduce slowly by binary fission. Mycobacteria cause a variety of diseases, including tuberculosis and leprosy. Also referred to as **tubercle bacilli** and **acid-fast/alcohol-fast bacilli (AFB)**.

Mycobacteriosis Human disease caused by non-tuberculous environmental mycobacteria, e.g. MAC.

Mycobacterium avium **complex (MAC)** A non-tuberculous (environmental) myco-bacterium that, along with *M. intracellulare*, causes severe disease in immunocompromised people. In the USA, it is frequently referred to as **MAI (*M. avium–intracellulare*)**. *See also* **mycobacteriosis**.

Mycobacterium intracellulare *See* *Mycobacterium avium* complex (MAC); mycobacteriosis.

Mycobacterium leprae Non-tuberculous environmental mycobacteria that causes leprosy (Hansen's disease).

Mycobacterium tuberculosis **complex** A group of mycobacteria (*M. tuberculosis, M. bovis, M. africaneum, M. canetti, M. microti*) that cause tuberculosis in humans and animals. *M. tuberculosis* is the most common cause of tuberculosis in humans. Sometimes abbreviated as **MTB complex** or, more usually, referred to as **tubercle bacilli**.

Mycosis Fungal disease.

Myopathy Loss of muscle due to wasting or disease.

Nadir Lowest out of a series of measurements, e.g. the lowest level to which the viral load falls after starting antiretroviral treatment. The opposite of **zenith**.

Nanometre A unit of linear measure composed of 10 angstrom units (Å) and equal to: one-billionth of a metre; 10^{-9} metre (m); one-millionth of a millimetre (mm); or, more commonly, one-thousandth (10^{-3}) of a micrometre (μm). *See also* **micrometre**.

Natural killer (NK) cells A type of lymphocyte involved in natural killing (apoptosis), especially targeting viral-infected cells and tumour cells. *See also* **killer cells**.

Neonatal The first 4 weeks of life after birth.

Neoplasm An abnormal and uncontrolled growth of tissues; a tumour.

Neopterin Protein molecules secreted principally by activated macrophages. An increased serum level of neopterin (e.g. more than 15 nanograms per millilitre) is associated with HIV disease progression. *See also* **beta-2 microglobulin**.

Neuralgia A sharp, stabbing pain along the path of a nerve.

Neuropathy A disease process of nerve degeneration and loss of function, especially **peripheral neuropathy**, commonly seen during the course of HIV disease. Patients experience a range of symptoms, from tingling sensation or numbness in the hands and feet to pain, immobility and paralysis.

Neutropenia *See* **granulocytopenia**.

Neutrophil A type of **granulocyte** that is involved in phagocytosis and protecting against infections.

Nucleic acids (DNA and RNA) Large molecules (macromolecules) found within the nucleus of cells that are made up of repeating **nucleotides** (*see also*). There are two types of nucleic acid. (1) **Deoxyribonucleic acid (DNA)** consists of two strands of nucleotides wound in a double helix held together by hydrogen bonds between purine and pyrimidine nucleotides. **Genes**, the basic units of heredity, are arranged within the DNA along the **chromosomes**. The DNA of chromosomes (and mitochondria) carries genetic information and DNA's capacity to replicate is the basis of hereditary transmission of genetically determined characteristics. (2) **Ribonucleic acid (RNA) nucleotides** consist of ribose (a pentose) and one of the following nitrogenous bases: cytosine, guanine, adenine or uracil. RNA is transcribed (made) from, and is a template of, DNA. Although it also holds genetic information (as in viruses) the principal function of RNA is to transfer information from DNA to the protein-synthesizing machinery of cells. RNA exists in three different forms: **messenger RNA (mRNA)**, which gives instructions for protein synthesis; **ribosomal RNA (rRNA)**, which makes more than half of all **ribosomes** (cell structures associated with mRNA which serve as factories for making new proteins); and **transfer RNA (tRNA)**, small RNA molecules that match and bind specific amino acids to mRNA codons (sites) during the translation (manufacturing) of larger proteins (polypeptide chains).

Nucleoside A deoxyribose or ribose sugar molecule bound to a nitrogen base consisting of either purine or pyrimidine. It becomes a **nucleotide** (*see also*) when a phosphate group becomes attached to its sugar.

Nucleotide The structural unit of **nucleic acids** (*see also*). Nucleotides are formed when a phosphate group becomes attached to a **nucleoside** (*see also*). Each nucleotide is composed of three parts: a nitrogen-containing base, a pentose (five-carbon) sugar called **deoxyribose** or **ribose**, and a phosphate group (phosphoric acid). Nucleotides containing ribose are known as **ribonucleotides** and those containing deoxyribose are known as **deoxyribonucleotides**.

Nucleus The central controlling body within a living cells which contains that cell's genetic codes and which is responsible for directing essential cell functions such as growth, reproduction and protein synthesis.

OI *See* **opportunistic infections**.

Oncogene (Greek *onkos* – tumour) A viral gene (often abbreviated as *onc*) present in some DNA viruses and some retroviruses that can cause cancer, e.g. they are **oncogenic** viruses. An example of an oncogenic retrovirus is the human T-cell lymphotropic virus type I (HTLV-I), which can cause adult T-cell leukaemia or lymphoma in some infected people.

Opportunistic infections Those infections caused by microorganisms which do not usually cause disease in people with competent immune systems but do take the 'opportunity' of a depressed immune system, such as the progressive immunosuppression caused by HIV disease, to cause clinical disease in immunocompromised people.

Oral hairy leucoplakia An unusual form of leucoplakia that is seen only in HIV-infected people. It consists of fuzzy (hairy) white patches on the tongue and, less frequently, elsewhere in the mouth. Hairy leucoplakia may be one of the first signs of infection with HIV.

Outbreak An epidemic limited to localized increase in the incidence of a disease, e.g. in a village, town or closed institution.

Pandemic An epidemic disease distributed or occurring widely throughout a country, region, continent or globally. *See also* **endemic**; **epidemic**.

Paraesthesia Abnormal sensations such as burning, tingling or a 'pins-and-needles' feeling. *See also* **circumoral paraesthesia**.

Parenteral Any route of drug administration apart from the alimentary canal, usually referring to intravenous injections and infusions and to intramuscular and subcutaneous injections of medications.

Pathogen, pathogenic Disease-causing, e.g. a pathogenic microorganism (a pathogen) can cause disease.

PCP *See* ***Pneumocystis carinii***.

PCR *See* **polymerase chain reaction tests**.

Pelvic inflammatory disease (PID) Gynaecological condition caused by a (usually) sexually transmitted infection that spreads from the vagina to the upper parts of a woman's reproductive tract in the pelvic cavity.

Pentamidine isethionate Antimicrobial agent used in the prophylaxis and treatment of pneumocystis pneumonia; injectable and nebulizer solutions are available (Pentacarinat®). *See also* ***Pneumocystis carinii.***

Perianal Around the anus.

PGL (persistent generalized lymphadenopathy) (in France: **LAS – lymphadenopathy syndrome**) Persistent and generalized swollen lymph glands in people infected with HIV, usually including cervical and axillary lymph nodes.

Phagocyte Cells capable of ingesting particulate matter, e.g. polymorphonuclear leucocytes, macrophages. This process is known as **phagocytosis** (as opposed to **pinocytosis**, the process whereby some cells engulf liquid).

Plasma cells Large antibody-producing cells that develop from activated B-lymphocytes following antigenic presentation.

Pneumocystis carinii Originally thought to be a protozoon, now known as a fungus belonging to *Ascomycetes* yeast; causes pneumonia (called **pneumocystosis, pneumocystis pneumonia** or **PCP**) in immunocompromised people.

Polymerase chain reaction (PCR) tests An extremely sensitive technique introduced in the late 1980s and used in the diagnosis of many illnesses, including HIV disease. In order to detect the presence of HIV, this technique amplifies viral DNA existing in very small quantities (as little as one copy of HIV per 100 000 cells) so that it can be detected. The technique can also be used to detect and amplify HIV RNA.

PPD Purified protein derivative of **tuberculin** used in tuberculin skin testing to identify previous exposure to *M. tuberculosis*. Available in various strengths, which are measured in **Tuberculin Units**. Undiluted PPD is used in the **Heaf test** and diluted PPD is used in the **Mantoux text**.

Prevalence The number of people who have a specific disease or condition that are present in a defined population at one specific point in time, e.g. the number of men and women between the ages of 14 and 65, residing in London, who are known to be infected with HIV and are alive by the end August 2002. *See also* **incidence**.

Progressive multifocal leucoencephalopathy (PML) A rare inflammatory disorder that leads to loss of myelin in multiple areas within the white matter of the brain. It is a virus-induced disease seen in people with poor immune function (immunocompromised). Symptoms and signs include loss of coordination, clumsiness, memory loss, progressively worsening weakness of the legs and, to a lesser extent, arms. Other signs may include language problems, visual field defects and headaches. It is caused by the **JC virus** (*see also*), a common resident in most adults, but it triggers loss of myelin in those whose immune function is deficient. It occurs in 4 per cent of adult individuals with AIDS.

Protease (abbreviated to **PR**) A viral enzyme in HIV (**p10**) that is responsible for cleaving (cutting, splitting) newly formed (nascent) polyproteins manufactured during viral replication.

Protease inhibitors (PIs) Antiretroviral drugs that work by inhibiting the protein-splitting action of protease.

Protozoa A group of single-celled animals, including amoebas. Pathogenic protozoan parasites include *Toxoplasma gondii*, *Isospora belli* and *Cryptosporidium parvum*, all of which cause opportunistic disease in immunocompromised people.

Pruritus Itching

Quasispecies Genetically diverse **viral variants**, e.g. synctium-inducing and non-synctium-inducing variants (*see* **syncytia**), produced as a result of errors in viral replication resulting in **mutation** of the HIV genome. This term is used to describe the virus population within an HIV-1-infected person (intra-host diversity), as opposed to HIV-1 **subtypes** or **clades** (*see also*).

Regimen A regulated system, programme or schedule (such as diet, therapy or exercise) intended to promote health or achieve another beneficial effect. Regimen is used in preference to **regime**, which more usually refers to a political system or structure.

Resistance A phenomenon whereby HIV develops resistance to one or more antiretroviral drugs.

Retrovirus (Greek *retro* – backward) RNA viruses (such as HIV) belonging to the *Retroviridae* family of viruses. These viruses possess a unique enzyme called **reverse transcriptase**, which uses the viral RNA as a template for making a DNA copy that is then integrated into the nucleus of the host cell it has infected and there serves either as a basis for further viral replication or as an oncogene. The name retrovirus was derived from the first two letters of the words **reverse transcriptase**. *See also* **reverse transcriptase; oncogene**.

Reverse transcriptase A retroviral enzyme that allows the viral RNA to be converted (transcribed) into complementary DNA (cDNA), which it can then integrate into the genome of the host cell it has infected. This process is known as **reverse transcription** and is an essential and unique characteristic of retroviruses such as HIV. It is called reverse because it reverses the usual direction of cellular information transfer, or transcription (DNA → RNA). This enzyme is often abbreviated as **RT**. It is a **heterodimer** (*see also*) and has two major subunits: **p66** and **p51**. The larger subunit (p66) has domains (homes) for additional enzymes involved in reverse transcription, i.e. **RNase H** and **DNA polymerase** (*see also*).

Ribonuclease H (RNase H) A hydrolase enzyme that splits the chemical bonds in ribonucleic acid (RNA); an enzyme present in HIV (p15) that, following reverse transcription, is responsible for degrading (destroying by digestion) the single-stranded RNA molecule that initially copies itself as a single strand of DNA.

RNA (ribonucleic acid) *See* **nucleic acids**.

RNase H *See* **ribonuclease H**.

R5 viruses Variants of HIV-1 that utilize the CCR5 chemokine receptor as a co-receptor for attaching to and infecting cells, e.g. M-tropic variants. *See also* **X4 viruses**.

Salvage therapy The antiretroviral regimen used following the failure (usually because of drug resistance) of previous regimens.

Sarcoma One of two types of cancer (the other being carcinoma). Malignant tumours consisting of embryonic-like connective tissue, composed of closely packed cells embedded in a fibrillar or homogeneous substances. *See also* **Kaposi's sarcoma**.

Seroconversion The period following HIV infection when anti-HIV IgG antibodies can be detected in the blood and the person's antibody status changes from negative to positive.

SIDA French/Spanish acronym for the acquired immunodeficiency syndrome, i.e. (Spanish) *Sindrome de Immunodeficiencia Adquirida*; (French) *Syndrome d'Immunodéficience Acquise*.

Slim disease *See* **AIDS wasting syndrome**.

Species A single kind of microorganism; a subdivision of **genus** (*see also*).

Stevens–Johnson syndrome A severe and sometimes fatal form of erythema multiforme that occurs as a result of an allergic reaction to some drugs (e.g. thiacetazone, sulphonamides, penicillins and barbiturates) and to some vaccines (e.g. vaccinia, BCG and poliomyelitis). This syndrome is characterized by fever and the occurrence of large, fluid-containing blisters (bullae) on the oral mucosa, pharynx, anogenital region and conjunctiva.

STI (sexually transmitted infection) A term now being used in preference to STD (sexually transmitted disease). *See also* **structured treatment interruption**.

Structured treatment interruption (STI) An antiretroviral drug regimen with carefully planned periods of intermittent therapy.

Subtypes Geographically diverse **variants** (*see also*) of HIV-1 (and, less commonly, of HIV-2), more usually referred to as **clades** (*see also*).

Syncytia Refers to the ability of one variant of HIV-1 (**syncytium-inducing**, or **SI**) to attract clumps of non-infected (and dysfunctional) CD4⁺ T-lymphocytes around a CD4⁺ T-lymphocyte infected with a SI variant of HIV-1. Those variants of HIV-1 that do not promote the formation of syncytia are referred to as **non-syncytium-inducing (NSI)** viral variants.

Syndrome A group of signs and symptoms that characterize a disease.

Teratogenesis (teratogenic) Congenital malformations of the fetus during pregnancy, e.g. caused by some drugs (especially when taken between the third and eleventh weeks of pregnancy) and infections.

Toxoplasmosis Infection caused by the protozoan parasite *Toxoplasma gondii*, which is carried by cats, birds and other animals, and is found in soil contaminated by cat faeces, and in meat, particularly pork. It can cause severe multi-system disease in immunocompromised people, including a life-threatening **encephalitis**.

Tropism (tropic) An affinity or attraction of one cell to another.

T-tropic HIV-1 variants Those variants of HIV-1 that preferentially seek out, infect and replicate in CD4⁺ T-lymphocytes. These variants generally form **syncytia** (*see also*), i.e. are syncytium inducing (SI), and use the CXCR4 chemokine receptor to bind to and infect cells. *See also* **X4 viruses**; **M-tropic variants**.

Tubercle A small nodule, also called a **granuloma** (*see also*).

Tubercle bacilli Another term for *Mycobacterium tuberculosis* complex. (N.B. All rod-shaped microorganisms are called bacilli.)

Tuberculin Heat-treated products of the growth and lysis of tubercle bacilli. *See also* **PPD**.

Tuberculosis (TB) Disease, especially pulmonary, caused by infection with *Mycobacterium tuberculosis* complex (*see also*). **Latent (dormant) TB** refers to a condition in which a person has been infected with tubercle bacilli but does not have active disease. **Reactivation (post-primary) disease** occurs when latent TB becomes active, and this condition may or may not be infectious. Sometimes people with latent TB become **re-infected** and may then develop active TB.

Tumour necrosis factor (TNF) A cytokine produced by macrophages which helps activate T-lymphocytes (and will also stimulate HIV replication).

UNAIDS Joint United Nations Programme on HIV/AIDS. Internet address on the worldwide web http://www.unaids.org

V3 loop The envelope glycoprotein 120 (gp120) of HIV has five disulphide-bonded loops made up of different amino acid sequences, one of which is known as V3 and is important in virus–cell fusion.

Variants (viral) A genetic variation or change in some characteristic of a virus; also called **isolates, phenotypes** or, less commonly, **strains**. Viral variants evolve as a result of mutation or genetic recombination. Genetic variations occurring in HIV-1 infected people are known as **quasispecies** (*see also*); HIV-1 genetic variations occurring in and associated with different geographical regions are known as **subtypes** or **clades** (*see also*).

Varicella zoster virus (VZV) A human herpesvirus that causes chickenpox during childhood and may reactivate later in life to cause shingles in immunocompromised people.

Vertical transmission Transmission of an infection from an infected mother to her newborn child during pregnancy, delivery or in the post-partum period from breast milk. Also called **perinatal** or **mother-to-child transmission**.

Viraemia The presence of virus in the blood.

Virion The complete, extracellular viral particle, i.e. the genome in the core surrounded by the capsid (and envelope, if present). *See also* **virus**.

Virus A group of minute (200–300 nm to 15 nm in size) infectious agents that cannot be visualized by light microscopy and are characterized by a lack of independent metabolism and an ability to replicate within living host cells. The term **virus** is used to describe the intracellular forms of the viral particle; the term **virion** is used to describe the extracellular form of the complete viral particle.

WHO World Health Organization, headquartered in Geneva. Internet address on the worldwide web http://www.who.int

X4 viruses Variants of HIV-1 that utilize the CXCR4 chemokine receptor as a co-receptor for attaching to and infecting cells, e.g. T-tropic variants. *See also* **R5 viruses**.

Zoonosis Any disease and/or infection that is naturally transmitted between animals (usually vertebrate animals, but may include invertebrates, e.g. shellfish) and humans, e.g. tuberculosis, lassa fever, rabies.

FURTHER READING

Dorland W.A. Newman (ed.). *Dorland's Illustrated Medical Dictionary*, 29th edn. Philadelphia: W.B. Saunders Co., 2000, ISBN 0-7216-6254-4.

HIV/AIDS Treatment Information Service (ATIS). *Glossary of HIV/AIDS-related Terms*, 4th edn. USA: Department of Health and Human Services. Available online at: http://www.hivatis.org or e-mail: atis@hivatis.org

MEDLINEplus Health Information from the National Library of Medicine (USA). *Dictionary, Encyclopedia, Drug Information* and *Health Topics* available online at: http://www.nlm.nih.gov/medlineplus/medlineplus.html

National AIDS Manual (NAM). UK Web-based *Glossary*. Available online at: http://www.aidsmap.com/main/glossary.asp

Weller B. (ed.). *Nurses' Dictionary*, 23rd edn. Edinburgh: Baillière Tindall, 2000, 568 pp, ISBN 0-7020-2557-7.

Index

Indexer: Dr Laurence Errington

Note: bold numbers indicate glossary references.